IACM
Clinical Medicine
Update 2022

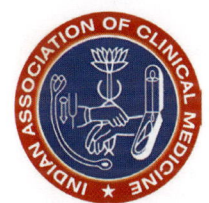

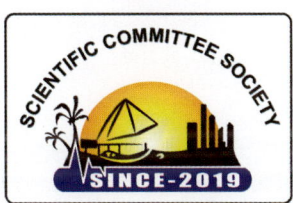

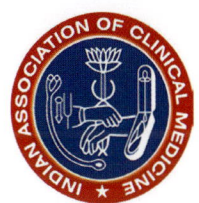 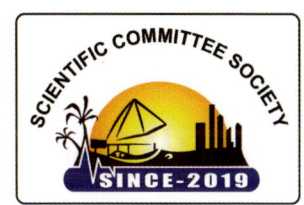

BLENDING TECHNOLOGY AND CLINICAL MEDICINE

IACM
Clinical Medicine Update 2022

Editor-in-Chief

KK Pareek
MD FICP FRCP (Glasg, Edin, Lond) FFIACM FGSI FRSSDI FACP

Senior Consultant in Medicine
President Elect—Indian Association of Clinical Medicine
Past President—Association of Physicians of India
Past Dean—Indian College of Physicians
Dr Jivraj Mehta Awardee
Director—SN Pareek Hospital and Research Center
Kota, Rajasthan, India

Foreword

MM Singh

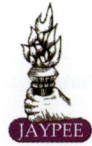

JAYPEE BROTHERS MEDICAL PUBLISHERS
The Health Sciences Publisher
New Delhi | London

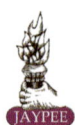 **Jaypee Brothers Medical Publishers (P) Ltd**

Headquarters
EMCA House
23/23-B, Ansari Road, Daryaganj
New Delhi 110 002, India
Landline: +91-11-23272143, +91-11-23272703
+91-11-23282021, +91-11-23245672
E-mail: jaypee@jaypeebrothers.com

Corporate Office
Jaypee Brothers Medical Publishers (P) Ltd.
4838/24, Ansari Road, Daryaganj
New Delhi 110 002, India
Phone: +91-11-43574357
Fax: +91-11-43574314
E-mail: jaypee@jaypeebrothers.com

Overseas Office
JP Medical Ltd.
83, Victoria Street, London
SW1H 0HW (UK)
Phone: +44-20 3170 8910
Fax: +44(0)20 3008 6180
E-mail: info@jpmedpub.com

Website: www.jaypeebrothers.com
Website: www.jaypeedigital.com

© 2023, Jaypee Brothers Medical Publishers

The views and opinions expressed in this book are solely those of the original contributor(s)/author(s) and do not necessarily represent those of editor(s) or publisher of the book.

All rights reserved by the author. No part of this publication may be reproduced, stored or transmitted in any form or by any means, electronic, mechanical, photocopying, recording or otherwise, without the prior permission in writing of the publishers.

All brand names and product names used in this book are trade names, service marks, trademarks or registered trademarks of their respective owners. The publisher is not associated with any product or vendor mentioned in this book.

Medical knowledge and practice change constantly. This book is designed to provide accurate, authoritative information about the subject matter in question. However, readers are advised to check the most current information available on procedures included and check information from the manufacturer of each product to be administered, to verify the recommended dose, formula, method and duration of administration, adverse effects and contraindications. It is the responsibility of the practitioner to take all appropriate safety precautions. Neither the publisher nor the author(s)/editor(s) assume any liability for any injury and/or damage to persons or property arising from or related to use of material in this book.

This book is sold on the understanding that the publisher is not engaged in providing professional medical services. If such advice or services are required, the services of a competent medical professional should be sought.

Every effort has been made where necessary to contact holders of copyright to obtain permission to reproduce copyright material. If any have been inadvertently overlooked, the publisher will be pleased to make the necessary arrangements at the first opportunity.

Inquiries for bulk sales may be solicited at: jaypee@jaypeebrothers.com

IACM Clinical Medicine Update 2022 / KK Pareek
First Edition: 2023
ISBN: 978-93-5465-869-3
Printed at: Samrat Offset Pvt. Ltd.

Dedication

To my honorable **Parents**
for everything they did for me and
making me who I am today.

My beloved **Wife**
Shashi for her constant support.

My wonderful **Children**
and grandchildren for their love.

Above all my **Institution**,
SMS Medical College Jaipur
and my **Teachers**
who gave me knowledge.

My **Colleagues**
who enrich me every day

and

My **Patients**
from whom I learned to be a better human being
and a good clinician.

FOUNDERS

THE GREAT VISIONARIES
The Founder Fathers
Who Nurtured the Dream of IACM

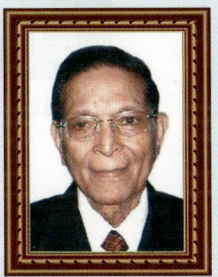

Late (Prof) Dr MC Gupta

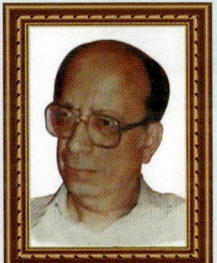

Late (Prof) Dr PK Wahal

Editor-in-Chief

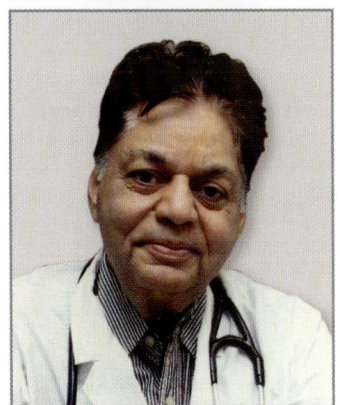

Dr KK Pareek

Editors

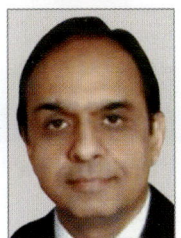

Dr Girish Mathur

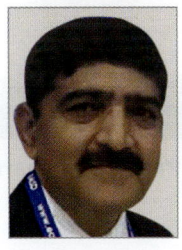

Dr GD Ramchandani

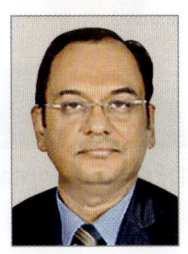

Dr Puneet Saxena

Advisors

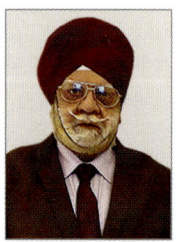 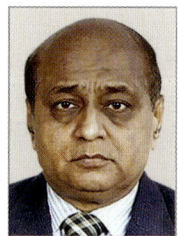 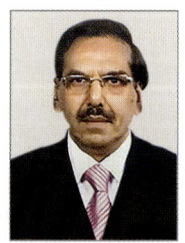

Dr MM Singh   **Dr AK Gupta**   **Dr Subhash Chandra**

Associate Editors

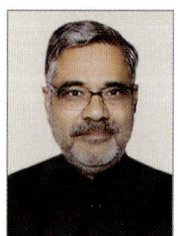 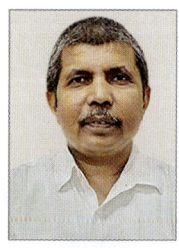 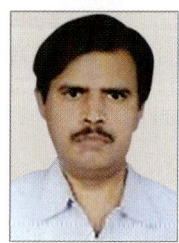

Dr Suresh Kushwaha   **Dr Sujit Kumar**   **Dr TP Singh**
(Organizing Secretary)

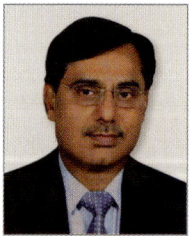 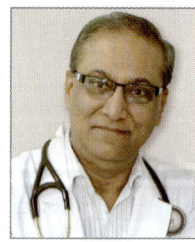 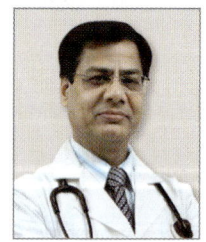

Dr Ajay Kumar   **Dr SK Sharma**   **Dr DC Sharma**

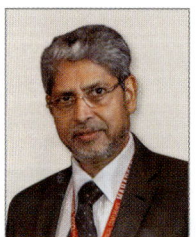 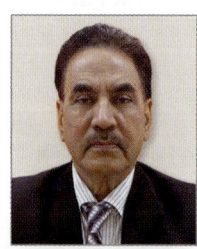 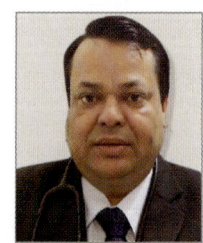

Dr Arvind Gupta   **Dr Pradyumn Sharma**   **Dr SS Dariya**

CONTRIBUTORS

Abhishek Goyal MD DM (Cardiology)
Associate Professor
Interventional Cardiology and
Electrophysiology
Dayanand Medical College and Hospital
Unit Hero DMC Heart Institute
Ludhiana, Punjab, India

Abhishek Kumar MD (Medicine) FICP
Consultant Medicine
Joint Pain and Arthritis Clinic
Patna, Bihar, India

Ajay Kumar MD FRCP
Consultant Physician and Diabetologist
Diabetes Care and Research Centre
Patna, Bihar, India

Ajit Singh Chahar MD
Associate Professor
Department of Medicine
SN Medical College
Agra, Uttar Pradesh, India

Ajoy Tewari MD (Medicine)
Director
Department of Diabetology
Jai Clinic and Diabetes Care Center
Lucknow, Uttar Pradesh, India

Akansha MD
Junior Resident
Department of General Medicine
SN Medical College
Agra, Uttar Pradesh, India

AK Gupta MD (Medicine)
Ex Director-Professor and Head
Postgraduate Department of Medicine
SN Medical College
Agra, Uttar Pradesh, India

Alladi Mohan MD
Dean, Professor (Senior Grade)
Department of Medicine
Sri Venkateswara Institute of Medical Sciences
Tirupati, Andhra Pradesh, India

Amit Aggarwal DNB (Gen Med) MNAMS
Senior Specialist, Department of Medicine
ABVIMS and Dr Ram Manohar Lohia Hospital
New Delhi, India

Amit K Adhikary MD
Assistant Professor
Department of Medicine
North Bengal Medical College
Darjeeling, West Bengal, India

Amrit Yog Datley MD
Senior Resident
Department of Gastroenterology and
Hepatology, Max Super Speciality Hospital
Shalimar Bagh, New Delhi

Anil Kumar Virmani MD DRM FICP FIACM
FACP FDI FRSSDI FICCMD FISH CCIO
Consultant Physician
Viru's Diabetes and Cardiac Care Centre
Jamshedpur, Jharkhand, India

Anirban Bhowmik MD
Assistant Professor
Department of Medicine
Tripura Medical College
Agartala, Tripura, India

Anju Dinkar MD (Microbiology) FICN
Associate Professor
Department of Microbiology
Institute of Medical Sciences BHU
Varanasi, Uttar Pradesh, India

AN Rai MD MRCP (UK) FRCP (Glasg) FICP FICC
FICN
Former Professor and Head
Department of Medicine
Principal of ANMMCH
Chairman of AIMS
Gaya, Bihar, India

Anuj Maheshwari MD FACP FRCP (Lond, Edin)
Professor in Medicine, Hind Institute of
Medical Sciences, Barabanki
Lucknow, Uttar Pradesh, India

Contributors

Anusha Singhania MBBS
Pre Resident
Department of Neurology
Christian Medical College and Hospital
Ludhiana, Punjab, India

Aradhana Sharma MD
Associate Professor
Department of General Medicine
SMS Medical College
Jaipur, Rajasthan, India

Arun Chaturvedi MD
Head, Department of Physiology
KD Medical College
Mathura, Uttar Pradesh, India

Arvinder Pal Singh MD
Professor and Head
Department of Emergency Medicine
Sri Guru Ram Das University of Health Sciences
Amritsar, Punjab, India

Arvind Gupta MD FRCP FACE FICP
Senior Consultant and Head
Department of Diabetes, Obesity and Metabolism, RHL-Rajasthan Hospital
Jaipur, Rajasthan, India

Ashish Gautam MD (Med) FRCP (Edin, Glasg)
Professor and Head
Department of Medicine
Rani Durgavati Medical College
Banda, Uttar Pradesh, India

Ashis Kumar Saha MD (Cal) DTM&H (Cal) FRCP (Edin and Glasg) FACP (USA) FICP (Ind) MNAMS (Ind) MBA
Professor and Head
Department of Medicine
MGM Medical College and LSK Hospital
Kishanganj, Bihar, India

Ashutosh Kumar MD
Assistant Professor
Department of Psychiatry
SN Medical College
Agra, Uttar Pradesh, India

Avik Chakraborty MD (Med) FICP FISH
Professor, Department of Medicine
Tripura Medical College and Dr BRAM Teaching Hospital
Agartala, Tripura, India

BB Rewari MD FRCP FICP MPH
Regional Advisor-Hepatitis/HIV/STIs
World Health Organization
Regional Office for South-East Asia
New Delhi, India

BK Singh MD FICP
Consultant Physician
Uttama Medicare and Research Centre
Aurangabad, Bihar, India

BL Bhardwaj MD (Med) MAMS FICP FIMSA FCCP
Ex Principal GMC, Patiala, Punjab
Principal, Adesh Medical College
Shahabad, Haryana, India

Daya Kishore Hazra MD PhD FICP FAMS FICNM FIACM PadmaShri
Emeritus Professor, National Academy of Medical Sciences
Consultant, Boston Medical Center
Agra, Uttar Pradesh, India

Debaprasad Chakrabarti MD (Med) FICP FIACM
Professor and Head
Department of Medicine
Tripura Medical College
Agartala, Tripura, India

Dipanjan Bandyopadhyay MD (Med) FICP FIACM Fellow IMA AMS
Professor and Head
Department of Medicine
North Bengal Medical College
Darjeeling, West Bengal, India

Dipankar Prakas Bhaumik MD DFID FICP FIACM
Associate Professor, Department of Medicine,
Tripura Medical College and Dr BRAM Teaching Hospital
Agartala, Tripura, India

Contributors   xi

Divyansh Mathur MBBS
Postgraduate Student
Department of Psychiatry
Geetanjali Medical College
Udaipur, Rajasthan, India

DP Singh MD DTCD FICP FACP FIAMS FCSI FICS
FRCP (Glasg and Edin)
Professor and Head
Department of Respiratory Medicine
JLN Medical College and Hospital
Bhagalpur, Bihar, India

G Bindhu Madhavi MBBS
Junior Resident
Department of Medicine
Sri Venkateswara Institute of Medical Sciences
Tirupati, Andhra Pradesh, India

Gaurav Ashish Khanna BFA
Medical Educator
Department of Medicine
Holy Family Hospital
Mawana (Meerut), Uttar Pradesh, India

GD Ramchandani MD FRCP (Lond, Ire, Glasg, Edin) FACE FACP FRSSDI FICP FIACM FDI FGSI
Professor, Department of Internal Medicine
Daswani Dental College
Senior Physician and Consultant
Diabetologist
Ramchandani Diabetes Care and Research Center
Kota, Rajasthan, India

G Narsimulu MD FICP FIACM
Head, Department of Rheumatology
ESIC Medical College and Hospital
Hyderabad, Telangana, India

Gurinder Mohan MD FICP FIACM
Professor and Head
Department of Medicine
Sri Guru Ram Das University of of Health Sciences
Amritsar, Punjab, India

Gursaran K Sidhu MD FIACM FICP FCCP
Physician (Gold Medalist)
Director Medical Division
Sidhu Hospital
Ludhiana, Punjab, India

Hem Shanker Sharma MD FICP MACP
Professor of Medicine
Department of Postgraduate Medicine
JLNMCH, Ashray Superspeciality Hospital
Bhagalpur, Bihar, India

Himanshu Jain MBBS
Resident Doctor Final Year
Department of Medicine
RD Gardi Medical College
Ujjain, Madhya Pradesh, India

Israrul Haque MD
Senior Resident
Department of Rheumatology
All India Institute of Medical Sciences
New Delhi, India

Jagga Sankalp Harish MBBS
Junior Resident
Department of Medicine
Sri Guru Ram Das University of Health Sciences
Amritsar, Punjab, India

Jitendra Singh MD (Gen Med) FICN CCCKD (Kidney Disease) PGDC (Cardiology) PGDRM PGDip
Assistant Professor
Department of General Medicine
Institute of Medical Sciences, BHU
Varanasi, Uttar Pradesh, India

Kamlesh Tewary MD FRCP (Glas and Edin) FACP (USA) FICP FFACM FIAMS
Ex Professor and HOD Medicine
SK Medical College, Muzaffarpur, Bihar
Director and Head
Deo Narayan Hospital and Maternity Centre
Muzaffarpur, Bihar, India

Kanika Agarwal MD (Med)
3rd Year Student
Department of Medicine
SN Medical College
Agra, Uttar Pradesh, India

KK Lohani MD
Associate Professor
Department of Medicine
ANMMCH
Gaya, Bihar, India

KK Pareek MD FICP FRCP (Glasg, Edin, Lond) FFIACM FGSI FRSSDI FACP
Senior Consultant in Medicine
President Elect—Indian Association of Clinical Medicine
Past President—Association of Physicians of India
Past Dean—Indian College of Physicians
Dr Jivraj Mehta Awardee
Director—SN Pareek Hospital and Research Center
Kota, Rajasthan, India

Madhuchanda Kar MD PhD
Clinical Director
Department of Oncology, Peerless Hospital
Kolkata, West Bengal, India

Mangesh Tiwaskar MD (Medicine)
Consultant Physician and Diabetologist
Shilpa Medical Research Centre
Mumbai, Maharashtra, India

Man Mohan Mehndiratta MD (Med) DNB (Med) DM (Neuro) FAAN FANA FAMS MNAMS FRCP FICP FIAN
Emeritus Professor
National Academy of Medical Sciences
Senior Director
Department of Neurology, BL Kapur Hospital (Max Health Care Group), Centre for Neurosciences
New Delhi, India

MPS Chawla MD FIACM FICP FACP FRCP FISC
Professor and Head
Department of Medicine
ABVIMS and Dr RML Hospital
New Delhi, India

Mritunjay Kumar Singh MD
Consultant Physician and Nephrologist
Chandraneel Clinic
Abhay Institute of Medical Sciences
Gaya, Bihar, India

Mudit Khurana MD DM (Nephro)
Assistant Professor
Department of Nephrology
SN Medical College
Agra, Uttar Pradesh, India

Mukesh K Sarna MD PGDHHM FACP FRCP (Edin and Glas) FICP FRSSDI FIACM
Professor and Unit Head
Department of General Medicine
Mahatma Gandhi Medical College and Hospital
Jaipur, Rajasthan, India

Mukut Roy MD DM FICP FIACM
Professor, Department of Medicine
Tripura Medical College and Dr BRAM Teaching Hospital
Agartala, Tripura, India

Nabanita De DNB (Pathology)
Senior Resident
Department of Pathology
ESI-PGIMSR, ESIC Medical College and Hospital
Kolkata, West Bengal, India

Naman Shukla MBBS
Junior Resident
Department of Medicine
Hind Institute of Medical Sciences
Lucknow, Uttar Pradesh, India

Nandini Chatterjee MD FRCP (Glasg) FICP
Professor
Department of Medicine
IPGMER/SSKM Hospital
Kolkata, West Bengal, India

Naval Chandra MD
Professor and Unit Head
Department of Medicine
Nizam's Institute of Medical Sciences
Hyderabad, Telangana, India

Navneet Agrawal MD PhD FCCP PGCD FIACM
Dip. Diabetology
Consulting Physician and Diabetologist
Department of Diabetes
Obesity and Thyroid Center
Gwalior, Madhya Pradesh, India

Niharikaa Sharma MD (Med)

Contributors

Niharika Sinha MBBS PGDM EULAR
Consultant Rheumatologist
Joint Pain and Arthritis Clinic
Patna, Bihar, India

Nikhil Pursnani MD (Med) MRCP (Glasg)
Associate Professor
Department of Medicine
SN Medical College
Agra, Uttar Pradesh, India

NK Singh MD FICP FACP
Director
Diabetes and Heart Research Centre
Dhanbad, Jharkhand, India

Padmamalika Khanna nee Hazra PhD
DPhil (Medical Biochemistry)
Assistant Professor, Chemistry
St John's College
Agra, Uttar Pradesh, India

Pallaavi Goel MBBS
Resident, Department of General Medicine
Mahatma Gandhi Medical College
and Hospital
Jaipur, Rajasthan, India

Partha Pratim Chakraborty MD DM (Endo)
DNB (Endo) FACE FICP FIACM
Assistant Professor
Department of Endocrinology and
Metabolism
Medical College Kolkata
Kolkata, West Bengal, India

Prabhat Agrawal MD MAMS FRCP (Edin and Glas) FICP FIACM FRSSDI Postgraduate Diploma of Diabetes (London)
Professor
Department of Medicine
SN Medical College
Agra, Uttar Pradesh, India

Pradip Bhaumik MD PhD
Professor
Department of Medicine
Agartala Govt Medical College
Agartala, Tripura, India

Pradyumn Sharma MD (Medicine) FICP
Fellow-Diabetes India Fellow RSSDI, Fellow-UAPM
Managing Director
Gopinath Hospital
Jaipur, Rajasthan, India

Prakhar Gupta MD MRCP (II)
Consultant
Ram Babu Gupta Heart and Medicine Centre
Agra, Uttar Pradesh, India

Prashant Prakash MD (Medicine)
MD (Respiratory Medicine)
Professor and Head
Super Specialty Department of
Pulmonary Medicine
SN Medical College
Agra, Uttar Pradesh, India

Priyanka MD (Chest)
Fellow
Department of Cardiology
Hero DMC Heart Institute
Unit of DMCH
Ludhiana, Punjab, India

Puneet Saxena MD FICP FRCP FRSSDI FIACM
Senior Professor and Unit Head
Department of General Medicine
SMS Medical College
Jaipur, Rajasthan, India

RN Tejaswini DNB
Resident
ESIC Medical College and Hospital
Hyderabad, Telangana, India

Rahin Mahata MD DM (Endo)
Senior Resident
Department of Endocrinology and
Metabolism
Medical College Kolkata
Kolkata, West Bengal, India

Rahul Ramchandani MBBS
Post Graduate Student
Department of Internal Medicine
IMS SUM Hospital
Bhubaneswar, Odisha, India

Rahul Yadati MBBS
Sri Ramachandra Institute of Health
Education and Research
Chennai, Tamil Nadu, India

Rajeev Gupta MD PhD
Director and Head
Department of Preventive Cardiology and
Medicine, Eternal Heart Care Centre and
Research Institute
Jaipur, Rajasthan, India

Rajesh Gopalakrishna MD DNB (Gastro)
MNAMS FIACM FICP FRCP (Edin) FISG
Professor
Department of Gastroenterology
Amrita Institute of Medical Sciences
Kochi, Kerala, India

Rajesh Upadhyay MD MRCP (UK) FRCP (Glasg)
FACP FICP FIAMS FISG
Senior Director and Head
Department of Gastroenterology and
Hepatology
Max Super Speciality Hospital
Shalimar Bagh, New Delhi, India

Rajnish Saxena MBBS PGCDM Dip Diabetology
FDFM FRSSDI F Diabetes India, FIPA
Diabetologist and Foot Care Specialist
Saxena Diabetes Care Centre (SDCC)
Ajmer, Rajasthan, India

Raman Puri DM (Card)
Senior Consultant Cardiologist
Apollo Hospital
Chairman, Lipid Association of India
New Delhi, India

Rashmi Nanda MD DFM Certification in
Lipidology (LAI)
Cardiologist, Cardiac Care Center
Secretary, Lipid Association of India
New Delhi, India

Reeja Antony MD
Academic Resident
JLNMCH, Ashray Superspeciality Hospital
Bhagalpur, Bihar, India

Rohit Tandon MD (Med)
Senior Consultant Physician Dayanand
Medical College and Hospital Unit Hero
DMC Heart Institute
Ludhiana, Punjab, India

SK Kushwaha MD (Med) FIACM
Senior Consultant Physician, Bodla Hospital
Agra, Uttar Pradesh, India

SN Yadav MD FCCS
Consultant
Ram Babu Gupta Heart and Medicine Centre
Agra, Uttar Pradesh, India

Sairam Yadati MBBS
Bhaskar Medical College, Moinabad
Hyderabad, Telangana, India

Samarth Loomba MBBS
Final year Student
Maharishi Markandeshwar Medical College
Solan, Himachal Pradesh, India

Santanu Hazra MD (Microbiology)
Assistant Professor
Department of Microbiology
North Bengal Medical College
Siliguri, West Bengal, India

Sarita Bajaj MD (Med) DM (Endo)
FRCP (Lond, Glasg, Edin)
Consultant Endocrinologist
Former Director-Professor and Head
Department of Medicine
MLN Medical College
Prayagraj, Uttar Pradesh, India

Saumya Ahluwalia MBBS Student
Dayanand Medical College and Hospital
Ludhiana, Punjab, India

Saurabh Srivastava MD (Gen Med) FRCP
(Edin) FRCP (Glasg) FICP FACP FIMSA FIACM FGSI
FISH FUDA FRSSDI F-Diab (Diabetes India)
Professor and Head
Chief Medical Superintendent
Department of Medicine
Government Institute of Medical Sciences
Greater Noida, Uttar Pradesh, India

Contributors

S Bhavana DNB
Resident, ESIC Medical College and Hospital
Hyderabad, Telangana, India

Shankar Dutta MD Internal Medicine
Senior Resident
Jalpaiguri Govt Medical College
Jalpaiguri, West Bengal, India

Shankha S Sen MD Medicine (Gold Medalist)
FACP FICP FIACM FIAMS FIMSA FISH
Fellow Diabetes India
Senior Consultant Physician
Siliguri, West Bengal, India

Shweta Yadav MBBS
Medical Student
Ram Babu Gupta Heart and Medicine Centre
Agra, Uttar Pradesh, India

Sidhant Sachdeva MD (Gen Medicine)
Fellow, Department of Cardiology
Hero DMC Heart Institute
Unit of DMCH
Ludhiana, Punjab, India

Sirshendu Pal MD (Med) FEAC FIACP FIAMS
FISH FIMSA
Senior Consultant Physician
Department of Medicine
Mitra's Multispeciality Hospital
Siliguri, West Bengal, India

SK Sharma MD (Med) DM (Endo)
Consultant Endocrinologist
Diabetes Thyroid and Endocrine Centre
Galaxy Speciality Centre
Jaipur, Rajasthan, India

Smarajit Banik MD (Medicine) FIACM FICP
Professor and Head
Department of Medicine Jalpaiguri
Jalpaiguri Govt Medical College
West Bengal, India

Soma Saha DNB FICP
Associate Professor
Department of Medicine
Tripura Medical College and
Dr BRAM Teaching Hospital
Agartala, Tripura, India

Srishta Hazra Freshman (UC Santa Cruz)
Information Technology Researcher
Biomolecular Engineering and Bioinformatics,
University of California
Santa Cruz, USA

Srishti Ahluwalia MBBS Student
Dayanand Medical College and Hospital
Ludhiana, Punjab, India

SS Dariya MD FGSI FDI PGDGM
Senior Physician and Consultant
Diabetologist
Department of Medicine
SMS Hospital
Jaipur, Rajasthan, India

Subhash Chandra MD (Hons) MRCP (UK)
DTM&H (UK) DTCD
President (IACM)
Director, Shri Ram Babu Gupta Heart and
Medicine Center
Agra, Uttar Pradesh, India

Sudhir Kumar MD (Medicine) FICP
Professor of Medicine
Department of Medicine
IGIMS
Patna, Bihar, India

Sugandha Sharma MS (Obst and Gynae)
Consultant Gynecologist
Global Heart and General Hospital
Jaipur, Rajasthan, India

Sukrati Maheshwari MD (Gen Med)
General Physician
Jai Prakash Hospital
Bhopal, Madhya Pradesh, India

Suresh Yadav MD
Assistant Professor
Department of General Medicine
SMS Medical College
Jaipur, Rajasthan, India

TP Singh MD (Medicine) FICP FIACM
Professor
Department of General Medicine
SN Medical College
Agra, Uttar Pradesh, India

Contributors

Tanuja Manohar MD (Med)
Associate Professor
Department of Medicine
NKP Salve Institute of Medical Sciences and
Research Centre (NKPSIMS and RC)
Nagpur, Maharashtra, India

Tarun Satija MD FIACM
Consultant Physician
Ludhiana, Punjab, India

Uma Kumar MD
Professor and Head
Department of Rheumatology
All India Institute of Medical Sciences
New Delhi, India

Vaibhav Saxena MBBS CDE
Junior Resident, Department of Medicine
Santokba Durlabhji Memorial Hospital
Jaipur, Rajasthan, India

Vasundhara Aggarwal DNB (Int Med)
DrNB (Neuro)
Assistant Professor (Neurology)
Department of Neurology, Janakpuri Super
Speciality Hospital
New Delhi, India

Vijaya Prasanna MD DM
Associate Professor
Department of Rheumatology
ESIC Medical College and Hospital
Hyderabad, Telangana, India

Vijay Garg MD FIAE FICP FCSI FICA (USA) FISE
FACC (USA) FACP (USA) FIMSA FISC FESC (EUROPE)
Professor, RD Gardi Medical College
Department of Medicine
Ujjain Charitable Trust Hospital
Ujjain, Madhya Pradesh, India

Vikas Loomba MBBS MD PGDGM FIACM FICP
Professor and Unit Head
Department of Medicine
Christian Medical College and Hospital
Ludhiana, Punjab, India

Vimlesh Patidar MD FIAE
Professor
Department of Medicine
RD Gardi Medical College
Ujjain, Madhya Pradesh, India

Vipin Mediratta DNB (Medicine)
Associate Professor and Consultant
Department of Medicine
Dr Ram Manohar Lohia Hospital
New Delhi, India

VS Gaurav Narayan MD
Senior Resident
Department of Gastroenterology and
Hepatology
Max Super Speciality Hospital
Shalimar Bagh, New Delhi, India

Y Sathyanarayana Raju MD FRCP (Edin)
FICP
Professor of Medicine
Department of Medicine
Nizam's Institute of Medical Sciences
Hyderabad, Telangana, India

FOREWORD

It is indeed a great honor and pleasure to write this foreword for "Clinical Medicine Update 2022"—an annual publication of the Indian Association of Clinical Medicine.

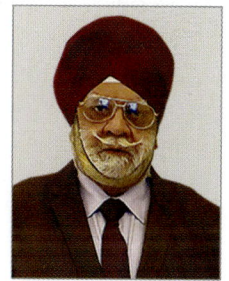

The Indian Association of Clinical Medicine was formed 30 years back in 1992 to establish the primacy of a logical clinical and rational approach to medical problems and to see that the art and science of clinical medicine and its methodology is not left out in the plethora of highly advanced scientific investigations.

The 20th century has witnessed many breakthrough in the field of medicine from artificial organ transplantation, functional MRIs (not to see the anatomical structure and abnormality but to see functions of human brain and neurons), bionic prosthetics, nanomedicine, targeted chemotherapy to surgical technique in form of cyber knife, 3D body part printing, laparoscopic surgery, completion of human genome draft, etc.

In this time when clinician feels lost in the plethora of these breakthrough and highly advanced investigations, Dr Pareek has chosen the most appropriate theme as. "Blending Technology and Clinical Medicine" for 28th annual conference of the Indian Association of Clinical Medicine.

Dr KK Pareek has been very closely associated with the Indian Association of Clinical Medicine. He has always taken active and keen interest in organizing various Continuing Medical Education (CME), workshops, and conferences in the past. Moreover Dr KK Pareek has gained lot of experience and expertise as President of the largest Association of Physicians—Association of Physicians of India. He has very ably selected the topics which impose an everyday challenge to the practicing physicians. He has not forgotten to include basic topics such as significance of general physical examination, tongue and tooth to highly advanced skills, and knowledge required for managing acute intensive care units—arterial blood gas (ABG) analysis, oxygen therapy, etc. He has also judiciously included topics of general interest like hypertension, diabetes, metabolic syndrome and coronary problems.

Dr Pareek has expeditiously edited the article and compiled them to prestigious Publication of the Indian Association of Clinical Medicine. I hope the book will be valuable equally to postgraduates and consultants.

Dr Pareek deserves appreciation and congratulations for the excellent work.
Dated: 19th Oct 2022

Prof (Dr) MM Singh
Founder Secretary—IACM
Past-President—IACM
Former Director Professor and Head
SN Medical College
Agra, Uttar Pradesh, India

PREFACE

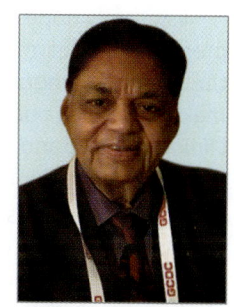

With the dawn of 28th annual conference of the Indian Association of Clinical Medicine Conference (IACMCON)-2020, Rajgir, we all members of Scientific Committee and editorial board have the pleasure and honour to present before all of you the "*IACM Clinical Medicine Update 2022*" book. This book will be delivered to all the delegates at the time of 28th annual conference of IACMCON-2022 at Rajgir.

You all know, the enormous responsibility of preparing an educative, meaningful, and exciting scientific program and publishing Clinical Medicine Update is not a small task. But with the support of wonderful editorial team and help of governing body members, this book becomes a small effort in pursuit of the larger motive and movement. The desire and endeavour of IACM to empower Indian physician with creative, continuous, and significant new knowledge in clinical medicine is being achieved through bringing out this book.

The chapters in this book contain all the lectures delivered by reputed faculty members of national repute and experts of their subjects who have applied the principles and theme of this conference "Blending Technology and Clinical Medicine" and then have written these chapters with their expertise on the subject. Every chapter has been written thoroughly to ensure that it reflects the cutting edge of the medical knowledge and practice in clinical medicine and pitched at a level of detail to meet the needs of a practising physician in their day to day practice.

In the last decade, clinical medicine has witnessed a rapid stride forward.

The pattern, profile, and presentations of the diseases are changing with a very rapid pace. Accordingly, every practising physician has a challenge of keeping abreast with these latest advances in diagnosis and the management of the disease.

Friends, education and knowledge are achieved by dissemination of the information and knowledge from many sources. Readers of these books can update their knowledge and this learning express can be complete by transforming this knowledge to clinical practice and the scientific program presented at the conference will be in continuation of this learning process. "Blending Technology and Clinical Medicine" is the theme of this 28th annual conference of IACM keeping in mind that technology has also become inseparable to clinical medicine. Technology has become as important as clinical medicine and helpful in diagnosis and management of diseases to our practising physicians in their day-to-day practices. Scientific program has been designed accordingly. I have requested all faculty members to start their presentation with case presentation.

We have tried to include six important workshops and hands on training on very common topics such as arterial blood gas (ABG) and fluid therapy, research methodology, diabetic foot, oxygen therapy and noninvasive ventilatory support, emergency echo for physicians and electrocardiogram (ECG) work shop for the delegates and PG students and will be conducted by the learner domain experts.

Preface

The journey as a president elect and Chairman Scientific Committee is difficult and challenging. It has taught me many new lessons, given me unique experiences and enhanced my knowledge to a great extent.

I sincerely hope that through this effort of the entire editorial team we will be able to present these learnings and much more in a very useful manner through this book and the scientific program which will be presented at the conference. Our endeavour is to make it useful to our readers/delegates in transforming this updated knowledge into their clinical practice and hope it will be a great source of dissemination of knowledge which is the important aim of every association.

We the members of editorial board extend our sincere thanks to all the members of the governing body of a IACM for their constant support and guidance from time to time and finally I welcome all the delegates to IACMCON-2022 Rajgir (Nalanda) at this annual conference which is filled with lot of opportunities for expanding your medical knowledge, sharing your clinical skills, and will also provide a great opportunity to network and build new relationship with your colleagues and legends of clinical medicine.

If this book is useful to our delegates, even in a small way in updating their knowledge, their clinical work, and their practice, our efforts will be greatly rewarded.

Jai HIND!
Jai IACM!

KK Pareek

ACKNOWLEDGMENTS

It is always a great pleasure to acknowledge and thank the contribution of legends who helped and supported me in publishing this "IACM Clinical Medicine Update 2022". I and my team of editorial board would like to express our deep appreciation and indebtedness particularly to all the eminent speakers from India who shared their learnings and knowledge through writing the chapters of this book. A special mention to our president of IACM Dr Subhash Chandra, Dr AK Gupta, pillar of strength to IACM, Dr Suresh Kushvaha, treasurer IACM, a very dynamic and dedicated GB member of IACM, Dr Sujit Kumar, sincere and resourceful organising Secretary of IACMCON-2022, and Dr TP Singh, energetic Hon'ble Secretary, for their guidance and endless support in publishing this book. The successful completion of this book could have not been possible without the collaborative efforts and support of the Scientific Committee and editorial board. I am grateful to all the members of the governing body for providing timely inputs which were very crucial in bringing everything together. I express my deepest thanks to my close associates Dr Girish Mathur, Dr GD Ramchandani, and Dr Puneet Saxena for being there for me in this and standing by me at every step in publishing this important document on proceedings of scientific program of IAMCON. Without their help, it would not have been possible to publish this Clinical Medicine Update 2022. A debt of gratitude to "Scientific Committee Society Trust" for providing financial support and unconditional education grant for publishing this book. On behalf of the editorial board, I express our appreciation and gratitude to the efforts of Shri Jitender P Vij (Group Chairman), Mr Ankit Vij (Managing Director), M/S Jaypee Brothers, Medical Publishers (P) Limited, New Delhi, India for printing this book in the present shape. Furthermore, I am thankful to Dr Richa Saxena (Director–Professional Publishing), Ms Upasana Kak (Developmental Editor) with Soumya Yadav (Content Development Editor) who have been instrumental in giving the final shape to the book. They have worked tirelessly and diligently as a team in collaboration with the office of editorial board. My special appreciation to the members of the editorial office Mr Vishal Pancholi in assisting me for scientific work, Mr Randhir Singh who is looking after the accommodation and transport of faculty members and other arrangements, Tirthankar Rai, from ICS GLOBAL a unit of ITS for scientific printing and event management. I sincerely thank to the members of the governing body of IACM for helping with their valuable suggestions and guiding me and structuring this book so beautifully. I am really grateful to the honourable members of IACM who gave me the opportunity to publish this book, as Chairman, Scientific Committee, IACMCON-2022 and President elect of the most prestigious Indian Association of clinical medicine.

My sincere thanks to all the members of my family for their never ending support and understanding, without their encouragement none of this would have been possible. Thanks for giving me the moral support and mental strength in compiling the book. The completion of this book "IACM Clinical Medicine Update 2022", could have not been possible without the participation and assistance of so many people whose name may not all be enumerated but their contributions are sincerely appreciated and gratefully acknowledged. In the end I would like to thank Almighty God for his blessings as without his blessings, I would not be able to do any of this.

KK Pareek
Chairman, Scientific Committee
IACMCON-2022 Rajgir

CONTENTS

SECTION 1: CARDIOLOGY

1. **Advances in Management of Heart Failure** — 1
   Debaprasad Chakrabarti, Anirban Bhowmik

2. **Microalbuminuria: A Risk Marker for CAD** — 9
   AN Rai

3. **Cardiomyopathy: Diagnosis and Management** — 16
   Subhash Chandra

4. **Echocardiography and Lung Ultrasound in the Emergency Room** — 41
   Rohit Tandon, Priyanka, Sidhant Sachdeva

5. **Electrocardiogram in Routine Practice** — 81
   Abhishek Goyal

SECTION 2: CLINICAL MEDICINE

6. **Hand Palmistry in Medicine** — 93
   Subhash Chandra, SN Yadav, Prakhar Gupta, Shweta Yadav

7. **General Physical Examination: A Window to Systemic Disease** — 107
   Y Sathyanarayana Raju, Rahul Yadati, Sairam Yadati

8. **Superior Vena Cava Syndrome: A Forgotten Clinical Entity** — 111
   Madhuchanda Kar, Amit K Adhikary

9. **Tongue is a Mirror of Systemic Diseases** — 117
   Smarajit Banik, Shankar Dutta

SECTION 3: CRITICAL CARE

10. **Metabolic Acidosis: Diagnosis and Management** — 125
    Subhash Chandra

11. **Hyponatremia** — 144
    Mukesh K Sarna, Pallaavi Goel

12. **Rational for Antibiotics: Guidelines** — 156
    Mangesh Tiwaskar, Tanuja Manohar

SECTION 4: DIABETOLOGY

13. **Surgery and Diabetes: Current Concepts** — 173
    BK Singh

14. **How Often Estimation of Urinary Albumin to Creatinine Ratio do Help to Identify Early DM Nephropathy?** — 178
    Dipankar Prakas Bhaumik, Mukut Roy, Soma Saha

15. **Difficult Case Scenarios in Diabetes Mellitus Management** — 184
    Anil Kumar Virmani

16. **Type 2 Diabetes Mellitus: Asian Indian Phenotype** — 191
    GD Ramchandani, Sugandha Sharma, Rahul Ramchandani, Divyansh Mathur

17. **Interpretation of Urine of a Diabetic Patient** — 194
    Prabhat Agrawal, Mudit Khurana, Nikhil Pursnani, Kanika Agarwal, Ashish Gautam

18. **Sulfonylureas in 2022: Are They Still Relevant?** — 201
    Abhishek Kumar, Sudhir Kumar, Niharika Sinha

19. **Remission and Reversal in Diabetes** — 206
    Navneet Agrawal

20. **Protecting the Diabetic Target Organs: Kidneys/Heart/Retina and the Liver** — 213
    Daya Kishore Hazra, Padmamalika Khanna nee Hazra, Gaurav Ashish Khanna, Srishta Hazra

21. **Gestational Diabetes Mellitus: A Window of Opportunity for Noncommunicable Disease Prevention** — 219
    Saurabh Srivastava

22. **Diabetes and Vaccination: The Need and Guideline** — 225
    Puneet Saxena, Aradhana Sharma, Suresh Yadav

23. **Prediabetes** — 230
    Vijay Garg, Himanshu Jain, Vimlesh Patidar, Sukrati Maheshwari

24. **Insulin: Initiation, Intensification, and Barriers** — 238
    Arvind Gupta, Rajeev Gupta, NK Singh

25. **Technology Transforming Diabetes Care** — 242
    Ajay Kumar

26. **Selection of Footwear in Patient with Diabetic Foot**   249
Vaibhav Saxena, Rajnish Saxena, SS Dariya

27. **Interplay between T2DM, Dyslipidemia and NASH**   255
Anuj Maheshwari, Naman Shukla, Ajoy Tewari

28. **Early Detections and Therapeutic Interventions in Diabetes Kidney Disease**   259
SK Sharma, Niharikaa Sharma

29. **Diabetes in Young: Current Concepts**   269
BK Singh

30. **Prediabetes: A Synopsis**   275
Sarita Bajaj

SECTION 5: ENDOCRINOLOGY

31. **Addison Disease, Clinical Challenges, and Treatment**   282
Gursaran K Sidhu

32. **Treatment Issues in Hypothyroidism**   293
Rahin Mahata, Partha Pratim Chakraborty

33. **Subclinical Hypothyroidism**   300
AK Gupta, Ajit Singh Chahar, Ashutosh Kumar

SECTION 6: EXERCISE AND GOOD HEALTH

34. **Physical Activity and Exercise Plan in a Patient with Type 2 Diabetes Mellitus**   314
Sirshendu Pal

35. **Physiology of Yoga and Its Effect on Body**   319
Arun Chaturvedi

36. **Enjoy Your Exercise**   323
KK Pareek

SECTION 7: GASTROENTEROLOGY

37. **Approach to a Patient of Dyspepsia**   334
Avik Chakraborty

38. **Recent Advances in Management of Acute Pancreatitis**   340
Gurinder Mohan, Arvinder Pal Singh, Jagga Sankalp Harish

39. **Chronic Pancreatitis: Newer Concepts in Management** 348
Rajesh Gopalakrishna

40. **Clinicopathological Approach in a Case of Chronic Diarrhea** 354
Ashis Kumar Saha

41. **Ascites: Diagnostic and Management Issues** 363
Rajesh Upadhyay, Amrit Yog Datley, VS Gaurav Narayan

SECTION 8: HEMATOLOGY

42. **Peripheral Blood Smear: Clues to Diagnosis** 371
Nandini Chatterjee, Nabanita De

43. **Approach to Lymphadenopathy** 379
Alladi Mohan, Srishti Ahluwalia, Saumya Ahluwalia, G Bindhu Madhavi

44. **Approach to Pancytopenia** 384
BL Bhardwaj

SECTION 9: HIV MEDICINE

45. **Updated Antiretroviral Therapy Guidelines: 2022 and Beyond** 391
BB Rewari

46. **Pre- and Post-exposure HIV Prophylaxis** 399
Naval Chandra

SECTION 10: HYPERTENSION

47. **What is New in Current Guidelines of Management of Hypertension?** 403
Hem Shanker Sharma, Reeja Antony

48. **Calcium Channel Blockers and Angiotensin Receptor Blockers: A Friendly Duo** 407
Kamlesh Tewary

49. **Management of Hypertension in Chronic Kidney Disease** 414
Mritunjay Kumar Singh

Contents xxvii

SECTION 11: INFECTIOUS DISEASE

50. **Antimicrobial Stewardship Program** 423
    Amit Aggarwal

51. **Systemic Fungal Infections** 430
    Vipin Mediratta

52. **Approach to Tropical Fever** 434
    Anusha Singhania, Vikas Loomba

53. **Sepsis Management: Current Update** 440
    Shankha S Sen

SECTION 12: METABOLIC MEDICINE

54. **Nonalcoholic Fatty Liver Disease: Current Understanding** 454
    Pradip Bhaumik

55. **Metabolic Syndrome: An Overview** 462
    KK Lohani

56. **Erectile Dysfunction** 467
    MPS Chawla

SECTION 13: NEUROLOGY

57. **The Untold Story of Acute Encephalitis Syndrome** 481
    Jitendra Singh, Anju Dinkar

58. **Management of Acute Ischemic Stroke: What is New?** 494
    TP Singh, Akansha

59. **Advances in Epilepsy Management and Current Perspectives** 505
    Man Mohan Mehndiratta, Vasundhara Aggarwal

SECTION 14: PULMONOLOGY

60. **Changing the Course of Allergic March** 518
    Pradyumn Sharma

61. **Recent Advances in Management of Interstitial Lung Disease** 527
    Prashant Prakash, SK Kushwaha

62. **Approach to Undiagnosed Pleural Effusion** 538
    DP Singh

SECTION 15: RHEUMATOLOGY

63. **A Clinical Approach to Patient with Joint Pain**   544
    Tarun Satija, Samarth Loomba

64. **New Concepts in Systemic Lupus Erythematosus**   550
    S Bhavana, RN Tejaswini, Vijaya Prasanna, G Narsimulu

65. **Changing Landscape of Rheumatoid Arthritis Management**   554
    Uma Kumar, Israrul Haque

SECTION 16: MISCELLANEOUS

66. **Familial Hypercholesterolemia**   558
    Raman Puri, Rashmi Nanda

67. **Antimicrobial Resistance: What the Clinician Should Know?**   566
    Dipanjan Bandyopadhyay, Santanu Hazra, Samarth Loomba

Index   575

CHAPTER 1

Advances in Management of Heart Failure

Debaprasad Chakrabarti, Anirban Bhowmik

■ INTRODUCTION

Heart failure (HF) is an increasing cause of cardiovascular mortality and morbidity in this present era. The figure touches around a humongous number of 26 million people being affected globally annually which contributes to increased healthcare costs worldwide.

The incidence of HF increases with aging from 20 per 1,000 in the age group of 60–69 years to >80 per 1,000 in the age group of more than 80 years. Mortality associated with HF is close to 50% after 5 years of diagnosis. Associated diabetes, hypertension, chronic obstructive pulmonary disease (COPD), coronary artery disease (CAD), and obesity add a poor prognostic outcome.

Hence, knowing about the updated management of HF is of paramount importance. HF has been traditionally classified into different stages according to clinical condition and subtypes based on left ventricular ejection fraction as shown in **Tables 1 and 2**.

As the space would not permit, here we will be discussing certain practice points for the treatment of HF only without referring to other aspects of the disease.

■ MANAGEMENT OF HEART FAILURE

Lifestyle modification and pharmacological therapy form the mainstay, which aims at improving the symptoms, reducing hospital admission, and improving survival. It is imperative that precipitants such as anemia, uncontrolled hypertension, CAD, arrhythmias, and thyrotoxicosis should be looked for and corrected to improve the outcome.

Pharmacological therapy of HF is mainly dependent upon the clinical stage at which the patient presents as well as the LV systolic function of the patient. Nevertheless, the therapy for HF in an acute decompensated stage mainly consists

TABLE 1: Heart failure stages definition and criteria.

Stages	Definition and criteria
Stage A: At risk for HF	At risk for HF but without symptoms, structural heart disease, or cardiac biomarkers of stretch or injury (e.g., patients with hypertension, atherosclerotic CVD, diabetes, metabolic syndrome, and obesity; exposure to cardiotoxic agents; genetic variant for cardiomyopathy; or positive family history of cardiomyopathy)
Stage B: Pre-HF	No symptoms or signs of HF and evidence of 1 of the following: Strutturot *heart disease* • Reduced left or right ventricular systolic function • Reduced ejection fraction, reduced strain • Ventricular hypertrophy • Chamber enlargement • Wall motion abnormalities • Valvular heart disease Evidence *for increased filling pressures* • By invasive hemodynamic measurements • By noninvasive imaging suggesting elevated filling pressures (e.g., Doppler echocardiography) *Patients with risk factors and* • Increased levels of BNPs or • Persistently *elevated cardiac troponin* In the absence of competing diagnoses resulting in such biomarker elevations such as acute coronary syndrome, CKD, pulmonary embolus, or myopericarditis
Stage 0: Symptomatic HF	Structural heart disease with current or previous symptoms of HF
Stage D: Advanced HF	Marked HF symptoms that interfere with daily life and with recurrent hospitalizations despite attempts to optimize GDMT

(BNP: brain natriuretic peptide; CKD: chronic kidney disease; CVD: cardiovascular disease; GDMT: guideline-directed medical therapy; HF: heart failure)

TABLE 2: Type of HF according to LVEF criteria.

Type of HF according to LVEF	Criteria
HFrEF (HF with reduced EF)	LVEF < 40%
HFimpEF (HF with improved EF)	Previous LVEF < 40% and a follow-up measurement of LVEF > 40%
HFmrEF (HF with mildly reduced EF)	LVEF 41–49%
	Evidence of spontaneous or provokable increased LV filling pressures (e.g., elevated natriuretic peptide, noninvasive and invasive hemodynamic measurement)
HFpEF (HF with preserved EF)	LVEF > 50%
	Evidence of spontaneous or provokable increased LV filling pressures (e.g., elevated natriuretic peptide, noninvasive and invasive hemodynamic measurement)

(EF: ejection fraction; HF: heart failure; LV: left ventricle; LVEF: left ventricular ejection fraction)

of drugs such as diuretics, which cause symptom relief. In cases with hemodynamic compromise, inotropes such as dopamine, dobutamine, and milrinone prove useful. In some selective cases with acute decompensated heart failure (ADHF) where intracardiac filling pressure and systemic vascular tone is elevated, vasodilators such as nitroglycerin are used.

Once the decongestion and primary symptom relief are achieved, the focus shifts toward careful transition to longitudinal HF management with the help of appropriate guideline-directed medical therapy (GDMT). Neurohormonal antagonism with renin–angiotensin–aldosterone system (RAAS) blockers such as angiotensin-converting enzyme inhibitors (ACEIs), angiotensin receptor blockers (ARBs), angiotensin receptor–neprilysin inhibitor (ARNi), and beta blockers have been shown to significantly reduce the mortality and risk of hospital admissions in HF. Addition of mineralocorticoid receptor antagonists (MRAs) is found to be useful in both heart failure with reduced ejection fraction (HFrEF) and heart failure with preserved ejection frdaction (HFdpEF). Newer drugs such as sodium-glucose cotransporter-2 inhibitors (SGLT-2i) and soluble guanylyl cyclase (sGC) inhibitors have shown a promising role in the treatment of HFrEF. These drugs work mainly by reversing the left ventricular (LV) remodeling and reduction in circulating natriuretic peptide concentration.

There have been certain recent developments and recommendations in the therapy of HF which is discussed below according to the recently published American College of Cardiology/American Heart Association (ACC/AHA) Guidelines for Heart failure 2022.

RECOMMENDATIONS CONSIDERED FOR PATIENTS AT RISK FOR HEART FAILURE STATES

Stage A: Primary Prevention

Healthy lifestyle habits such as regular physical activity, maintaining normal weight, following healthy dietary patterns, and avoiding smoking should be encouraged to reduce the future risk of HF. Blood pressure should be controlled in accordance with GDMT for hypertension to prevent symptoms of impending HF. An SGLT-2i should be used to prevent recurrent hospitalizations for HF in patients having type 2 diabetes mellitus (T2DM) with either established cardiovascular diseases or at high risk for cardiovascular diseases.

Management of Stage B: Preventing the Syndrome of Clinical HF in Patients with Pre-HF

In patients who have LVEF ≤ 40%, ACEIs/ARBs are preferred to prevent symptomatic HF and reduce mortality. Cardio-selective beta blockers are proven to reduce mortality in patients with antecedent history of myocardial infarction (MI) or acute coronary syndrome (ACS) and LVEF ≤ 40% and are used to prevent symptomatic HF in such patients.

Management of Stage C Heart Failure

Diuretics and Decongestion Strategies in Patients with HF

Diuretics, preferably IV loop diuretics, are recommended to relieve congestive symptoms in HF patients with fluid overload. Patients who fail to respond to high doses of oral furosemide may benefit from transition to torsemide due to greater oral bioavailability. Addition of a thiazide (e.g., metolazone) to treatment with a loop diuretic should be reserved for patients who do not respond to moderate- or high-dose loop diuretics to minimize electrolyte abnormalities.

Pharmacological Treatment for HFrEF: Renin–Angiotensin System Inhibition with ACEI or ARB or ARNi

Sacubitril–valsartan has been approved for patients with symptomatic HF. In the PARADIGM-HF, a randomized controlled trial, patients with HFrEF treated with GDMT were randomly allocated to treatment with either enalapril or sacubitril–valsartan. Compared to those assigned to enalapril, patients assigned to sacubitril–valsartan experienced a dramatic 20% reduction in the composite primary endpoint of cardiovascular death or HF hospitalization and a 16% reduction in all-cause mortality. In patients with HFrEF and New York Heart Association (NYHA) class II to III symptoms, the use of ARNi is recommended to reduce morbidity and mortality. ACEI is preferred when use of ARNi is not feasible due to nonaffordability.

In chronic symptomatic HFrEF paitents (NYHA class II or III) who can tolerate an ACEI or ARB, ARNi is recommended to further reduce morbidity and mortality. ARNi should not be administered concomitantly with ACEI or within 36 hours of the last dose of an ACEI. ARNI and ACEIs should not be administered to patients with any history of angioedema.

Beta Blockers

Beta blocker use in HFrEF should ideally be restricted to carvedilol, bisoprolol, and metoprolol succinate—agents tested and proven to improve survival in clinical trials. Cardiac Insufficiency Bisoprolol Study (CIBIS) III revealed that outcomes did not vary with the sequence of initiation between beta blockers and ACEIs.

Mineralocorticoid Receptor Antagonists

Elevated aldosterone levels in HFrEF promote sodium retention, endothelial dysfunction, and may directly contribute to myocardial fibrosis. In patients with HFrEF and NYHA class II to IV symptoms, an MRA (spironolactone or eplerenone) is recommended, if estimated glomerular filtration rate (eGFR) is >30 mL/min/1.73 m^2 and serum potassium is <5.0 mEq/L. Addition of MRAs to treatment with ACEIs/ARBs and beta blockers in class II-IV patients of HFrEF is associated with further reductions in mortality.

Sodium-Glucose Cotransporter-2 Inhibitors

Sodium-glucose cotransporter-2 inhibitors such as dapagliflozin and empagliflozin are recommended in patients with symptomatic chronic HFrEF, to reduce hospitalization for HF and cardiovascular mortality, irrespective of the presence of T2DM.

Several trials have been done to examine the efficacy of SGLT-2i on outcomes in patients with HF, irrespective of the presence of T2DM. The DAPA-HF trial and EMPEROR-Reduced demonstrated the benefit of SGLT-2i (dapagliflozin and empagliflozin, respectively) compared to placebo in reducing the composite of cardiovascular death or HF hospitalization by approximately 25%. Therapy with SGLT-2i as a class showed a reduction in all-cause mortality and cardiovascular death irrespective of the baseline diabetes status. The rate of decline in eGFR was also slower in patients treated with SGLT-2i.

During SGLT-2i use, caution has to be warranted for euglycemic ketoacidosis, and genital and soft-tissue infections.

Hydralazine and Isosorbide Dinitrate

This combination improves survival in HFrEF but to a lesser extent than ACEIs. The combination of hydralazine and isosorbide dinitrate is recommended for patients with NYHA class III–IV HFrEF to improve symptoms and reduce morbidity and mortality, especially in whom first-line agents such as ARNi, ACEI, or ARBs cannot be given, because of drug intolerance or renal insufficiency.

Other Drug Treatment

Ivabradine

Ivabradine can be beneficial to reduce HF cardiovascular death in patients with symptomatic stable chronic HFrEF (LVEF ≤ 35%) who are receiving GDMT, including a beta blocker at maximum tolerated dose with a heart rate of ≥70 bpm at rest, still in sinus rhythm seen in SHIFT trial.

Digoxin

The Digitalis Investigation Group (DIG) trial, a large-scale randomized controlled trial (RCT) of digoxin in patients with HF, showed a modest decrease in hospitalization and death risk but no significant mortality benefit.

Soluble Guanylyl Cyclase Stimulators

Vericiguat is a novel oral sGC stimulator that enhances cyclic guanosine monophosphate (GMP) and nitric oxide (NO) signaling by directly stimulating sGC and sensitizing sGC to endogenous NO. In selected high-risk patients with HFrEF, vericiguat may be considered to reduce HF hospitalization and cardiovascular death seen in VICTORIA trial.

Myosin Activation

Omecamtiv mecarbil, a selective myosin activator, prolongs the ejection period and increases fractional shortening without altering the force of contraction as a consequence. It showed a 14% reduction in the primary composite endpoint of death from cardiovascular causes or first HF event in patients with symptomatic chronic HF and ejection fraction of 35% or less in GALACTIC-HF trial.

Implantable Cardioverter Defibrillator and Cardiac Resynchronization Therapy

Implantable cardioverter defibrillator (ICD) is recommended in patients with nonischemic dilated cardiomyopathy (DCM) or ischemic heart disease at least 40 days post-MI with LVEF ≤ 35% and NYHA class II or III symptoms or 40 days post MI with LVEF < 30% and NYHA I symptoms, receiving GDMT who have reasonable expectation of meaningful survival for >1 year, for primary prevention of sudden cardiac death (SCD) to reduce total mortality.

Cardiac resynchronization therapy (CRT) is recommended in patients with LV systolic dysfunction (LVEF ≤ 35%), sinus rhythm, left bundle branch block (LBBB)/non-LBBB with a QRS duration ≥ 150 ms, and NYHA class II, III, or ambulatory IV symptoms on GDMT, to reduce total mortality and hospitalizations and to improve symptoms seen. For patients who have LVEF ≤ 35%, sinus rhythm, a non-LBBB pattern with a QRS duration of 120–149 ms, and NYHA class III or ambulatory class IV on GDMT, CRT may be considered to reduce total mortality, reduce hospitalizations, and improve symptoms.

Other devices such as MitraClip, cardiac contractility modulation, baroreflex activation therapy, and phrenic nerve stimulation therapy have been found to improve the functional class and reduce hospitalization.

Mechanical Circulatory Support and Transplantation

Left ventricular assist device (LVAD) supports the function of failing heart partially or completely making it a choice for bridge to transplantation. Last, patients with end-stage HF with refractory symptoms on GDMT should be assessed for heart transplantation.

HEART FAILURE WITH PRESERVED EJECTION FRACTION

Sodium-glucose cotransporter-2 inhibitors can be beneficial in decreasing hospitalizations and cardiovascular mortality in patients with HFpEF. In selected patients, MRAs, ARBs, and ARNIs may be considered to decrease hospitalizations, particularly among patients with LVEF on the lower end of this spectrum.

Management of Stages C and D of Heart Failure

Because of space constraint, the treatment of stages C and D is presented here in an algorithmic chart **(Fig. 1)**.

CONCLUSION

With the advent of universal definition and classification, the management of HF is expected to become more standardized. While conventional GDMT in optimal dosage remains the standard of care, the newer drugs and devices appear promising if introduced in a sequential manner to offer maximum benefit.

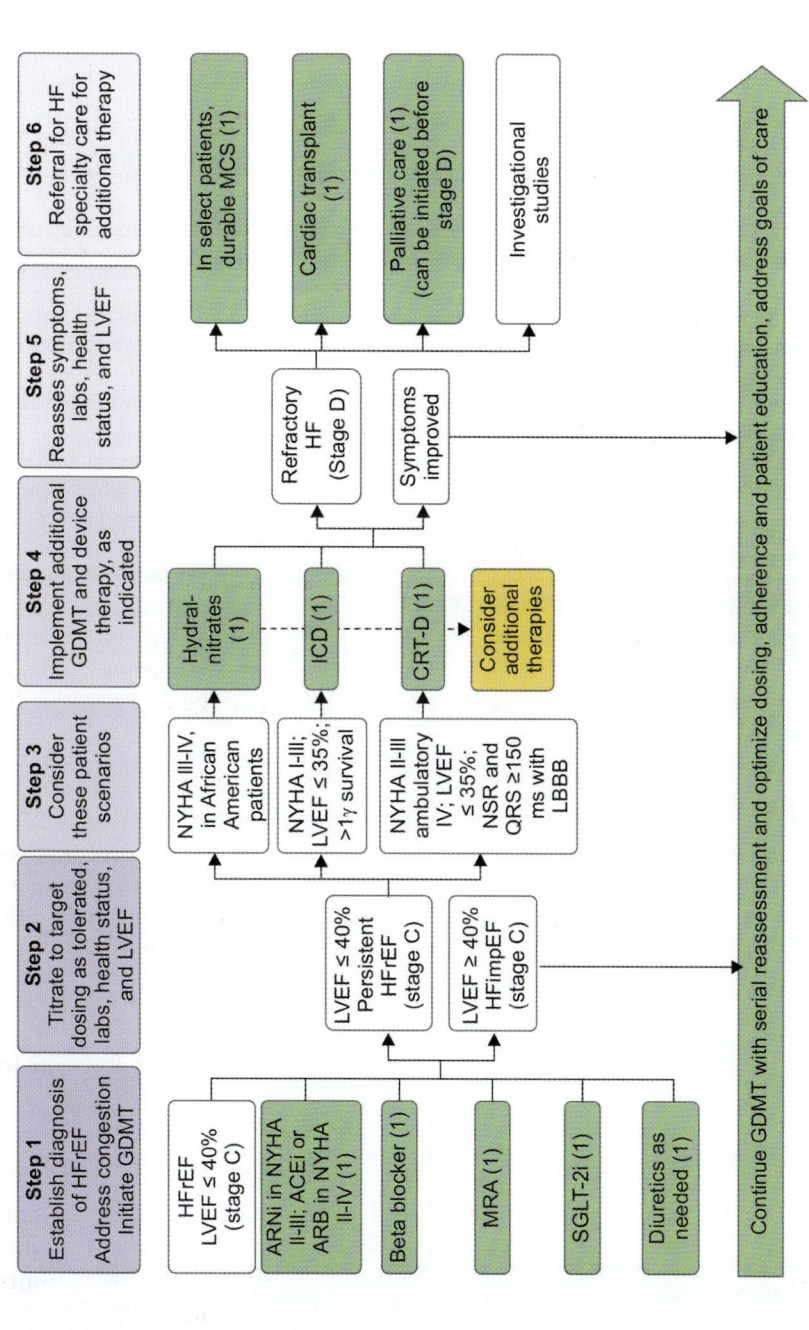

FIG. 1: Management of stages C and D of heart failure.

SUGGESTED READINGS

1. Savarese G, Lund LH. Global public health burden of heart failure. Card Fail Rev. 2017;3(1):7-11.
2. Heidenreich PA, Bozkurt B, Aguilar D, et al; 2022 AHA/ACC/HFSA Guideline for the Management of Heart Failure: A Report of the American College of Cardiology/American Heart Association Joint Committee on Clinical Practice Guidelines. J American Coll Cardiol. 2022;79(17):e263-e421.
3. SOLVD Investigators. Effect of enalapril on mortality and the development of heart failure in asymptomatic patients with reduced left ventricular ejection fractions. N Engl J Med. 1992;327:685-91.
4. McMurray JJ, Packer M, Desai AS, et al. Angiotensin neprilysin inhibition versus enalapril in heart failure. N Engl J Med. 2014;371:993-1004.
5. Wachter R, Senni M, Belohlavek J, et al. Initiation of sacubitril/valsartan in haemodynamically stabilised heart failure patients in hospital or early after discharge: primary results of the randomised TRANSITION study. Eur J Heart Fail. 2019;21:998-1007.
6. Pitt B, Zannad F, Remme WJ, et al. The effect of spironolactone on morbidity and mortality in patients with severe heart failure. Randomized Aldactone Evaluation Study Investigators. N Engl J Med. 1999;341:709-17.
7. McMurray JJV, Solomon SD, Inzucchi SE, et al. Dapagliflozin in patients with heart failure and reduced ejection fraction. N Engl J Med. 2019;381:1995-2008.
8. Packer M, Anker SD, Butler J, et al. Cardiovascular and renal outcomes with empagliflozin in heart failure. N Engl J Med. 2020;383:1413-24.
9. Swedberg K, Komajda M, Böhm M, et al. Ivabradine and outcomes in chronic heart failure (SHIFT): a randomised placebo-controlled study. Lancet. 2010;376:875-85.
10. Wagner BR, Frishman WH. Devices for autonomic regulation therapy in heart failure with reduced ejection fraction. Cardiol Rev. 2018;26:43-9.

CHAPTER 2

Microalbuminuria: A Risk Marker for CAD

AN Rai

"One can obtain considerable information concerning the general health by examining the urine."

—Hippocrates

■ INTRODUCTION

Coronary artery disease (CAD) is a major cause of mortality and morbidity in both developed and now in developing countries. Atherosclerosis is responsible for almost all cases of CAD. CAD is a multifactorial disorder with several classical risk factors—namely blood pressure, smoking, cholesterol, diabetes, and obesity. Subsequent studies and meta-analyses have identified other factors to better identify patients potentially at risk of CAD, including inflammatory markers, hemostatic factors, left ventricular hypertrophy, metabolic syndrome, and markers of kidney dysfunctions such as decreased GFR and microalbuminuria (MAU). MAU is gaining recognition as a simple marker of an atherogenic milieu, owing to its association with several atherosclerotic risk factors and early systemic vascular (endothelial) damage. MAU is also a marker of subclinical organ damage and cost-effective and useful tool for screening of high risk persons and helps in modifying and optimizing the treatment strategy.

■ MICROALBUMINURIA: MEASUREMENT AND DEFINITION

- **A 24-hour timed urine sample** has long been the gold standard for measuring albuminuria, but the collection is cumbersome and time-consuming, and the test is prone to laboratory error.
- **Dipstick measurements** are more convenient but they have low sensitivity and high interobserver variation.
- **The albumin-to-creatinine ratio (ACR)** is consistent with the 24-hour timed collection (the gold standard) and is the recommended method of assessing albuminuria

Microalbuminuria is defined as persistent increased urinary albumin excretion (UAE) in the range of 20–200 µg/minute or 30–300 mg/24 hours. Persistent MAU is defined as the presence of MAU in two or three consecutively collected samples preferably within a period of 6 months.

Microalbuminuria can also be defined in terms of the urinary albumin to creatinine ratio. A ratio greater than 30 mg/g in the first voided, clear, and midstream morning urine sample is considered abnormal.

■ LINK BETWEEN ALBUMINURIA AND CORONARY ARTERY DISEASE

The endothelium, once considered a simple, inert semipermeable barrier between the bloodstream and the outer vascular wall, is now recognized to mediate vasoactivity, maintains blood fluidity, and contributes to the local balance between pro and anti-inflammatory activity as well as pro and anticoagulant activity.

Thus endothelial dysfunctions are considered to be the first stage of atherosclerosis and precede structural disorder, plaque buildup and clinical events such as CAD **(Fig. 1)**.

It was shown that imaging technique for endothelial dysfunction (ED) such as flow-mediated vasodilation, was impaired in individuals with diabetes mellitus as compared with those without and also was impaired in individuals with microalbuminuria as compared with those without, regardless of whether they had diabetes or not.

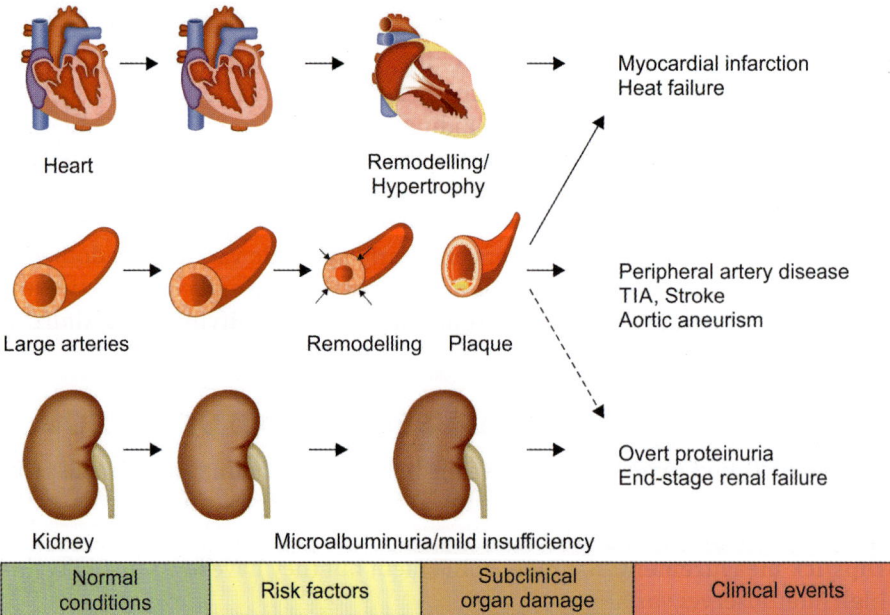

FIG.1: Schematic representation of the cardiovascular continuum from normal physiologic condition (left) to the presence of cardiovascular risk factors, subclinical organ damage, and eventually cardiovascular, cerebrovascular, and renal events (right).

In view of these considerations, endothelial dysfunction with an impaired nitric oxide (NO) balance, activation of local mediators, and increased activity of the renin-angiotensin–aldosterone system (RAAS) system possibly explain the association between microalbuminuria and various diseases including cardiovascular disease (CVD) **(Fig. 2)**.

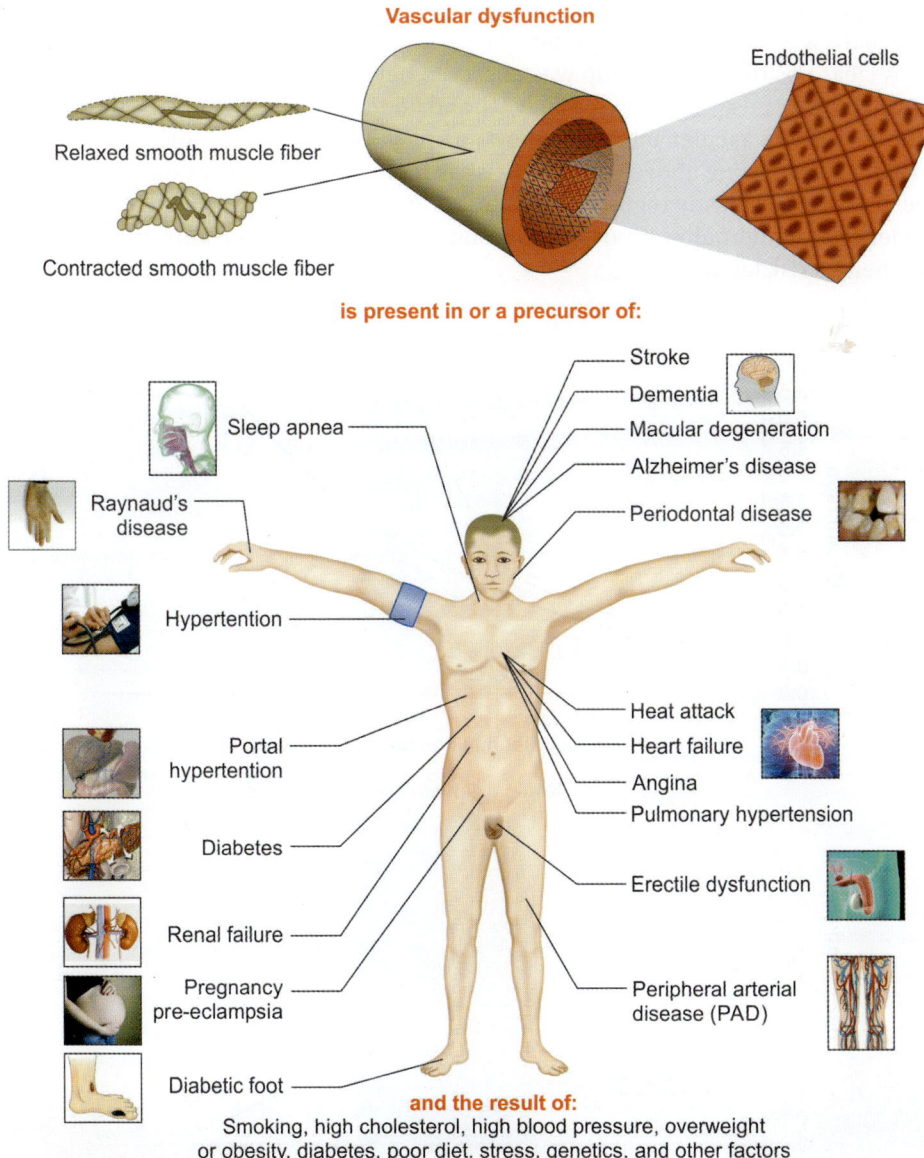

FIG. 2: Microalbuminuria and cardiovascular complications.

PREVEND: To Assess the Impact of Microalbuminuria in General

The **P**revention of **Re**nal and **V**ascular **En**d-stage **D**isease (PREVEND) study aims to study the natural course of an elevated urinary albumin loss in general population. The prevalence of microalbuminuria in a select sample ($n = 40{,}856$) of the mostly Caucasian population of 28–75 years in the city of Groningen is 7.2% ($n = 2{,}918$). Of the 2,918 subjects, that were found to be microalbuminuric (defined as a morning urinary albumin concentration of 20–200 mg/L) only 6.2% was known to be diabetic and 18.9% was known to be hypertensive.

A clear positive relationship was observed between urinary albumin excretion (UAE) and all-cause, cardiovascular (CV), and noncardiovascular death. The hazard ratio for cardiovascular mortality shows a splay as shown in **Figure 3**, without a specific cut-off value above which the risk is increased. For every doubling of UAE the risk of CV death is increased by almost 30%. The results provide compelling evidence that microalbuminuria is a strong predictor of CV mortality, independent of other CV risk factors.

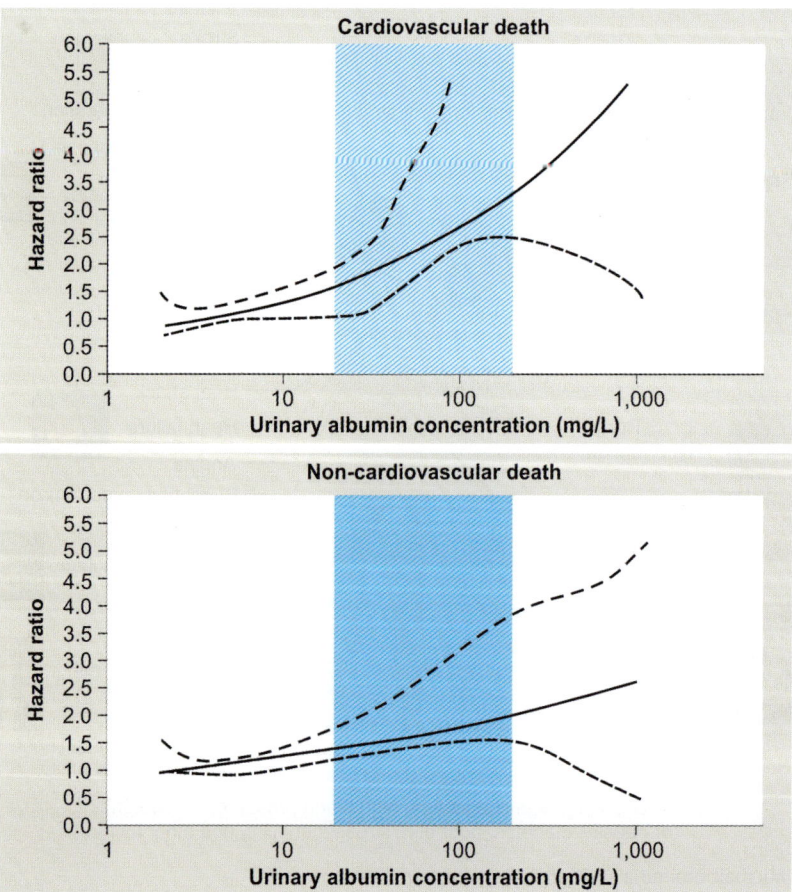

FIG. 3: Concentrations of microalbuminuria and cardiovascular and non-cardiovascular complications.

The LIFE Study: To Assess the Impact of Albuminuria in Hypertensive Patients with Left Ventricular Hypertrophy

The Losartan Intervention for Endpoint reduction in hypertension (LIFE) study aims to determine the albuminuria level at which CV morbidity and mortality are increased in a large group ($n = 8,106$) of hypertensive patients with left ventricular hypertrophy.

A clear positive relationship was observed between UACR and primary composite endpoint (CV death, fatal and non-fatal MI, fatal and non-fatal stroke) **(Fig. 4)**. Moreover it has been shown that MAU is independently associated with CV mortality with such a relationship maintained even within normal range of UACR. Investigators also suggested that detecting microalbuminuria would help clinicians decide when to initiate antihypertensive therapy, since it represents target organ damage.

HOPE: To Assess the Impact of Microalbuminuria in High Risk Patients

In a Heart Outcomes Prevention Evaluation (HOPE) substudy, UAE predicted mortality in patients who were at high CV risk (55 years of age with CVD or diabetes plus at least one other CV risk factor). A linear relationship was also observed between the level of microalbuminuria and CV events, even extending below the traditional microalbuminuria threshold.

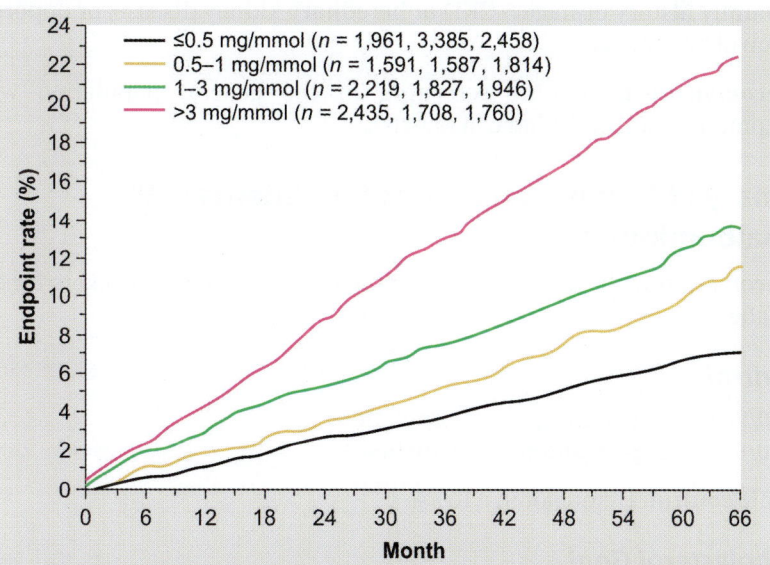

FIG. 4: Composite end point stratified by time-varying albuminuria. The numbers in parentheses are the numbers of at-risk patients in each range of UACR at baseline, year 2, and year 4.

CV RISK STRATIFICATION

Cardiovascular risk assessment in the clinical practice is mostly based on risk charts, such as Framingham risk score and Systemic Coronary Risk Estimation (SCORE). Based on these individuals are classified at low risk (<1% of CVD death at 10 years with SCORE), intermediate risk (1–5% in SCORE), or high risk (>5% with SCORE). These scoring systems guide the appropriate clinical management.

Sehestedt et al. investigated, whether inclusion of marker of subclinical organ damage such as MA and LVH could improve the CV risk prediction beyond SCORE. Based on their findings the authors concluded that the most efficient approach would be only to measure MA in subjects with SCORE between 1–5% rather than in subjects with SCORE <1%. In fact, these patients in the presence of MAU would become at high CV risk by having CV death odds more than three-fold higher compared to those patients without MAU.

GUIDELINES ON SCREENING

KDIGO: People with diabetes, hypertension, CVD, family history of CKD, obesity, hyperlipidemia, metabolic syndrome, smoking, treatment with potentially nephrotoxic drugs, some chronic infectious diseases, and cancers, age >60.

ADA: Patients with type 1 diabetes mellitus with a duration ≥5 years and in all patients with type 2 diabetes mellitus at the time of diagnosis.

NICE: People at risk—e.g., those with diabetes, hypertension, CVD, structural renal tract disease, renal calculi, prostatic hypertrophy, multisystem diseases such as SLE, a family history of stage 5 CKD or hereditary kidney disease, or opportunistic detection of hematuria.

Not recommended: Routine screening in the general population who are asymptomatic or are considered at low risk.

Summary of Recommendations for Patients with Microalbuminuria

Reno protection with ACE inhibitors or angiotensin receptor blockers for patients with diabetes.

BP Control
- <140/90 mm Hg for the general population.
- <130/80 mm Hg for patients with diabetes.

Glycemic control: Hemoglobin A1c 7%

LDL Cholesterol Goal
- <100 mg/dL for patients with advanced renal disease or diabetes.
- <70 mg/dL is patients with diabetes and CVD HDL levels.
- Consider screening in patients with diabetes.
- Smoking cessation.

- Dietary limitation of salt (3 g/day) and saturated fat.
- Regular exercise and weight control.
- Antiplatelet therapy.

CONCLUSION

- MAU is a risk marker of both renal and CVD.
- MAU and CVD linked by a common pathophysiological process (generalized endothelial dysfunction).
- MAU is most effective tool to measure target organ damage in hypertensive patients.
- Risk of adverse clinical outcomes starts below the traditional MAU threshold.
- It is a treatable marker, and blood pressure control is most effective means to reduce MAU.

SUGGESTED READINGS

1. Johnson RJ, Feehily J, Floege J. Comprehensive Clinical Nephrology, 5th edition. Elsevier Saunders; 2014.
2. Versari D, Daghini E, Virdis A, et al. Endothelial dysfunction as a target for prevention of cardiovascular disease. Diabetes Care. 2009;Suppl 2(Suppl 2):S314-21.
3. Hillege HL, Fidler V, Diercks GF, et al. Urinary albumin excretion predicts cardiovascular and Non cardiovascular mortality in general population. Circulation. 2002;106(14):1777-82.
4. Ibsen H, Olsen MH, Wachtel K, et al. Reduction in albuminuria translates to reduction in cardiovascular events in hypertensive patients: losartan intervention for endpoint reduction in hypertension study. Hypertension. 2005;45(2):198-202.
5. Gerstein HC, Mann JF, Pogue J, et al. Prevalence and determinants of microalbuminuria in high risk diabetes determinants of microalbuminuria in high risk diabetes and non-diabetic patients in the heart outcomes prevention evaluation study. The HOPE study investigators. Diabetes Care. 2000;23 (Suppl 2):B35-9.
6. Sehestedt T, Jeppesen J, Hansen TW, et al. Risk prediction is improved by adding markers of subclinical organ damage to SCORE. Eur Heart J. 2010;31(7):883-91.
7. Weir MR. Microalbuminuria and cardiovascular disease. Clin J Am Soc Nephrol. 2007;2(3):581-90.

CHAPTER 3

Cardiomyopathy: Diagnosis and Management

Subhash Chandra

■ DEFINITION

A heterogeneous group of diseases of the myocardium associated with mechanical and/or electrical dysfunction that usually (but not invariably) exhibit inappropriate ventricular hypertrophy or dilatation and are due to a variety of causes that frequently are genetic. Cardiomyopathies either are confined to the heart or are part of generalized systemic disorders, often leading to cardiovascular death or progressive heart failure-related disability.
(Ref: American Heart Association, Clinical Cardiology Current Practice Guidelines by OXFORD 2016, pp. 427)

■ FRANK–STARLING LAW

The *Frank–Starling law* represents the relationship between stroke volume and end-diastolic volume. The law states that the stroke volume of the heart increases in response to an increase in the volume of blood in the ventricles, before contraction (the end-diastolic volume), when all other factors remain constant. As a larger volume of blood flows into the ventricle, the blood stretches cardiac muscle, leading to an increase in the force of contraction.

With increase in right atrial pressure/end-diastolic volume will increase cardiac volume. At certain level, cardiac volume will not increase and will come to stationary point. After this with further increase in right atrial pressure, the patient will go into LVF. So, our aim is to reduce end-diastolic volume to this point where we can get maximum contractibility and "cardiac output".

Cardiomyopathy: Diagnosis and Management

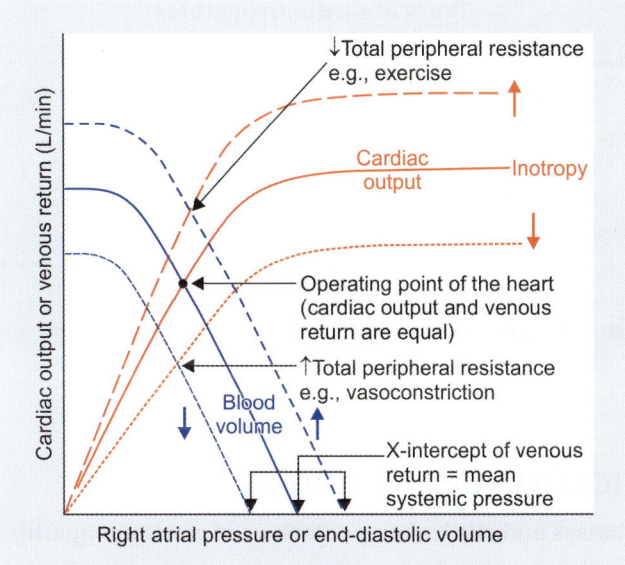

TYPES OF CARDIOMYOPATHIES

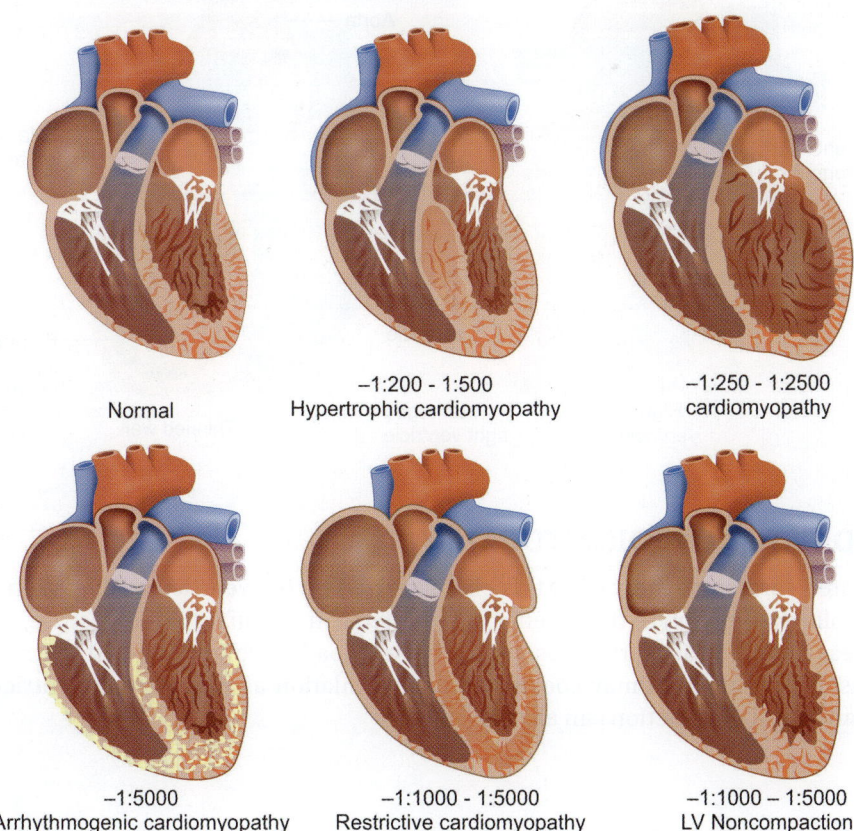

Normal

−1:200 - 1:500
Hypertrophic cardiomyopathy

−1:250 - 1:2500
cardiomyopathy

−1:5000
Arrhythmogenic cardiomyopathy

−1:1000 - 1:5000
Restrictive cardiomyopathy

−1:1000 − 1:5000
LV Noncompaction

18 Cardiomyopathy: Diagnosis and Management

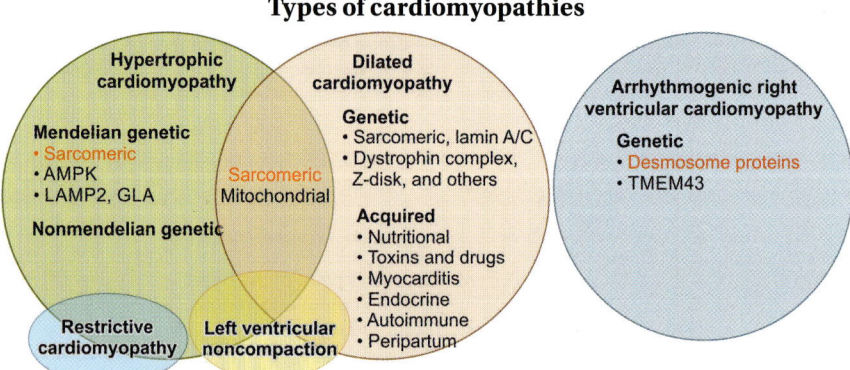

■ CLASSIFICATION OF CARDIOMYOPATHIES

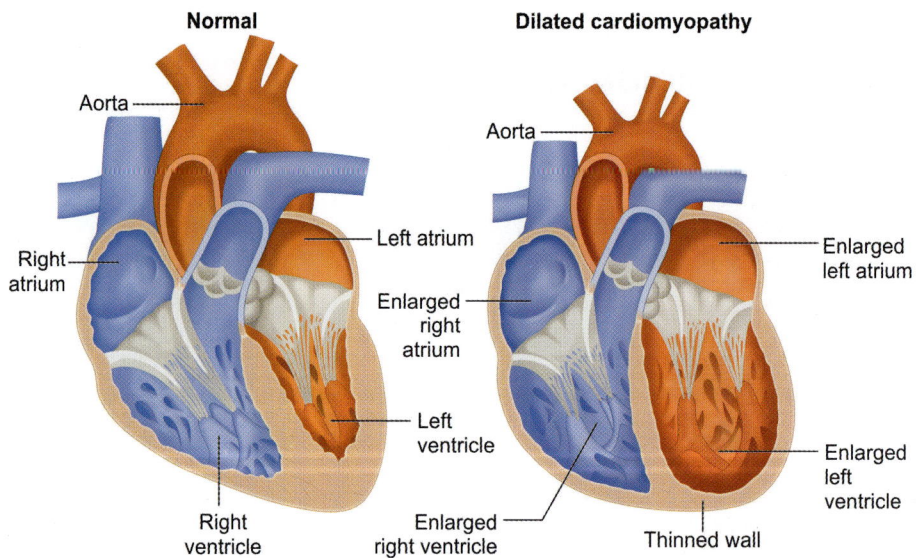

■ DILATED CARDIOMYOPATHY

Dilated cardiomyopathy (DCM) is characterized by left ventricular dilatation and systolic dysfunction in the absence of hypertension, coronary artery disease, valve disease, congenital heart disease, and other overloading conditions. Left ventricular diastolic dysfunction may coexist, and atrial dilation as well as right ventricular dilation and dysfunction can also develop.

MAJOR CAUSES OF DILATED CARDIOMYOPATHY

Inflammatory Myocarditis

Infective
- Viral (coxsackie, an adenovirus, an HIV, and hepatitis C)
- Parasitic (*T. cruzi*—Chagas' disease, trypanosomiasis, and toxoplasmosis)
- Bacterial (diphtheria)
- Spirochetal (Borreliaburgdorferi—Lyme disease)
- Rickettsial (Q fever)
- Fungal (with systemic infection)

Noninfective
- Granulomatous inflammatory disease
- Sarcoidosis
- Giant cell myocarditis
- Eosinophilic myocarditis
- Polymyositis, dermatomyositis
- Collagen vascular disease

Toxic
- Alcohol
- Catecholamines: Amphetamines, cocaine
- Chemotherapeutic agents (anthracyclines, trastuzumab)
- Interferon
- Other therapeutic agents (hydroxychloroquine, chloroquine)
- Drugs of misuse (emetine, anabolic steroids)
- Heavy metals: Lead, mercury
- Occupational exposure: Hydrocarbons, arsenicals

Metabolic
- Nutritional deficiencies: Thiamine, selenium, and carnitine
- Electrolyte deficiencies: Calcium, phosphate, and magnesium
- Endocrinopathy
- Thyroid disease
- Pheochromocytoma
- Diabetes
- Obesity
- Hemochromatosis
- Inherited metabolic pathway defects

Familial
- Skeletal and cardiac myopathy
- Dystrophin-related dystrophy (Duchenne's, Becker's)
- Mitochondrial myopathies (e.g., Kearns–Sayre syndrome)
- Arrhythmogenic ventricular dysplasia

- Hemochromatosis
- Associated with other systemic diseases
- Susceptibility to immune-mediated myocarditis

Overlap with Nondilated Cardiomyopathy: Minimally Dilated Cardiomyopathy
- Hemochromatosis
- Amyloidosis
- Hypertrophic cardiomyopathy ("burned-out")
- Idiopathic

Coronary Artery Occlusion
Ischemic Dilated cardiac myopathy.

Peripartum Cardiomyopathy

TakotSubo (Stress Cardiomyopathy)

IDIOPATHIC DILATED CARDIOMYOPATHY (PATHOLOGIC FINDINGS)

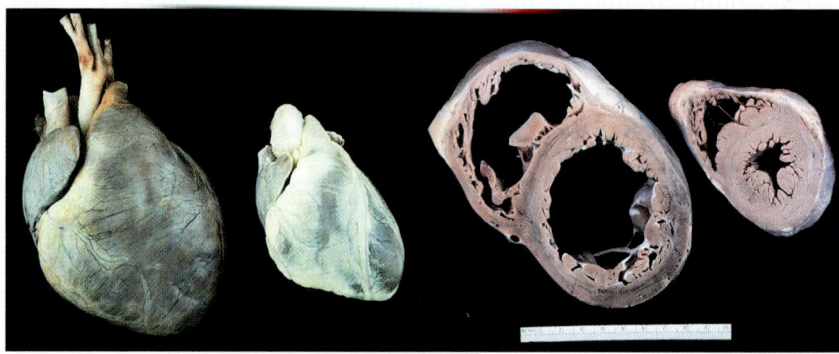

DILATED CARDIOMYOPATHY: CLINICAL FEATURES
- Highest incidence in middle age
- Symptoms may be gradual in onset.
- Acute presentation
- Misdiagnosed as viral URTI in young adults
- Symptoms/Signs of heart failure
- Pulmonary congestion (left heart failure) dyspnea (rest, exertional, nocturnal), orthopnea
- Systemic congestion (right heart failure) edema, nausea, abdominal pain, nocturia
- Low cardiac output

- Hypotension, tachycardia, and tachypnea
- Fatigue and weakness
- Arrhythmia
- Atrial fibrillation, conduction delays, sudden death

■ INCIDENCE OF SYMPTOMS

- Heart failure symptoms   75–85%
- Anginal chest pain   8–20%
- Emboli (systemic or pulmonary) 1–4%
- Syncope   <1%
- Sudden cardiac death   <1%

■ DILATED CARDIOMYOPATHY: INCIDENCE AND PROGNOSIS

- Prevalence is 36 per 100,000 population
- Third most common cause of heart failure
- Most frequent cause of heart transplantation
- Complete recovery is rare.
- 50% die within 2 years and 25% survive longer than 5 years

■ THE NEW YORK HEART ASSOCIATION CLASSIFICATION

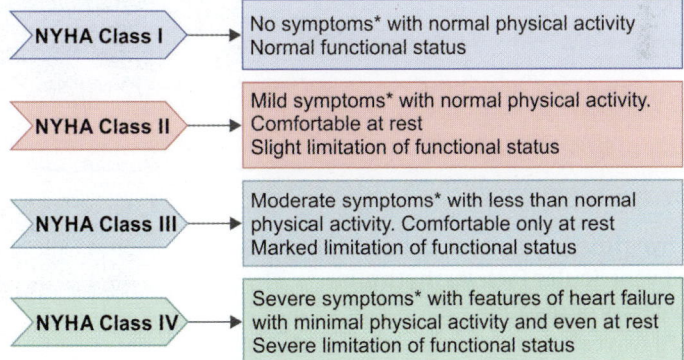

New York heart association (NYHA) classification of severity of heart failure

NYHA Class I → No symptoms* with normal physical activity. Normal functional status

NYHA Class II → Mild symptoms* with normal physical activity. Comfortable at rest. Slight limitation of functional status

NYHA Class III → Moderate symptoms* with less than normal physical activity. Comfortable only at rest. Marked limitation of functional status

NYHA Class IV → Severe symptoms* with features of heart failure with minimal physical activity and even at rest. Severe limitation of functional status

Symptoms: Fatigue, palpitations, chest pain, dyspnea, syncope

■ DILATED CARDIOMYOPATHY: LABORATORY FINDINGS

- Red cell distribution width (RDW)
- Kidney function test
- Chronic kidney disease is another poor prognostic factor in heart failure and may limit certain treatment options.
- Serum electrolytes may disclose hypokalemia, which increases the risk of arrhythmias; hyperkalemia, which may limit the use of inhibitors of the renin-angiotensin system; or hyponatremia, an indicator of marked activation of the renin-angiotensin system and a poor prognostic sign.

- Thyroid function should be assessed to detect occult thyrotoxicosis or myxedema and iron studies should be checked to test for hemochromatosis.
- In unexplained cases, appropriate biopsies may lead to a diagnosis of amyloidosis. Myocardial biopsy may exclude specific causes of dilated cardiomyopathy but rarely reveals specific reversible diagnoses.
- Serum BNP is a powerful prognostic marker that adds to clinical assessment in differentiating dyspnea due to heart failure from noncardiac causes. *Two markers—BNP and NT-proBNP—provide similar diagnostic and prognostic information.* BNP is expressed primarily in the ventricles and is elevated when ventricular filling pressures are high.
- However, there is no proven value in using serial natriuretic peptide measurements to guide therapy, as shown in the *GUIDE-IT trial*. Elevation of serum troponin, and especially of high-sensitivity troponin, is common in both chronic and acute heart failure, and it is associated with higher risk of adverse outcomes.

ECG

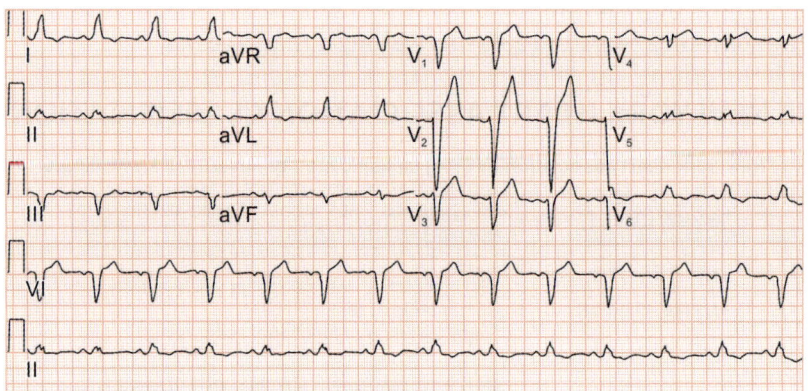

- Sinus tachycardia in presence of heart failure
- Atrial and ventricular tachyarrhythmia
- Poor "r wave" progression
- Anterior "q waves"
- Intraventricular conduction defects—mostly LBBB
- Left atrial abnormality
- Hypertensive changes by voltage criteria not evident

CHEST RADIOGRAPHY

Pleural effusions are common and tend to be bilateral or right-sided.

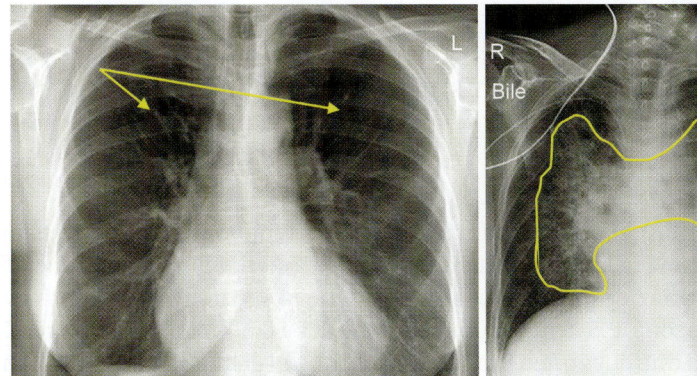

ECHOCARDIOGRAPHY

- Dilated chambers
- Left atrium is usually enlarged.
- Left ventricle is enlarged. Normal 3.8–5.0 cm
- Mitral and tricuspid regurgitation on Doppler flow
- Stress testing—tachyarryhthmias
- Dobutamine stress echocardiography is helpful in assessing the clinical prognosis.

CARDIAC CATHETERIZATION

Clinical examination and noninvasive tests can determine LV size and function and valve function to support and refine the diagnosis. Left heart catheterization may be helpful to define the presence and extent of CAD, although CT angiography may also be appropriate, especially when the likelihood of coronary disease is low.

Evaluation for coronary disease is particularly important when LV dysfunction may be partially reversible by revascularization.

The combination of angina or noninvasive evidence of significant myocardial ischemia with symptomatic heart failure is often an indication for coronary angiography if the patient is a potential candidate for revascularization.

Right heart catheterization may be useful to select and monitor therapy in patient's refractory to standard therapy.

DILATED CARDIOMYOPATHY: TREATMENT

Correction of Reversible Causes

The major reversible causes of heart failure with reduced EF, also called chronic systolic heart failure, include *valvular lesions, myocardial ischemia, uncontrolled hypertension, arrhythmias (especially persistent tachycardias), alcohol- or drug-induced myocardial depression, hypothyroidism, intracardiac shunts, and high-output states.*

Calcium-channel blockers with negative inotropy (specifically verapamil or diltiazem), antiarrhythmic medications, thiazolidinediones, and nonsteroidal anti-inflammatory drugs (NSAIDs) may be important contributors to worsening the heart failure.

DILATED CARDIOMYOPATHY: PROVEN THERAPEUTIC OPTION

Diuretic Therapy

Diuretics are the most effective means of providing symptomatic relief to patients with moderate to severe heart failure with dyspnea and fluid overload. When fluid retention is mild, thiazide diuretics or a similar type of agent (hydrochlorothiazide, 25–100 mg; metolazone, 2.5–5 mg; chlorthalidone, 25–50 mg; etc.) may be sufficient. Thiazide or related diuretics often provide better control of hypertension than short-acting la agents.

Metolazone maintains its efficacy down to a glomerular filtration rate of approximately 20–30 mL/min. Adverse reactions include hypokalemia and intravascular volume depletion with resulting prerenal azotemia, skin rash neutropenia and thrombocytopenia, hyperglycemia, hyperuricemia, and hepatic dysfunction.

Patients with more severe heart failure should be treated with one of the oral loop diuretics. These include furosemide (20–320 mg daily), bumetanide (1–8 mg daily), and torsemide (20–200 mg daily). These agents have rapid onset and a relatively short duration of action. Torsemide may be effective when furosemide is not, related to better absorption and a longer half life. Larger doses (up to 500 mg of furosemide or equivalent) may be required with severe renal impairment. The major adverse reactions include intravascular volume depletion, prerenal azotemia, and hypotension. Hypokalemia, particularly with accompanying digitalis therapy, is a major problem. Less common side effects include skin rashes, gastrointestinal distress, and ototoxicity (the latter more common with ethacrynic acid and possibly less common with bumetanide).

The oral potassium-sparing agents are often useful in combination with the loop diuretics and thiazides. Triamterene (37.5–75 mg daily) and amiloride (5–10 mg daily) act on the distal tubule to reduce potassium secretion.

Spironolactone (12.5–100 mg daily) and eplerenone (25–100 mg daily) are specific inhibitors of aldosterone, which is often increased in heart failure. Combinations of potassium supplements or ACE inhibitors and potassium-sparing medications can increase the risk of hyperkalemia, but have been used with success in patients with persistent hypokalemia. Patients with refractory edema may respond to combinations of a loop diuretic and thiazide-like agents. Metolazone, because of its maintained activity with chronic kidney disease, is the most useful agent for such a combination.

Inhibitors of Renin Angiotensin-Aldosterone system

Angiotensin-converting Enzyme Inhibitors

Kidney dysfunction is more frequent in patients with diabetes, older patients, and those with low systolic pressures, and these groups should be monitored more closely.

The most common side effects of ACE inhibitors in heart failure patients are dizziness (often not related to the level of BP) and cough, though the latter is often due as much to heart failure or intercurrent pulmonary conditions as to the ACE inhibitor.

ACE inhibitor-induced cough is more common in women than in men.

Angiotensin II Receptor Blocker

Angiotensin receptor blockers, specifically candesartan or valsartan, provide important benefits as an alternative to ACE inhibitors in chronic heart failure with reduced LVEF.

(A large trial of patients with chronic heart failure and preserved LVEF found no benefit from the ARB irbesartan.) While they have the same level of recommendation in the guidelines, generally ACE inhibitors are preferred over ARBS for patients who tolerate them.

Spironolactione and Eplerenone

The RALES trial compared spironolactone 25 mg daily with placebo patients with advanced heart failure (current or recent class IV) already receiving ACE inhibitors and diuretics and showed a 29% reduction in mortality as well as similar decreases in other clinical endpoints.

Based on the EMPHASIS-HF trial, the efficacy and safety of aldosterone antagonism—in the form of eplerenone, 25–50 mg orally daily—is established for patients with mild or moderate heart failure. Hyperkalemia was uncommon in severe heart failure clinical trial patients who received high doses of diuretic as maintenance therapy; however, hyperkalemia in patients taking spironolactone appears to be common in general practice. Potassium levels must be monitored closely during initiation of spironolactone (after 1 and 4 weeks of therapy) and periodically thereafter, particularly for patients with even mild degrees of kidney injury, and in patients receiving ACE inhibitors.

Combination of Sacubitril and Valasartan

The most recently approved medication to improve clinical outcome in patients with heart failure and reduced LVEF is the combination of valsartan and sacubitril, called an angiotensin receptor-neprilysin inhibitor (ARNI).

Compared to the ACE inhibitor enalapril, the ARNI was shown to reduce cardiovascular death and hospitalization for heart failure by 20% for patients with heart failure and reduced LVEF in a large randomized trial (PARADIGM HF) of patients who had been taking an ACE inhibitor or ARB.

Cardiovascular death itself was also reduced by 20%. This has led to a class I recommendation by the American College of Cardiology (ACC), the American Heart

Association (AHA), and the European Society of Cardiology (ESC) guidelines for the use of sacubitril/valsartan as a replacement for ACE inhibitors for patients with heart failure with reduced EF who remain symptomatic on an ACE inhibitor, beta-blocker, and mineralocorticoia inhibitor.

For some patients, cost will be a barrier to use, although analyses have shown that sacubitril/valsartan is cost effective.

Patients with baseline systolic blood pressure < 100 mm Hg were not included in the PARADIGM trial, and symptomatic hypotension is more common with sacubitril/valsartan than ACE inhibitor. Sacubitril/valsartan can be safely started in the hospital for patients admitted with decompensated failure, once they are stable with systolic blood pressure of at least 100 mm Hg.

While there was some evidence of benefit, sacubitril/valsartan did not result in significant improvement in the primary outcome of total heart failure hospitalizations and cardiovascular death in the *PARAGON-HE trial* studying a population of patients with heart failure and preserved LVEF (45% or greater).

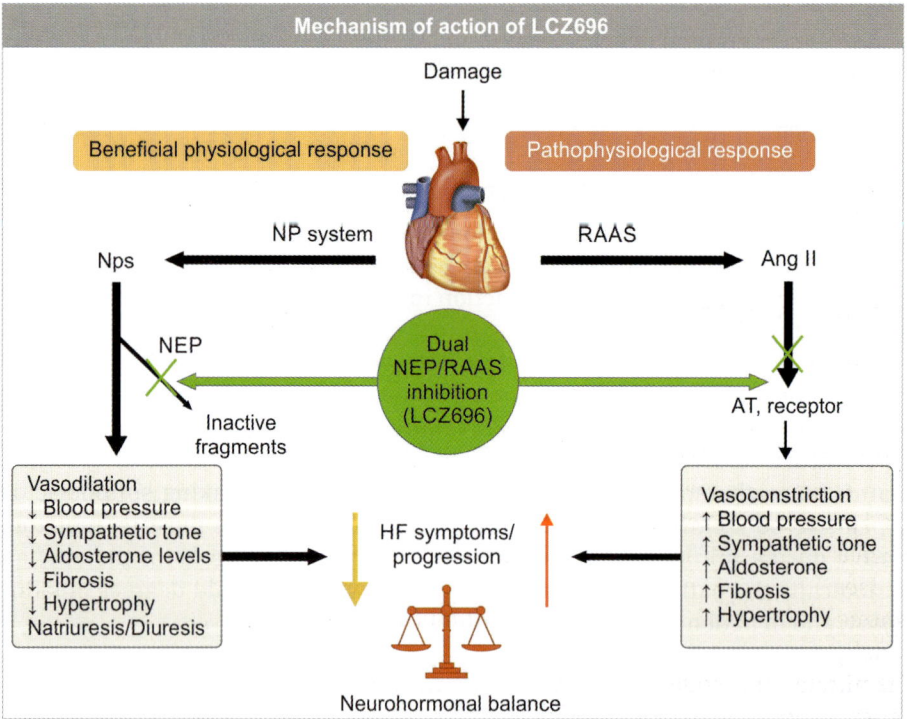

Beta Blocker

Carvedilol (a nonselective beta-1- and beta-receptor blocker), the beta-1-selective extended-release agent metoprolol succinate (but not short-acting metoprolol tartrate), and bisoprolol (beta-1-selective agent).

Stable patients (defined as having no recent deterioration or evidence of volume overload) with mild, moderate, and even severe heart failure should be treated with a beta-blocker unless there is a noncardiac contraindication.

In the COPERNICUS trial, carvedilol was both well tolerated and highly effective in reducing both mortality and heart failure hospitalizations in a group of patients with severe [the New York Heart Association (NYHA class III or IV)[symptoms, but care was taken to ensure that they were free of fluid retention at the time of initiation.

In this study, one death was prevented for every 13 patients treated for 1 year—as dramatic an effect as has been seen with a pharmacologic therapy in the history of cardiovascular medicine.

One trial comparing carvedilol and (short-acting) metoprolol tartrate (*COMET*) found significant reductions in all-cause mortality and cardiovascular mortality with carvedilol. Thus, patients with chronic heart failure should be treated with extended-release metoprolol succinate, bisoprolol, or carvedilol but not short-acting metoprolol tartrate.

Patients should be instructed to monitor their weight at home as an indicator of fluid retention and to report any increase or change in symptoms immediately.

Digitalis Glycosides

Digoxin should be considered for patients who remain symptomatic when taking diuretics and ACE inhibitors as well as for patients with heart failure who are in atrial fibrillation and require rate control.

In most patients with chronic heart failure it is sufficient to begin with the expected maintenance dose (usually 0.125–0.25 mg daily). Amiodarone, quinidine, propafenone, and verapamil are among the medications that may increase digoxin levels up to 100%.

Nitrates and Hydralazine

The combination of hydralazine and isosorbide dinitrate has been shown to improve outcomes in African Americans, but the effect is less clear than the well-established benefits of ACE inhibitors. ARBs or ARNIs have largely supplanted the use of the hydralazine-isosorbidedinitrate combination in ACE-intolerant patients.

Nitrates—Intravenous vasodilators (sodium nitroprusside or nitroglycerin) are used primarily for acute or severely decompensated chronic heart failure, especially when accompanied by hypertension or myocardial ischemia.

Isosorbidedinitrate, 20–40 mg orally three times daily. and nitroglycerin ointment, 2%, 15–16 mg (1.4 inches 1 inch 15 mg) every 6–8 hours, appear to be equally effective, although the ointment is generally reserved for inpatient use only. The nitrates are moderately effective in relieving shortness of breath, especially in patients with mild to moderate symptoms.

Ivabradine

Ivabradine inhibits the I-channel in the sinus node and has the specific effect of slowing sinus rate. lvabradine is approved by the Food and Drug Administration (FDA) for use in stable patients with heart failure and heart rate of 70 beats/min who are taking the maximally tolerated dose of beta-blockers or in patients in whom beta-blockers are contraindicated.

In a trial of patients with chronic angina, ivabradine did not reduce cardiovascular events, and there may have been more events with ivabradine (than placebo) in patients with symptomatic angina.

Sodium-glucose Cotransporter-2 Inhibitors

Large clinical trials of patients with type 2 diabetes mellitus have shown that inhibitors of sodium-glucose cotransporter-2 (SGLT-2) reduce the risk of hospitalization for heart failure.

One trial showed that one SGLT-2 inhibitor *dapagliflozin* reduced the risk of hospitalization for heart failure and cardiovascular death for patients with heart failure and reduced ejection fraction, with or without diabetes. Thus, for patients with diabetes at risk for heart failure, SGLT-2 inhibitors may be a good choice.

Combination of Medical Therapies

Optimal management of chronic heart failure involves using combinations of proven life-saving therapies. In addition to ACE inhibitors and beta-blockers, patients who remain symptomatic should be considered for mineralocorticoid (aldosterone) receptor antagonists and for sacubitril/valsartan.

Treatments that may Cause Harm in Heart Failure with Reduced Left Ventricular Ejection Fraction

Several therapies should be avoided, when possible, in patients with systolic heart failure.

These include thiazoladinediones (glitazones) that cause worsening heart failure, most calcium-channel blockers (with the exception of amlodipine and felodipine), nonsteroidal anti-inflammatory medications, and cyclooxygenase-2 inhibitors that cause sodium and water retention and renal impairment, and the combination of an ACE inhibitor, ARB, and aldosterone blocker that increases the risk of hyperkalemia.

Anticoagulation

In general, these patients should receive warfarin for 3 months following the MI. Other patients with heart failure have embolic rates of approximately two per 100 patient-years of follow-up which approximates the rate of major bleeding, and routine anticoagulation is not warranted except in patients with prior embolic events or mobile LV thrombi. A clinical trial of low-dose rivaroxaban failed to show substantial benefit in patients with heart failure with reduced LVEF.

Antiarrhythmic therapy

Patients with moderate to severe heart failure have a high incidence of both symptomatic and asymptomatic arrhythmias.

Less than 10% of patients have syncope or presyncope resulting from ventricular tachycardia, ambulatory monitoring reveals that up to 70% of patients have asymptomatic episodes of nonsustained ventricular tachycardia.

These arrhythmias indicate a poor prognosis independent of the severity of LV dysfunction, but many of the deaths are probably not arrhythmia related. Beta-blockers, because of their marked favorable effect on prognosis in general and on the incidence of sudden death specifically, should be initiated in these as well as all other patients with heart failure (see beta-blockers).

Other evidence-based therapies for heart failure, including ACE inhibitors, ARBs, mineralocorticoid receptor antagonists, and ARNIs, have all been shown (to reduce sudden cardiac death. Empiric antiarrhythmic therapy with amiodarone did not improve outcome in the SCD-HeFT trial, and most other agents are contraindicated because of their proarrhythmic effects in this population and their adverse effect on cardiac function. For patients with systolic heart failure and atrial fibrillation, a rhythm control strategy has not been shown to improve outcome compared to a rate control strategy and thus should be reserved for patients with a reversible cause of atrial fibrillation or refractory symptoms. Then, amiodarone is the medication of choice.

Statin Therapy

Even though vascular disease is present in many patients with chronic heart failure, the role of statins has not been well defined in the heart failure population. The CORONA and the GISSI-HF trials show no benefits of statins in the chronic heart failure population.

DILATED CARDIOMYOPATHY—NONPHARMACOLOGICAL TREATMENT

- Implantable cardioverter defibrillators (ICDs)
- Biventricular pacing
- Case management, diet and exercise training
- Coronary revascularization
- Cardiac transplantation
- Other surgical options
- Palliative care

Treatment of Heart Failure with Preserved Ejection Fraction

Although half of all heart failure occurs among patients with normal LVEF, often with diastolic dysfunction, no therapies have been shown to improve survival in this population. The mainstay of management of patients with heart failure with preserved EF is to manage fluid overload with diuretic therapy and to treat comorbidities like hypertension, diabetes, and arrhythmias.

Correction of Reversible Causes

Hypertension, pericardial disease, and atrial tachycardias are potentially reversible factors that can contribute to heart failure with preserved EF. Since tachycardia is associated with shorter overall diastolic filling time, controlling accelerated heart rate may be important. Now that there is effective treatment available for familial and wild-type transthyretin amyloid cardiomyopathy, this diagnosis should be considered for patients with unexplained heart failure with preserved EF.

Pharmacologic Treatment

Diuretic Therapy
Diuretics are important to control symptoms of fluid overload in patients with heart failure with preserved EF, similar to symptoms from systolic heart failure.

Inhibitors of the Renin-angiotensin-aldosterone System
ACE inhibitors and ARBs have not been shown to improve outcome in patients with heart failure and preserved EF, despite being good therapies for the comorbidity of hypertension. Sacubitril/valsartan does not substantially improve outcome in patients with heart failure and preserved EF.

Spironolactone has not been shown to improve outcome in a large trial of patients with heart failure and. preserved EF, but there may have been some benefit in patients enrolled in the Americas who had more clearly defined heart failure. Spironolactone should remain a therapeutic option, especially for patients who also have hypertension.

Nonpharmacologic Treatment
Unlike in patients with heart failure and reduced EF, ICD, and resynchronization device treatments do not have a role in patients with preserved EF. Revascularization for patients with heart failure and preserved EF should be guided by the same considerations as for patients with heart failure with reduced EF.

Peripartum Cardiomyopathy

Definition: Four Criteria
Three clinical and one echocardiographic:
1. Development of heart failure during last trimester of pregnancy or first 6 months postpartum
2. Absence of any identifiable cause for cardiac failure
3. Absence of any recognizable heart disease prior to last trimester of pregnancy
4. Echocardiographic criteria: Demonstrable echocardiographic proof of left ventricular systolic dysfunction. Ejection fraction <45%, left ventricular fractional shortening < 30% or left ventricular end-diastolic dimension > 2.7 cm/m^2 of body surface area.

Hypertropic Cardiomyopathy

This is the most common form of cardiomyopathy, with a prevalence of approximately 100 per 100,000. It is characterized by inappropriate and elaborate left ventricular hypertrophy with malalignment of the myocardial fibers and myocardial fibrosis caused by mutation of genes encoding sarcomeric proteins. The hypertrophy may be generalized or confined largely to the interventricular septum or other regions.

Cardiomyopathy: Diagnosis and Management

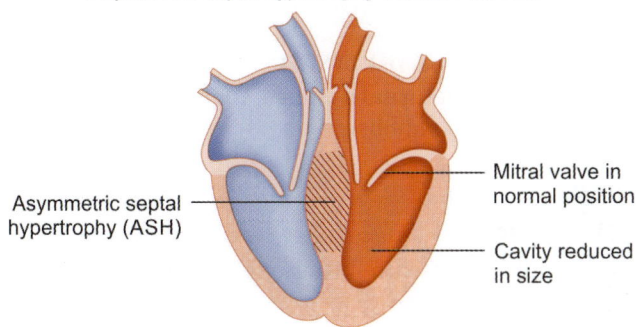

Hypertrophic cardiomyopathy
Asymmetric septal hypertrophy without obstruction

- Asymmetric septal hypertrophy (ASH)
- Mitral valve in normal position
- Cavity reduced in size

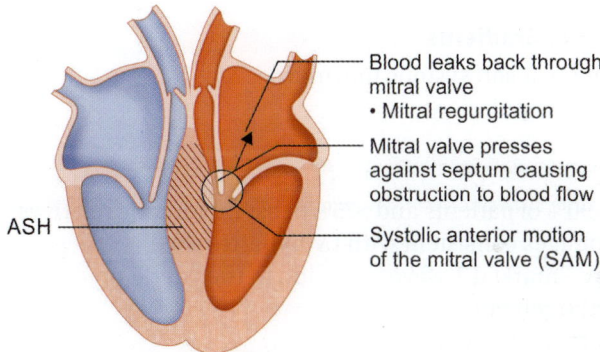

Hypertrophic cardiomyopathy
Asymmetric septal hypertrophy with obstruction

- ASH
- Blood leaks back through mitral valve
  • Mitral regurgitation
- Mitral valve presses against septum causing obstruction to blood flow
- Systolic anterior motion of the mitral valve (SAM)

Pathogenesis
- Autosomal dominant with variable penetrance
- Remaining are sporadic.
- Mutations are mostly missense.
- Mutations causing HCM found in genes encoding β-MHC, cardiac TnT, α-tropomyosin, myosin-binding protein C.

The major abnormality of the heart in HCM—excessive thickening of the muscle. Thickening usually begins during early adolescence and stops when growth has finished. Uncommon for thickening to progress after this age left ventricle almost always affected. Hypertrophy is usually greatest in the septum, associated with obstruction to the flow of blood into the aorta.

Asymmetric septal hypertrophy with obstruction to the outflow of blood from the heart may occur. The mitral valve touches the septum, blocking the outflow tract. Some blood is leaking back through the mitral valve causing mitral regurgitation.

Clinical Features
- Asymptomatic
- Echocardiographic finding only
- Symptomatic

- Dyspnea in 90%
- Harsh systolic ejection murmur
- Angina pectoris in 75%
- Fatigue, presyncope, syncope, risk of SCD
- Palpitation, paroxysmal nocturnal dyspnea, CHF, dizziness
- Atrial fibrillation, thromboembolism

Physical Findings
With Outflow Obstruction
- Arterial pulses rapid rise—with bisferiens contour double or triple apical impulses may be palpable.
- Outward systolic thrust—ventricular contraction
- Presystolic accentuated atrial contraction
- Medium-pitch ESM at the lower left sternal border and apex
- Loud murmurs—LV outflow gradients >30 mm Hg

Without Subaortic Gradients
- Subtle—with no or soft systolic murmur
- Forceful apical impulse

ECG
- *Abnormal*: >90% of patients and >75% of asymptomatic relatives
- Increased voltages consistent with LV hypertrophy
- ST-T changes—marked T wave inversion in the lateral precordial leads
- Left atrial enlargement
- Deep and narrow Q waves
- Diminished R waves in the lateral precordial leads.

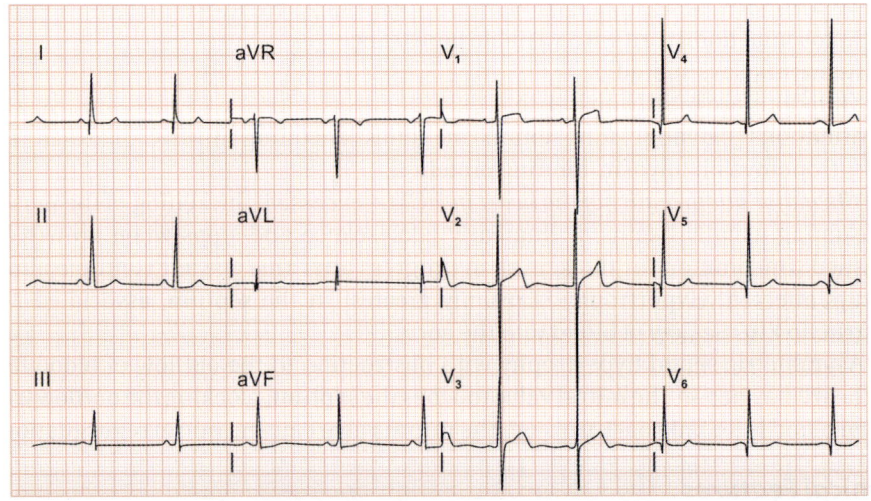

Normal ECG: 5% of Patients
- Less severe phenotype and favorable course
- Not predictive of future sudden death

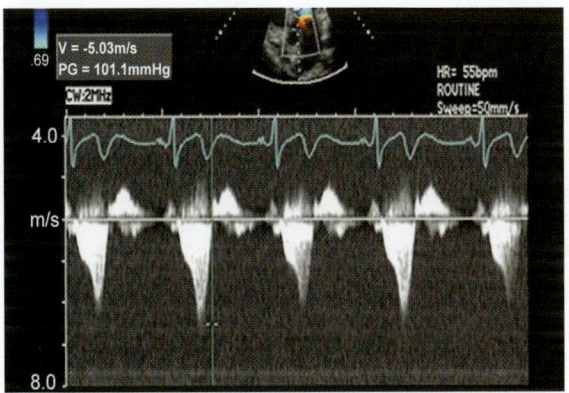

Increased Voltages
- Weakly correlated with the magnitude of LV hypertrophy
- Do not distinguish the obstructive and nonobstructive forms

Holter
- Supraventricular tachycardia (46%)
- Premature ventricular contractions (43%)
- Nonsustained ventricular tachycardia (26%)
- Atrial fibrillation (25–30%)
- Preexcitation has also been associated with HCM.

Serum C-terminal Propeptide of Type Iprocollagen (PICP)
Elevated levels PICP indicated increased myocardial collagen synthesis in sarcomere-mutation carriers without overt disease. Profibrotic state preceded left ventricular hypertrophy or fibrosis visible on MRI.

Echocardiography
- Diffuse hypertrophy of the ventricular septum and anterolateral free wall (70–75%)
- Basal septal hypertrophy (10–15%)
- Concentric hypertrophy (5%)
- Apical hypertrophy (<5%)
- Hypertrophy of the lateral wall (1–2%)
- Mitral annulus velocity, Ea - status of myocardial relaxation—reduced in most patients with HCM

Mimicking Hypertrophic Cardiomyopathy
- Chronic hypertension
- RV hypertrophy

- Cardiac amyloidosis
- Athlete's heart
- Pheochromocytoma
- Long-term hemodialysis
- Fabryl disease
- Friedreich ataxia
- Apical hypertrophy—apical cavity obliteration caused by hypereosinophilic syndrome or noncompaction

MANAGEMENT
General Guidelines
- Screening all first-degree relatives is recommended.
- Echocardiography
- Children and participating in competitive athletics every 12–18 months
- Adults no competitive athletics—every 5 years
- Counseled against engaging in competitive athletics
- Maintain hydration

Sudden Death and Risk stratification
- Primary ventricular tachycardia and ventricular fibrillation
- Adolescents and young adults <30–35 years of age
- Most common cause of athletic field deaths
- Death most commonly occurs at rest.

HIGH RISK
Primary Prevention
- One or more of the following
- Family history of one or more premature HCM-related deaths, particularly if sudden and multiple
- Unexplained syncope, especially if recent and in the young
- Hypotensive or attenuated blood pressure response to exercise
- Multiple, repetitive (or prolonged) nonsustained ventricular tachycardia (NSVT) on Holter
- Massive LVH (wall thickness, ≥30 mm), particularly in young patients

Secondary prevention
- Prior cardiac arrest
- Sustained ventricular tachycardia

Potential Arbitrators
- When level of risk judged—ambiguous on the basis of conventional markers
- CMR—delayed enhancement

- Thin-walled akinetic LV apical aneurysms
- End-stage phase
- Percutaneous alcohol septal ablation
- Very limited prognostic significance can be attributed to specific HCM-causing mutations

PREVENTION OF SCD
CD Implantation
- As primary prevention following cardiac arrest
- As secondary prevention if one or more high risk factors
- Empirical pharmacological therapy with amiodarone is now obsolete.

MEDICAL TREATMENT
Empirical and highly variable.

Beta-blockers
- Slowing heart rate
- Reducing force of LV contraction
- Augmenting ventricular filling and relaxation
- Decreasing myocardial oxygen consumption
- Long-acting preparations—propranolol, atenolol, metoprolol, or nadolol
- Blunt LV outflow gradient triggered by physiologic exercise
- Target resting heart rate—60 beats/min
- May require up to 400 mg equivalent of metoprolol.

Verapamil
- Improves symptoms and exercise capacity (patients without marked obstruction to LV outflow)
- Beneficial effect on ventricular relaxation and filling
- Better angina control than beta-blocker
- Hemodynamic deterioration with CCB agents—lowering of the afterload in the presence of severe outflow tract gradients and high-diastolic filling pressures

Disopyramide (Sodium-channel Blocker)
- Negative inotropic effect decreases the gradient and improve symptoms.
- Concomitant beta-blockade may be important to prevent rapid.
- Atrioventricular node conduction between 300 and 600 mg/day
- The corrected QT interval must be monitored anticholinergic side effects in older patients.
- Diuretic agents may be judiciously administered either beta-blockers or verapamil initially
- No advantage by combinations of BB and CCB disopyramide may be combined with BB or CCB.

Agents that modulate myocardial metabolic efficiency and their major mechanism(s) for potentially improving energetics.	
Agent	Mechanisms of action
Perhexiline	CPT1/CPT2 inhibition
	NAD(P)H oxidase inhibition
	NO potentiation
Amiodarone	CPT, inhibition
	β-adrenoceptor blockade
Trimetazidine	PFOX inhibition
	? CPT, inhibition
Ranolazine	PFOX inhibition
	? Late Na current inhibition
Metformin	AMPK stimulation

(AMPK: 5' adenosine monophosphate-activated protein kinase; CPT: carnitine palmitoyltransferase; NAD(P)H: nicotinamide adenine dinucleotide phosphate; PFOX: partial fatty acid oxidation)

SURGICAL MYECTOMY

- Drug-refractory heart failure symptoms
- NYHA Classes III (Marked limitation of physical activity. Comfortable at rest. Less than ordinary activity causes fatigue, palpitation, or dyspnea) and IV (Unable to carry on any physical activity without discomfort. Symptoms of heart failure at rest. If any physical activity is undertaken, discomfort increases).
- LV outflow obstruction
  - Rest—gradient ≥ 30 mm Hg
  - Physiologic exercise—gradient ≥ 50 mm Hg
- Transaortic resection of muscle from the proximal to mid-septal region. Operative mortality <1%
- Maintain long-lasting improvement in symptoms and exercise capacity
- Mortality may be improved after septal myectomy.

DDD PACING (DUAL-CHAMBERED PACING)

- Objective measurements of exercise capacity did not differ significantly.
- Overall decrease in outflow tract gradient (25–40% of baseline)
- Role of dual-chamber pacing—patients at high risk for other therapeutic modalities
- Candidates for dual-chamber pacing
- Significant bradycardia in which pacing may allow an increased dosage of medication
- Patients who need ICD as a primary treatment.

ALCOHOL SEPTAL ABLATION

- Outflow tract gradient is reduced from a mean of 60-70 mm of mercury often to <20 mm of mercury
- 80-85% symptomatic improvement
- Complications:
  - Complete heart block < 10%
  - Coronary dissections
  - Large myocardial infarctions
  - Ventricular septal defects
  - Myocardial perforations
- Ventricular fibrillation

RESTRICTIVE CARDIOMYOPATHY

In this rare condition, ventricular filling is impaired because the ventricles are "stiff". This leads to high atrial pressures with atrial hypertrophy, dilatation and later, atrial fibrillation.

Causes

Myocardial

- Idiopathic cardiomyopathy
- Familial cardiomyopathy
- Scleroderma
- Pseudoxanthoma elasticum
- Diabetic cardiomyopathy
- Infiltrative amyloidosis *
- Sarcoidosis *
- Gaucher's disease
- Mucopolysaccharidoses
- Fatty infiltration
- Storage diseases
- Fabry disease
- Iron overload cardiomyopathy

Endomyocardial

- Endomyocardial fibrosis
- Radiation
- Cardiotoxicity of anthracyclines
- Hypereosinophilic syndrome
- Carcinoid heart disease
- Metastatic cancers
- Drugs causing fibrous endocarditis (serotonin and methysergide, ergotamine, mercurial agents, and busulfan)

Clinical Manifestations
- *Symptoms of right and left heart failure*
- *Echo-Doppler*
    - Abnormal mitral inflow pattern
    - Prominent E wave (rapid diastolic filling)
    - Almost invariably progresses to congestive heart failure, 10% survive for 10 years.

Amyloidosis
- Cardiac enlargement without ventricular dilatation
- Ventricular walls are thickened and rubbery.
- Amyloid deposition is the most prominent in interstitial, perivascular, and endocardial regions.

ENDOMYOCARDIAL DISEASES
- Endomyocardial fibrosis
- Loeffers endomyocarditis:
    - Inherited disease of cardiac muscle
    - RVF, rhythm disturbances, ventricular tachycardia, fibrillation
    - Right ventricular wall is thinned, extensive fatty infiltration and fibrosis
    - Autosomal dominant inheritance

TAKOTSUBO (STRESS CARDIOMYOPATHY)

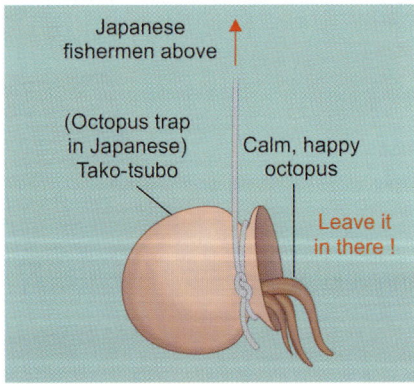

Also called "transient apical ballooning" and stress cardiomyopathy. It is a reversible cardiomyopathy featuring symptoms and signs of acute myocardial infarction without demonstrable coronary artery stenosis or spasm, in which the heart takes on the appearance of a Japanese octopus fishing pot called a 'takotsubo" *(Takatsubo = Octopus Trap)*.

It is characterized by transient systolic ventricular dysfunction with regional wall motion abnormalities beyond a single vascular territory and in the absence of significant epicardial coronary artery obstruction.

Often, there is an acute emotional or physical stress or immediately preceding the presentation. Classical apical ballooning is seen on ventriculography or echocardiography.

Catecholamine excess and cardiotoxicity is the most compelling putative mechanism.

The long-term prognosis is excellent but serious complications including cardiogenic shock and arrhythmias may occur acutely. Supportive treatment is the mainstay of therapy.

■ TAKOTSUBO: CLINICAL PRESENTATION

The clinical presentation of TTC is often identical to acute myocardial infarction (AMI).

Most patients with TTC present with typical anginal chest pain, dyspnea, ischemic changes on electrocardiogram (ECG), and elevated cardiac markers, whereas syncope and out-of-hospital cardiac arrest are rare.

Emotional stress, such as news of the death of a family member, divorce, or public speaking, is implicated as the trigger in approximately two-thirds of patients.

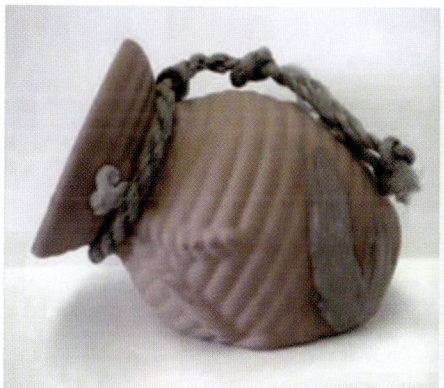 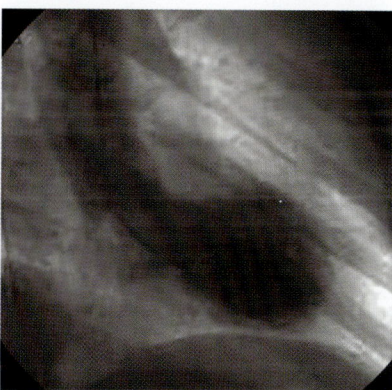

Management

- Takotsubo cardiomyopathy is a temporary condition and hence the goals of treatment are usually *conservative, supportive care.*
- The therapy is guided by the patient's clinical presentation and hemodynamic status.
- Despite the supposed causative role of catecholamines in the disorder, patients who present in cardiogenic shock, and in the absence of LVOT obstruction, may be treated with inotropes.
- Alternatively patients may derive further benefit from mechanical hemodynamic support with intra-aortic balloon pump or rarely, left ventricular assist devices.
- If LVOT obstruction is present with cardiogenic shock, inotropes should be avoided and phenylphrine is the pressor agent of choice often combined with beta-blockade.

- Most experts advocate guideline-directed medical therapy for patients with left ventricular dysfunction.
- This includes cardioselective beta-blockers and ACE inhibitor for a short period of time (3–6 months).
- Full anticoagulation is usually reserved for those with documented ventricular thrombus or evidence of embolic events.

CHAPTER 4

Echocardiography and Lung Ultrasound in the Emergency Room

Rohit Tandon, Priyanka, Sidhant Sachdeva

■ INTRODUCTION

- Echocardiography has emerged as an important noninvasive tool for improving the efficiency in the diagnosis of serious conditions in the medical emergency department.
- Lung ultrasonography allows for rapid assessment of numerous conditions, including pulmonary edema, pleural effusion, and pneumothorax.
- Over-reliance of traditional clinical findings and symptoms can cause potential delay in various cardiac and noncardiac emergencies.
- The use of echocardiography and lung ultrasonography can help to improve diagnostic accuracy and monitor responses to interventions in these patients.

■ CONSIDERATIONS PRIOR TO SCANNING

Setting

Preparation
- Appropriate transducer selection
- Appropriate preset selection

Ultrasound Protocol
- Focused examination
- Diagnostic examination

■ CARDIAC PROBE SELECTION
- Small round footprint for scan between ribs
- 2.5 MHz: Above average sized patient
- 3.5 MHz: Average sized patient
- 5.0 MHz: Below average sized patient or child

VASCULAR PROBE FOR LUNG USG

- Long foot print
- 3–12 MHz range
- Good resolution

CLINICAL INDICATION

- *Hemodynamic instability and/or hypoxemia of unclear etiology*
  - Suspected tamponade
  - Pulseless electrical activity (PEA) can be the presenting symptom for:
    - Tamponade
    - Massive pulmonary embolism
    - Acute massive internal hemorrhage
    - Tension pneumothorax

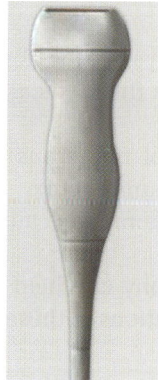 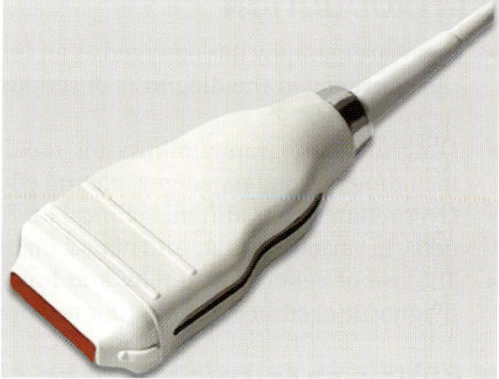

FIG. 1: Sector probe for echocardiography.   **FIG. 2:** Vascular probe for lung USG.

TABLE 1: Major causes of cardiac and cardiac like emergencies and their common clinical presentation in emergency.

	ACS	AoD	PE	P	Ptx	ADHF	T	AVR/PVD
Acute chest pain	+++	+++	++	+++	+++	+	+	+
Acute dyspnea	++	+	+++	0	++	++++	++++	++++
Hemodynamic instability/shock	++	++	+++	+	+	++++	++++	++++
New murmur	+	+	+	+	0	+	0	++++
Cardiac sources of embolism/syncope	+	+	+	0	0	+	0	+
Chest trauma	+	+++	0	+	++	0	+++	+
Cardiac arrest/CPR	++++	+	+++	+	+	+	+++	+

Echocardiography and Lung Ultrasound in the Emergency Room

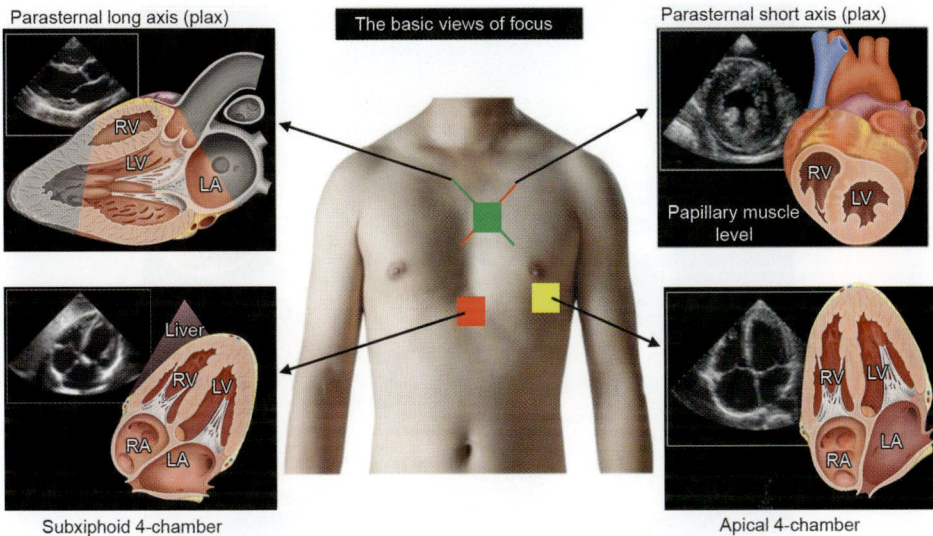

FIG. 3: Focus-assessed transthoracic echocardiography (FATE).

- Aortic dissection
- Acute coronary syndromes
- Acute valvular pathology, prosthetic valve malfunction
- Infective endocarditis
- Massive pulmonary embolism
- Acute embolic event
- Critically ill patients due to noncardiac illness: Cardiac function and left ventricular (LV) filling may be crucial to guide fluid-resuscitation: (a) Septic shock, and (b) Diabetic ketoacidosis
  Major causes of cardiac and cardiac like emergencies and their common initial clinical presentation in the emergency room.

PARASTERNAL LONG AXIS VIEW

- Most echocardiography studies begin with this view.
- Transducer position: Left sternal edge; 3rd–4th intercostal space.
- Marker dot direction: Points toward right shoulder.

Purpose

- Overview of LV inflow, outflow, aortic root
- LV dimensions
- Perimembranous ventricular septal defect (VSD)
- Measurements:
  - Mandatory: LV systolic and diastolic diameters; interventricular septal and posterior wall thickness.

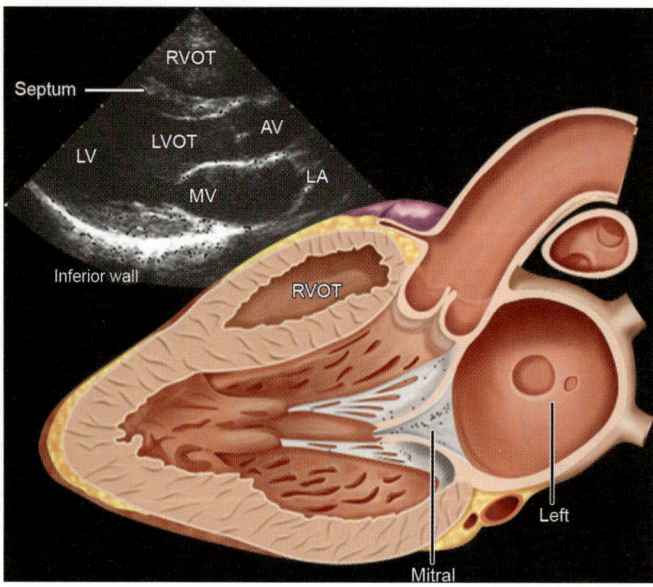

FIG. 4: Parasternal long-axis view.

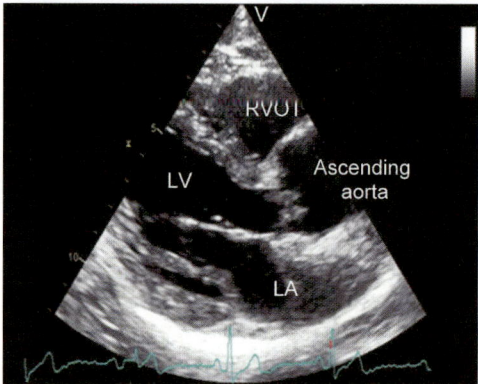

FIG. 5: Parasternal long-axis view.

PARASTERNAL LONG-AXIS MITRAL VALVE ZOOM TWO-DIMENSIONAL AND COLOR

- *Purpose:*
    - 2D: Mitral leaflet motion and pathology
    - Color: Detection of mitral regurgitation (MR), measurement of MR jet vena contracta
- *Measurements:*
    - 2D: Mitral annulus anteroposterior diameter
    - Color: Vena contracta, proximal isovelocity surface area (PISA)

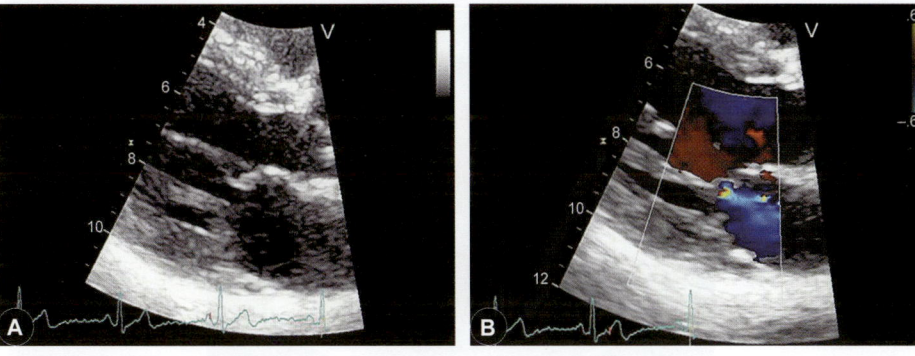

FIGS. 6A AND B: PLAX mitral valve zoom 2D and color.

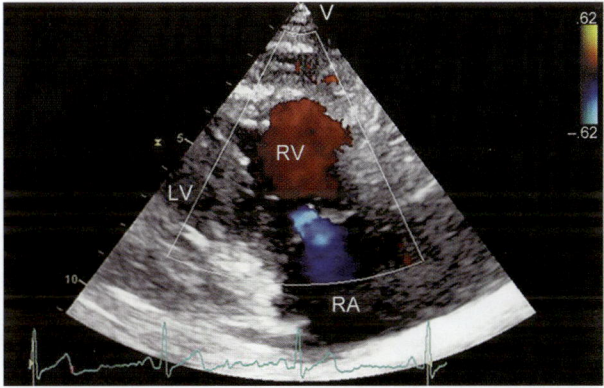

FIG. 7: Right ventricular (RV) inflow view.

■ RIGHT VENTRICULAR INFLOW VIEW

- Obtained by angling the transducer medially, toward the right hip
- RA, TV, and RV can be visualized.
- Ostium of the inferior vena cava, including Eustachian valve, is seen draining into the RA.
- *Purpose:*
    - Tricuspid leaflet pathology
    - Tricuspid regurgitation (TR) mechanism and severity
- *Measurements:*
    - Qualitative for TR, also CW for estimation of TR gradient

■ PARASTERNAL SHORT AXIS VIEW (SEMILUNAR VALVES)

- Obtained from the PLAX view by rotating the transducer orientation mark by 90° in the clockwise direction, such that it points to the patient's left shoulder.

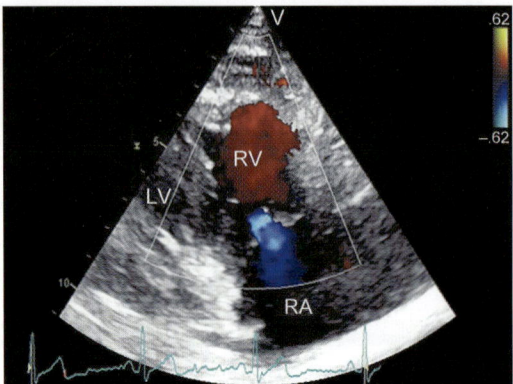

FIG. 8: Right ventricular (RV) inflow view.

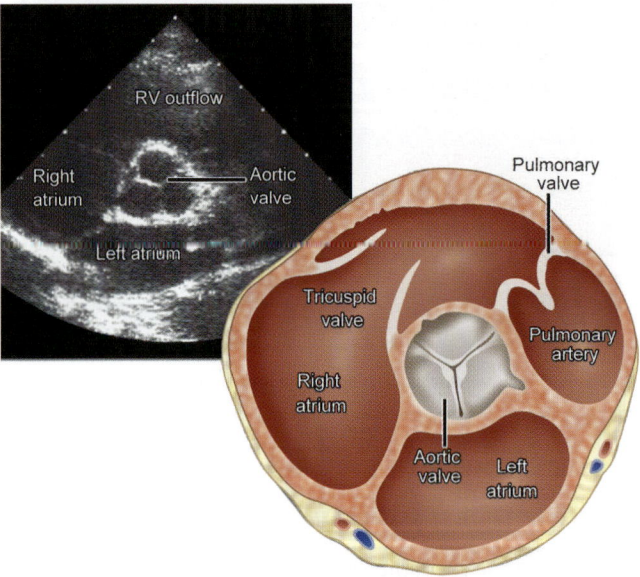

FIG. 9: Parasternal short-axis view aortic valve level.

- Moving the transducer superiorly with a slight cranial angulation provides a cross-section of the aortic root (commonly referred to "circle and sausage" view)
- Coronary arteries are best visualized using a higher transducer frequency.
- *Purpose:*
    - 2D: Aortic valve, RVOT, pulmonary valve pathology
    - Color: To detect perimembranous/supracristal VSD, RVOT stenosis, TR
- *Measurements:*
    - Pulmonary valve annulus size

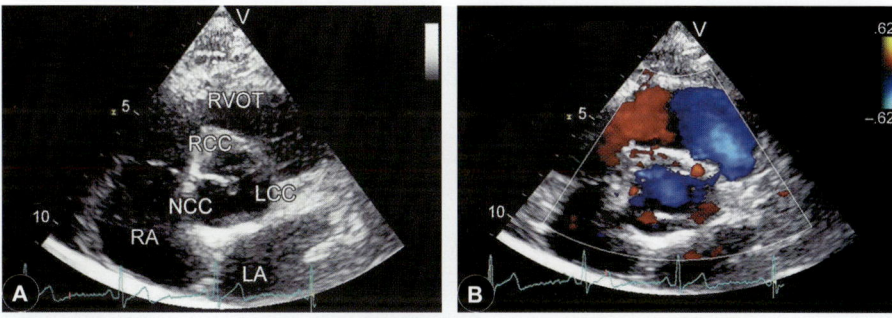

FIGS. 10A AND B: Parasternal short-axis view (semilunar valves).

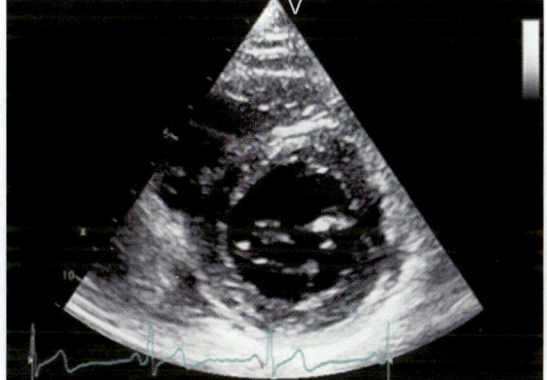

FIG. 11: Parasternal short-axis view (mitral valve level).

PARASTERNAL SHORT AXIS VIEW (MITRAL VALVE LEVEL)

- Characterized by a "fish mouth" appearance of the anterior and posterior mitral leaflets
- *Purpose:*
  - RWMA
  - Mitral valve end-on view for the assessment of mitral valve pathologies such as prolapse, MS (planimetry, commissures, etc.)
- *Measurements:*
  - Mitral valve area in those with MS
  - Optional: 2D circumferential and radial strain, basal rotation

PARASTERNAL SHORT AXIS VIEW (PAPILLARY MUSCLE LEVEL)

- *Purpose:*
  - Assessment of LVEF
  - RWMA-LV mass estimation
  - Papillary muscle geometry and morphology

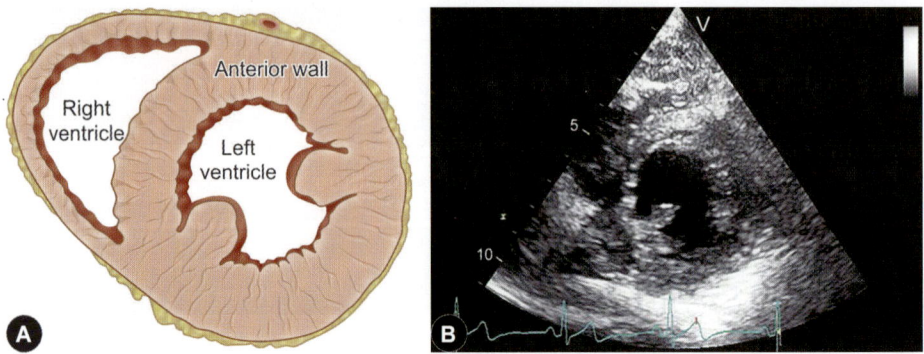

FIGS. 12A AND B: Parasternal short-axis view (papillary muscle level).

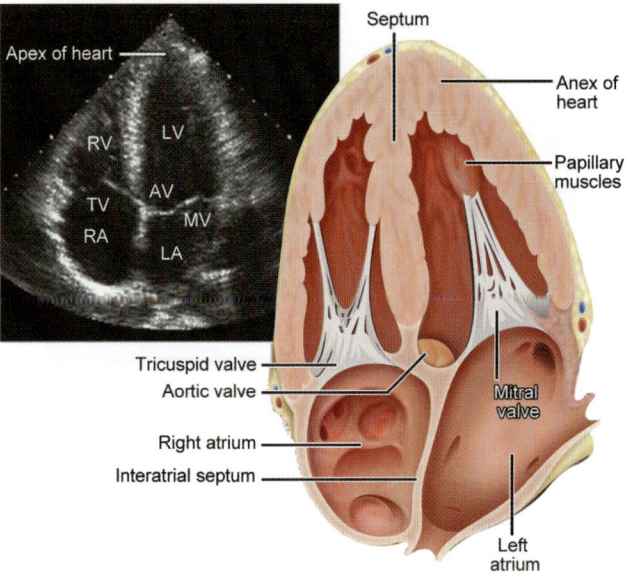

FIG. 13: Apical four-chamber view.

- *Measurements:*
  - Optional: LV mass calculation
  - 2D circumferential and radial strain, basal rotation

APICAL FOUR-CHAMBER VIEW

- Acquired with the patient positioned in the steep left lateral decubitus position.
- Apical pulse is palpated and the probe positioned slightly lateral to this position.
- Orientation marker is positioned at the 5 o'clock position to image the four chambers of the heart.
- Patient may be requested to suspend respiration at end-expiration to reduce translational disturbances.

Echocardiography and Lung Ultrasound in the Emergency Room

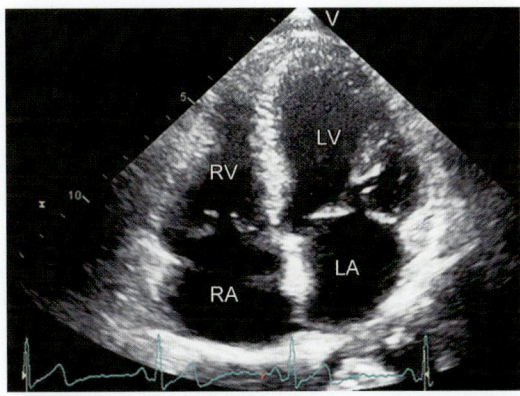

FIG. 14: Apical four-chamber view.

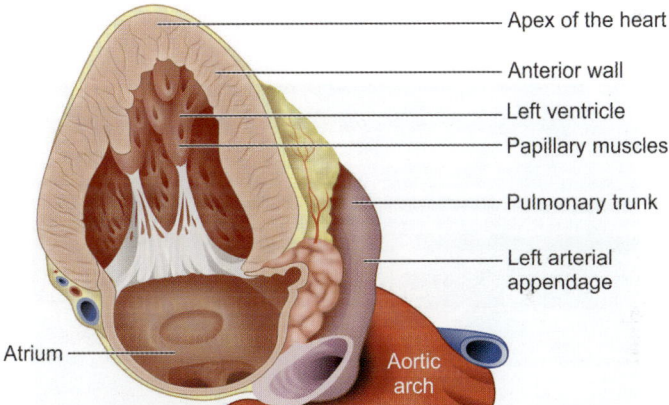

FIG. 15: Apical four-chamber view.

- *Purpose:*
  - Overview of chambers
  - Pericardial or extracardiac pathology
  - ASD
- *Measurements:*
  - Mandatory: LV volume and EF by Simpson's method
  - LA, RA, RV diameters; LA area
  - Optional: RA area, RV fractional shortening; LV length; 2D longitudinal strain

APICAL TWO-CHAMBER VIEW

- Obtained from the focused four-chamber view by rotating the transducer counterclockwise by approximately 60°.
- Provides a complete visualization of the anterior wall to the right of the display and the inferior wall to the left.
- *Purpose:*
  - RWMA in anterior and inferior wall

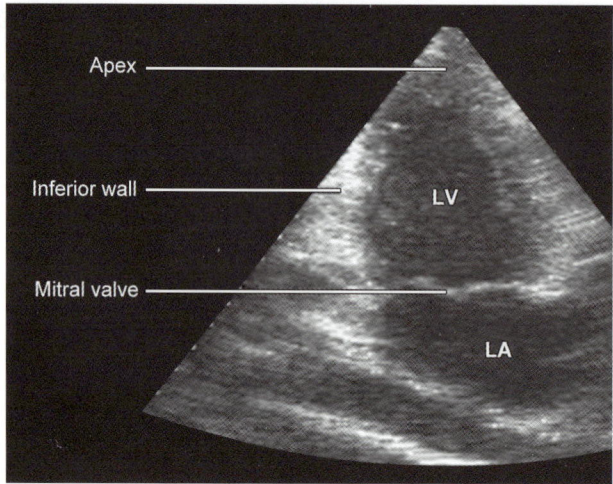

FIG. 16: Apical two-chamber view.

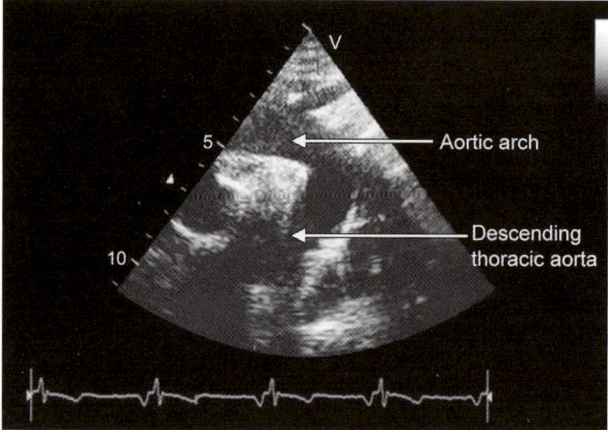

FIG. 17: Suprasternal view.

- *Measurements:*
    - Mandatory: LV volume and EF by Simpson's method
    - Optional: 2D longitudinal strain

SUPRASTERNAL VIEW

- Obtained by placing the transducer in the suprasternal notch with the orientation marker pointing toward the patient's left shoulder.
- With a slight anterior angulation, the aortic arch and branch vessels are seen.
- Moving from proximal to distal arch, the aortic arch first gives rise to the brachiocephalic artery, followed by the common carotid and the left subclavian artery, respectively.
- *Purpose:*
    - Linear measurements of aortic arch and isthmus

Echocardiography and Lung Ultrasound in the Emergency Room

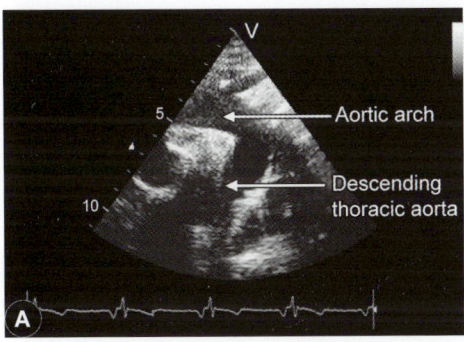
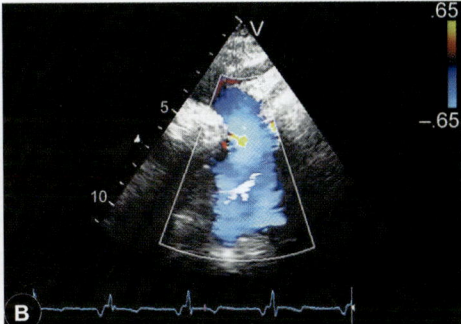

FIGS. 18A AND B: Suprasternal view.

> **BOX 1: Frequent causes of acute chest pain in patients presenting in the emergency room.**
>
> - Acute coronary syndrome
> - Aortic dissection
> - Pulmonary embolism
> - Pericarditis
> - Myocarditis
> - Pneumothorax
> - Aortic stenosis
> - Hypertrophic cardiomyopathy
> - Takotsubo cardiomyopathy
> - Mitral valve prolapse

- *Color:*
  - Color M-mode for qualitative assessment of diastolic flow reversal in case of AR
  - Descending aorta PW for diastolic flow reversal
  - CW Doppler for coarctation gradient

ROLE OF ECHOCARDIOGRAPHY IN ACUTE CHEST PAIN SYNDROMES

- Chest pain accounts for about 8% of all emergency room visits. The major life-threatening cardiovascular emergencies presenting as chest pain are:
  - Acute coronary syndrome
  - Aortic dissection
  - Acute pulmonary embolism

REGIONAL WALL MOTION ABNORMALITY

- Normal left ventricular wall motion consists of simultaneous myocardial thickening and endocardial excursion so as the cavity size decreases in a symmetrical manner.

TABLE 2: Regional wall motion abnormality scoring.

Score	Wall motion	Endocardial motion	Wall thickening
1	Normal	Normal	Normal (>30%)
2	Hypokinesis	Reduced	Reduced (<30%)
3	Akinesis	Absent	Absent
4	Dyskinesis	Outward	Thinning
5	Aneurysmal	Diastolic deformity	Absent or thinning

BOX 2: Conditions other than coronary artery disease presenting with regional wall motion abnormalities on the resting echocardiographic study.
- Acute myocarditis
- Cardiomyopathies
- Left bundle branch block
- Pacemaker
- Right ventricular pressure or volume overload
- Takotsubo cardiomyopathy

- Interruption of normal myocardial contraction due to ischemia (reduced blood supply) or infarction (complete cessation of blood supply) results in abnormality in systolic endocardial thickening termed as "wall motion abnormality".

DEFINITIONS

COMPLICATION OF ACUTE MYOCARDIAL INFARCTION
- Hemodynamic states:
  - Globally reduced LV contractility
  - Right ventricular infarction
  - Hypovolemia
  - Ischemic MR
- Mechanical complications:
  - Papillary muscle rupture
  - Ventricular septal rupture
  - Free wall rupture and tamponade
  - Left ventricular aneurysm
  - Mural thrombus

ISCHEMIC MITRAL REGURGITATION (FIGS. 19A AND B)

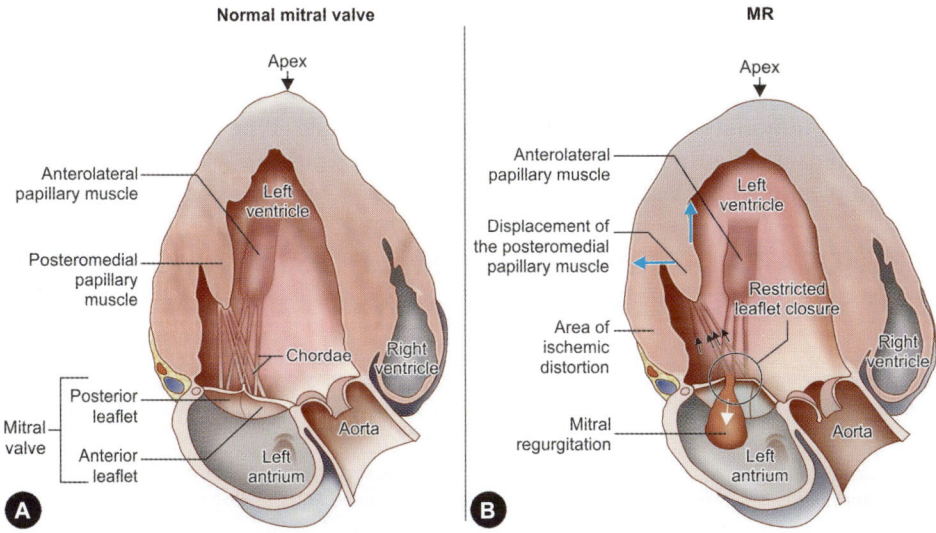

FIGS. 19A AND B: Ischemic mitral regurgitation.

PAPILLARY MUSCLE RUPTURE

- About 1% of all MIs
- Sudden development of apical systolic murmur and CHF/shock
- Bimodal peak: Within 24 hours and 3–5 days (Range 1–14 days)
- Posteromedial papillary muscle most often involved
- Infarct usually involves the RCA or LCX.

VENTRICULAR SEPTAL RUPTURE

- 1–3% in patients with reperfusion therapy
- Bimodal peak: Within 24 hours and 3–5 days (Range 1–14 days)
- Equal frequency between IWMI and AWMI
- Seen commonly in elderly women without previous MI (single vessel CAD).
- New systolic murmur with abrupt and progressive hemodynamic deterioration.

FREE-WALL RUPTURE

It is one of the most feared complications which usually occurs in acute lateral wall myocardial infarction. Free-wall rupture is suspected when a patient of myocardial infarction develops sudden hypotension preceded by diaphoresis, vomiting, and chest pain. Echocardiography shows mobile pericardial hematoma, torn ends of left ventricular free-wall endocardium usually at junction of normal hypercontractile basal segments and infarct segments.

HYPOTENSION

Types of Shock
- Hypovolemic shock-inadequate circulating volume
- Cardiogenic shock-failure of pump function
- Obstructive shock-obstruction to blood flow
- Acute pulmonary embolism, pericardial; tamponade, Type A aortic dissection, and Tension pneumothorax
- Vasoplegic shock—loss of vascular tone

ECHOCARDIOGRAPHY ABNORMALITIES IN VARIOUS TYPES OF SHOCK (TABLE 3)

TABLE 3: Echocardiography abnormalities in various types of shock.

Echocardiographic measurement	Hypovolemic	Obstructive shock – Tamponade	Obstructive shock – Increased RV afterload	Cardiogenic	Distributive
Cardiac volumes	Very small; kissing ventricles	Small; systolic collapse RA; diastolic collapse RV	Dilated RV cavities; paradoxical septal movement	Often dilated	Variable
Contractility	Preserved or increased	Preserved or increased	Impaired RV function	Decreased LV or RV function*	Variable**
Vena cava size	Small size; respiratory variations (collapsed)	Dilated	Dilated	Variable	Variable, often small size; respiratory variations if fluid responsive
Intravascular pressures	Very low; respiratory variations	Impaired diastolic function; respiratory variations	Increased PAP; clots sometimes seen; short PA acceleration time; biphasic PA flow	Elevated filling pressures (left and/or right)	Variable but low in most cases
Pericardial space	Empty	Markedly filled; may be focal	Empty or minimally filled	Empty or minimally filled	Empty or minimally filled
Other		Check for aortic dissection or cardiac rupture		Check valves and/or abnormal flows (interventricular communication)	Check for endocarditis

* Left ventricular volume and contractility are often preserved or increased in aortic stenosis.
** Left ventricular contractility is impaired in up to 30% of patients on admission, but cardiac output is often preserved.

Echocardiography and Lung Ultrasound in the Emergency Room

CARDIAC ABNORMALITIES IN SEVERE SEPSIS
- Left ventricular dilatation
- Left ventricular contraction impairment Global/Segmental

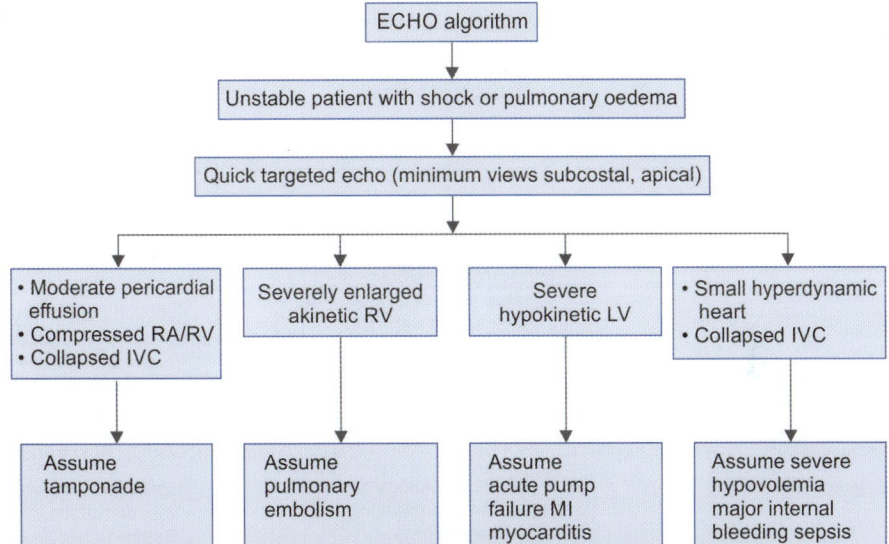

FLOWCHART 1: ECHO algorithm for unstable patient with shock or pulmonary edema.

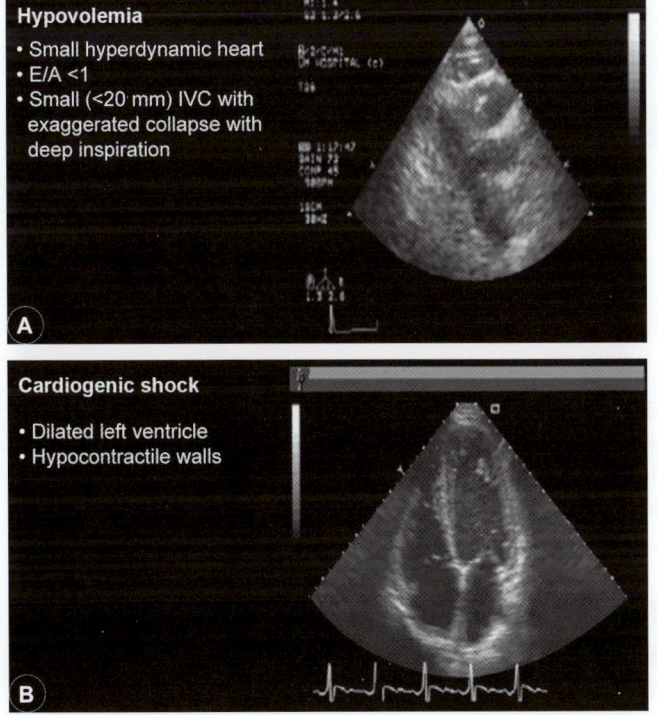

FIGS. 20A AND B: ECHO in hypovolemic and cardiogenic shock.

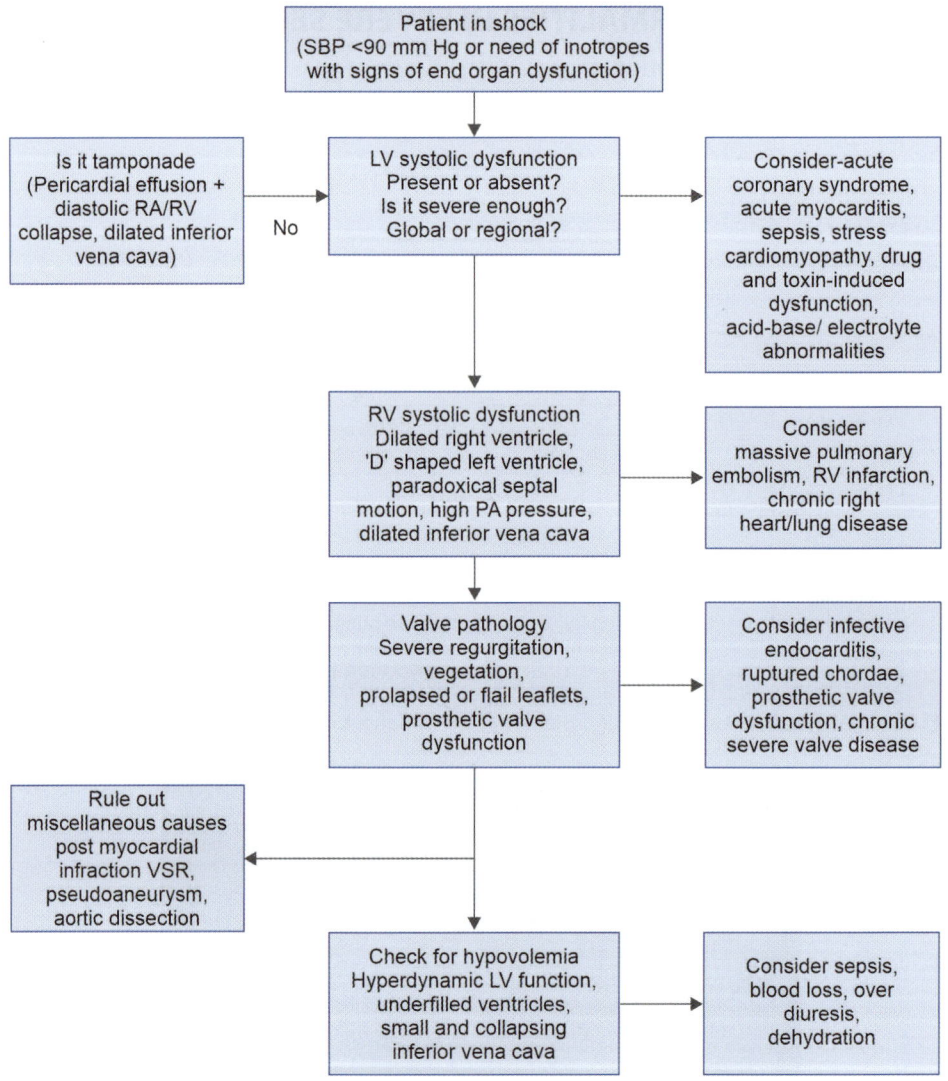

FLOWCHART 2: ECHO algorithm for patient in shock.

- Left ventricular diastolic dysfunction
- Right ventricle systolic/diastolic
- Dysfunction
- Valvular lesions
- Functional/Endocarditis

ECHOCARDIOGRAPHY FREE SPACE AROUND THE HEART

- Pericardial effusion
- Pleural effusion

- Epicardial fat (posterior and/or anterior)
- Less common causes:
  - Aortic aneurysm
  - Pericardial cyst
  - Dilated pulmonary artery

Size of the Pericardial Effusion

- Small: Confined to posterior space, <0.5 cm
- Moderate: Anterior and posterior, 0.5–2 cm (diastole)
- Large: >2 cm

Clinical Features of Pericardial Effusion

- Pericardial fluid accumulation may be clinically silent.
- Symptoms are due to:
  - Mechanical compression of adjacent structures
  - Increased intrapericardial pressure

Cardiac Tamponade

- Increased intracardiac pressures
- Limitation of ventricular diastolic filling
- Reduction of stroke volume and cardiac output

PERICARDIAL TAMPONADE: PATHOPHYSIOLOGY (FLOWCHART 3)

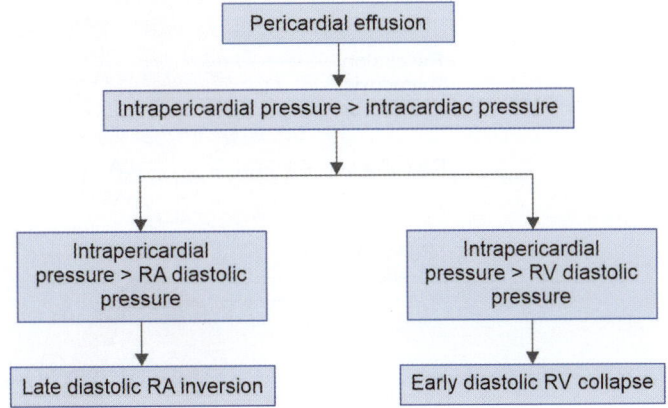

FLOWCHART 3: Pericardial tamponade-pathophysiology.

MASSIVE PULMONARY EMBOLISM OR RIGHT VENTRICULAR INFARCT

- Dilated right ventricle
- RV hypokinesis
- Normal left ventricle function
- Dilated noncollapsing IVC

ACUTE PULMONARY EMBOLISM (BOX 3)

- Focused echocardiography in emergency life support (FEEL)

> **BOX 3: Echocardiography in PE: To identify RV overload.**
> - RV dilatation
> - Abnormal right ventricular wall motion (McConnells sign)
> - Systolic flattening of the interventricular septum
> - Tricuspid valve insufficiency
> - Increased pulmonary arterial pressure
> - Inferior vena cavga congestion
> - Dilated pulmonary artery
> - Right-sided cardiac thrombus

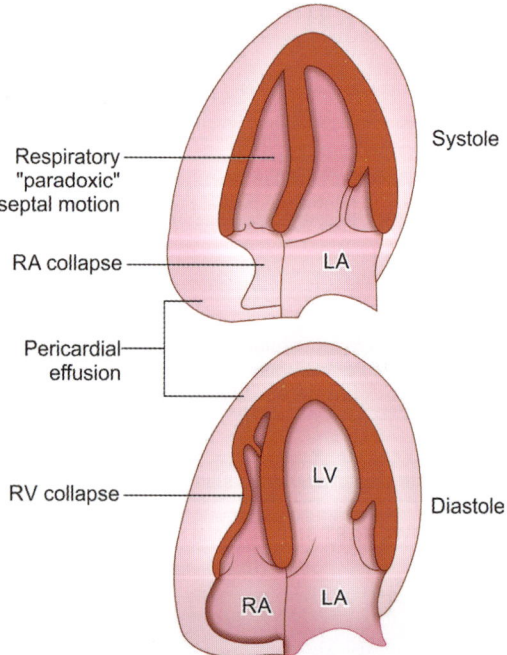

FIG. 21: Echocardiography signs in pericardial tamponade.

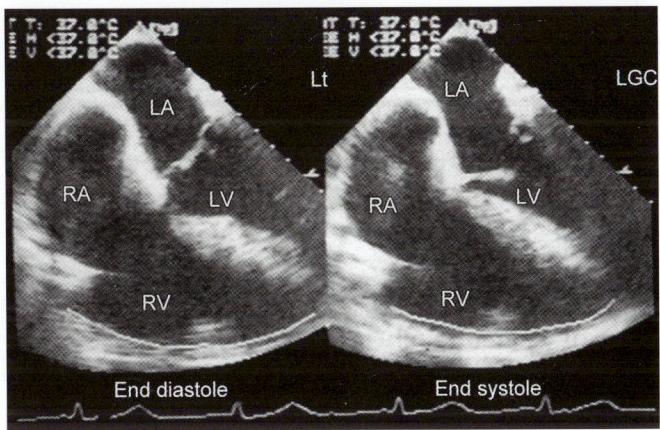

FIG. 22: Dilated and dysfunction right ventricle secondary to RV infarct.

NONTRAUMATIC RESUSCITATION

Direct Visualization

Is there effective myocardial contractility?
- Asystole
- Myocardial "twitch"
- Hypokinesis
- Normal
  Is there a pericardial effusion?

ECHO in pulseless electrical activity:
- Perform ECHO during "quick look" and in pulse checks
- Change management based on "Positive" findings
- Pericardial tamponade
  - Pericardiocentesis
  - Hyperdynamic cardiac wall motion
  - Volume resuscitate

RV dilatation:
- Hypoxic? Likely PE
- ECG—IMI with RV infarct?

Profound hypokinesis:
- Inotropic support:
  - Asystole
- Follow ACLS protocols (for now)
- Early data suggesting poor prognosis

False positive cardiac motion:
- Transthoracic pacemaker
- Positive pressure ventilation

BOX 4: The BLUE Protocol combined with simple echocardiography.
- The BLUE Protocol applies LUS and venous ultrasound for drawing profiles
- A simplified echocardiography without Doppler can be associated with the BLUE protocol
- The BLUE protocol can be adapted to multiple clinical settings:
  - Trauma
  - Neonate
- Acute Respiratory Distress Syndrome (ARDS)

CHEST TRAUMA

Focused Assessment with Sonography for Trauma (FAST).

Penetrating Chest trauma

Physician's ability to determine whether there is a hemodynamically significant effusion is poor Beck' Triad.
- Dependent on patient cardiovascular status
- Findings are often late.

Determinants of hemodynamic compromise:
- Size of the effusion
- Rate of formation

Technical Problems

- Subcutaneous air
- Pneumopericardium
- Mechanical ventilation
- Scanning limited by:
  - Pain/tenderness
  - Spinal immobilization
  - Ongoing procedures
- Narrow intercostal spaces
- Obesity
- Muscular chest
- Chronic obstructive pulmonary disease
- Calcified rib cartilages
- Abdominal distention

Sonographic Pitfalls

- Pericardial versus pleural fluid
- Pericardial clot
- Pericardial fat

Pericardial or Pleural Fluid

- Left parasternal long axis:
  - Pericardial fluid does not extend posterior to descending aorta or left atrium
- Subcostal:
  - No pleural reflection between liver and right-sided chambers
  - A pleural effusion will not extend between to RV free wall and the liver

Blunt Cardiac Trauma

- Cardiac contusion
- Cardiac rupture
- Valvular disruption
- Aortic disruption/dissection
- Pericardial effusion
- Assess for wall motion abnormality
  - RV dyskinesis (takes the first hit)
- Assess thoracic aorta:
  - Hematoma
  - Intimal flap
  - Abnormal contour
- Valvular dysfunction or septal rupture

Cardiac Contusion

- Akinetic anterior RV wall
- Small pericardial effusion
- Diminished ejection fraction

■ AORTIC DISSECTION (FLOWCHART 4)

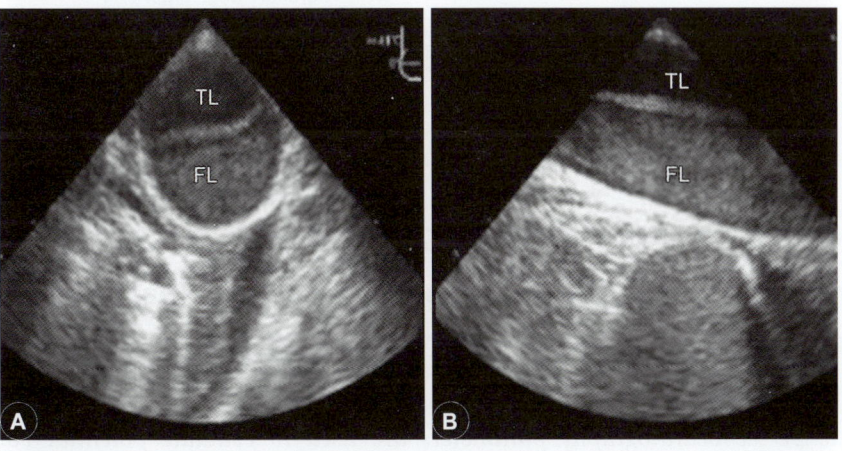

FIGS. 23 AND B: True versus false lumen.

TABLE 4: Differentiating true and false lumen in aortic dissection.

	True lumen	False lumen
Size	True < false	Most often; false true lumen
Pulsation	Systolic expansion	Systolic compression
Flow direction	Systolic antegrade flow	Systolic antegrade
Flow reduced or	Absent, or retrograde	Flow
	Communication	From true to false
Flow	lumen in systole	
Contrast echo	Early and fast	Delayed and slow
Flow		

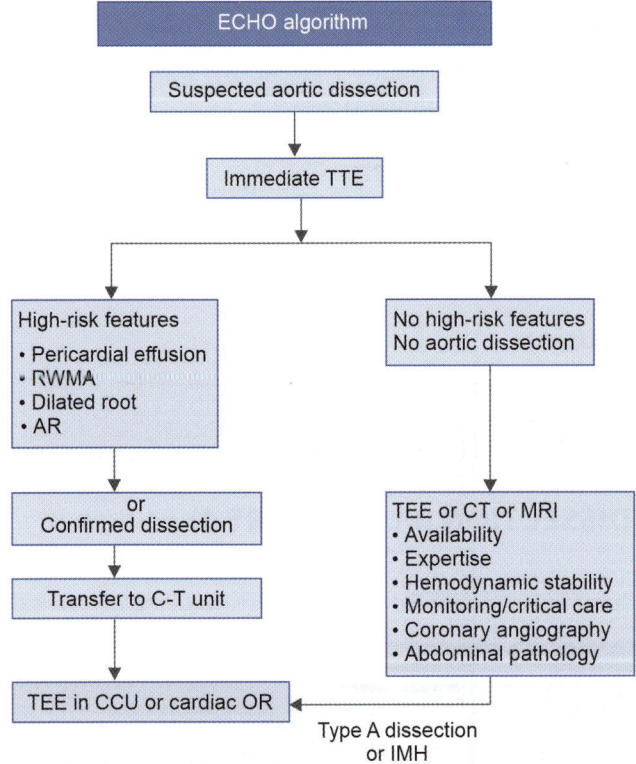

FLOWCHART 4: Echocardiography algorithm in aortic dissection.

■ HEMODYNAMICS BY ECHOCARDIOGRAPHY

Echocardiographic Methods to Estimate Left Atrial Pressure

Echocardiographic Features in Patients Presenting with Severe Hemodynamic Impairment

Static 2D echocardiography parameters are used to evaluate potential volume responsiveness.

Echocardiography and Lung Ultrasound in the Emergency Room

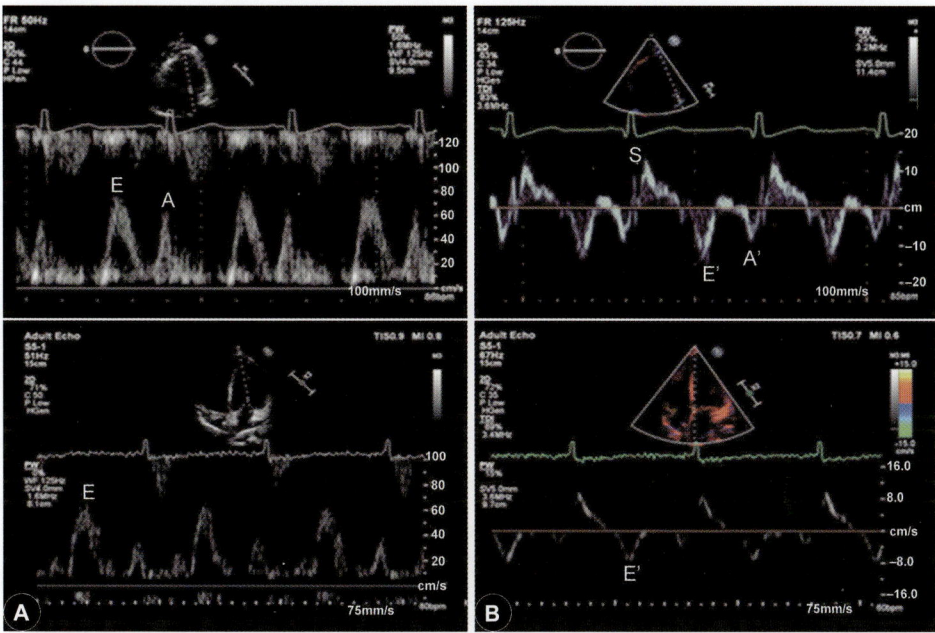

FIGS. 24A AND B: Echocardiographic methods to estimate left atrial pressure.

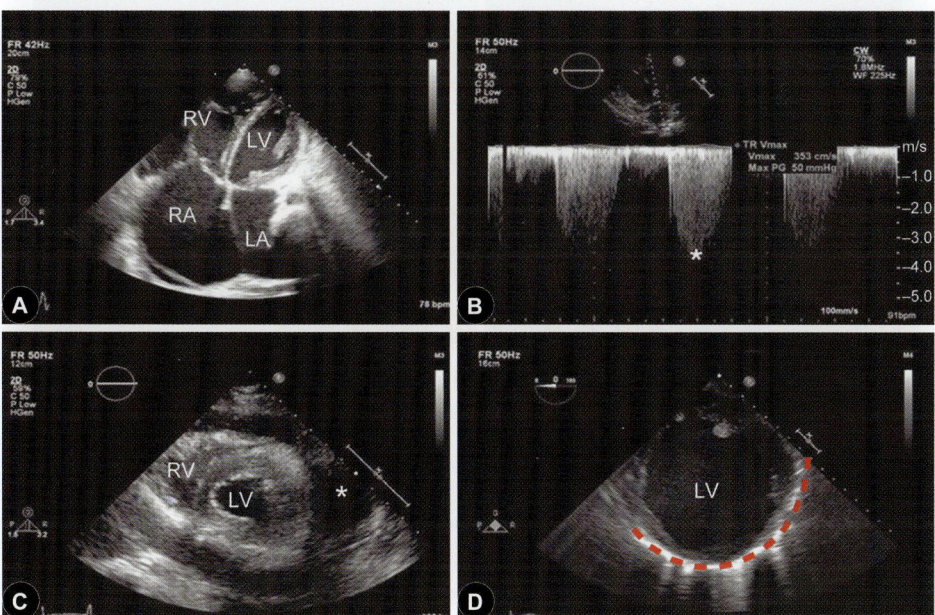

FIGS. 25A TO D: Echocardiographic features in patients presenting with severe hemodynamic impairment.

TABLE 5: Estimation of right atrial pressure using Inferior vena cava size and collapsibility on inspiration. Comparison of 2005 and 2010 ASE guidelines.

Measurement	eRAP
2005 ASE guidelines	
0–5 mm Hg	IVC maximum ≤ l.7 cm and collapsibility index ≥ 50%
6–10 mm Hg	IVC maximum > 1.7 cm and collapsibility index ≥ 50%
11–15 mm Hg	IVC maximum > 1.7 cm and collapsibility index < 50%
>15 mm Hg	IVC maximum> 1.7 cm and collapsibility index < 25%
2010 ASE guidelines	
Normal	IVC maximum ≤ 2.1 cm and collapsibility index > 50%
Intermediate	IVC maximum ≤ 2.1 cm and collapsibility index < 50%
High	IVC maximum > 2.1 cm and collapsibility index < 50%

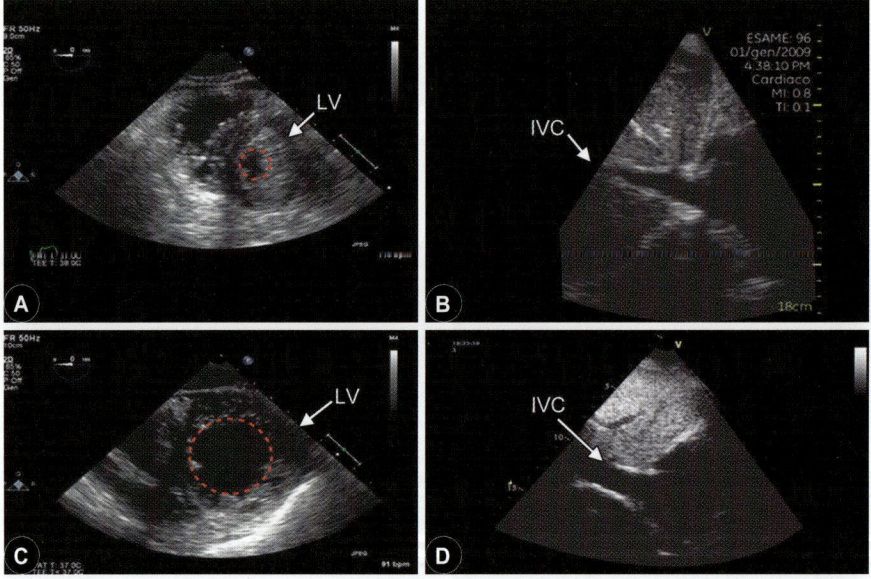

FIGS. 26A TO D: Static two-dimensional (2D) echocardiography parameters are used to evaluate potential volume responsiveness.

Echocardiography-guided cardiac output optimization using pulsed-wave Doppler imaging
Hemodynamic effects of coronary and pulmonary thrombosis
- For practical purposes, in the acute setting for the spontaneously breathing patient in shock, the IVC diameter is measured within 0.5–3 cm from the caval-right atrial junction in the subcostal view
- When IVC diameter is <10 mm the patient is likely to respond to fluid
- When >20 mm—unlikely.
- Collapse of >50 % between the diameters of 10–20 mm should result in a trial of fluid.

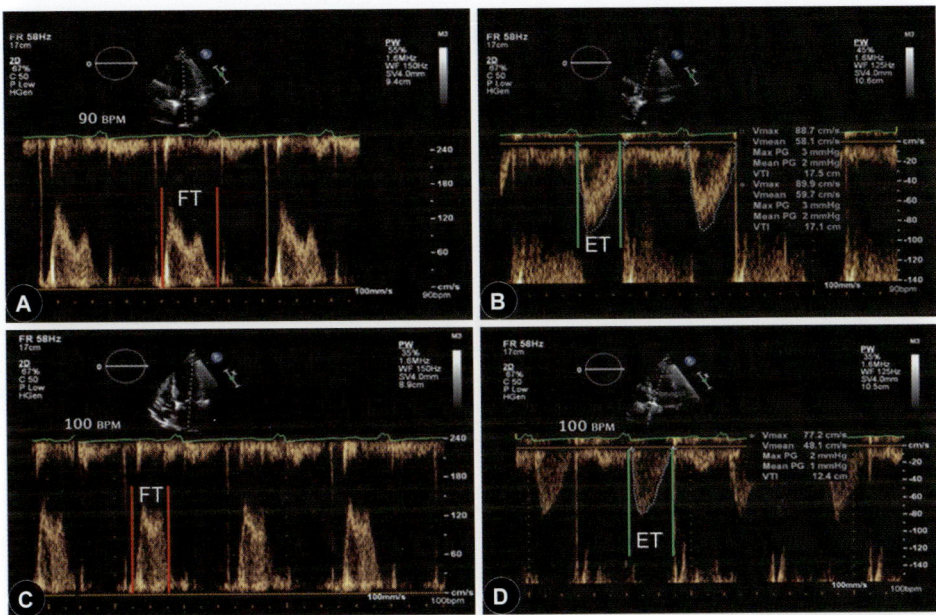

FIGS. 27A TO D: Echocardiography-guided cardiac output optimization using pulsed-wave Doppler imaging.

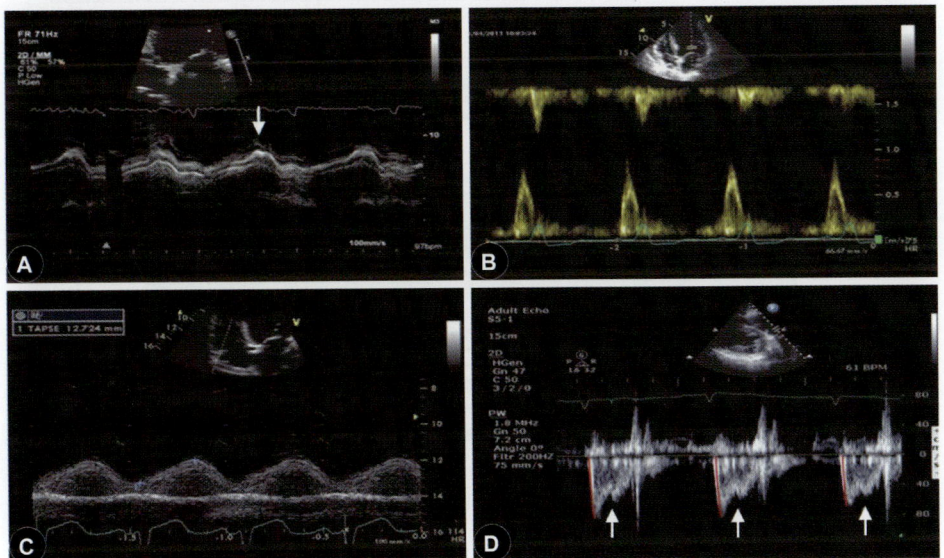

FIGS. 28A TO D: Hemodynamic effects of coronary and pulmonary thrombosis.

- Fluid responsiveness is determined if there is, on average, a >15% increase in SV or CO after fluid administration
- Or a change in VTI of >10% after the infusion of first 100 mL of colloid solution predicted fluid responsiveness

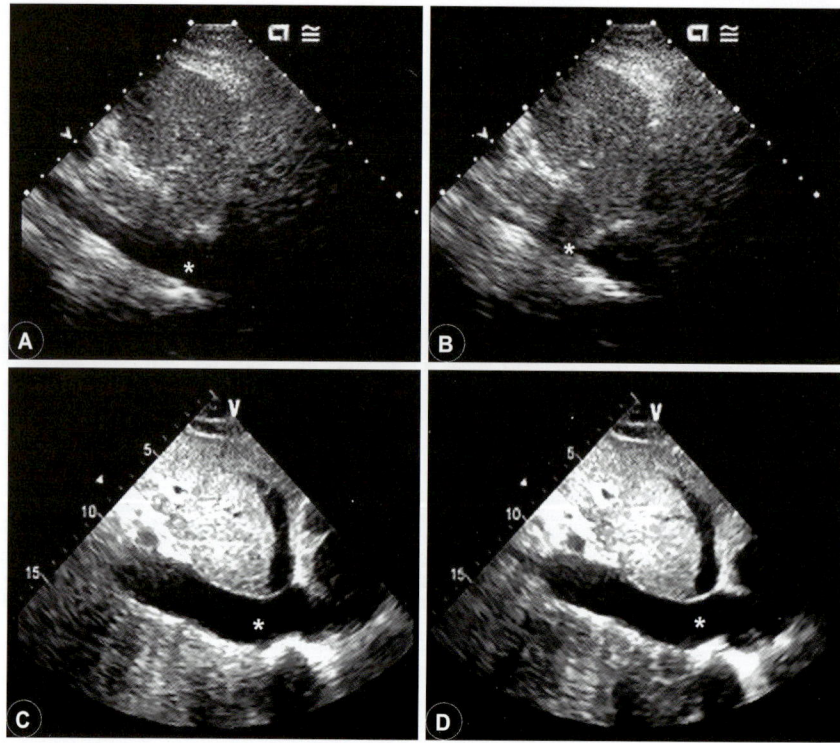

FIGS. 29A TO D: Estimated right atrial pressure by echocardiography (A to D), The inferior vena cava (IVC) (*) during normal respiration (A) and inspiratory sniff (B) in a patient with estimated right atrial pressure of 5 mm Hg. Conversely, the IVC in a patient with estimated right atrial pressure of 20 mm Hg is dilated during normal respiration (C) and does not collapse with inspiratory sniff (D).

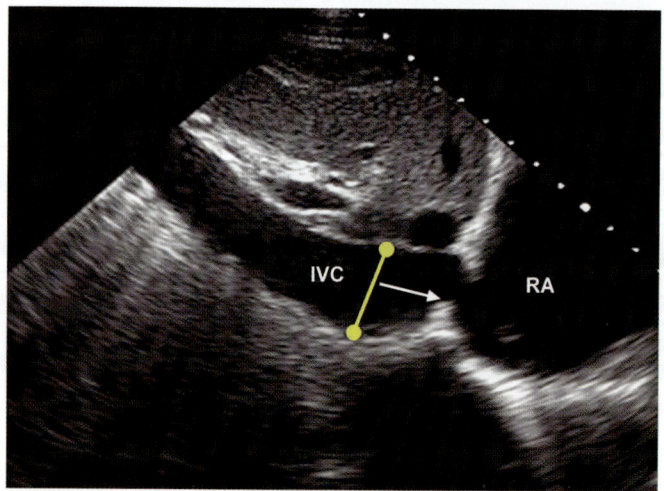

FIG. 30: In mechanically ventilated patients IVC <1.2 cm has 100% specificity for a RA pressure <10 mm Hg.

- In a patient on fully supported positive pressure ventilation, the distensibility index (dIVC) is a good guide to fluid responsiveness.
- dIVC is calculated as the ratio of $(D_{max} - D_{min})/D_{min}$, with a threshold of 18% discriminating between responders and nonresponders with 90% sensitivity and specificity
- Aggressive fluid resuscitation consists of a bolus of 20 mL/kg of body weight, followed by 3 mL/kg/h.
- Moderate fluid resuscitation consists of a bolus of 10 mL/kg of body weight in patients with hypovolemia, or
- No bolus in patients with normovolemia, followed by 1.5 mL/kg/h

ACUTE RESPIRATORY SYMPTOMS IN THE ED
- Decompensated HF
- Pneumonia
- COPD exacerbation
- Large pleural effusion
- Pneumothorax

BASIC PRINCIPLES IN LUNG USG
- When the ultrasound beam is directed to image the lungs, most (99%) of the waves are reflected back on striking the soft tissue and air interface.
- This implies that structures beneath the pleura (soft tissue) in an air-filled lung will only be sparsely visualized, and mostly artifacts will be seen.
- Appearance of these artifacts will change depending on the relative amount of air and fluid in the lungs/pleural
- Normal lung—98% air
- Interstitial syndromes—90% air
- Alveolar syndromes—10% air, and
- Atelectasis—5% air
- LUS relies on the direct visualization of structures and artifact interpretation.

CARDIOGENIC PULMONARY EDEMA IN THE EMERGENCY DEPARTMENT (FIGURES 31A TO I)

PERFORMANCE OF LUNG ULTRASONOGRAPHY IN THE CRITICAL CARE (TABLES 6 AND 7)
- Upper BLUE-point is at the middle of the upper hand
- Lower-BLUE-point is at the middle of the lower hand
- PLAPS-point (posterolateral alveolar or pleural syndromes), which is indicated by the intersection of a horizontal line at the level of the lower BLUE-point and a vertical line at the posterior axillary line.

The probe should be moved as posteriorly as possible, along this line to get more information in supine patients.

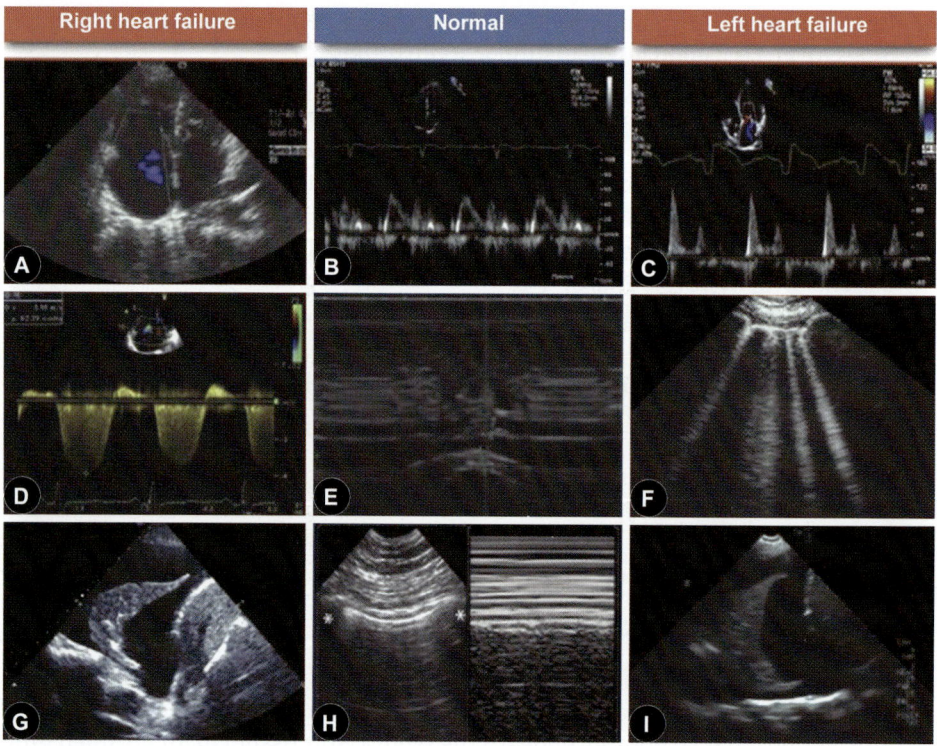

FIGS. 31A TO I: Echocardiography, Doppler and lung ultrasound findings in heart failure.

TABLE 6: Sensitivity and specificity of clinical examination, chest X-ray (CXR) and lung ultrasound in various clinical settings.

Clinical examination	CXR
Sens: 85.3% (81.8–88.4%)	Sens: 69.5% (65.1–73.7%)
Spec: 90.0% (87.2–92.4%)	Spec: 82.1% (78.6–85.2%)
NT-pro-BNP	FLUS
Sens: 85.0% (80.3–89.0%)	Sens: 97.0% (95.0–98.3%)
Spec: 61.7% (54.6–68.3%)	Spec: 97.4% (95.7–98.6%)

TABLE 7: Accuracy of lung ultrasound (LUS) in the critical ill compared with computed tomography.

Ultrasound	Sensitivity	Specificity
Pleural effusion	94%	97%
Alveolar consolidation	90%	98%
Interstitial syndrome	93%	93%
Pneumothorax	95%	94%
Complete pneumothorax	100%	96%
Occult pneumothorax	79%	100%

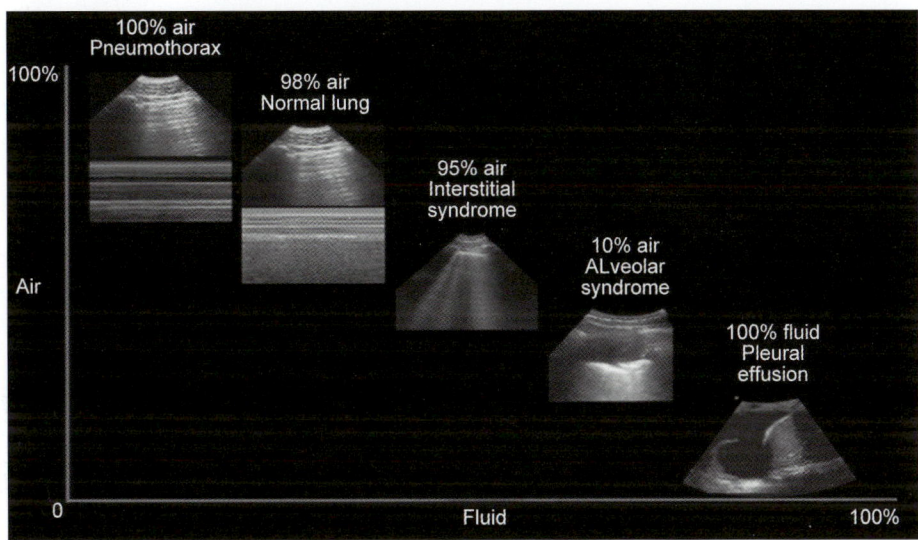

FIG. 32: Air and fluid on lung ultrasound.

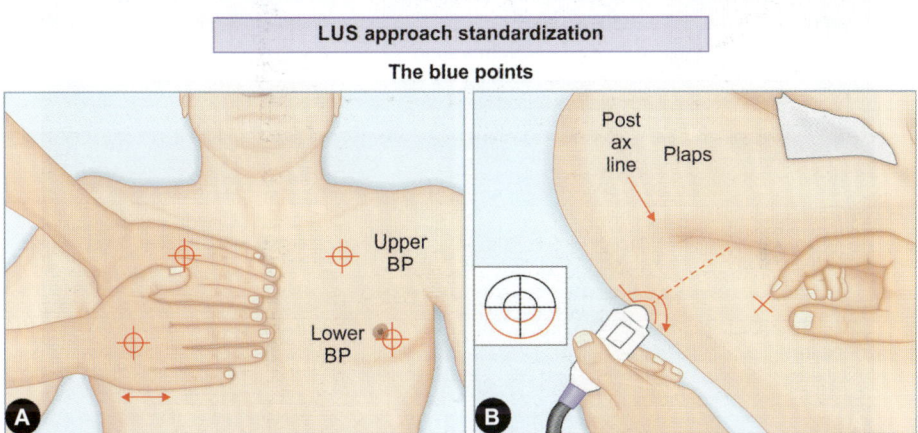

FIGS. 33A AND B: Each point shows a standardized for a given disorder

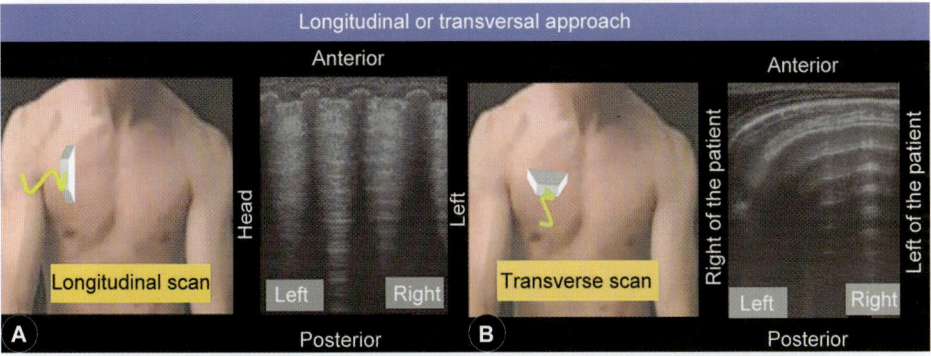

FIGS. 34A AND B: The longitudinal approach has the advantages of locating the pleural line in all circumstances.

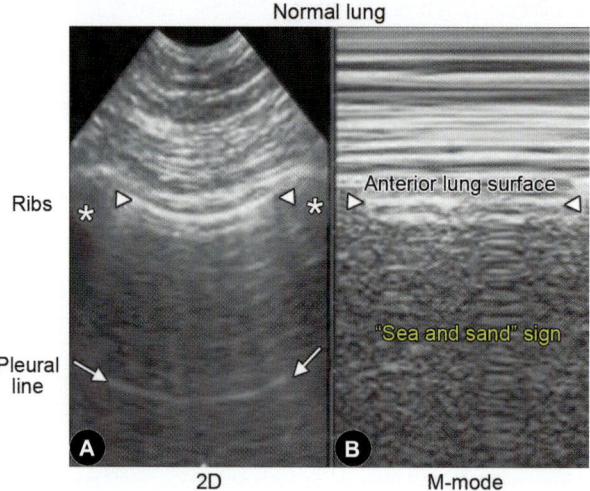

FIGS. 35A AND B: Normal lung ultrasound.

1. Lung Ultrasound (LUS): The A lines

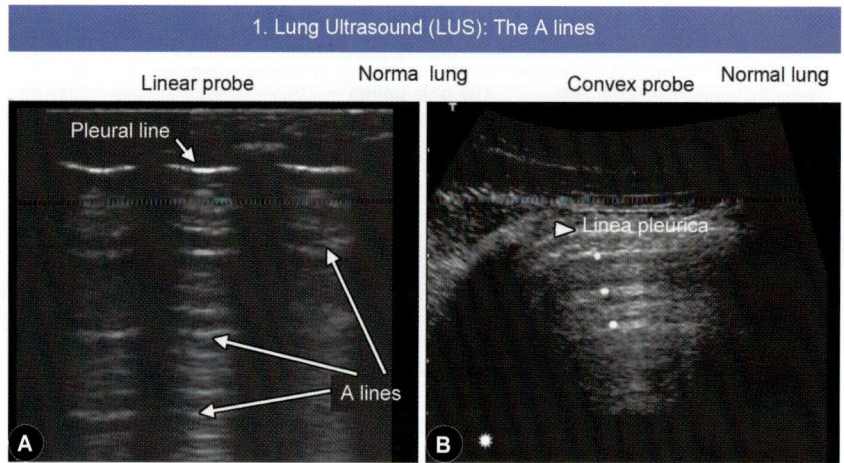

FIGS. 36A AND B: 'A' line on USG using linear and convex probe.

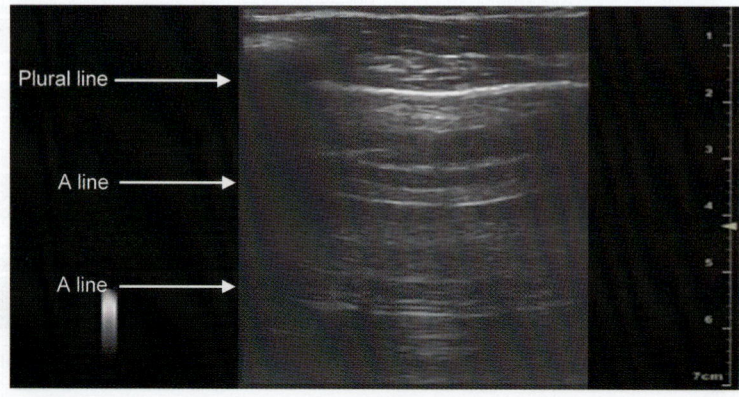

FIG. 37: 'A' line on USG.

A profile is when we see A lines with normal lung sliding
A-lines are better appreciated with the linear transducer
- A-lines are echogenic, gradually fading horizontal lines arranged at equal intervals below the pleural line.
- They represent the repetition artifact of the parietal pleura.
- Their presence indicates that air/gas is present below the pleura, which reflects the ultrasound waves back to the probe.
- The distance between A-lines is almost the same as the distance between the skin surface and the pleural line.

On M-mode, a sinusoid pattern is seen which is due to the movement of the lung line toward the pleural line on inspiration, and back on expiration

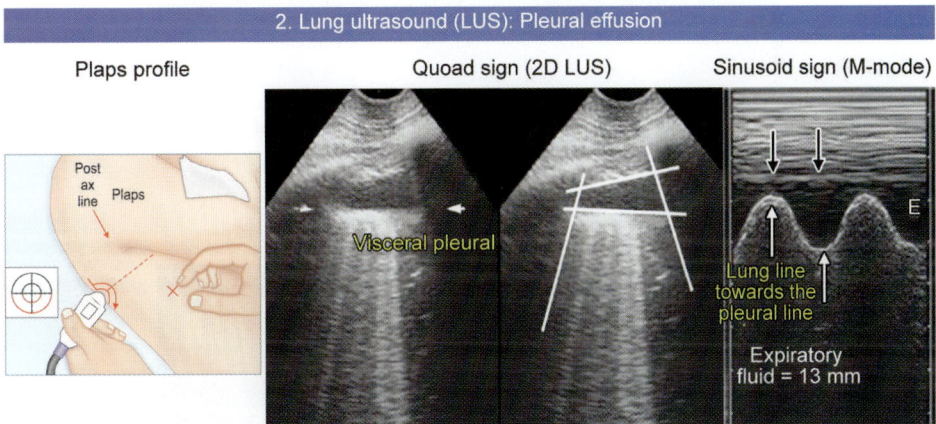

FIGS. 38A TO C: A 15-mm distance is our minimum required for safe diagnostic of therapeutic puncture.

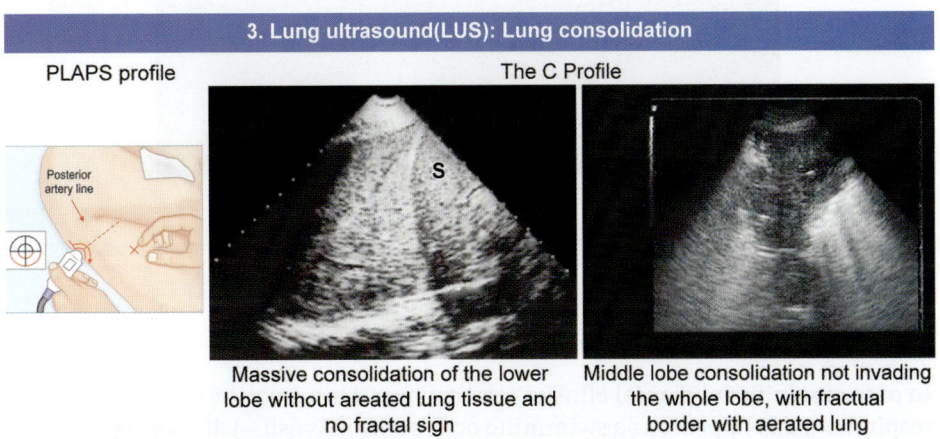

FIGS. 39A AND B: lung USG: Lung consolidation.

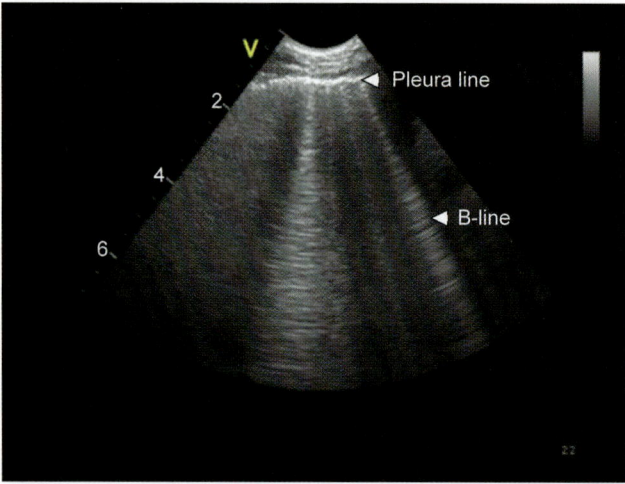

FIG. 40: B line on USG.

Note: Definition of the B-line are defined as discrete laser-like vertical hyperechoic reverberation artifacts that arise from the pleural line (Previously described as "comet tails"), extend to the bottom of the screen without fading, and move synchronously with lung sliding.

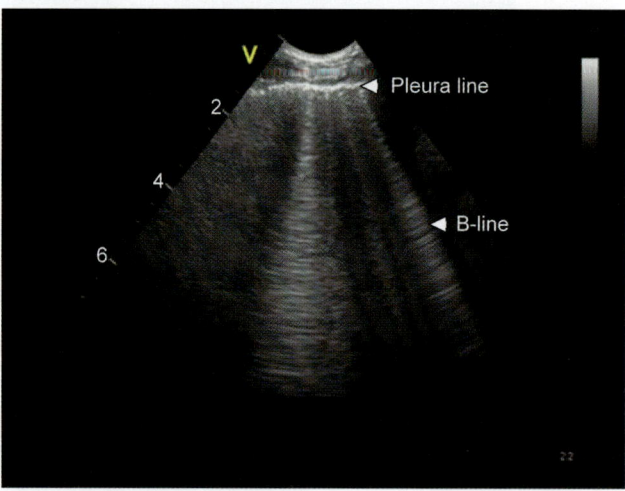

FIG. 41: B line on USG.

Note: The B-line artifact visible when the density of the interstitial lung tissue has been increased (e.g., pulmonary edema, lung fibrosis).

JELLY FISH SIGN

In case of significant pleural effusion, the collapsed lung may be seen moving with respiration, and appears as a swimming or flapping jellyfish—jellyfish sign.

Visualization of this sign implies the absence of consolidation and pleural adhesions in the region.

Echocardiography and Lung Ultrasound in the Emergency Room

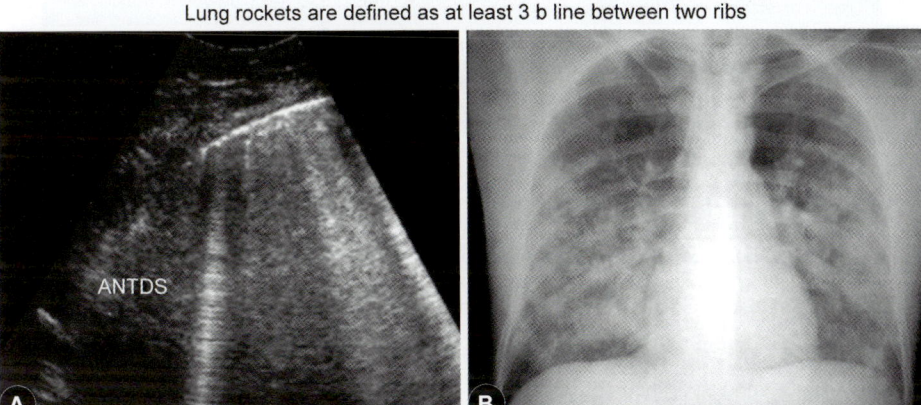

FIGS. 42A AND B: Lung USG: Interstitial syndrome.

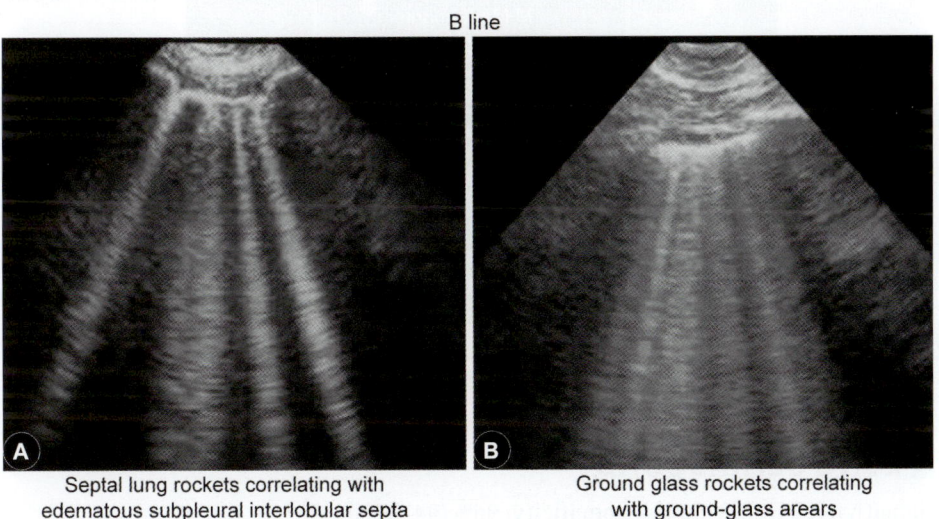

FIGS. 43A AND B: B lines on USG.

Free movement indicated by this sign means that low viscosity fluid is present, which suggests that the pleural effusion is of transudative type (as opposed to high viscosity associated with exudative effusion which may obstruct the free movement of the collapsed lung).

- B-lines are not observed in pneumothorax, as they are seen only at pleura/tissue acoustic interface (for which the apposition of both pleural layers is required)
- In pneumothorax both layers are separated by air in-between pleural layers.
- Up to two B-lines can be seen in normal lungs (commonly at the bases).
- They are considered significant if three or more B-lines are seen in a single image between two ribs.

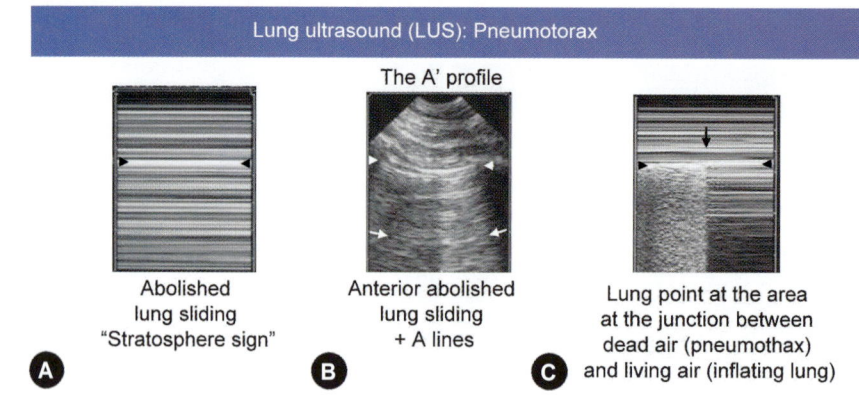

FIGS. 44A TO C: Lung USG: Pneumothorax.

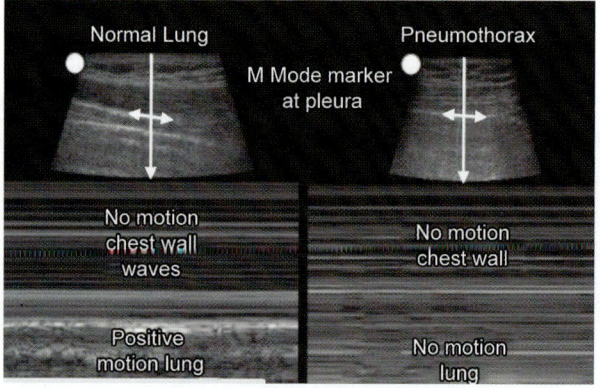

FIG. 45: Lung ultrasound showing pneumothorax.

LUNG ULTRASOUND

Sensitivity: 94% (92–96%) – Specificity: 96% (94–97%)

"ABCD APPROACH" IN PERFORMING EMERGENCY ECHOCARDIOGRAPHY

A Awareness Fight against routine. Think beyond apparent explanations
B Be suspicious Referral diagnosis may be misleading. Never trust, confirm
C Comprehensiveness Do as complete examination as a suitable. Careful interpretation
D Double R. The study should be recorded and reviewed. Team work is crucial.

Echocardiography and Lung Ultrasound in the Emergency Room

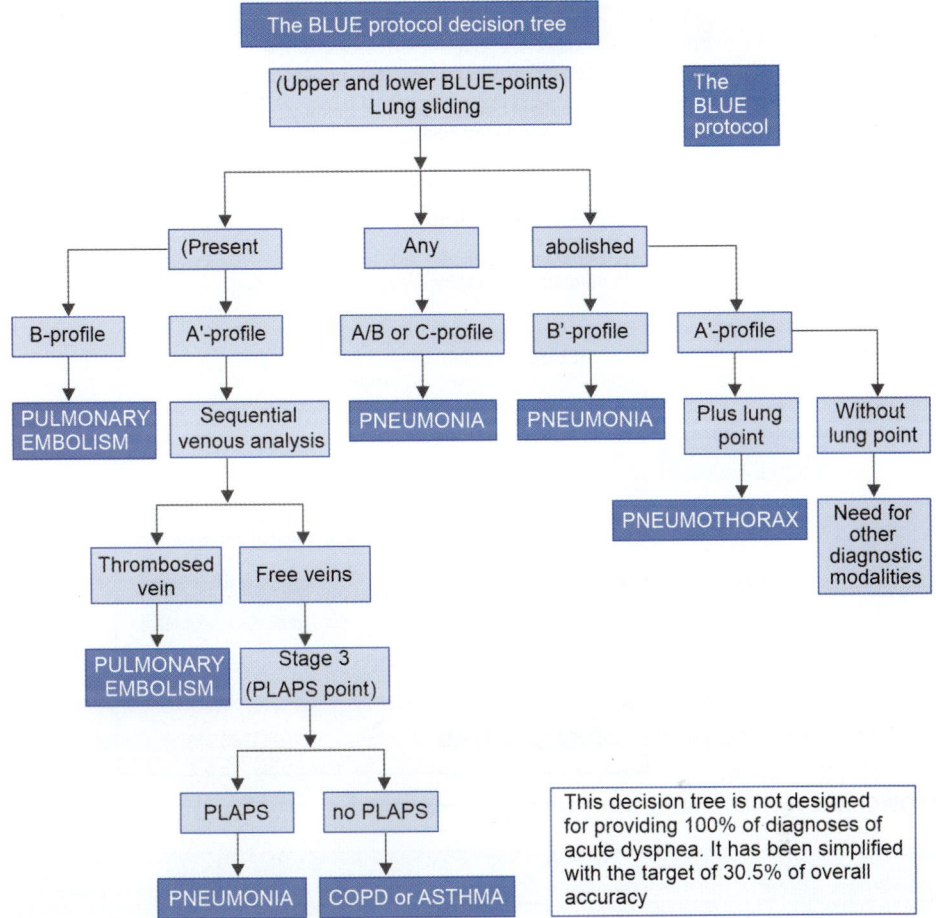

FLOWCHART 5: The BLUE protocol decision tree.

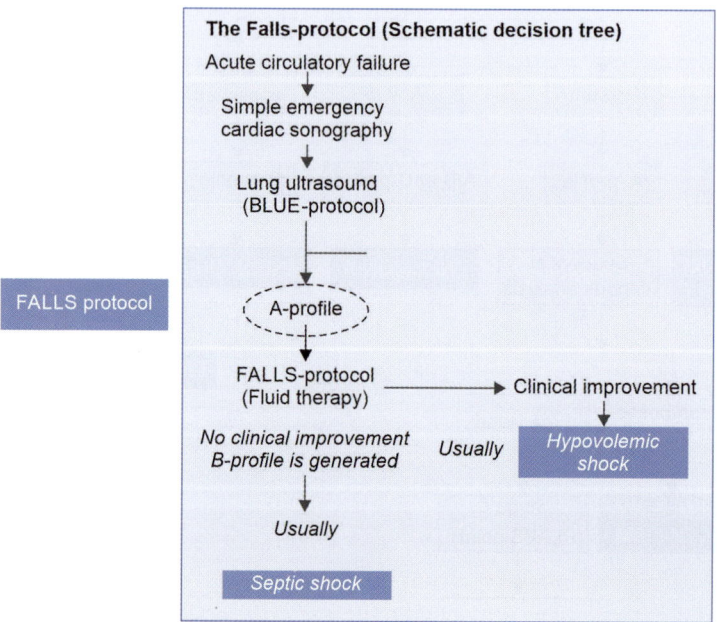

FLOWCHART 6: Fluid administration limited by LUS protocol.

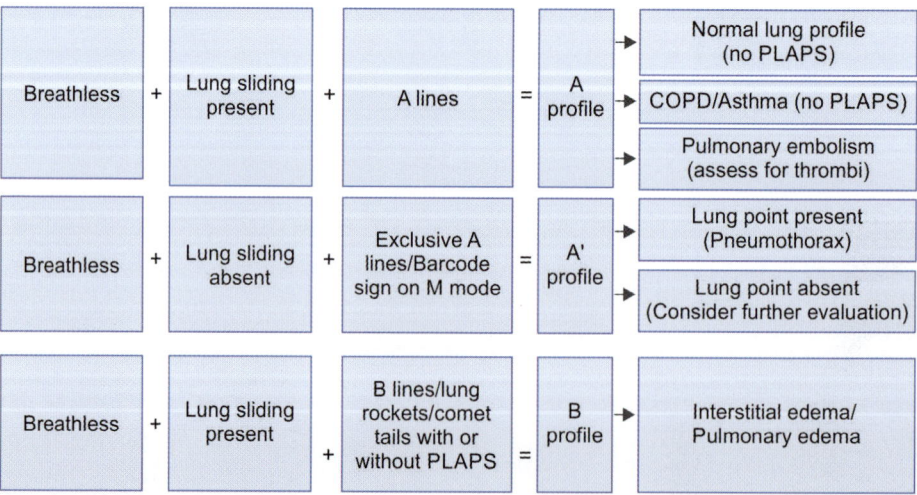

FIG. 46: Approach to respiratory failure patient.

Echocardiography and Lung Ultrasound in the Emergency Room

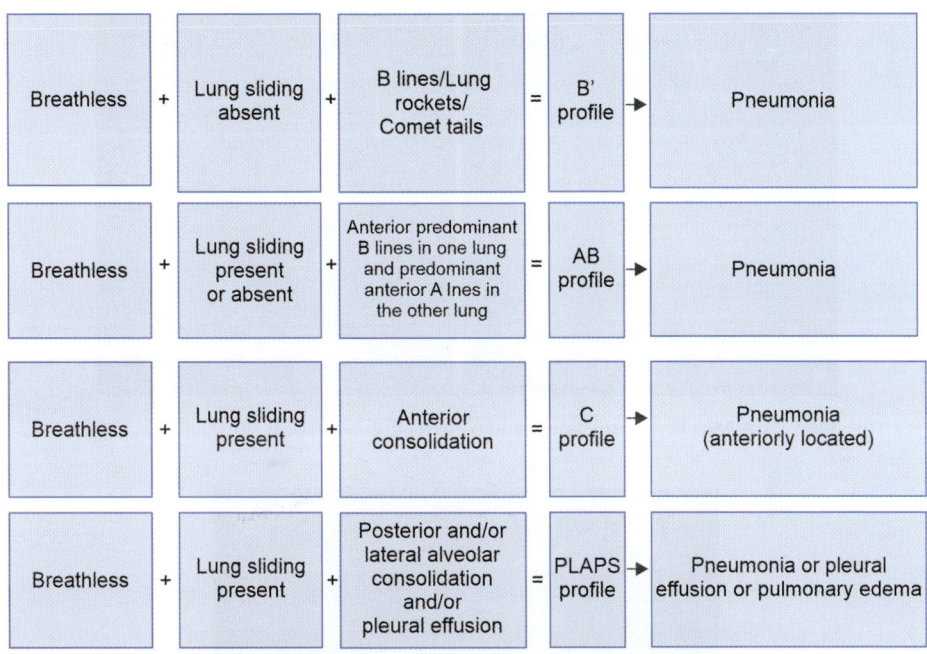

FIG. 47: Approach to respiratory failure patient.

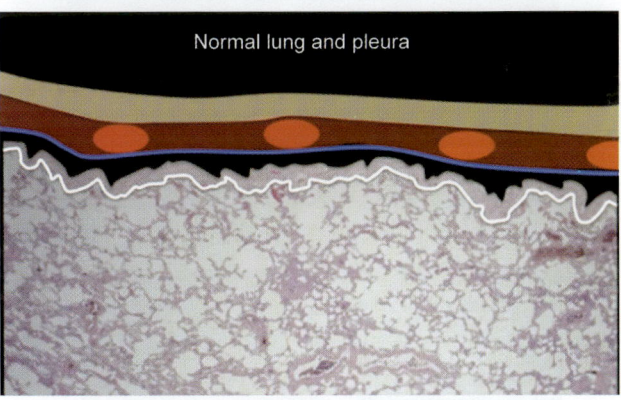

FIG. 48: Normal lung and pleura.

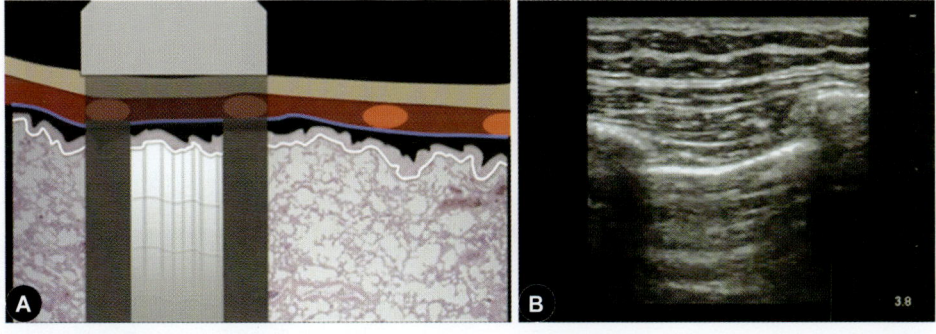

FIGS. 49A AND B: Normal lung and pleura on USG.

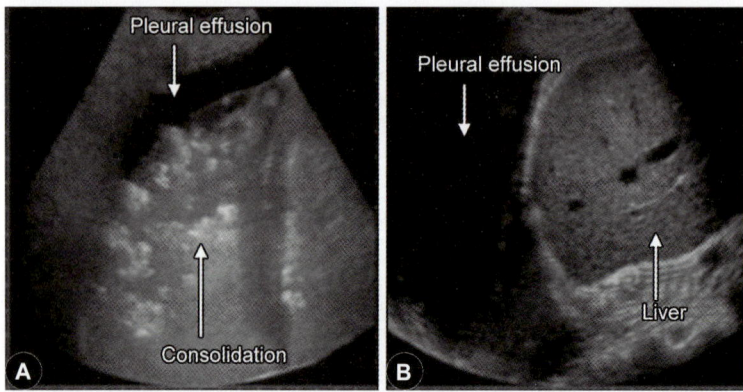

FIGS. 50A AND B: Consolidation and pleural effusion on USG.

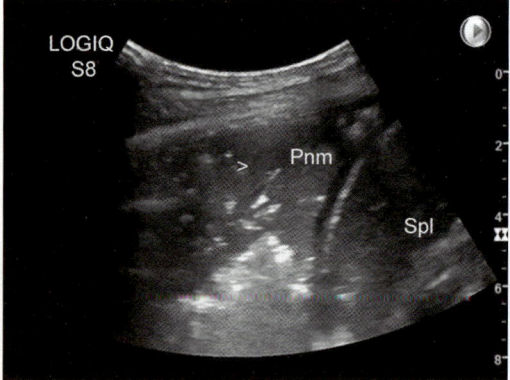

FIG. 51: Consolidation on USG.

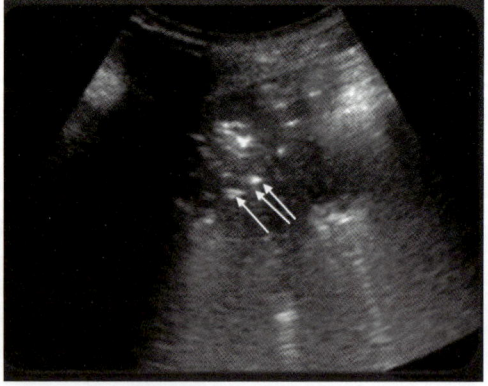

FIG. 52: Consolidation on USG.

Note: Pneumonia posterior intercostal scan shows a hypoechoic consolidated area that contains multiple echogenic lines that represent an air bronchogram.

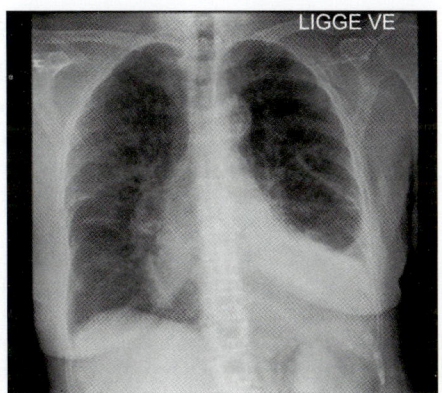

FIG. 53: X-ray of atelectasis.

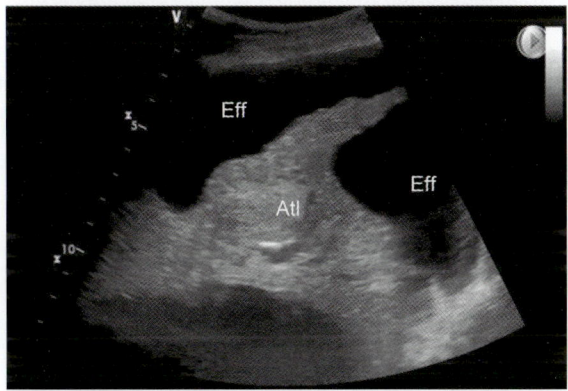

FIG. 54: Obstructive atelectasis.

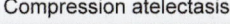

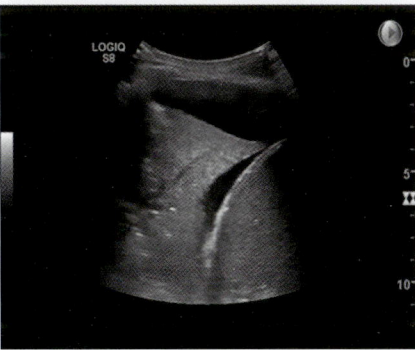

FIG. 55: Compression atelectasis.

CONCLUSION

Bedside echocardiography combined with lung ultrasound provides one of the easiest, radiation free and low cost investigation for the emergency physician. Its availability and short-term training should be made mandatory in every emergency care providing facility.

SUGGESTED READING

1. Bhoil R, Ahluwalia A, Chopra R, Surya M, Bhoil S: Signs and lines in lung ultrasound. J Ultrason 2021;21: e225–e233.
2. Jambrik Z, Monti S, Coppola V, Agricola E, Mottola G, Picano E. Usefulness of ultrasound lung comets as a nonradiologic sign of extravascular lung water. Am J Cardiol. 2004;93:1265-70.
3. Nazerian P, Vanni S, Zanobetti M, et al. Diagnostic accuracy of emergency Doppler echocardiography for identification of acute left ventricular heart failure in patients with acute dyspnea: comparison with Boston criteria and N-terminal prohormone brain natriuretic peptide. Acad Emerg Med. 2010;17:18-26.
4. Ponikowski P, Voors AA, Anker SD, et al. ESC guidelines for the diagnosis and treatment of acute and chronic heart failure: the Task Force for the Diagnosis and Treatment of Acute and Chronic Heart Failure of the European Society of Cardiology. Eur J Heart Fail. 2016;18:891-975.

CHAPTER 5

Electrocardiogram in Routine Practice

Abhishek Goyal

■ INTRODUCTION

Electrocardiogram (ECG) is a graphic recording of the electrical properties of the heart on a standardized piece of paper. Information given by ECG is immense and quite useful in clinical practice. It is often the first investigation in a suspected cardiac patient. Its role in various cardiac conditions such as ST-elevation myocardial infarction (STEMI) is paramount.

Current manuscript highlights important concepts in ECG reading, which are useful in day-to-day clinical practice.

■ GENESIS OF VARIOUS WAVEFORMS

Electrical activity is spontaneously generated in sinoatrial (SA) node and propagated in an orderly fashion through a specialized conduction system to the rest of the heart.

From the ECG, we can identify origin of impulse, its frequency, where and how the impulse is traveling, and the tissue response.

- *Primary pacemaker*: The fastest spontaneous impulse generator in the heart is the primary pacemaker. It is the SA node which is located at the junction of the superior vena cava (SVC) and right atrium. This has the steepest spontaneous diastolic depolarization curve.
- *Secondary pacemaker*: When the primary pacemaker fails, other pacemakers which are called secondary pacemakers take over to prevent cardiac standstill, by producing an escape rhythm. These are atrioventricular (AV) junction, His bundle, and ventricles, in whom the rate is much slower.
- *Sinus rate*: 60–100 beats/min
- *AV junction*: 40–60 beats/min
- *Ventricle*: 30–40 beats/min

STANDARDIZATION AND NOMENCLATURE (FIGS. 1A AND B)

A properly recorded ECG should include a standardization deflection. 1 mV of current will result in a 1-cm deflection, and standard speed of recording is 25 mm/s.

Nomenclature of waves is as follows:
- "q": First negative wave of the QRS complex
- "r": First positive wave
- "s": Second negative wave, which follows "r" wave
- "r′": "r dash"; a second r wave following s wave.

Small letters denote small amplitude waves (<5 mm), and capital letters denote taller waves (>5 mm), as shown in **Figure 1B**. **Table 1** summarizes various waveforms, their origin, and abnormalities in various pathological conditions.

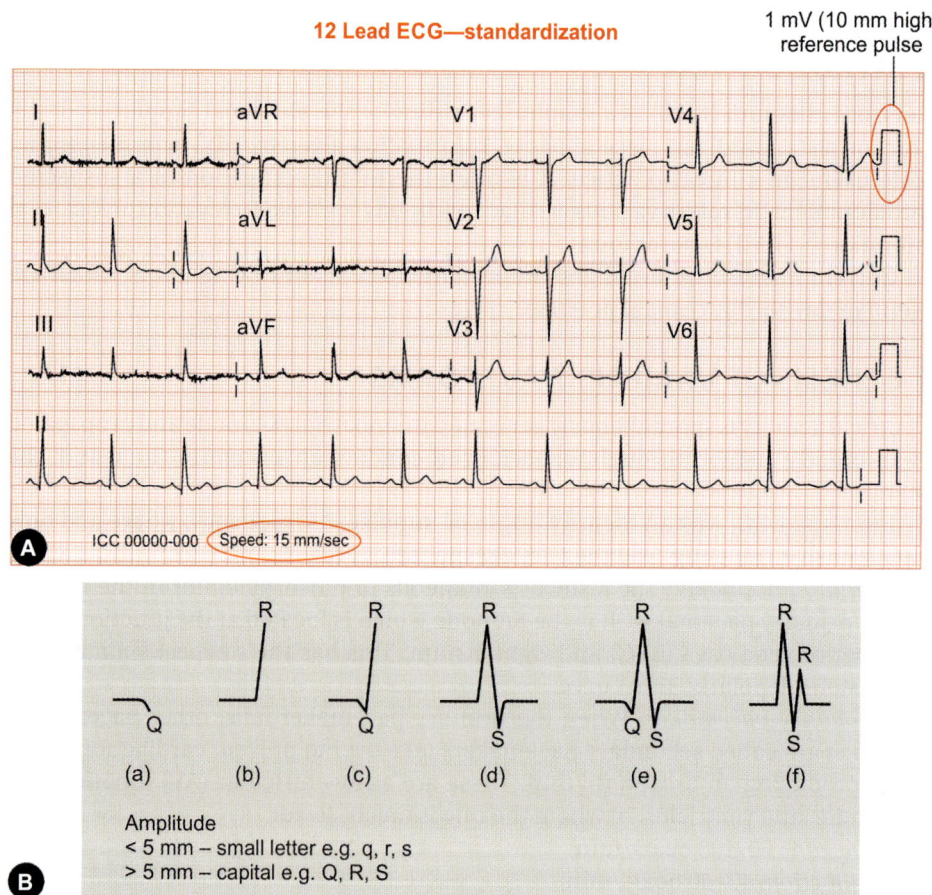

FIGS. 1A AND B: (A) 12-lead ECG; (B) Nomenclature.

TABLE 1: Various waveforms, their origin, and abnormalities in various pathological conditions.

Wave/segment	Genesis	Normal values	Abnormal values, findings	Clinical conditions
P	Atrial depolarization	2.5 small squares, horizontally, vertically	>2.5 vertically >2.5 horizontally	• Tall P: Right atrial enlargement • Wide P: Left atrial enlargement
PR interval	Atrioventricular conduction time	0.12–0.21 s	<0.12 short PR, >0.12 long PR	• Short PR: Preexcitation • Long PR: first-degree AV block
QRS	Ventricular depolarization	Higher amplitude is suggestive of increased ventricular mass (refer to text for various criteria)	• LVH • RVH	• LVH: Hypertension/AS/HCM • RVH: Pulmonary stenosis/PHT
T	Ventricular repolarization	20–40% of preceding QRS	• <20% low voltage • >40% tall T waves	• Low voltage: Hypokalemia • Tall T wanes: Hyperkalemia, acute ischemia
QT interval	Sum of ventricular depolarization, ST interval, and ventricular repolarization	0.36–0.46 s (to be corrected for HR–QTc)	• Long QTc >0.46 s • Short QTc < 0.36 s	• Congenital (Long QT syndrome), drugs, electrolytes; • Digoxin, hypocalcemia

(AS: aortic stenosis; AV: atrioventricular; HCM: hypertrophic cardiomyopathy; LVH: left ventricular hypertrophy; PHT: pulmonary hypertension; RVH: right ventricular hypertrophy)

Commonly used ECG criteria for diagnosing LVH include the following:

Sokolow-Lyon criteria: Left ventricular hypertrophy (LVH) is diagnosed if either of the two criteria is present:
- Sum of S wave in V1 and R wave in V5 or V6 ≥ 3.5 mV (35 mm).

or

- R wave in aVL ≥ 1.1 mV (≥1.3 mV in the presence of concurrent left anterior fascicular block)

Romhilt-Estes point score system: This index gives different scores to specific findings. A score of five or more indicates "definite" LVH; a score of four indicates "probable" LVH. Reader is referred to specific text for further details.

Cornell voltage criteria:
- *Males*: S in V3 plus R in aVL > 2.8 mV (28 mm)
- *Females*: S in V3 plus R in aVL > 2.0 mV (20 mm)

RHYTHM DISORDERS

Bradycardia

Classification of bradyarrhythmia is shown in **Box 1**. Sinus bradycardia can be physiological and asymptomatic. This does not require any treatment. The other two sets of conditions are usually pathological and need active management. These are sinus node dysfunction (sick sinus syndrome) and AV blocks. Patients of sick sinus syndrome have abnormality in impulse initiation from the sinus node. They have severe sinus bradycardia, sinus pauses, and sinus arrests. Patients who present with Stokes–Adams attacks (syncope due to bradyarrhythmia) need pacemaker after ruling out reversible factors such as drugs (beta blockers, nondihydropyridine calcium channel blockers etc.).

Atrioventricular blocks involve block in the conduction system from the AV node to the His bundle and the left and right bundles. First-degree AV block and Mobitz type I block are usually benign. Mobitz type II block, high-grade AV block, and complete heart block require permanent pacemaker implantation after ruling out the reversible causes **(Box 2)**.

BOX 1: Classifications of bradyarrhythmias.

Sinus node dysfunction
- Sinus bradycardia and chronotropic incompetence
- Sick sinus syndrome
    - Sinus pause
    - Arrest
    - Sinoatrial exit block

Atrioventricular (AV) conduction abnormalities
- First-degree heart block
- Second-degree heart block (Mobitz type I and Mobitz type II)
- High-grade AV block
- Third-degree (complete) heart block

BOX 2: Common causes of bradyarrhythmias.

- Degenerative fibrosis of conduction system
- Ischemic heart disease (IHD)
- Infiltrative diseases
- Postradiation fibrosis
- Drugs
- Hypothyroidism
- Electrolytes (K^+ and Ca^{2+})
- Postoperative blocks after cardiac surgeries
- Congenital

Diagnostic Evaluation

Bradyarrhythmias can be diagnosed by ECG when they are persistent. In those with intermittent blocks, Holter monitoring is useful. In patients with infrequent syncope, when the cause of syncope is not obvious, long-term monitoring with loop recorders is required. Each of these investigations is discussed below.

- *Holter monitors*: Ambulatory Holter recording is useful in patients with frequent symptoms suggestive of arrhythmias. These devices continuously record the ECG for 24–48 hours. Prolonged monitoring may increase the diagnostic yield. The recorded events require correlation with symptoms.
- *Loop recorders*: The loop recorders may be categorized as external loop recorders (ELRs) or implantable loop recorders (ILRS). These devices are useful in less frequent symptoms. ELR does not require electrodes and can monitor rhythm for 30 days. ILR is implanted in chest wall subcutaneously and can monitor rhythm for 3 years.
- *Postevent recorders*: The patient is advised to place the device on chest as soon as he/she experiences the symptoms.
- *Electrophysiological studies*: This is an invasive procedure and is recommended in patients with unexplained symptoms when noninvasive assessment is noncontributory.

Ventricular Tachyarrhythmias

Clinically, the first task in a tachycardia ECG is to differentiate ventricular tachyarrhythmia (VT) from supraventricular tachyarrhythmia (SVT) with aberrancy. One can resort to various algorithms such as Brugada algorithm or Vereckei algorithm **(Flowchart 1)**. Besides these algorithms, there are important clinical pointers which are quite useful **(Box 3)**.

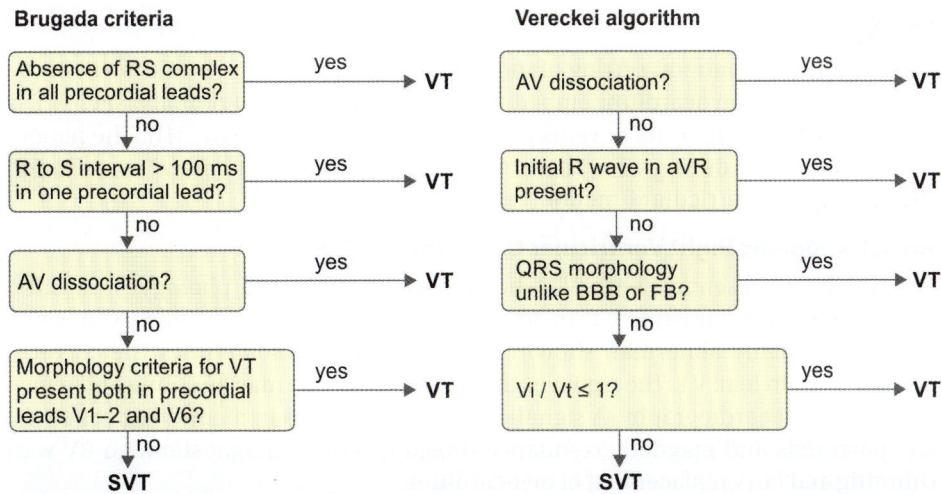

FLOWCHART 1: Brugada and Vereckei criteria.

(AV: atrioventricular; BBB: bundle branch block; FB: fasicular block; SVT: supraventricular tachycardia; VT: ventricular tachycardia)

> **BOX 3: Features favoring VT over SVT with abberancy.**
> - AV dissociation
> - Fusion and capture beats
> - Concordance
> - QRS duration > 150 ms
> - Discordant axis, e.g., RRBB with LAD
> - *Morphology criteria*: Absence of typical RBBB or LBBB
> - Superior/NW axis
> - Presence of LV dysfunction
>
> (AV: atrioventricular; LAD: left anterior descending artery; LBBB: left bundle branch block; LV: left ventricular; RBBB: right bundle branch block; SVT: supraventricular tachyarrhythmia; VT: ventricular tachyarrhythmia)

The three different morphologies of VT are:
- Monomorphic
- Pleomorphic
- Polymorphic

Monomorphic VT has a single morphology throughout, with the QRS complex showing either a right bundle branch block (RBBB) pattern or a left bundle branch block (LBBB) pattern. Typically, the complex is broad (QRS more than 0.12 s), and the rhythm is regular. Pleomorphic VT has more than one morphologically distinct QRS complex occurring during the same episode of VT, but the QRS morphology is not continuously changing. Polymorphic VT has a continuously changing QRS morphology and rhythm from beat to beat. In the presence of a baseline prolonged QT (QTc more than 440 ms), it is referred to as "torsades de pointes" where the QRS complexes appear to twist around the baseline.

Classification of ventricular arrhythmia is shown in **Box 4**.

Special Scenarios

Scar VT
This is the most common setting of monomorphic VT. Reentry circuits form in the islands of viable myocardium embedded in fibrous tissue. Commonly, such VT is seen to start a few months to years after a myocardial infarction (MI). The patient may be very stable during VT or there may be hemodynamic collapse, depending on the underlying ventricular function.

Arrhythmogenic Right Ventricular Cardiomyopathy
Young adults presenting with VT showing a LBBB-like morphology. It is often misdiagnosed as idiopathic VT. In 30% of the cases, it is familial. The ECG in sinus rhythm is usually abnormal, showing T inversions and sometimes the classical epsilon wave in lead V1. The right ventricular (RV) disease may be subtle and hence missed at echocardiography. A signal-averaged ECG helps in identifying abnormal late potentials and magnetic resonance imaging is often diagnostic with RV wall thinning and fatty replacement of myocardium.

> **BOX 4: Ventricular arrhythmias: Clinical scenario.**
>
> - Structural heart disease
> - Ischemic heart disease
> - Dilated cardiomyopathy
> - Hypertrophic cardiomyopathy
> - Arrhythmogenic right ventricular cardiomyopathy
> - *Idiopathic VT (in normal heart)*
> - Right ventricular outflow tract VT
> - Fascicular VT
> - Others
> - *Primarily electrical disease*
> - Long QT and torsades
> - Brugada syndrome
> - Idiopathic VF
> - Specific VT
> - Bundle branch reentrant VT
> - Bidirectional VT
>
> (VF: ventricular fibrillation; VT: ventricular tachycardia)

Idiopathic VT

Idiopathic VT in patients with a structurally normal heart is a unique entity. The tachycardia's QRS morphology on surface ECG is useful in predicting the site of origin of tachycardia. Most cases of idiopathic ventricular tachycardia carry good prognosis, although patients should be on regular cardiac follow-ups as few idiopathic VT may be a marker of latent progressive heart disease such as arrhythmogenic RV dysplasia or other forms of cardiomyopathies, which manifest later. Two patterns are commonly seen—one arising from the outflow tract (RV or left ventricular) and the other from the left ventricular posterior fascicle, known as fascicular VT. The RV outflow tract VT shows a LBBB-like morphology and a vertical QRS axis and is either repetitive, ill-sustained, or could be sustained. It is exercise-induced and responds well to beta blockers. The left posterior VT shows a RBBB-like morphology with left superior QRS axis deviation. It is relatively narrow, as it arises from the left posterior fascicle.

Polymorphic VT

This is a life-threatening arrhythmia since it can degenerate into ventricular fibrillation (VF). The underlying abnormalities include long QT syndrome and acute ischemia.

Long QT Syndrome

This could be either congenital or acquired. The congenital long QT syndrome is a genetic defect, whereas the acquired form is due to hypokalemia or potassium channel blocking cardiac or noncardiac drugs. The characteristic arrhythmia, torsades de pointes is triggered by a ventricular premature beat (VPB), which occurs while the ventricles are still depolarizing. The torsades is often self-terminating, but is fatal in the event it is sustained. The most common presentation is unexplained syncope, and the ECG must be carefully assessed for QT prolongation. Beta blockers with pacemaker are the treatment of choice for the congenital long QT syndrome. Left cervical stellate ganglionectomy and implantable cardioverter–defibrillator (ICD) implantation are other options for the resistant variety. Removal of the offending agent and correcting electrolyte imbalance is the mainstay for the acquired long QT variety.

LOCALIZATION OF MYOCARDIAL INFARCTION

In patients with acute STEMI, the ECG evolves through a sequence of changes. "STEMI in ECG" can be defined as new ST-elevation at the J-point in two contiguous leads of more than 0.1 mV in all leads other than leads V2–V3. For leads V2–V3, the following cut points apply: ≥0.2 mV in men ≥ 40 years, ≥0.25 mV in men aged < 40 years, or ≥0.15 mV in women. Other conditions which are treated as a STEMI are: (1) New or presumed new LBBB and (2) isolated posterior MI. The early and accurate identification of the infarct-related artery on the ECG can help predict the amount of myocardium at risk, and guide decisions regarding the urgency revascularization in STEMI.

Acute Inferior Wall Myocardial Infarction

Inferior wall MI (IWMI) may be caused by occlusion in the course of either the right coronary artery (RCA) or the left circumflex (LCx) artery. The important features favoring RCA rather than the LCx artery as the culprit artery in IWMI are ST-segment elevation in lead III more than lead II, and more than 1 mm ST-segment depression in leads I and aVL **(Table 2)**. In IWMI caused by RCA occlusion, injury vector is directed toward right (lead III); hence, ST-segment elevation in lead III is greater than that in lead II. An illustrative example of a patient with IWMI due to RCA occlusion is shown in **Figure 2**. One of the important clues that suggests proximal occlusion of the RCA with associated RV infarction in a case of IWMI is the additional finding of ST-segment elevation in lead VI **(Fig. 3)**. Associated ST-segment depression in leads VI and V2 in a case of IWMI suggests concomitant posterior wall MI, which is usually caused by LCx occlusion but may also be seen in dominant RCA occlusion.

Right Ventricular Myocardial Infarction

When RCA occlusion occurs proximal to the RV branch, the right ventricle will be in jeopardy and subsequently infarcted. This concept is the basis for using the ECG findings of RV infarction as an indicator of proximal RCA occlusion. Hence, right

TABLE 2: Localization of IWMI.

RCA occlusion	Circumflex occlusion
• STE in lead III > lead II • Presence of reciprocal ST depression in lead I, aVL • Signs of RVMI: STE in V1 and V4R	• STE in lead II ≥ lead III • Absence of ST ↓ in I, aVL • STE in I and aVL or V5–6 • ST ↓ in V1–3 greater than ST ↑ in inferior leads

(IWMI: Inferior wall myocardial infarction; RVMI: right ventricular myocardial infarction; STE: ST elevation)

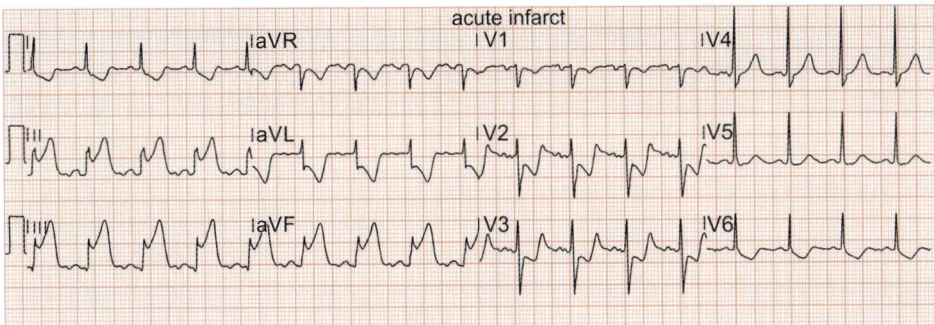

FIG. 2: IWMI due to RCA occlusion: ST elevation in lead III>II and significant ST depression in lead I and aVL.
(IWMI: inferior wall myocardial infarction; RCA: right coronary artery)

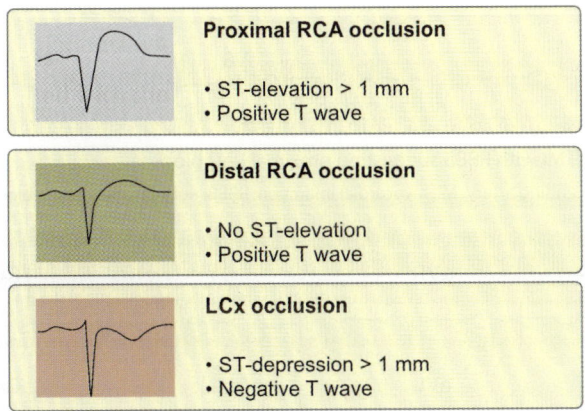

FIG. 3: Changes in lead V4R to localize infarct-related artery in IWMI.
(IWMI: inferior wall myocardial infarction; LCx: left circumflex; RCA: right coronary artery)

ventricular MI (RVMI) is always associated with occlusion of the proximal RCA. ST-segment elevation of more than 1 mm in lead V4R with an upright T wave in that lead is the most sensitive ECG sign of RVMI. This is an early sign and is rarely seen after 12 hours.

Anterior Wall Myocardial Infarction

Determining the site of left anterior descending artery (LAD) occlusion is of great help to the treating physician to know prognosis and on planning further management. LAD has two major branches—first septal (S1) and first diagonal (D1). Proximal LAD occlusion (proximal to first S1 and D1) has the following features on ECG:
- Complete RBBB **(Fig. 4)**
- ST ↑ in V1 > 2.5 mm **(Fig. 5)**
- ST ↑ in lead aVR (<V1)
- ST ↓ in V5

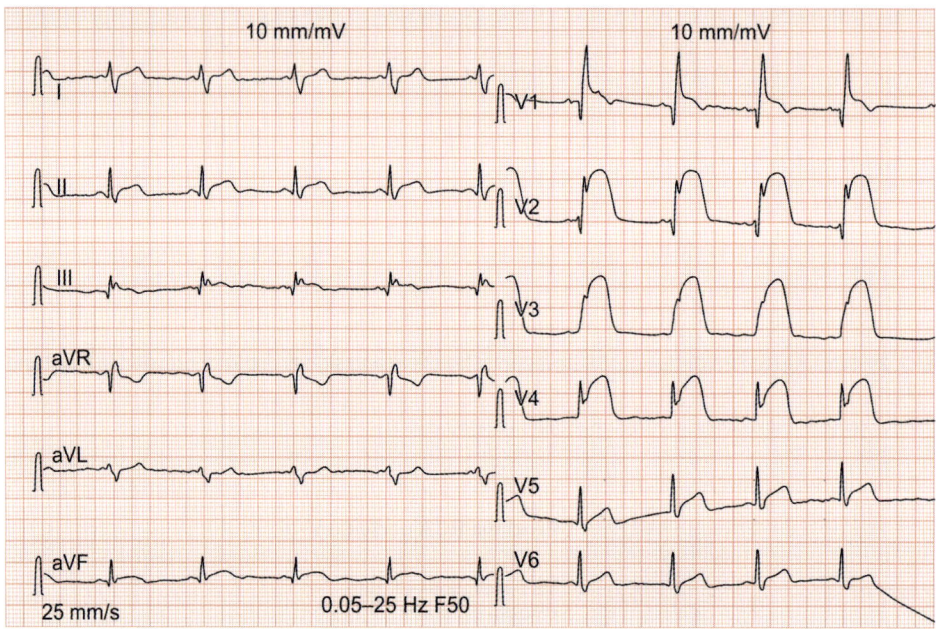

FIG. 4: Anterior wall MI with RBBB suggesting proximal LAD block.
(LAD: left anterior descending artery; MI: myocardial infarction; RBBB: right bundle branch block)

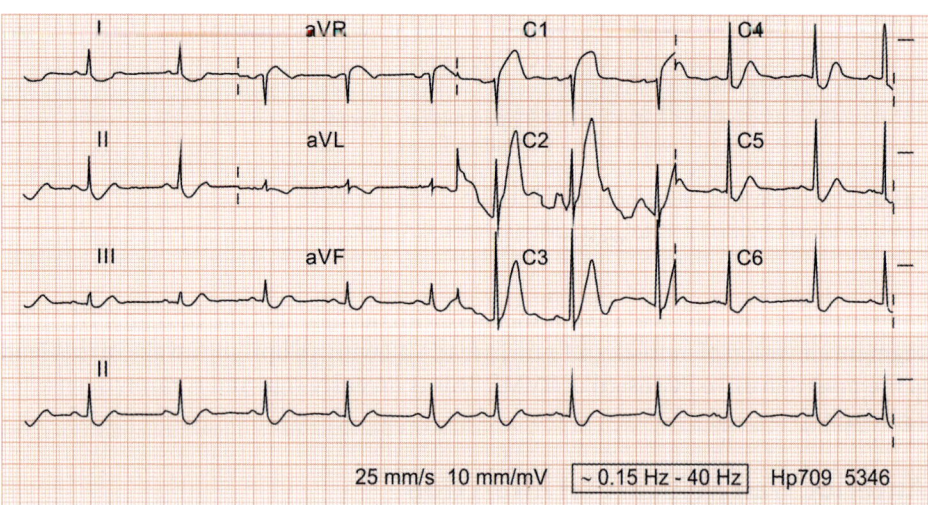

FIG. 5: Anterior wall MI with V1 showing ST elevation (>2.5 mm) suggesting proximal LAD block.
(LAD: left anterior descending artery; MI: myocardial infarction)

- ST ↓ in lead II, lead III > 1 mm
- ST ↓ in lead aVF > 2 mm

The most powerful predictors of proximal LAD occlusion include ST-segment elevation in aVL or aVR, concomitant ST-segment depression in inferior leads,

ST-segment depression in V5, and disappearance of preexistent septal Q waves in lateral leads. New RBBB with a Q wave preceding the R wave in lead V1 is a specific but insensitive marker of proximal LAD occlusion in association with anterior wall MI (AWMI).

Features suggestive of occlusion before D1 are:
- ST ↑ lateral wall (I, avL, V5, V6)
- ST ↓ in lead II, III, aVF > 1 mm
- *Typical feature*: Q waves in left lateral leads (V4–V6)
- Q in aVL (85% specific)

ST-segment elevation in leads V1, V2, and V3 without significant inferior ST-segment depression suggests occlusion of the LAD beyond the origin of the first diagonal branch.

ST-segment elevation in leads V1, V2, and V3 with concomitant elevation in the inferior leads suggests LAD occlusion distal to the origin of the first diagonal branch, in a vessel that wraps around the apex to supply the inferoapical region of the left ventricle (wrap around LAD).

Posterior Wall Myocardial Infarction

Routine ECG leads are relatively insensitive for detecting posterior wall MI (PWMI). This is due to the lack of standard leads facing the posterior wall of LV. In up to 50% of patients with PWMI, ST-segment elevation is not seen on the standard 12-lead ECG. During acute inferior infarction or when PWMI is suspected, it is imperative to record ST-segment elevation in the posterior chest leads V7 through V9. PWMI can be caused by lesions in the RCA or LCx, which may be indirectly recognized by reciprocal ST-depression in precordial leads V1–V3. Similar ST changes can also be the primary ECG manifestation of unstable angina or non-STEMI (NSTEMI). Findings suggestive of PWMI are:
- Presence of ST-segment elevations in posterior leads (V7–V9), although these are not routinely recorded
- Abnormal R wave in V1 (0.04 in duration and/or R/S ratio ≥ 1 in the absence of preexcitation or RV hypertrophy), with inferior or lateral Q waves

Acute Myocardial Infarction with Left Bundle Branch Block or Ventricular Paced Rhythm

Certain ST changes can be used to diagnose acute MI in the setting of LBBB mainly called "concordant changes." The three criteria used to diagnose infarction in patients with LBBB also known as Sgarbossa's criteria are:
1. Concordant ST-elevation more than 1 mm in leads with a positive QRS complex (score 5)
2. Concordant ST-depression more than 1 mm in V1–V3 (score 3)
3. Excessively discordant ST-elevation more than 5 mm in leads with a negative QRS complex (score 2) **(Fig. 6)**

The third criterion is sensitive, but not specific for ischemia in LBBB.

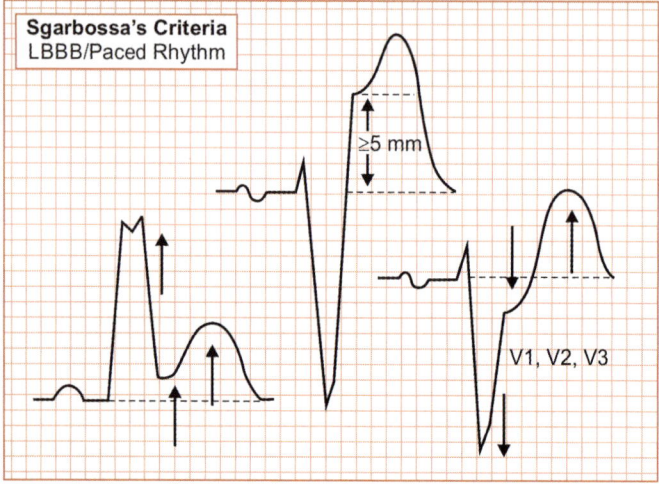

FIG. 6: Sgarbossa's criteria.

CONCLUSION

ECG reading in routine practice is based on understanding of normal waveforms and changes which occur in various pathologies. There are very well described ECG abnormalities which not only help in accurate diagnosis, but also have significant prognostic implications. There are numerous derivations of ECG which are quite useful. Holter is ECG recorded over extended period of time which can diagnose infrequent entities such as arrhythmias. Various life-threatening conditions such as long QT syndrome, brugada syndrome are primarily ECG based diagnosis. Use of ECG in STEMI has saved millions of lives. Detailed knowledge and practice of ECG is a clinical tool which should be considered as sine qua non of good clinical practice.

SUGGESTED READINGS

1. Surawicz B, Knilans T. Chou's Electrocardiography in Clinical Practice: Adult and Pediatric, 6th edition. Amsterdam: Elsevier Health Sciences; 2008.
2. Klimczak A, Wranicz JK, Cygankiewicz I, et al. Electrocardiographic diagnosis of acute coronary syndromes in patients with left bundle branch block or paced rhythm. Cardiol J. 2007;14(2): 207-13.

CHAPTER 6

Hand Palmistry in Medicine

Subhash Chabdra, SN Yadav, Prakhar Gupta, Shweta Yadav

1. **Clubbing**
   - Angle between nail bed and nail >180°
   - Swelling of subcutaneous tissues (parrot beak)
   - Peripheral/transverse diameter increases
   - Nail changes with wrist swelling

   Causes: Lung abscess, empyema, endocarditis, bronchiectasis, carcinoma of bronchus, and Eisenmenger's syndrome.

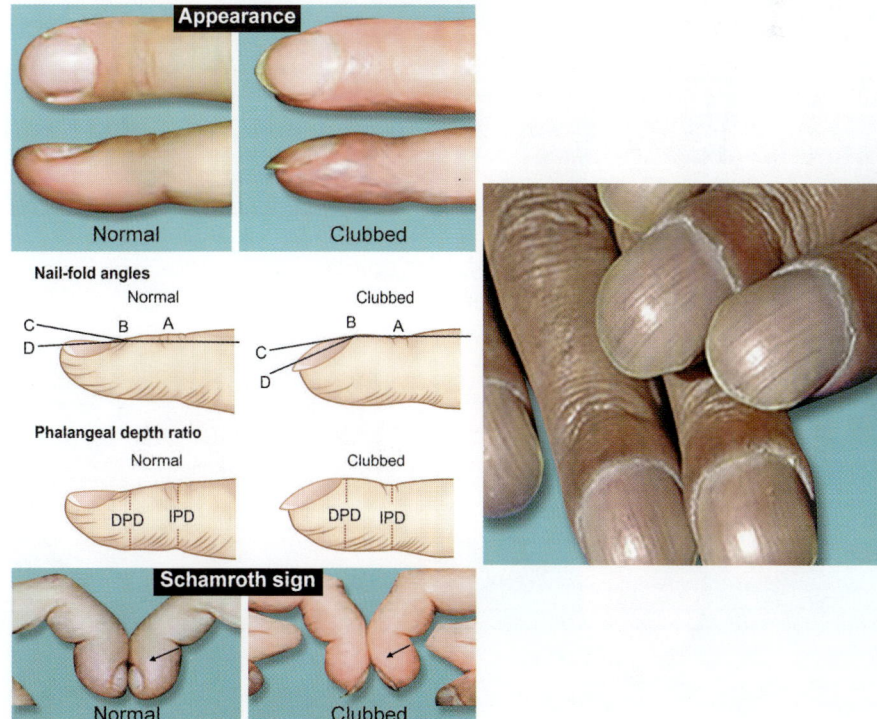

2. **Leukonychia**
   White nails as dot/lines due to lack of albumin.

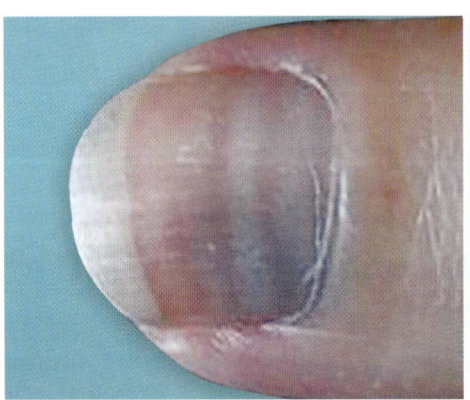
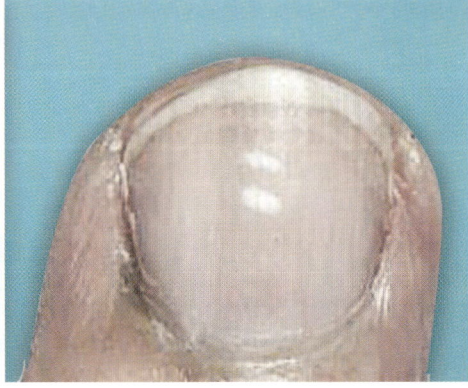

3. **Terry's nails**
   Ground glass appearance due to reduced vascularity and increased connective tissue.
   Causes: Liver disease, congestive heart failure (CHF), and kidney failure.

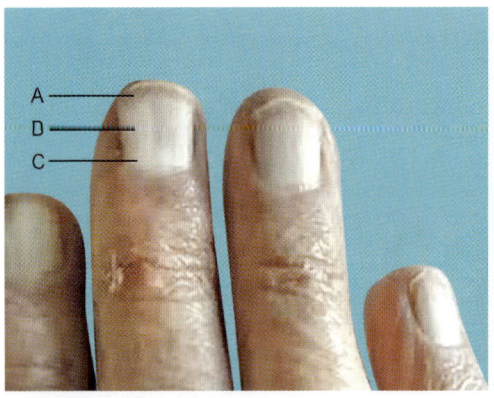
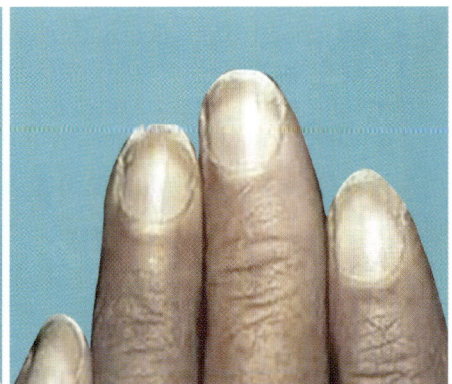

4. **Koilonychia**
   Spoon-shaped nails due to iron deficiency.

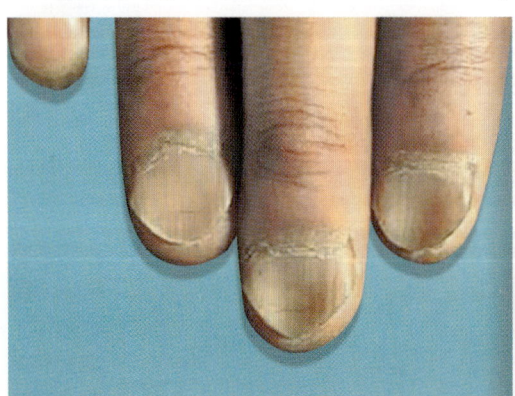
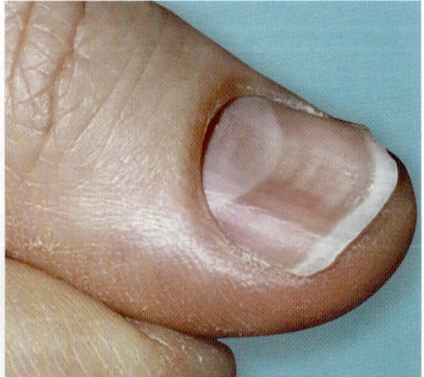

5. **Onycholysis**
   Nail destruction and separation from underlying skin.
   Causes: Palmer erythema, psoriasis, and fungal infection.

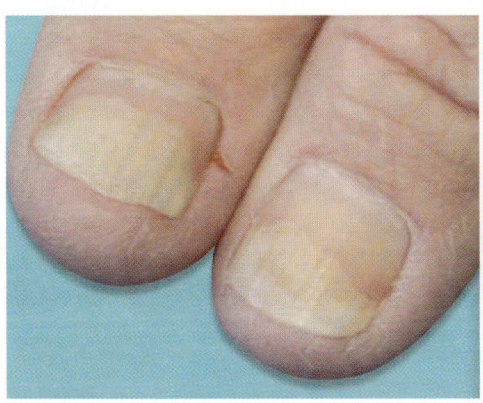
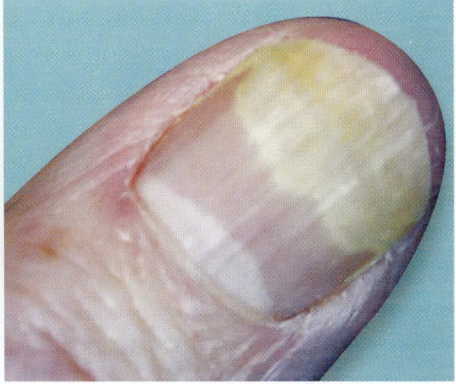

6. **Splinter hemorrhage**
   Punctate hemorrhage due to autoimmune diseases/vitamin C deficiency/vasculitis/lupus.

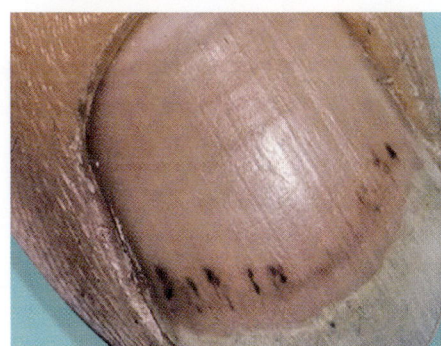
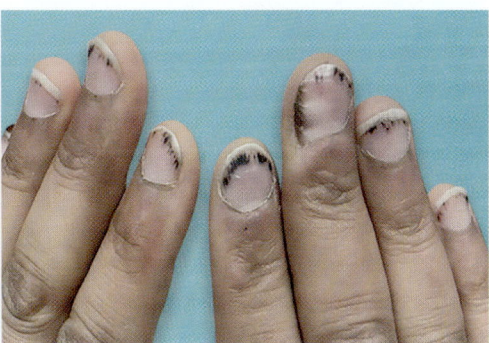

7. **Dupuytren's contracture**
   Connective tissue in palm thickens and restrict movement.
   Causes: Genetic, smoking, alcohol, chronic liver disease (CLD), and chronic phenytoin use.

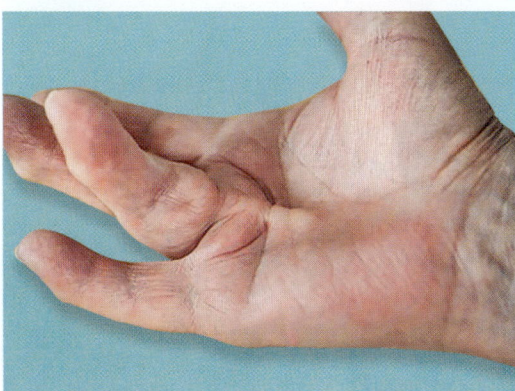
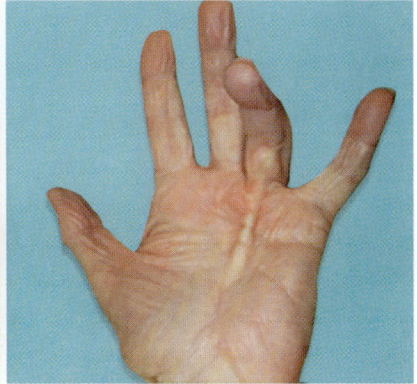

8. **Paronychia**
   Infection of tissue fold around the nail.

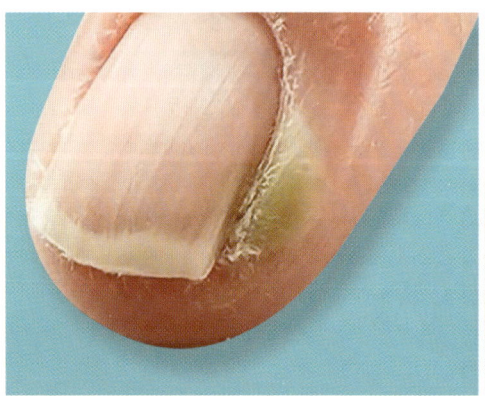
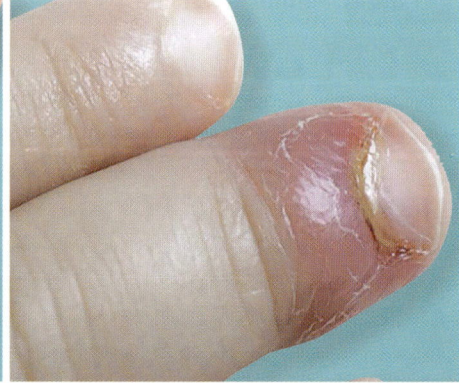

9. **Beau's lines**
   Causes: Any life-threatening condition, malnutrition, myocardial infarction, and infections such as mumps and measles.

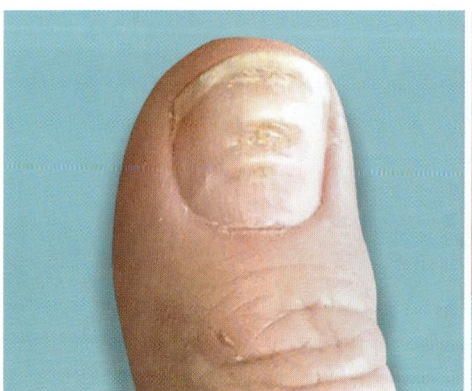
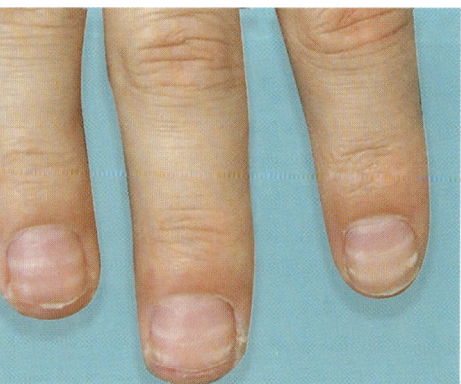

10. **Pitting nails**
    Causes: Psoriasis and joint inflammation.

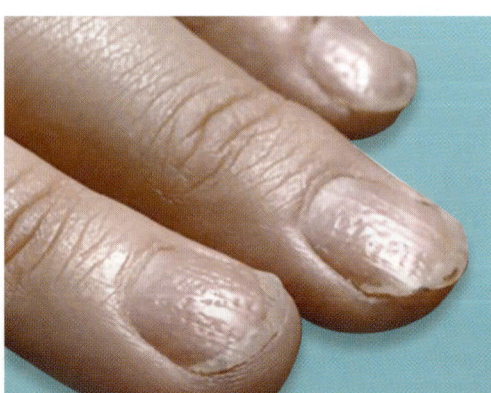
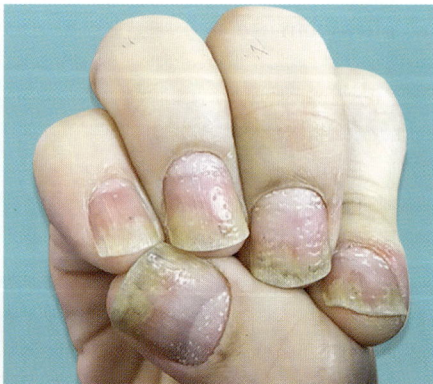

11. Sclerodactyly
Thickening of skin of digits of hands and feet.
Causes: Systemic scleroderma and autoimmune diseases.

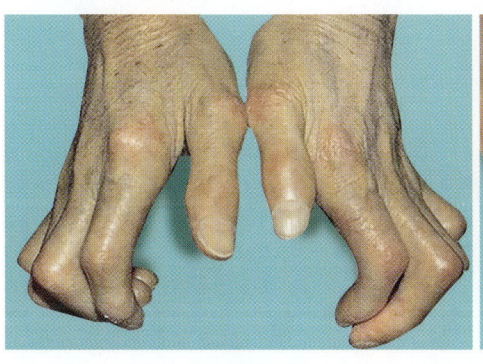
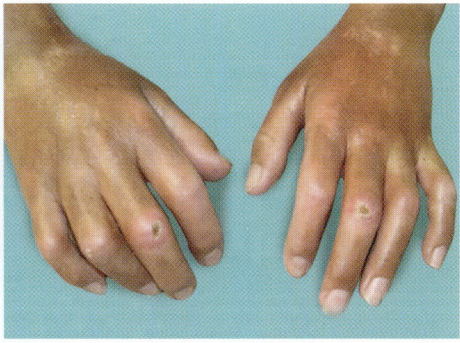

12. Involvement of terminal interphalangeal joint
Causes: Osteoarthritis and psoriasis.

13. Proximal interphalangeal joint
Causes: Osteoarthritis and rheumatoid arthritis.

14. Metacarpophalangeal joint
Cause: Rheumatoid arthritis.

15. Wasting of thenar compartment
Seen in amyotrophic lateral sclerosis, abductor pollicis, opponens pollicis, and opponens brevis.

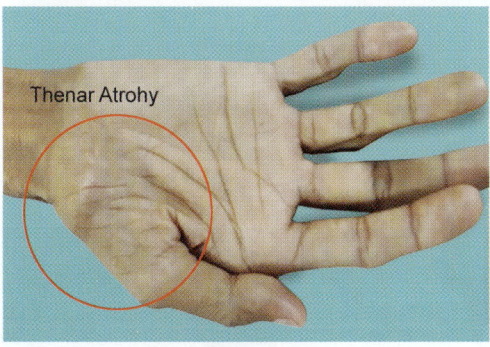
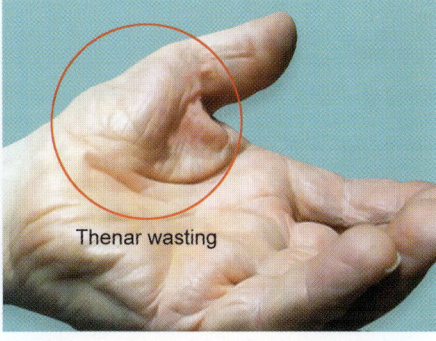

16. Carpal tunnel syndrome
Median nerve syndrome affected.

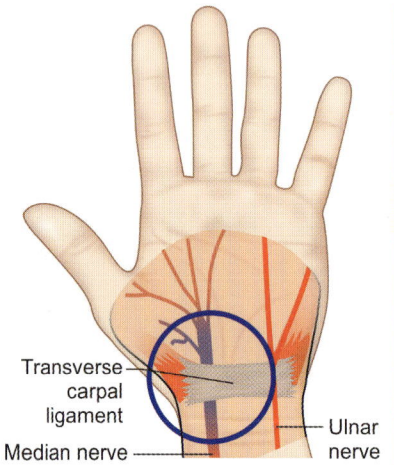
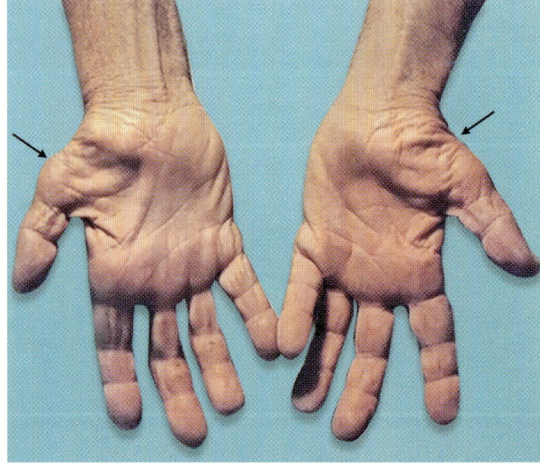

17. Rheumatoid nodules
Seen in rheumatoid arthritis.

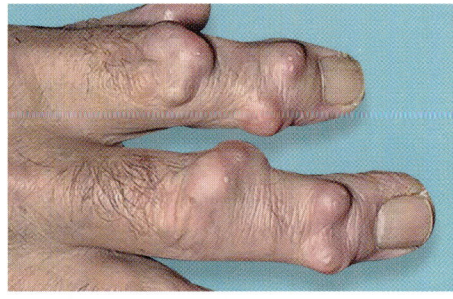
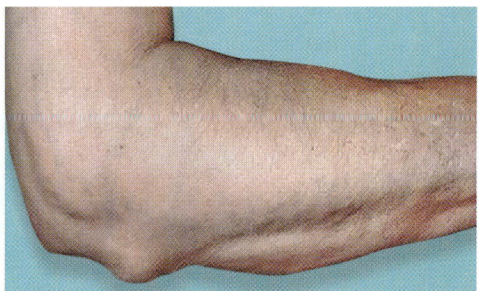

18. Tendon xanthomas
Cholesterol deposits in tendon due to hypercholesterolemia.

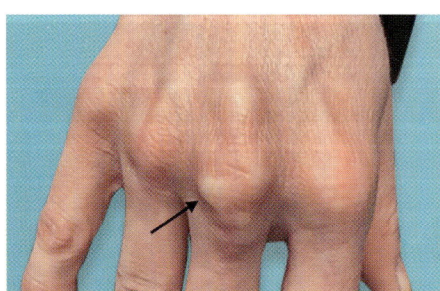
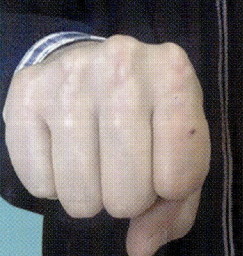
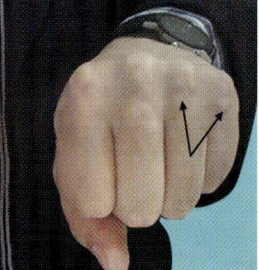

Hand Palmistry in Medicine 99

19. Wrist drop
Brachioradialis weakness due to radial nerve paralysis (Saturday nerve palsy).

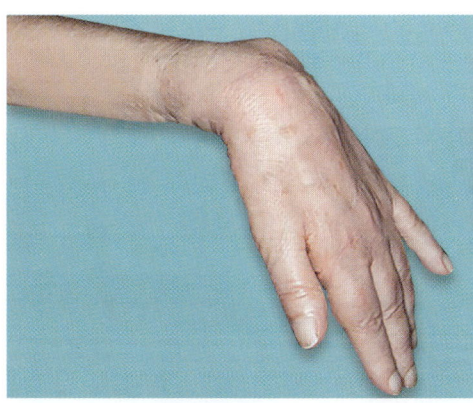
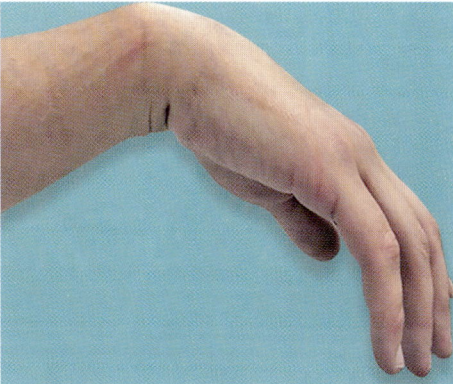

20. Darkening of creases/dark knuckles
- Addison's disease
- Acanthosis nigricans

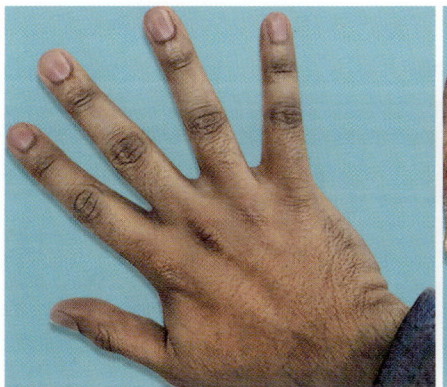
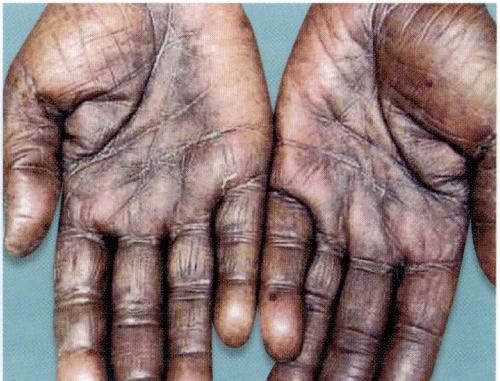

21. Senile keratosis
Skin ageing due to too much sun exposure.

22. Spade-like hands
Seen in acromegaly

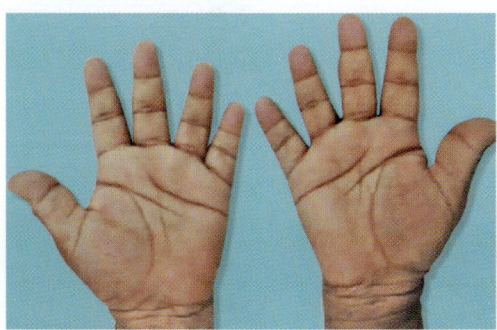
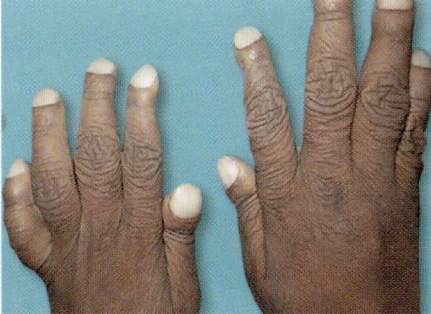

23. Apert syndrome

24. X-ray of terminal phalanges
    - Acro-osteolysis—scleroderma and psoriatic arthritis
    - Pencil-like terminal phalanges—hyperparathyroidism
    - Tufting of terminal phalanges—acromegaly

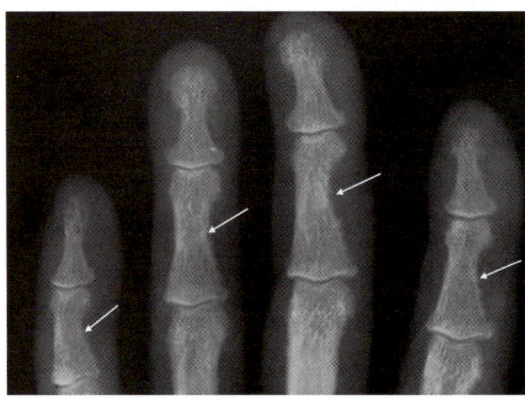
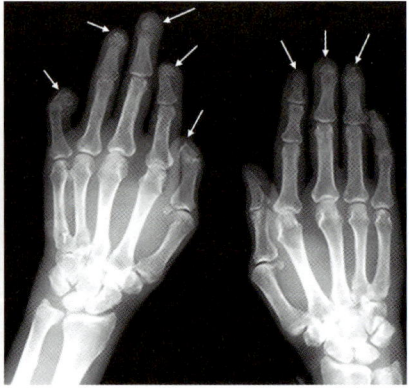

25. Cystic lesion of terminal phalanges
    Sarcoidosis, trauma, and benign conditions

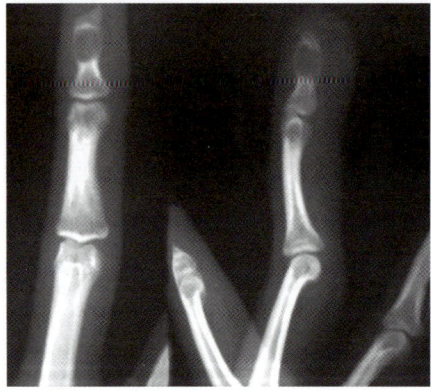
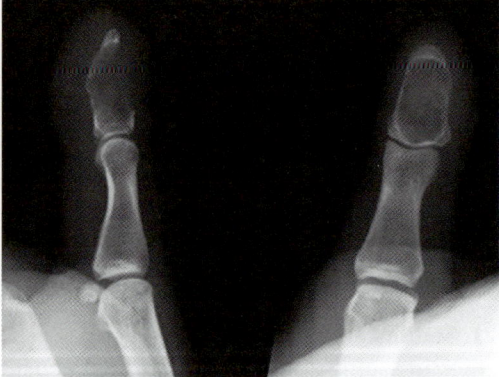

26. Subcutaneous calcification
    Infection, calcium metabolic disorder, scleroderma, genetic, and autoimmune

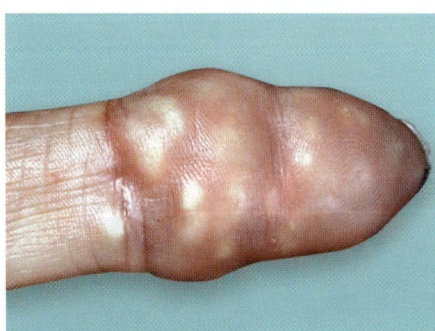
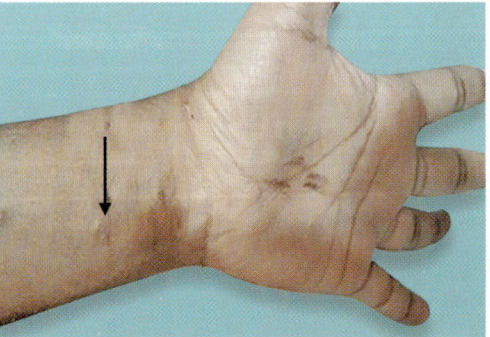

Hand Palmistry in Medicine

27. Osler's nodes
Painful
Causes: Bacterial endocarditis and immune complex deposition

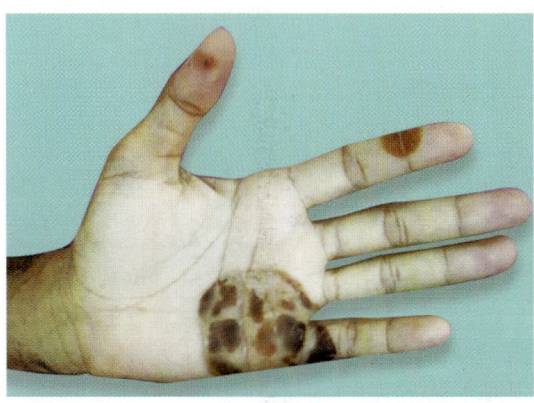
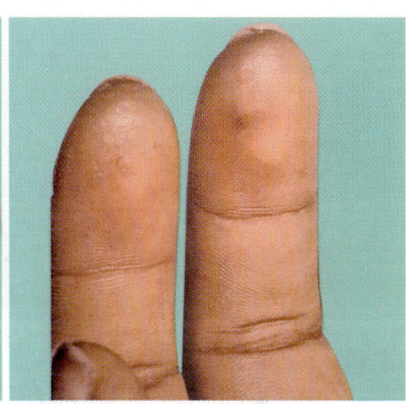

28. Raynaud's phenomenon
- Bluish discoloration
- Spasm of blood vessels due to cold or stress
- May be primary (idiopathic) or secondary

Causes: Lupus and scleroderma

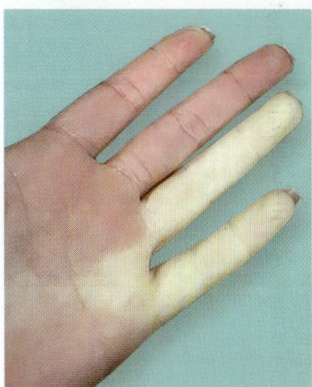
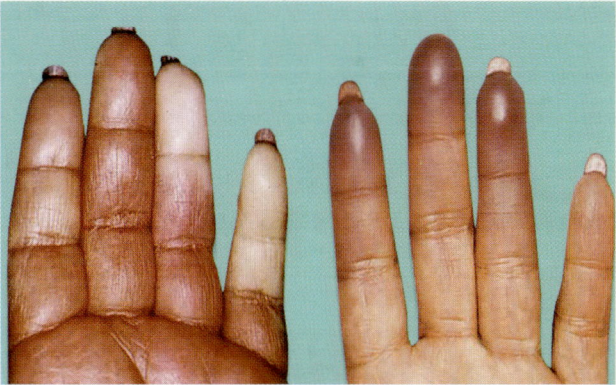

29. Lac phalanges
Sarcoidosis

30. Granuloma annulare
Diabetes, thyroid, and viral infection

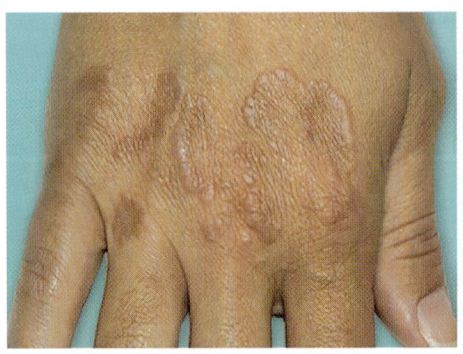
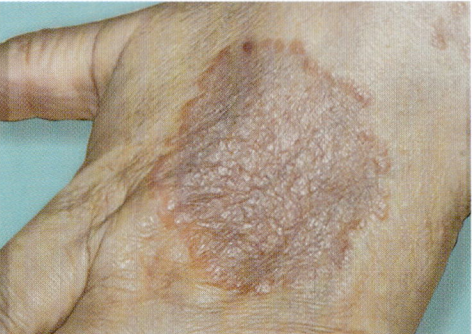

31. Lichen planus
- Inflammatory condition—itchy and purplish
- Hepatitis C

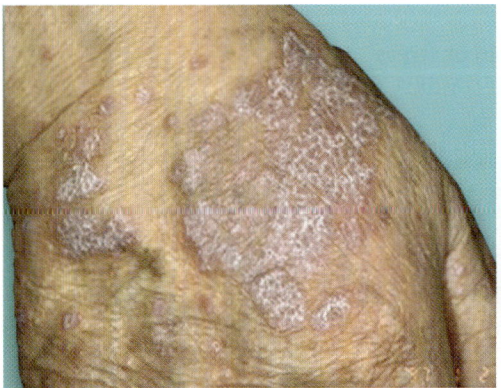
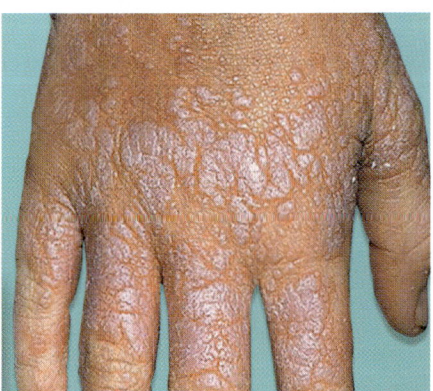

32. Tophi
Gout

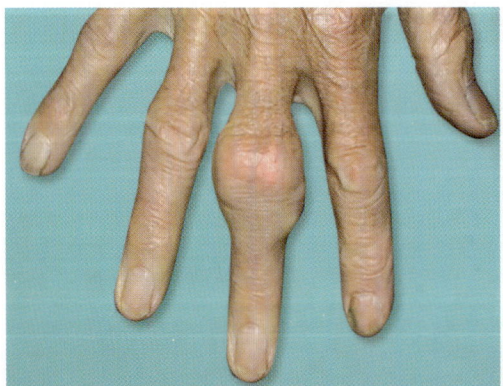
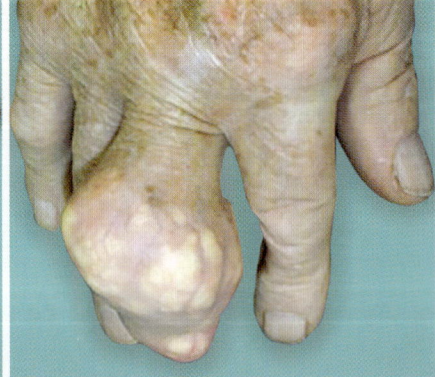

Hand Palmistry in Medicine

33. Marfan syndrome
Connective tissue disorder, muscles relax, and finger touches the dorsal part.

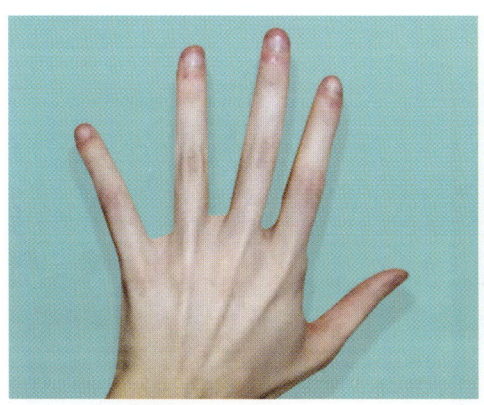
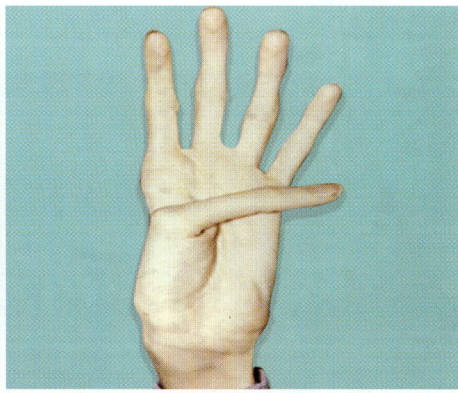

34. Absent radial artery

35. X-ray wrist
Rickets

36. Prayer's hand/diabetic hand syndrome
Diabetes

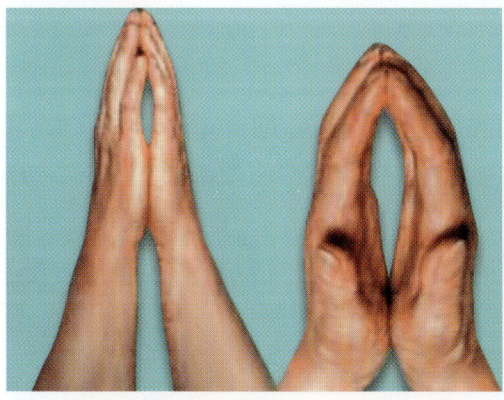
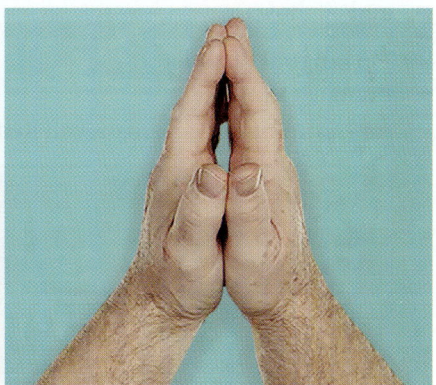

37. Secondary syphilis
Maculopapillary rashes on distal/dorsal part

38. Janeway lesion
- Nontender, small erythematous, hemorrhagic macular/nodular lesion on palms
- Seen in infective endocarditis

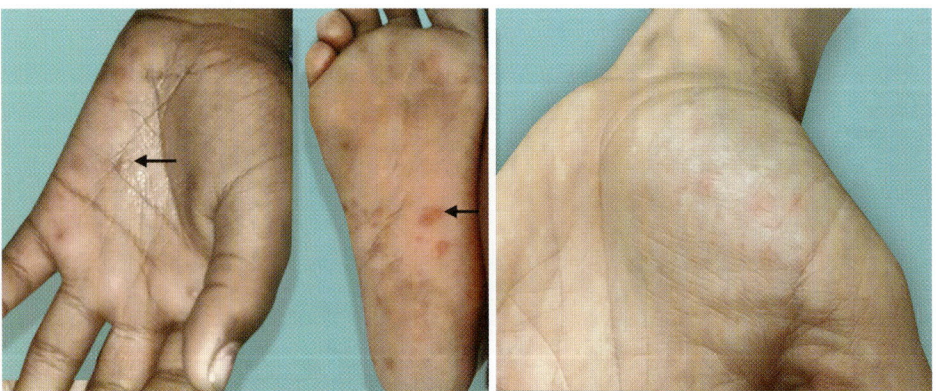

39. Flapping tremors/asterixis
- Loss of muscle tone or contraction
- Due to thalamus and motor cortex affect

Causes: Hepatic encephalopathy, Wilson's disease, hepatic failure, CO_2 narcosis, and cirrhosis.

40. Periungual fibroma
Benign lesion

Causes: Tuberous sclerosis/von Recklinghausen's disease

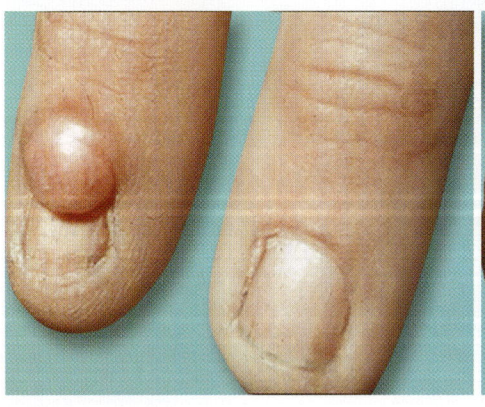
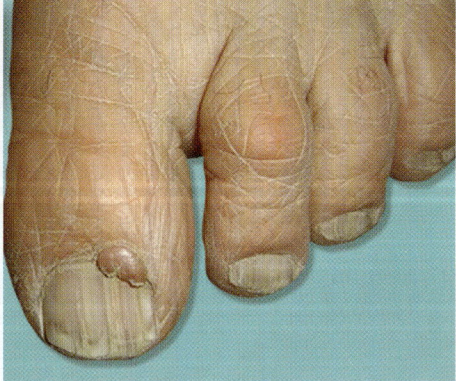

41. Fine tremor
Involuntary and rhythmic shaking

Cause: Hyperthyroidism

Hand Palmistry in Medicine

42. Cerebellar tremor
- Intentional tremors
- Slow, high amplitude, and mostly on extremities
- Due to stroke/tumor
- Perform finger nose test, heel-shin test

43. Pill-rolling tremor
Parkinson's disease

44. Trigger finger
- Finger stuck in bent position
- Due to inflammation within tendon sheath thereby reducing movement

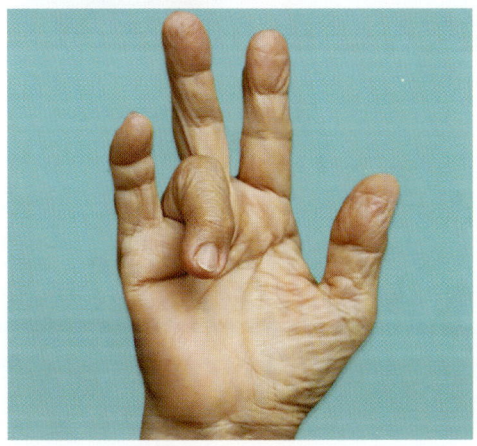
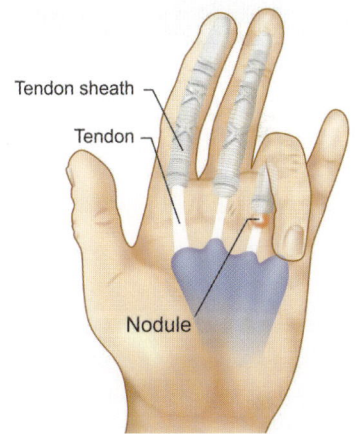

45. Tenosynovitis
- Direct tendon injury
- Inflammatory arthritis

46. Swan neck deformity
- Flexion of base of finger and extension of middle joint
- Due to rheumatoid arthritis

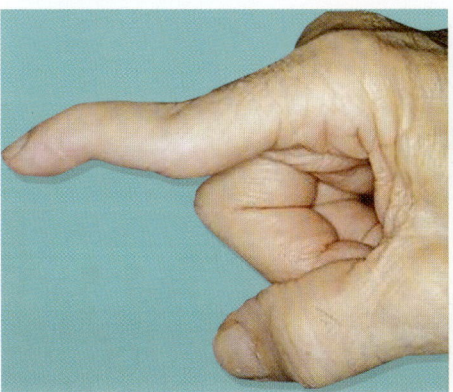
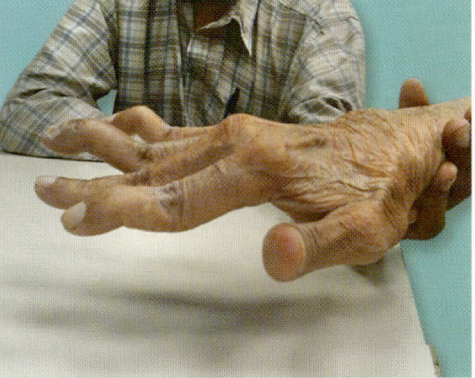

47. Boutonniere deformity

Injury to tendon that straightens the middle joint of finger.

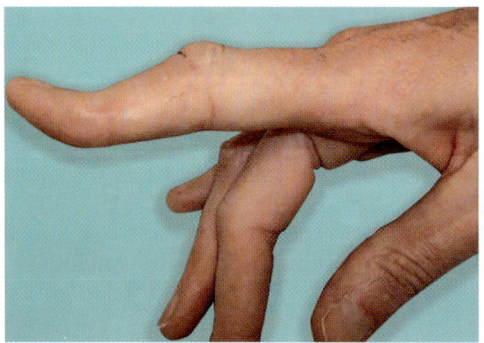 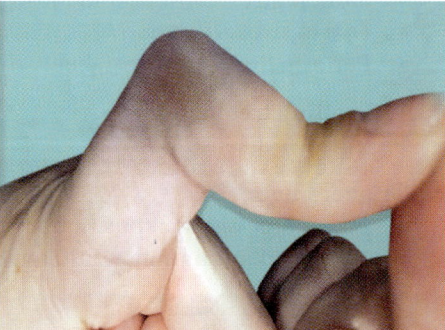

CHAPTER 7

General Physical Examination: A Window to Systemic Disease

Y Sathyanarayana Raju, Y Rahul, Y Sairam

■ INTRODUCTION

Physical examination is a systematic and structured approach to clinical diagnosis. General physical examination is carried out prior to detailed physical examination of each of the systems based on a well-structured sequence systematically looking for diagnostic clues. Based on the history obtained, the general physical examination not only provides clues to differential diagnosis related to the system(s) involved, it also facilitates identification of additional diagnostic clues as well.

The topic is exhaustive and a detailed narrative of general physical examination is beyond the scope of this chapter. Some physical signs on general physical examination are manifestations of certain diseases. However, presence of certain general physical examination findings gives a diagnostic clue to an underlying systemic disease. Rather than go about providing a list-of-lists of causes of "pallor, icterus, cyanosis, clubbing, koilonychia, lymphadenopathy, and edema (PICKLE)" which can be found in standard textbooks of clinical examination, this chapter focuses on providing an overview regarding the "clinical method" and diagnostic approach for looking for "clues suggestive of systemic disease" from general physical examination.

■ GENERAL PHYSICAL EXAMINATION CLUES SOME COMMONLY SEEN SYSTEMIC DISEASES

Diabetes Mellitus

Several general physical examination findings may indicate the presence of diabetes mellitus. These include vitiligo, necrobiosis lipoidica diabeticorum, diabetic dermopathy, scleredema diabeticorum (diffuse, waxy, and nonpitting induration of skin over back of neck and upper trunk), evidence of infections such as furuncle, carbuncle, balanoposthitis, intertrigo, vaginitis, *Candida* paronychia, and among others.

Internal Malignancy

The clinical presentation of internal malignancy is often atypical. While symptoms, signs related to a particular system involvement may point to the diagnosis on physical examination, some of the general physical examination findings may alert the physician to the possibility of an underlying internal malignancy. Some of these classical examples are listed below. Palmoplantar keratoderma (bronchogenic carcinoma), acanthosis nigricans (adenocarcinomas of the gastrointestinal tract), necrolytic migratory erythema (glucagonoma), pityriasis rotunda (hepatocellular carcinoma), migratory thrombophlebitis, also called *Trousseau's syndrome* or *thrombophlebitis migrans* (carcinoma pancreas), sign of Leser–Trelat (sudden eruption of intensely pruritic multiple seborrheic keratosis) (carcinoma stomach), digital clubbing, hypertrophic osteoarthropathy, and indicate the presence of internal malignancy.

Other general physical examination findings suggesting internal malignancy include—acrokeratosis paraneoplastica (Bazex syndrome) (squamous cell carcinoma of upper aerodigestive tract), Sweet syndrome (leukemias and lymphomas), necrobiotic xanthogranulomas, scleromyxedema (multiple myeloma), and among others.

Erythema gyratum repens is a paraneoplastic manifestation presenting as annular erythema with a distinctive figurate "wood-grain" appearance in patient with internal malignancy. Left supraclavicular node enlargement, (Virchow node), leading to a clinically palpable abdominal mass (Troisier sign) is a well-known general physical examination clinical sign of gastric cancer metastasis.

Gastrointestinal and Hepatic Disease

Bilateral parotid enlargement, spider naevi, palmar erythema, loss of secondary sexual characters, Dupuytren's contracture, asterixis, digital clubbing, and indicate the presence of chronic liver disease. Extraintestinal manifestations of inflammatory bowel disease (IBD) (ulcerative colitis and Crohn's disease) discovered on general physical examination such as erythema nodosum, pyoderma gangrenosum, episcleritis, scleritis, scleromalacia, digital clubbing, acrodermatitis enteropathica (ulcerative colitis), may sometimes clinch the diagnosis. Hepatitis C virus infection is associated with cutaneous manifestations such as cutaneous vasculitis (leucocytoclastic, urticarial, and cryoglobulinemic), lichen planus, and necrolytic acral erythema.

Chronic Kidney Disease

Presence of uremic frost, erythema papulatum uraemicum (over palms, soles, and forearm), nail changes (half-and-half nails and Mees' lines) on general physical examination, may point to chronic kidney disease (CKD).

Rheumatological and Connective Tissue Disorders

While there are several clues to rheumatological disorders, some commonly useful diagnostic clues include: Purpura (e.g., Henoch–Schönlein purpura) butterfly rash over the face, photosensitivity, noncicatricial alopecia, and oral ulcers indicate systemic lupus erythematosus (SLE). Heliotrope rash, Gottron's papules [papules with a violaceous hue seen at the dorsal-lateral interphalangeal (IP) and/or metacarpophalangeal (MCP) joints] are seen in dermatomyositis. Raynaud's phenomenon, livedo reticularis, erythromelalgia indicate the presence of underlying connective tissue disorders.

Cardiovascular

A prominent crease seen over the lobule of the pinna is considered a marker for coronary artery disease. Other general physical examination clues include: Erythema marginatum, subcutaneous nodules (acute rheumatic fever), Janeway lesions, Osler's nodes (infective endocarditis), ectopia lentis, arachnodactyly (Marfan's syndrome and aortic regurgitation), blue sclera, brittle bones (osteogenesis imperfecta and mitral valve prolapse), thumb with extra phalanx (Holt–Oram syndrome and atrial septal defect).

Endocrine Disorders

Classical appearances of Cushing's syndrome (moon face, buffalo hump, and hirsutism) are easily recognized. Generalized hyperpigmentation of the skin is evident in hemochromatosis, endocrine disorders such as Addison's disease and Cushing's syndrome. Macroglossia (myxedema), digital clubbing, thyroid acropachy (Graves' disease) are also valuable clues.

Neurological Disorders

Café-au-lait spots (significant when six or more of these hypopigmented macules, each >1.5 cm in diameter are present) point to neurofibromatosis. Adenoma sebaceum, shagreen patch, and ash leaf macules are seen in tuberous sclerosis. The presence of a tuft of hair or a lipoma over the lower lumbar region may indicate the presence of a spina bifida. While peripheral nerve thickening can be a manifestation of hereditary sensorimotor neuropathies, thickened peripheral nerves on general physical examination may indicate the presence of Hansen's disease, sarcoidosis as well.

Human Immunodeficiency Virus/Acquired Immunodeficiency Syndrome

Hairy leucoplakia and Kaposi's sarcoma are practically diagnostic of human immunodeficiency virus (HIV) infection/acquired immunodeficiency syndrome (AIDS). Other commonly seen manifestations in HIV/AIDS include recurrent herpes zoster and oral candidiasis.

▮ SKIN SIGNS OF SYSTEMIC DISORDERS

Some skin signs indicate the presence of systemic disease. These include: Erythema nodosum (sarcoidosis, tuberculosis, connective tissue diseases, poststreptococcal infection, and drugs), rheumatoid arthritis, dermatitis herpetiformis (gluten-sensitive enteropathy), dermatitis artefacta (personality disorders), generalized purpura [immune thrombocytopenic purpura (previously called idiopathic thrombocytopenic purpura)], telangiectasias (Osler–Rendu–Weber syndrome), tendon xanthomas (hyperlipidemias), cicatricial alopecia (discoid lupus erythematosus and sarcoidosis), and telogen effluvium (typhoid fever).

OTHERS

Generalized absence of skin pigmentation seen in albinism could point to Chédiak-Higashi syndrome or phenylketonuria. Circumscribed hypopigmented patches are seen in Hansen's disease (where they may be anesthetic), tinea versi color. Patchy hyperpigmentation as in patchy hyper pigmentation in sunexposed areas could point to pellagra. Knuckle pigmentation in a patient with anemia can point to megaloblastic anemia.

CONCLUSION

General physical examination provides a valuable window to underlying systemic diseases. The diagnostic clues obtained on general physical examination not only prompt physicians as to what to look for (classic manifestations of disease), they also facilitate the physician to look further and formulate a diagnostic workup to exclude underlying systemic disease. Further, as in the case of general physical examination findings in internal malignancy, these findings also serve a reminder to physicians so that underlying systemic disease is not missed out.

SUGGESTED READINGS

1. Lee A. Skin manifestations of systemic disease. Aust Fam Physician. 2009;38(7):498-505.
2. Cahill J, Sinclair R. Cutaneous manifestations of systemic disease. Aust Fam Physician. 2005;34(5):335-40.
3. Trost LB, McDonnell JK. Important cutaneous manifestations of inflammatory bowel disease. Postgrad Med J. 2005;81(959):580-5.
4. Pagani K, Lukac D, Bhukhan A, et al. Cutaneous manifestations of inflammatory bowel disease: A basic overview. Am J Clin Dermatol. 2022;23(4):481-97.
5. Silva JA, Mesquita Kde C, Igreja AC, et al. Paraneoplastic cutaneous manifestations: concepts and updates. An Bras Dermatol. 2013;88(1):9-22.
6. Sontheimer RD. Skin manifestations of systemic autoimmune connective tissue disease: diagnostics and therapeutics. Best Pract Res Clin Rheumatol. 2004;18(3):429-62.

CHAPTER 8

Superior Vena Cava Syndrome: A Forgotten Clinical Entity

Madhuchanda Kar, Amit K Adhikary

■ INTRODUCTION

Superior vena cava (SVC) syndrome is a collection of clinical signs and symptoms resulting from either partial or complete obstruction of blood flow through the SVC. This obstruction is most commonly a result of thrombus formation or tumor infiltration of the vessel wall or due to external compression or constriction. Clinically it is not difficult to pick up by a trained eye. A careful clinician can notice the localization of edema and congestion in the face, trunk, and neck region, and the distinct sparing of the lower limbs and arrive at the diagnosis of SVC obstruction (SVCO). Earlier the signs are picked up by a doctor; the better is the prognosis for the patient. Thrombosis of the SVC due to infiltration by a malignant tumor is the most common cause of this syndrome so any clinical suspicion must set the ball rolling for a rapid radiological and pathological diagnosis, thus giving the patient a chance for disease free survival with improved quality of life.

■ HISTORY

William Hunter a Scottish physicist first described SVCS in a 39-year-old man who died of syphilitic aortitis in 1757. For two centuries—aortic aneurysms, syphilitic aortitis, and chronic tuberculosis (TB) mediastinitis were the predominant etiologic factors of SVC syndrome. Malignancy became the most common cause (90%) by the 1980s. Thrombosis has raised the incidence of SVCs due to the use of intravascular devices like catheters and pacemakers. Benign causes now account for only 10–20% of SVCs.

■ ANATOMY

The superior vena cava is formed by the junction of the left and right brachiocephalic veins and returns blood from the head, neck, upper limbs, and trunk back to the heart. The SVC is 6–8 cm long and 1.5–2 cm wide and extends between the first and third costal cartilages. Azygos vein joins SVC from the right side, at its mid length, above the right bronchus just before entering the pericardial sac. SVC is surrounded by rigid structures (i.e., mediastinum, sternum, right main bronchus, and lymph nodes). Being thin walled it is easily compressible. As obstruction develops, several venous collaterals are established as alternate pathways for venous return to the right atrium.

Four distinctive collateral systems have been identified. They were first described in 1949 by McIntire and Sykes.
- Azygos venous system is the only direct collateral path into the SVC.
- Internal thoracic vein is the connection between SVC and inferior vena cava (IVC) via epigastric and iliac veins.
- Vertebral veins with intercostals, lumbar, and sacral veins represent the posterior network between SVC and IVC.
- External thoracic vein system is the most superficial and it is represented by axillary, lateral thoracic and superficial epigastric veins.

PATHOPHYSIOLOGY

Primary pathophysiologic event is the intraluminal or extraluminal obstruction of SVC. Extraluminal obstruction is often caused by malignant tumors such as lung cancer, lymphoma, sarcoma, metastatic cancer, leiomyosarcoma, and plasmacytoma. Mediastinitis, cardiovascular, or pulmonary trauma and some benign tumors are the nonmalignant causes of extraluminal obstruction. Intraluminal causes of obstruction include long-term indwelling catheters (chemoport and Hickman catheter) or pacemaker/defibrillators leads, hypercoagulable states and infections such as tuberculosis and syphilis. Symptoms and signs of SVC obstruction depend upon the rate at which obstruction of the SVC occurs in relation to the recruitment of venous collaterals. In malignant disease the symptoms develop in weeks to months as the rapidly growing tumor does not allow adequate time for development of collaterals. In contrast, fibrosing mediastinitis due to an infection like histoplasmosis may not become symptomatic even after passing of few years. Narrowing of the lumen of the nasal passages, pharynx, and larynx due to the edema give rise to symptoms such as dyspnea, stridor, cough, hoarseness, and dysphagia. In extreme cases cerebral edema occurs, which results in cerebral ischemia, herniation and can even lead to death.

CLASSIFICATION OF SUPERIOR VENA CAVA SYNDROME

There are three main classifications which are as follows:
1. Doty and Standford's classification (anatomical)
2. Yu's classification (clinical)
3. Bigsby's classification (operative risk)

Anatomic Classification

It is to three levels of obstruction are as follows:
1. Obstruction of the upper SVC, proximal to the azygos entry point.
2. Obstruction with azygos involvement.
3. Obstruction of the lower SVC, distal to the azygos entry point.

Clinical Classification

It is based on the severity of symptoms ranging from early asymptomatic cases with only radiological evidence to the extreme end of death from progressive cerebral and laryngeal edema.

Grade	Category	Incidence	Definition
0	Asymptomatic	10%	Radiographic SVC obstruction in the absence of symptoms.
1	Mild	25%	Edema in head or neck (vascular distention), cyanosis, and plethora
2	Moderate	50%	Edema in head or neck with functional impairment (mild dysphagia, cough, mild or moderate impairment of head, jaw or eyelid movements, and visual disturbances)
3	Severe	10%	Mild or moderate cerebral edema (headache and dizziness) or mild/moderate laryngeal edema or diminished cardiac reserve (syncope after bending)
4	Life-threatening	5%	Significant cerebral edema or significant laryngeal edema or significant hemodynamic compromise
5	Fatal	<1%	Death

■ CLINICAL FEATURES OF SUPERIOR VENA CAVA SYNDROME

Common symptoms include facial swelling, shortness of breath, chest pain, cough, and headache. Other symptoms such as dizziness, tinnitus, bursting of head sensation, nasal congestion have also been reported. Very often the first complain among affected men has been an increase in collar size of shirts.

Signs in SVC syndrome are edema and plethora of face, neck, arm, and anterior chest wall (**Fig. 1A**). Neck vein distension (nonpulsatile), venous collaterals over anterior chest wall, cyanosis, conjunctival congestion, and proptosis. Papilledema needs to be searched in patient's complaining of visual disturbances. Esophageal varices should be ruled out by endoscopy. Pleural and pericardial effusions are also common findings. Pemberton's sign is one of the earliest signs that can be elicited even in subclinical asymptomatic patients.

■ ETIOLOGY AND WORKUP

Etiology of SVC syndrome includes malignant causes (90%) such as lung cancer, lymphoma, thymoma, metastatic cancers, and germ cell tumors. Benign tumor, aortic aneurysm, goiter, thrombosis, Behcet's syndrome, and fibrosing mediastinitis (due to tuberculosis, histoplasmosis, blastomycosis, aspergillosis, or filariasis) are some of the nonmalignant causes of SVCO. Invasive procedures such as central venous catheterization and pacemaker implantation, parenteral nutrition lines, central venous line for chemotherapy and dialysis catheter placement are some of the emerging causes. Since 20th century leading cause for SVCO is bronchogenic carcinoma. Squamous and small cell cancer of lung accounts for >85% of all the

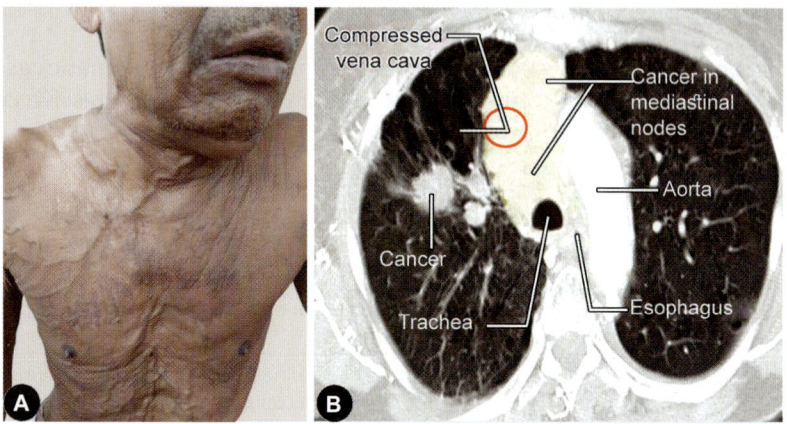

FIG. 1: (A) Engorged neck veins with multiple collaterals in anterior chest wall, axillary, and epigastric region; (B) CT scan – recurrent small cell carcinoma with superior vena cava syndrome

SVCO cases. Non-Hodgkin's Lymphoma, metastatic cancers from breast, germ cell tumors, thymoma, mesothelioma, and primary angiosarcoma also form a major chunk of the remaining cases. Rarely diffuse adenopathy in cystic fibrosis, Castleman's disease and Hemophagocytic lymphohistiocytosis can present with SVCO.

Superior vena cava syndrome is the presenting feature in as many as 4% of all lung cancer and 12% of small cell carcinoma of lungs. As many as 21% of all mediastinal B cell lymphomas present with features of SVCO. This data obtained over years of observation has changed the approach in management. While previously all cases of SVCO were treated as oncologic emergencies and managed with palliative radiotherapy, nowadays the histopathological diagnosis prior to initiation of radio/chemotherapy is prioritized.

Differential diagnosis of SVC syndrome includes congestive heart failure, cor pulmonale, Cushing's syndrome, cardiac tamponade, mediastinitis, thoracic aortic aneurysm, and tuberculosis.

Diagnosis of the etiology often needs evaluation by chest radiograph, duplex ultrasound, chest computed tomography (CT) scan, venogram, and sometimes radionuclide studies.

Mediastinal mass or widening, hilar lymphadenopathy and pleural effusions are the most common chest radiographic findings in SVCOs, however, it is worth remembering that a normal chest X-ray does not exclude SVCO.

Contrast enhanced computerized tomography (CECT) **(Fig. 1B)** thorax is the most useful tool in the evaluation of the mediastinal syndromes as they help to assess the level of obstruction and differentiate between thrombosis and tumor. It also helps to differentiate between compression and infiltration. Contrast flow can also help to assess the extent of collateral networks.

Venogram is the most conclusive test. It not only defines the SVC obstruction and collaterals, it also identifies the thrombus, extent and degree of obstruction and patency of vessels.

MANAGEMENT OF SUPERIOR VENA CAVA OBSTRUCTION

Superior vena cava syndrome always warrants treatment by an interdisciplinary team. Treatment is guided by severity of symptoms, etiology, and prognosis. Treatment goal is to relieve symptoms and attempt cure of the primary process. Supportive therapy, chemotherapy, radiotherapy, surgery, and interventional procedure, e.g., stenting are the available modalities. Older concept was that SVCO is an oncologic emergency as it can cause cerebral venous thrombosis, so very high dose radiotherapy of 3,000–4,000 rads for 4 days was the standard practice. Nowadays, tissue diagnosis is given due importance before starting cytotoxic or radiation therapy as these can distort the histopathological findings.

Supportive treatment consists of upright positioning with oxygen by mask. Injection dexamethasone (8–16 mg daily) and low molecular weight heparin for proven thrombus. Diuretics have also used as an effective treatment for the edema. A general rule is to avoid injections in peripheral veins of upper limbs.

Radiotherapy is associated with improvement of signs and symptoms in most patients, but majority patients have no measurable increase in vena cava blood flow. Development of collaterals probably contributes to clinical improvement in some patients. Overall, 50–70% patients achieve symptomatic improvement within 2 weeks.

Chemotherapy is targeted against the underlying pathological diagnosis. A Cochrane systematic review by Rowell and Gleeson in 2001 concluded that chemotherapy and radiotherapy were equally effective at relieving SVCO secondary to lung cancer, whereas stent insertion provided higher rates of response at least more rapidly. Platinum based chemotherapy and concurrent radiotherapy is the standard treatment, if performance status is good, and disease is localized to the thorax. Relief of symptoms is generally seen by 7 days and complete resolution occurs in 14 days. The syndrome recurs in up to 25% of patients. Chemotherapy is the first line of management in lymphomas. Radiotherapy is indicated after completion of chemotherapy in large cell lymphoblastic lymphoma if size of the mediastinal mass is >10 cm, as in these cases the chances of recurrence is very high.

Open surgical repair through bypass grafting with spiral saphenous vein, femoral vein, polytetrafluoroethylene (PTFE) graft, or Dacron graft have traditionally been considered to overcome SVC obstruction. However, this is now reserved only for cases in which recanalization through endovascular repair is either not possible or has previously failed. Self-expanding, intravascular stents often offer relief within 24–48 hours. Z-stent, wall stent, Palmaz stent are some of the commonly used stents. Magnetic resonance imaging (MRI) compatible nickel–titanium (Nitinol) alloy metallic stent is popular nowadays. Complications occur in 3–7% of stenting procedure. Early complications include Infection, pulmonary embolism, stent migration, hematoma at the insertion site, bleeding and rarely, perforation or rupture of the SVC. Late complications are bleeding (1–14%), death (1–2%) from anticoagulation and stent failure with reocclusion.

Iatrogenic SVCS are managed by thrombolysis with streptokinase or urokinase followed by anticoagulants (heparin/oral anticoagulants). Removal of the catheter is an option and should be combined with anticoagulation to prevent embolization.

OUTCOME

The prognosis of patients with SVCS depends on the cause. For patients with a benign cause of SVCS, the life expectancy is not changed, but for malignant cases, there is a significant drop in survival. Sudden death can occur in patients who develop features of cerebral or laryngeal edema. Patients with SVCS due to lung cancer usually live <24 months. For those who do not respond to radiation treatment, the survival is dismal, usually <1 year in most of the cases.

CONCLUSION

SVCO is not a forgotten clinical entity but is still observed in our day to day clinical practice. Physicians need to be aware of this clinical entity and intervene as early as possible for the best outcome.

SUGGESTED READINGS

1. Seligson T, Surowiec SM. Superior Vena Cava Syndrome. In: StatPearls [Internet]. Treasure Island (FL): StatPearls Publishing; 2022.
2. MedlinePlus. (2022). SVC obstruction. [online] Available from https://medlineplus.gov/ency/article/001097.htm [Last accessed October, 2022].
3. Rice TW, Rodriguez RM, Light RW. The superior vena cava syndrome: clinical characteristics and evolving etiology. Medicine (Baltimore). 2006;85(1):37-42.
4. Cheng S. Superior vena cava syndrome: a contemporary review of a historic disease. Cardiol Rev. 2009;17(1):16-23.
5. Kent MS, Port JL. Superior Vena Cava Syndrome. In: Chang AE, Ganz PA, Hayes DF, et al (Eds). Oncology: An Evidence-based Approach. Germany: Springer Science & Business Media; 2007. pp. 1291-9.
6. Wilson LD, Detterbeck FC, Yahalom J. Clinical practice. Superior vena cava syndrome with malignant causes. N Engl J Med. 2007;356(18):1862-9.
7. Gibson CM, Villarreal FM. (2019). Superior vena cava syndrome pathophysiology. [online] Available from https://www.wikidoc.org/index.php/Superior_vena_cava_syndrome_pathophysiology [Last accessed October, 2022].
8. Lepper M, Ott SR, Hoppe H, et al. Superior Vena Cava Syndrome in Thoracic Malignancies. Respiratory Care. 2011;56(5):653-66.
9. Cohen R, Mena D, Carbajal-Mendoza R, et al. Superior vena cava syndrome: A medical emergency? Int J Angiol. 2008 Spring;17(1):43-6.
10. Kim HJ, Kim HS, Chung SH. CT diagnosis of superior vena cava syndrome: importance of collateral vessels. AJR Am J Roentgenol. 1993;161(3):539-42.
11. Yu JB, Wilson LD, Detterbeck FC. Superior vena cava syndrome--a proposed classification system and algorithm for management. J Thorac Oncol. 2008;3(8):811-4.
12. Yim CD, Sane SS, Bjarnason H. Superior vena cava stenting. Radiol Clin North Am. 2000;38(2):409-24.
13. Kalra M, Sen I, Gloviczki P. Endovenous and Operative Treatment of Superior Vena Cava Syndrome. Surg Clin North Am. 2018;98(2):321-35.
14. Baker GL, Barnes HJ. Superior vena cava syndrome: etiology, diagnosis, and treatment. Am J Crit Care. 1992;1(1):54-64.

CHAPTER 9

Tongue is a Mirror of Systemic Diseases

Smarajit Banik, Shankar Dutta

■ INTRODUCTION

Tongue is a vital and often neglected organ during clinical examination. Although in the past, examination of the tongue used to hold a major part in general examination of the patient such that many adult patients reflexly used to stick out their tongues as soon as the examiner displays a flashlight or tongue blade.
This discussion refers to examination of the anterior two-thirds of the tongue visible on routine examination.
- Color: The oral tongue is moist and pink-red on dorsal and ventral surfaces. The ventral surface may have some visible vasculature.
- Texture: Filiform, fungiform, and circumvallate papillae give a rough texture to the dorsal surface. There is neither localized nor diffuse discoloration or ulceration. There is normally a very thin "coat."
- Size: The tongue should fit comfortably within the mouth with the tip against lower incisors.
- Apart from local diseases of the tongue and buccal mucosa, several systemic diseases may manifest as changes in the tongue.

■ SMOOTH TONGUE

Tongue in pernicious anemia is beefy-red, sore, and smooth with papillary atrophy **(Fig. 1)**. The tongue appears shiny, smooth with shallow, reddened ulcers flanked by desquamating tissue.

Atrophy may be associated with xerostomia, iron-deficiency anemia, and pellagra as well.

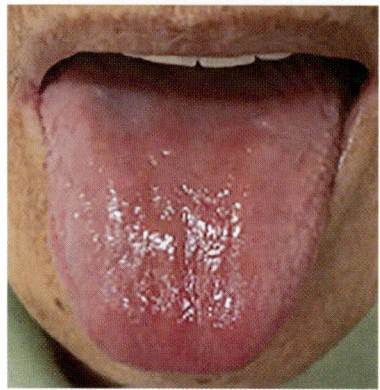 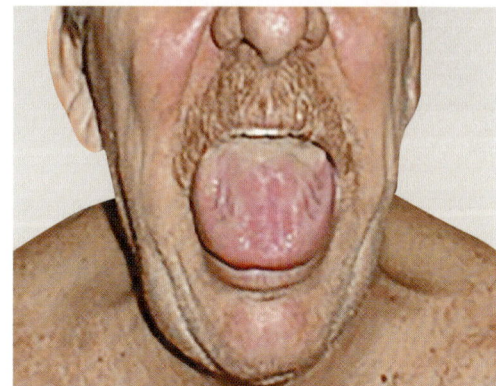

FIG. 1: Red beefy tongue in pernicious anemia. **FIG. 2:** Macroglossia in acromegaly patient.

■ MICROGLOSSIA

Microglossia may result from pseudobulbar palsy where is damage to bilateral upper motor neurons of the corticobulbar tracts that innervate the tongue. The presentation is a small stiff tongue often called as "nut in an open shell" tongue lying in the floor of the mouth, its surface little altered, but almost incapable of protrusion and with gross disturbance of speech. The jaw jerk will be exaggerated.

In newborns, there may be an apparent microglossia due to a congenitally short frenulum.

■ MACROGLOSSIA

Macroglossia is enlarged tongue with marks of teeth indentation that may be seen in:
- As a part of a syndrome like Down syndrome, Simpson–Golabi–Behmel syndrome or Beckwith–Weidemann syndrome
- Tumor as hemangioma or lymphangioma
- Metabolic disease as primary amyloidosis
- Endocrine disease as acromegaly or cretinism **(Fig. 2)**
- May occur when all teeth are removed.

■ FISSURED TONGUE

Also often this condition is described as "scrotal tongue". Dorsal surface and sides of tongue covered by painless shallow or deep fissures that may collect debris and become irritated. It is mostly a benign condition **(Fig. 3)**.

■ GEOGRAPHIC TONGUE

Asymptomatic inflammatory condition of tongue with rapid loss and regrowth of filiform papillae leading to appearance of denuded red patches "wandering" across surface. It is a benign condition and often called as "benign migratory glossitis" **(Fig. 4)**.

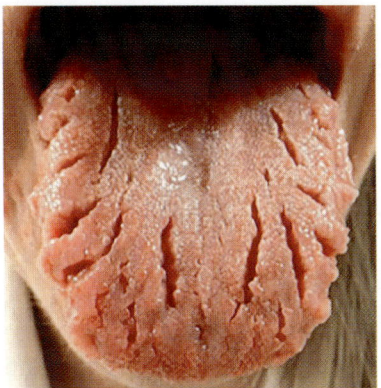

FIG. 3: Fissured tongue.

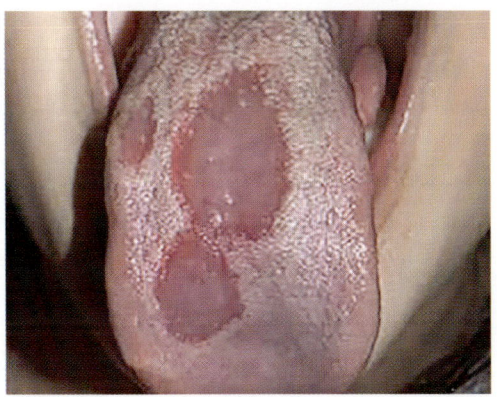

FIG. 4: Geographic tongue.

HAIRY TONGUE

Elongation of filiform papillae of medial dorsal surface area due to failure of keratin layer of papillae to desquamate normally; brownish-black coloration may be due to staining by tobacco, food, or chromogenic organisms.

White hairs along the sides of the tongue is the classic appearance of oral hairy leukoplakia as a result of EBV infection in HIV positive patients. It responds to acyclovir, but recurs.

ULCERS

Aphthous ulcers are frequently encountered painful form of ulcers which usually heal spontaneously but may be distressing if it is recurrent and often associated with Crohn disease, Behçetsyndrome, and pemphigus or herpes simplex virus.

A single nonhealing, painful, and erythematous ulcer may be suggestive of malignancy particularly if the patient has history of tobacco and/or alcohol addiction. There may be associated dysphagia or dysarthria. Biopsy or Fnac can guide toward diagnosis.

CANDIDIASIS

Oral candidiasis or oral thrush is a common finding and it occurs as a result of *Candida albicans*. It is typically seen in immunocompromised individuals as HIV patients, diabetics, hematological malignancy, chronic alcoholics, long course systemic steroid use, etc.

The patients present with painless, creamy white, curd-like plaques on the tongue and oropharynx which can be easily scraped off leaving behind a raw bleeding surface.

The diagnosis is made by direct examination of a scraping for pseudohyphal elements. Culturing is of no diagnostic value, as patients with HIV infection may have a positive throat culture for *Candida* in the absence of thrush.

Treatment includes topical and/or systemic antifungal agents.

LICHEN PLANUS

Striae such as white plaques and purplish papules may be asymptomatic, sore, or painful. It has a protracted course and responds to topical glucocorticoids **(Fig. 5)**.

CORROSIONS

Tongue will show corrosion after ingestion of caustic fluids as acids, paraquat **(Fig. 6)**, etc.

ABNORMAL MOVEMENTS

- A coarse, trombone-like tremor on protrusion may be seen in neurosyphilis and some cases of Parkinsonism.
- An up and down flapping movement with alternate protrusion and retraction is common in chorea.
- Dystonic movements of the tongue follow high and prolonged doses of chlorpromazine derivatives.
- Fine tremor may be seen in thyrotoxicosis.
- Fasciculations are seen in motor neuron disease affecting the hypoglossal nerve nucleus.

HEMATOLOGICAL DISORDERS

- Anemia: Iron-deficiency anemia often presents as atrophy and pallor of the mucosa and atrophic glossitis. Patients with pernicious anemia may present with erythema of the tongue (either focal or diffuse) along with atrophy. This condition is often referred to as magenta tongue.
- Leukemia: Petechiae, mucosal bleeding, and ulcerations are findings within the oral cavity that are suggestive of leukemia.
- Thrombocytopenia: Hemorrhages can range from petechiae to hemorrhagic bullae and hematomas. Bleeding can occur with minor trauma or occur spontaneously.
- Multiple myeloma: Deposition of amyloid that leads to macroglossia can occur **(Fig. 7)**.

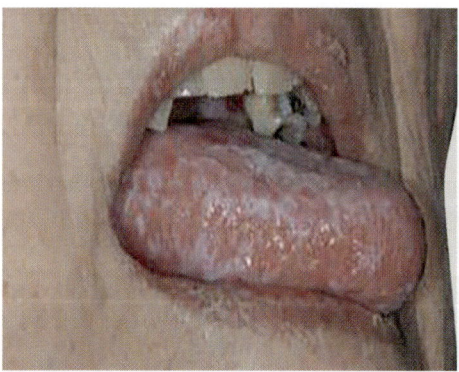

FIG. 5: Lichen planus of tongue.

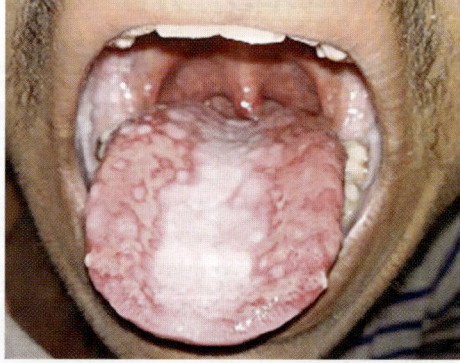

FIG. 6: Paraquat ingestion corroded tongue.

ENDOCRINE DISORDERS

- Thyroid disease: In patients with hypothyroidism, glycosaminoglycan deposition in the lips and tongue leads to associated swelling. In thyrotoxicosis, fine tremor may be visible in protruded tongue.
- Adrenal disease: Addison disease results from destruction of the adrenal cortex **(Fig. 8)**. The etiology can be variable, but often is autoimmune in nature. Hyperpigmentation of the oral mucosa and tongue, although nonspecific, may be the initial presentation.
- Diabetes mellitus: Higher susceptibility to infections such as *Candida* and *Mucormycosis*, often secondary to poor glucose control.

NEUROLOGICAL DISORDERS

- Ipsilateral lower motor neuron lesion manifests as unilateral muscle wasting, exaggerated longitudinal folds on that side and deviation of the tip toward the affected side on protrusion. There may be fasciculations if the lesion is nuclear.
- Bilateral lower motor neuron lesion shows severe wasting of whole tongue with difficulty in protrusion and grossly disturbed speech **(Figs. 9 and 10)**.

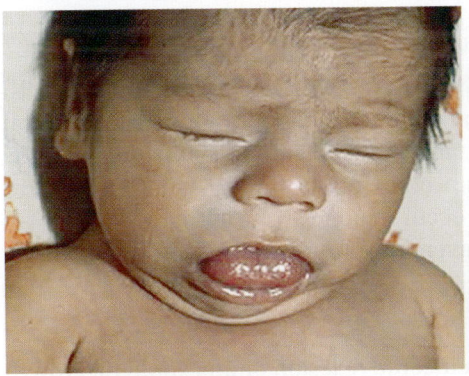

FIG. 7: Cretinism with macroglossia.

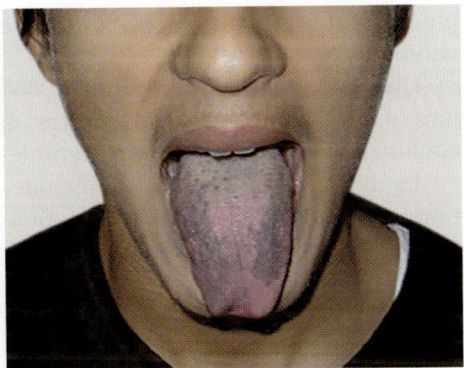

FIG. 8: Addison disease.

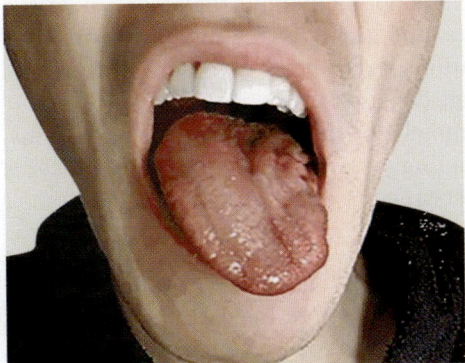

FIG. 9: Left hypoglossal nerve palsy.

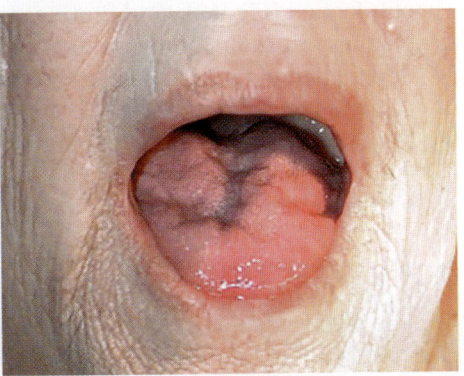

FIG. 10: Bilateral hypoglossal nerve palsy.

- Bilateral upper motor neuron lesion presents with a small stiff tongue lying in the floor of the mouth, its surface little altered, but almost incapable of protrusion and with gross disturbance of speech.

AUTOIMMUNE DISEASES

- Sjögren's syndrome is characterized by xerostomia and xerophthalmia and more commonly affects females. The tongue may be atrophic or fissured with deep grooves and malodorous due to food trapping. The oral mucosa may be dry, red, and wrinkled.
- Amyloidosis can be classified as two types: organ-limited or systemic. The oral soft tissues are rarely affected in organ-limited amyloidosis. Systemic amyloidosis can lead to macroglossia due to amyloid deposition in the tongue. Tongue lesions present as nodular or diffuse enlargement with subsequent ulcerations or hemorrhages. Biopsy can confirm the diagnosis. Treatment depends on the type of amyloidosis and the source of amyloid production.

KAWASAKI DISEASE

Kawasaki disease predominantly affects children younger than 5 years of age. It is also known as mucocutaneous lymph node disease. It is a medium vessel predominant systemic vasculitis and one of the important cause of heart disease in children.

Diagnosis is based on a fever of 38.5°C with a duration of 5 days along with four of five principal clinical features: oral changes, polymorphous rash, bilateral conjunctivitis, changes in the extremities, and cervical lymphadenopathy.

Findings in the oral cavity include lip cracking, erythema, and "strawberry tongue" **(Fig. 11)**. The oral manifestations occur in up to 96.5% of cases.

Treatment is done with high-dose intravenous immunoglobulin and aspirin.

NEOPLASTIC LESIONS

- Tongue malignancy may present as an ulcerative lesion or an exophytic growth in individuals with history of tobacco addiction.
- Oral Kaposi sarcoma occurs in up to 25% of HIV cases and may be the initial sign of infection **(Fig. 12)**. Oral findings include nonpigmented, violet, or brown-red plaques or tumors of the tongue, palate, and gingiva. Treatment involves focal destruction of the lesions with medications, excision, or cryotherapy as well as radiation or chemotherapy for later-stage disease.
- Metastatic tumors constitute approximately 1% of oral malignant neoplasms. Patients typically complain of pain, tingling, or swelling. In men, lung cancer is most common and in females it is breast cancer.

HIV INFECTION

Tongue involvement is a common feature of HIV infection. They are most frequently due to secondary infections like *Candida* and viruses.

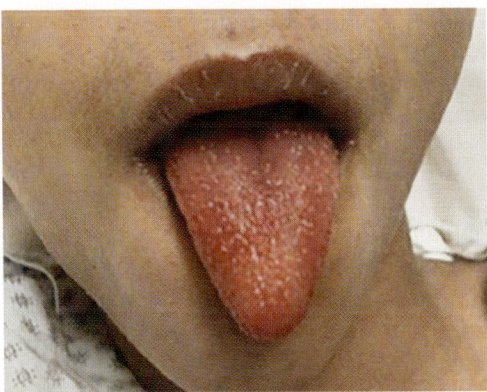
FIG. 11: Strawberry tongue in Kawasaki disease.

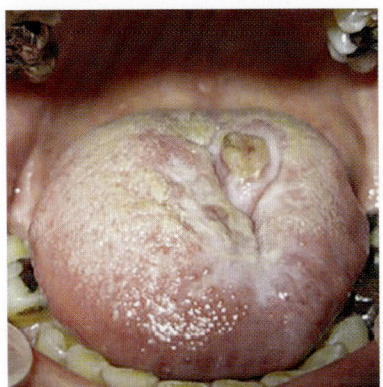
FIG. 12: Kaposi sarcoma in an HIV patient.

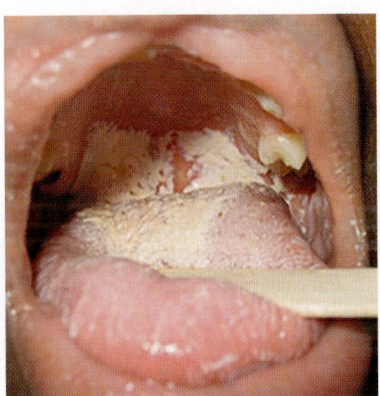
FIG. 13: Oral thrush in HIV patient.

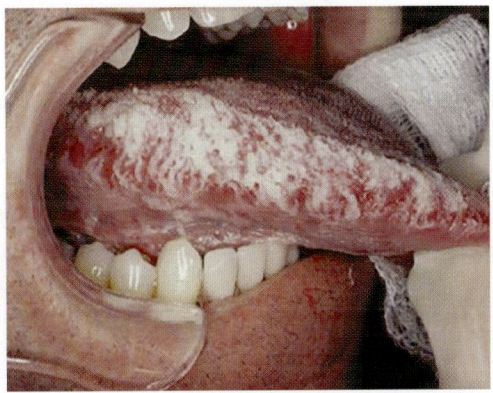
FIG. 14: Oral hairy leukoplakia.

- Oral thrush caused by *Candida* infection is common and indicative of fairly advanced immunological decline, generally seen in patients with CD4+ T cell count < 300/μL **(Fig. 13)**.
- Oral hairy leukoplakia is caused due to EBV and also marks advanced disease. It presents as white, frond-like lesions, generally along the lateral borders of the tongue and sometimes on the adjacent buccal mucosa. Oral hairy leukoplakia is not considered a premalignant condition **(Fig. 14)**. Severe cases have been reported to respond to topical podophyllin or systemic therapy with anti-herpesvirus agents.
- Aphthous ulcers may also be seen with regularity in patients with untreated HIV infection. These lesions are of unknown etiology and can be quite painful and interfere with swallowing. Topical anesthetics provide immediate symptomatic relief of short duration. Glossal ulcers may also result from cryptococcal disease or histoplasmosis.
- Kaposi sarcoma

Numerous systemic conditions, including some autoimmune, hematologic, endocrine, and neoplastic diseases as well as chronic illnesses, cause pathognomonic changes in the tongue. Hence, tongue remains as a vital examination point in general survey and may provide clues toward further evaluation and diagnosis.

CONCLUSION

Numerous systemic conditions, including some autoimmune, hematologic, endocrine, and neoplastic diseases as well as chronic illnesses, cause pathognomonic changes in the tongue. Hence, tongue remains as a vital examination point in general survey and may provide clues toward further evaluation and diagnosis. Thus it is said that tongue is the mirror of clinical medicine.

SUGGESTED READINGS

1. Huguley CM. The Tongue, 3rd edition. In: Walker HK, Hall WD, Hurst JW (eds). Clinical Methods: The History, Physical, and Laboratory Examinations. Boston: Butterworths; 1990.
2. Spillane J, Bickerstaff E. Bickerstaff's neurological examination in clinical practice. Oxford, OX: Blackwell Science; 1996.
3. Loscalzo J, Fauci A, Kasper D, et al. Harrison's principles of internal Medicine, 20th edition. USA: McGraw Hill Education; 2018.
4. Lamey PJ, Lewis M. The tongue: 1. Normal appearance and clinical examination. Dent Update. 1985;12(1):269-71.
5. Douglas G, Nicol E, Robertson C, et al. Macleod's clinical examination, 13th edition. Edinburgh: Churchill Livingstone Elsevier; 2013. p. 451.
6. Benedictis FM, Jorini M, Palumbo P. Black tongue due to adrenocortical insufficiency. Arch Dis Childhood. 2012;97:1033.

CHAPTER 10

Metabolic Acidosis: Diagnosis and Management

Subhash Chandra

Acid-base disorders are common in the critically ill patient, and assessment of acid-base status may indicate specific diagnoses and/or therapeutic interventions. The presence of a metabolic acidosis should suggest hypoperfusion and prompt further assessment of the adequacy of the oxygen balance.

An appropriate evaluation of acid-base status requires accurate interpretation of simultaneous measurements of electrolytes, albumin, and arterial blood gases (ABGs), as well as knowledge of compensatory physiologic responses.

WHAT IS pH?

It is the negative logarithm of H^+ ion concentration in the extracellular fluid (ECF).
- pH decreases as H^+ concentration increases:
  - pH > 7.45 alkalemia/alkalosis
  - pH < 7.35 acidosis/acidemia

HENDERSON–HASSELBALCH EQUATION

The H^+ ion concentration in ECF is determined by balance between partial pressure of CO_2 (PCO_2) and the concentration of bicarbonate [HCO_3^-] ion in the fluid.

$$pH \propto \frac{HCO_3^-}{PCO_2}$$

From this equation, one can see that pH increases as HCO_3^- increases and pH decreases as $PaCO_2$ increases.

HOW TO READ AN ABG?

pH	7.40 (7.35–7.45)
PO_2	80–104 mm Hg
PCO_2	40 mm Hg (35–45)
HCO_3^- (act)	24 ± 2 mEq/L
HCO_3^- (std)	24 ± 2 mEq/L
BE	± 2
O_2 sat	96–98%
Na^+	135–148 mmol/L
K^+	3.5–5.5 mmol/L
Ca^{++}	1.13–1.32 mmol/L
Cl^-	98–106 mmol/L
Anion gap	$(Na^+ K^+) - (Cl^- + HCO_3^-)$

Step 1

First look at pH:
- Acidemia = Decrease pH.
- Alkalemia = Increase pH.
- Normal pH.

Step 2

If acidemia is there—Check $PaCO_2$:
- Normal or low = Metabolic acidosis.
- High = Primary respiratory acidosis.

Step 3

If alkalemia is there—Check $PaCO_2$:
- If pH is alkalemic and $PaCO_2$ is normal or high, it indicates primary metabolic alkalosis.
- If pH is alkalemic and $PaCO_2$ is low, it indicates primary respiratory alkalosis.

Step 4

If normal pH—Check $PaCO_2$:
- High $PaCO_2$ = Mixed respiratory acidosis with metabolic alkalosis.
- Low $PaCO_2$ = Mixed respiratory alkalosis + Metabolic acidosis.

Step 5

If metabolic acidosis is diagnosed:
- Check—Anion gap (AG)
- Anion gap = $(Na^+ K^+) - (Cl^- + HCO_3^-)$

Metabolic Acidosis: Diagnosis and Management

NORMOGRAM

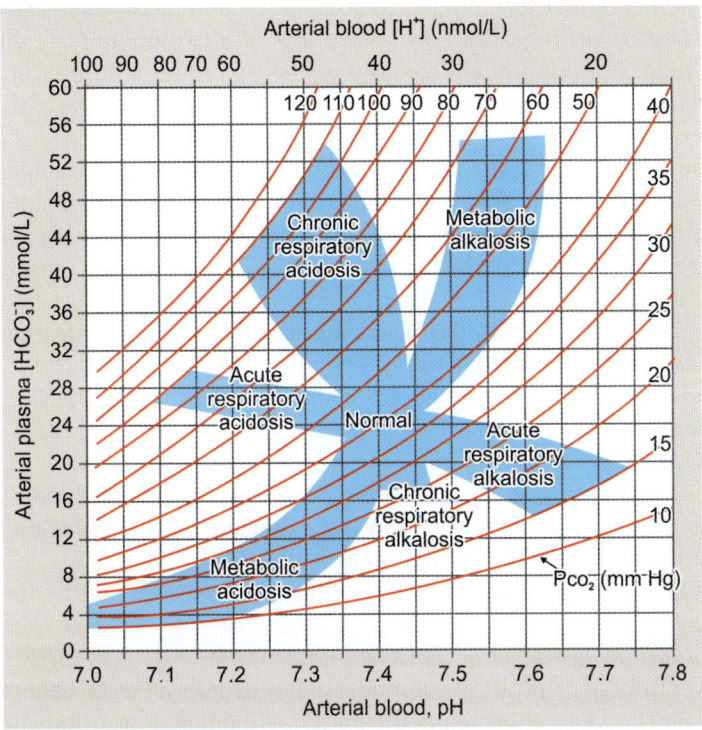

METABOLIC ACIDOSIS

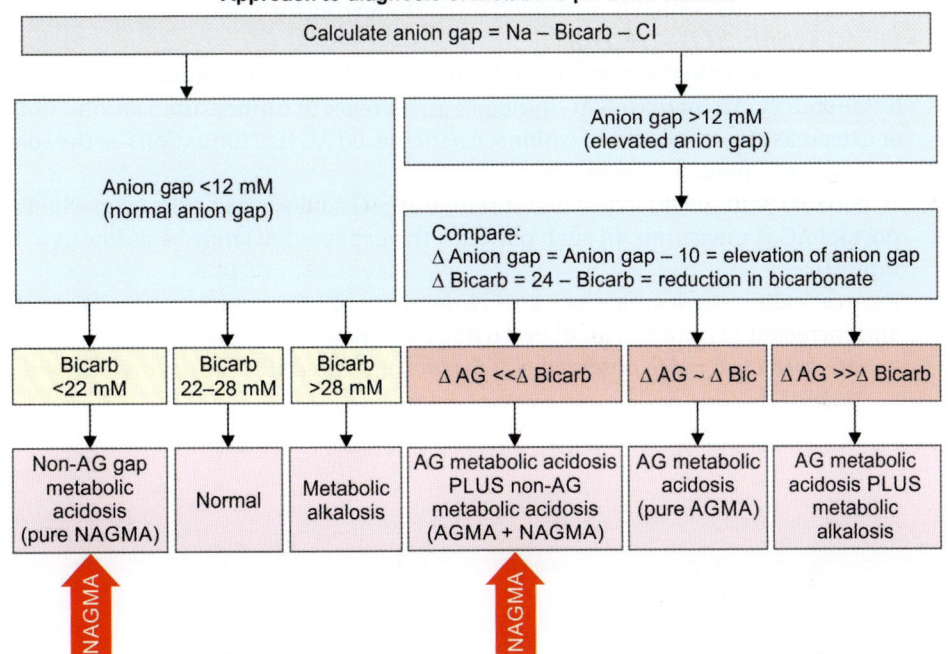

Metabolic Acidosis: Diagnosis and Management

Metabolic acidosis results from an increase in endogenous acid production that overwhelms renal excretion (e.g., ketoacidosis and lactic acidosis), exogenous acid input (e.g., toxin ingestion), excessive loss of bicarbonate (e.g., diarrhea), or decreased renal excretion of endogenous acids (e.g., renal failure). Compensation is achieved primarily by increasing minute ventilation to eliminate carbon dioxide (CO_2).

- In seriously ill patients, the most common causes of metabolic acidosis with an increased AG are lactic acidosis, renal failure, and diabetic ketoacidosis.
- Metabolic acidosis with a normal AG, often called hyperchloremic acidosis, may result from gastrointestinal or renal loss of HCO_3 or volume resuscitation with normal saline.
- Primary change is decreased HCO_3^- or increased H^+ leading to decreased pH.
    - For each decrease in HCO_3^- of 7–7.5 mmol/L, pH decreased by 0.1.
- Compensatory change for metabolic acidosis is a decrease in $PaCO_2$
    - Expected compensatory $PaCO_2$ = (1.5 × HCO_3^-) + 8 ± 2 or expected CO_2 level = HCO_3^- + 15.
- If $PaCO_2$ is higher than the expected, then there is an associated respiratory acidosis and if $PaCO_2$ is lower than the expected, then there is an associated respiratory alkalosis with the metabolic acidosis.
- The adequacy of respiratory compensation can be estimated by the following formulas:
    - Appropriate $PaCO_2$ = 1.5 × (HCO_3) + 8 ± 2; or $\Delta PaCO_2$ = 1.2 × $\Delta(HCO_3)$.
- The lower limit of respiratory compensation is usually a $PaCO_2$ of approximately 10 mm Hg (1.3 kPa). This means the $PaCO_2$ will not go lower than 10 mm Hg to compensate for a metabolic acidosis.

Metabolic acidosis is further characterized by a normal or increased AG. Normally, unmeasured anions exceed unmeasured cations, and the difference results in the AG, which is estimated by the following formula:
- AG = (Na) − [(Cl) + (HCO_3)]

The normal AG value is approximately 10 ± 4 mmol/L but the normal range varies by laboratory. An increased AG indicates an increase in unmeasured anions and/or a decrease in unmeasured cations. An increased AG has limitations as the sole indicator of a metabolic acidosis.

- In patients with severe hypoalbuminemia, an AG acidosis can exist even when a normal AG is measured. In such patients, the expected AG may be as low as 4–5 mmol/L.
- For every albumin decrease of 1 g/dL, a decrease of 2.5–3 mmol in AG will occur. The corrected AG can be calculated using the following formula:
    - AG corrected = AG observed + 2.5 ×[normal albumin − measured albumin (in g/dL)]

Anion Gap

It is an acid-base parameter that is used to evaluate patients with a metabolic acidosis to determine whether the problem is due to accumulation of H⁺ ions or due to loss of HCO_3^-.

Normal anion gap = 12 (±4) mEq/L

When organic acids such as lactic acids, keto acids, and ethanol accumulate, they cause increased anion gap.

Causes of Normal Anion Gap Acidosis
Gastrointestinal Loss of Bicarbonate
- Diarrhea
- Ureterosigmoidostomy

Renal Bicarbonate Loss (Proximal Renal Tubular Acidosis Type 2)
- Fanconi's syndrome
- Carbonic anhydrase inhibitors
- Ileal bladder

Reduced Renal H⁺ Secretion Distal Renal Tubular Acidosis (Type 1)

Causes of normal anion gap metabolic acidosis	
With a tendency to hyperkalemia	With a tendency to hypokalemia
Subsiding diabetic ketoacidosis	Renal tubular acidosis, type I (classical distal acidosis)
Early uremic acidosis	Renal tubular acidosis, type II (proximal acidosis)
Early obstructive uropathy	Acetazolamide
Renal tubular acidosis, type IV	Acute diarrhea with losses of HCO_3^- and K⁺
Hypoaldosteronism (Addison's disease)	Ureterosigmoidostomy with increased resorption of (H⁺) and (Or) and losses of HCO_3^- and K⁺
Infusion or ingestion of HCl, NH₄Cl, lysine-HCl, or arginine-HCl	Obstruction of artificial ileal bladder
Potassium-sparing diuretics	Dilution acidosis (may occur with 0.9% NaCl infusion)

Source: Tintinalli J, Stapczynski J, Ma OJ, et al. Tintinalli's Emergency Medicine: A Comprehensive Study Guide, 8th edition. US: McGraw-Hill Education/Medical; 2015.

Familial, hypercalcemia/hypercalciuric states, Sjogren's syndrome, autoimmune diseases, amphotericin, and renal transplant.

Type IV Renal Tubular Acidosis

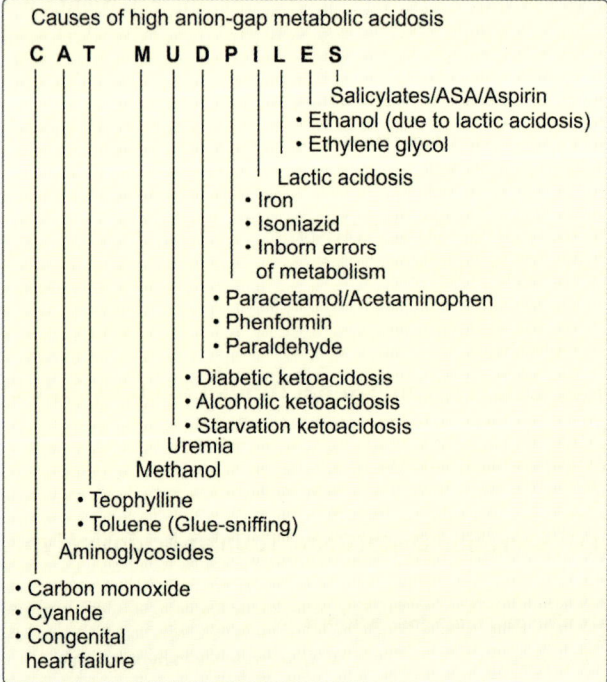

- Hyporeninemic-hypoaldosteronism, diabetes mellitus (DM), nonsteroidal anti-inflammatory drug (NSAIDs)
- Defective mineralocorticoid synthesis—Addison's disease, chronic heparin therapy
- Inadequate renal response to mineralocorticoids—Systemic lupus erythematosus (SLE), K^+ sparing diuretics.
- Early uremia

I/HCl Precursor Ingestion

HCl, NH_4Cl, NaCl, and arginine HCl.

Others

- Postchronic hyperventilation
- Recovery from diabetic ketoacidosis (DKA)
- Toluene inhalation

Mnemonic for non-anion-gap metabolic acidosis (NAGMA)	An updated and improved mnemonic	
USED CARP		
U – Ureteroenterostomy	• Glycols	• Rhabdomyolysis
S – Small bowel fistula	• Oxoproline	• Toluene intoxication
E – Extra chloride (K^+ normal or ↑)	• L-lactate	• Type B lactic acidosis

D – Diarrhea C – Carbonic anhydrase inhibitor A – Addison's disease (K*↑) R – Renal tubular acidosis (RTA) P – Pancreatic fistula	• D-lactate • Methanol • Aspirin • Renal failure • Ketoacidosis	• Malignancy • Liver failure • Thiamine deficiency • Drugs (metformin, NRTI, linezolid) • Toxins (CO, cyanide)

Source: Mehta AN, Emmett JB, Emmett M, et al. GOLD MARK: an anion gap mnemonic for the 21st century. Lancet. 2008;372(9642):892.

Example 1

pH	7.213
PCO_2	31.5 mm Hg
PO_2	172 mm Hg
Na^+	140 mmol/L
K^+	3.0 mmol/L
HCO_3^-	14.7 mEq/L
BE(ecf)	−15
BE	−2.6
CO_2	14
O_2 sat	99%

Metabolic acidosis:
Expected $PaCO_2$: $(HCO_3 \times 1.5) + 8\ (\pm 2)$
$= (14.7 \times 1.5) + 8\ (\pm 2)$
$= 22 + 8 + 2$
$= 32$

Example 2

pH	7.25
PO_2	104 mm Hg
PCO_2	50 mm Hg
HCO_3^-	15 mEq/L
BE	−8
O_2 sat	95%
Na^+	140 mmol/L
K^+	4.5 mmol/L
Cl^-	105 mmol/L
Anion gap	20

High anion gap metabolic acidosis with respiratory acidosis:
Expected PaCO$_2$: (HCO$_3$ × 1.5) + 8 (±2)
      = (15 × 1.5) + 8 (±2)
      = 22.5 + 8 + 2
      = 32.5

Example 3

pH	7.31
PCO$_2$	16.2 mm Hg
PO$_2$	110.5 mm Hg
Na$^+$	137 mmol/L
K$^+$	4.8 mmol/L
Cl$^-$	110.5 mmol/L
HCO$_3^-$	8.3 mEq/L
BE(ecf)	−17.8
BE	−14.9
CO$_2$	8.8

High anion gap metabolic acidosis with respiratory alkalosis:
Expected PaCO$_2$: (HCO$_3$ × 1.5) + 8(±2)
      = (8.3 × 1.5) + 8 + 2
      − 22.45

Example 4

pH	7.31
PCO$_2$	16.2 mm Hg
PO$_2$	110.5 mm Hg
Na$^+$	137 mmol/L
K$^+$	4.8 mmol/L
Cl$^-$	110.5 mmol/L
HCO$_3^-$	8.3 mEq/L
BE(ecf)	−17.8
BE	−14.9
CO$_2$	8.8

Metabolic acidosis with uncompensated respiratory alkalosis (normal anion gap):
Expected PaCO$_2$: (HCO$_3$ × 1.5) + 8 (±2)
      = (12.8 × 1.5) + 8 + 2
      = 27.2 + 2
      = 29.2

MIXED ACID BASE DISORDERS
Mixed Metabolic Acidosis and Metabolic Alkalosis
Essential clue to mixed disorders is:
- Anion gap—HCO_3 relationship
- Change in anion gap above 12 is called ΔAG.
- Change of HCO_3 below 24 is called ΔHCO_3.
- AG excess/HCO_3 deficit = (AG $-12/24 - HCO_3$)
- Or $\Delta AG/\Delta HCO_3$ is called Gap—Gap.

For anion gap acidosis: $\Delta AG/\Delta HCO_3$? 1
For hyperchloremic (normal) AG acidosis: $\Delta AG/\Delta HCO_3$? 0
For metabolic acidosis with metabolic alkalosis: $\Delta AG/\Delta HCO_3 \geq 1.5$, i.e., change in AG excess is greater than change in HCO_3 deficit.

Causes of Mixed Disorders
- Diabetic ketoacidosis with nasogastric (NG) suction/vomiting.
- Sepsis with lactic acidosis with NG suction/vomiting or patient on steroids.
- ARF with sepsis on steroids and NG suction.

Example 1

pH	7.23
PCO_2	37.6 mm Hg
PO_2	189.7 mm Hg
Na^+	140 mmol/L
K^+	3.0 mmol/L
Cl^-	126 mmol/L
HCO_3^-	16.0 mEq/L
BE(ecf)	−11.5
BE	−10.7
CO_2	17.1
Anion gap	1
O_2 sat	99.5%
Lactate	1.63 mmol/L

Metabolic acidosis with respiratory acidosis:
Expected $PaCO_2$ = ($HCO_3 \times 1.5$) + 8 (±2)
$\qquad\qquad\quad$ = (16 × 1.5) + 8
$\qquad\qquad\quad$ = 24 + 8
$\qquad\qquad\quad$ = 32

Example 2

pH	7.42
PCO$_2$	6.4 mm Hg
PO$_2$	63.6 mm Hg
Na$^+$	136 mmol/L
K$^+$	4.2 mmol/L
Cl$^-$	122 mmol/L
HCO$_3^-$	4.2 mEq/L
BE(ecf)	−20.1
BE	−17.9
CO$_2$	<5
Anion gap	14
O$_2$ sat	93.8%
Lactate	2.29 mmol/L

Compensated respiratory alkalosis with metabolic acidosis:
Expected PaCO$_2$ = (HCO$_3$ × 1.5) + 8 (±2)
$\qquad\qquad\quad$ = (4.2 × 1.5) + 8 + 2
$\qquad\qquad\quad$ = 6.3 + 8 = 14.3

■ TRIPLE DISORDERS

These are combination of metabolic acidosis, metabolic alkalosis combined with either respiratory acidosis or respiratory alkalosis.

Example 1

pH	7.40
PO$_2$	60 mm Hg
PCO$_2$	28 mm Hg
HCO$_3^-$	15 mEq/L
BE	−9
O$_2$ sat	90%
Na$^+$	140 mmol/L
K$^+$	3.5 mmol/L
Cl$^-$	98 mmol/L
Anion gap	27

High anion gap metabolic acidosis with metabolic alkalosis and respiratory alkalosis —*"Triple Disorder"*
ΔAG/ΔHCO$_3$ = (27 − 12/24 − 15)
$\qquad\qquad\;$ = 15/9 = 1.66

Expected $CO_2 = 15 \times 1.5 + 8 = 22 + 8 = 30$
CO_2 reduction = 40 − 28 = 12
For each 10 mmHg decrease in $PaCO_2$, HCO_3 reduces by 4 mEq/L
Expected $HCO_3 = 24 − 4 = 20$

Example 2

pH	7.32
PCO_2	23.7 mm Hg
PO_2	94.9 mm Hg
Na^+	144 mmol/L
K^+	4.1 mmol/L
Cl^-	103.8 mmol/L
HCO_3^-	13.3 mEq/L
BE (ecf)	−12.2
BE(B)	−10.2
CO_2	14.0
Anion gap	31
O_2 sat	97.3%
Lactate	9.58 mmol/L

High anion gap metabolic acidosis with metabolic alkalosis and respiratory alkalosis—"*Triple Disorder*"
$\Delta AG/\Delta HCO_3 = (31 − 12)/(24 − 13.3)$
$\qquad\qquad = 19/10.7 = 1.77$
Expected $CO_2 = 13.3 \times 1.5 + 8 = 27.95$
Decrease in CO_2 is 16.3
Expected decrease in $PaCO_2 = 1.6 \times 2 = 3.2$

Example 3

pH	7.36
PO_2	100 mmHg
PCO_2	38 mmHg
HCO_3^-	16 mEq/L
BE	8
Na^+	140 mmol/L
K^+	3.5 mmol/L
Cl^-	98 mmol/L
Anion gap	26
pH	7.36

High anion gap metabolic acidosis with metabolic alkalosis and respiratory Acidosis—"*Triple Disorder*"

$\Delta AG/\Delta HCO_3 = (26 - 12/24 - 16)$
$= 14/8 = 1.75$
Expected $CO_2 = 16 \times 1.5 + 8$
$= 24 + 8$
$= 32$

■ CASE 1

A 26-year-old man arrives at the emergency department with multisystem trauma following a motorcycle collision. He is somnolent with a Glasgow Coma Scale score of 13. The primary survey reveals an open airway with equal breath sounds bilaterally.

pH	7.31
PO_2	163 mm Hg
PCO_2	32 mm Hg
HCO_3^-	15 mEq/L
Na^+	140 mmol/L
Cl^-	105 mmol/L

His vital signs are:
- Temperature 36.2°C (97.2°F)
- Heart rate 116 beats/min
- Respiratory rate 20 breaths/min
- Blood pressure 100/50 mm Hg
- Oxygen saturation on pulse oximetry 99% with a nonrebreather mask in place.

The patient undergoes diagnostic radiological evaluations that reveal left rib fractures without hemothorax or pneumothorax.

Laboratory values are as follows:
Q. 1a. Which acid-base disorder is present?
Ans: Anion gap metabolic acidosis.
- The pH is acidemic. The low bicarbonate concentration is consistent with a metabolic process. The next step is to determine if appropriate respiratory compensation is present.
  - Appropriate $PaCO_2$ compensation = $1.5 \times (HCO_3) + 8 \pm 2$
- In this case, the appropriate compensation would yield $PaCO_2$ 30.5 ± 2 mm Hg. Thus, respiratory compensation is appropriate. The next step is to calculate the anion gap.
  - AG = [Na] − [(Cl) + (HCO_3)]
  - AG for this case = (140) − [(105 + 15)] = 20 mmol/L
- This patient has an elevated anion gap metabolic acidosis. With an anion gap acidosis, the Δ gap should be calculated to determine if additional metabolic processes are present.
  - Δ gap = (deviation of AG from normal) − [deviation of (HCO_3) from normal]
  $= (20 - 12) - (24 - 15) = -1$ mmol/L

- This is within the normal range of 0 + 6, indicating that no additional metabolic process is present.

Q. 1b. What is the suspected cause of the acid-base disorder?
Ans: Lactic acidosis.
The causes of elevated anion gap metabolic acidosis can be remembered with the following mnemonic *MUDPILES*, which stands for methanol, uremia, diabetic ketoacidosis, paracetamol/acetaminophen, isoniazid, lactic acidosis, ethylene glycol or methanol, and salicylates.
   This case depicts a trauma patient in shock with hypoperfusion, resulting in lactic acidosis.

Q. 1c. Which of the following is the most appropriate intervention?
Ans: Fluid and blood product administration.
   The goal is restore perfusion to the tissues. This patient is experiencing hypovolemic hemorrhagic shock. The treatment is fluid and blood product administration and control.

■ CASE 2

A 55-year-old man is admitted to the surgical intensive care unit (ICU) after elective laparoscopic cholecystectomy. An iatrogenic injury to the hepatic artery required conversion to an open cholecystectomy and fluid resuscitation with normal saline and blood products.

pH	7.32
PCO_2	36 mm Hg
HCO_3^-	18 mEq/L
Na^+	146 mmol/L
K^+	3.8 mmol/L
Cl^-	117 mmol/L

His vital signs are:
- Heart rate 115 beats/min
- Respiratory rate 12 breaths/min (ventilator rate)
- Blood pressure 105/68 mm Hg
- Oxygen saturation on pulse oximetry 99% at fraction of inspired oxygen of 50%.

Laboratory values are as follows:
Q. 2a. Which acid-base disorder is present?
Ans: Nonanion gap metabolic acidosis.
- The pH is academic and the change in HCO_3 concentration would indicate a metabolic process. The next step is to evaluate whether the respiratory compensation is appropriate.
    - *Respiratory compensation: $1.5 \times (HCO_3) + 8 \pm 2$*
    - *Respiratory compensation: $1.5 \times (18) + 8 \pm 2 = 35 \pm 2$*

- In this case the patient has appropriate respiratory compensation. The next step is to determine if the anion gap is elevated.
  - $AG = (Na) - [(Cl) + (HCO_3)]$
  - $146 - (117 + 18) = 11$ mmol/L
- There is no elevation in the anion gap, so this patient has a nonanion gap metabolic acidosis.

Q. 2b. Which of the following is the most likely cause of the acid-base disorder in this patient?
Ans: Normal saline administration.
- Metabolic acidosis with a normal anion gap, which is a hyperchloremic acidosis, may result from gastrointestinal or renal loss of HCO_3 or volume resuscitation with normal saline.
- In this case, the patient received excess fluid resuscitation due to hemorrhage in surgery. This patient has metabolic acidosis as a result of hyperchloremia from normal saline resuscitation.
- Cardiogenic shock and hemorrhagic shock would result in metabolic acidosis with an elevated anion gap.
- Hypoventilation would be associated with a respiratory acidosis.
- The appropriate intervention is to change to an intravenous fluid with lower chloride content, such as Ringer lactate

CASE 3

A 58-year-old woman with hypertension and chronic kidney disease is admitted to the hospital with alcohol intoxication. She is somnolent and arouses to painful stimuli.

pH	7.32
PCO_2	38 mm Hg
HCO_3^-	15 mEq/L
Na^+	134 mmol/L
K^+	6.1 mmol/L
Cl^-	117 mmol/L
PaO_2	78 mm Hg
Blood urea	62 mg/dL
Creatinine	3.7 mg/dL
Glucose	125 mg/dL

Her vital signs are:
- Heart rate 110 beats/min
- Respiratory rate 10 breaths/min (ventilator rate)
- Blood pressure 142/88 mm Hg
- Temperature 37° (98.6° F)
- Oxygen saturation on pulse oximetry 94%

Laboratory values are as follows:
Q.3. Which one of the following best describes the acid-base disorder?
Ans: Anion gap metabolic acidosis and respiratory acidosis.
- The pH is acidemic and the low (HCO_3) indicates a metabolic process. The formula for determining the expected respiratory compensation is:
  - $PaCO_2 = 1.5 \times (HCO_3) + 8 \pm 2$
- The expected $PaCO_2$ would be approximately 30 mm Hg (4.0 kPa). Thus, the finding of a higher $PaCO_2$ than expected indicates another acid-base process of respiratory acidosis.
- The respiratory acidosis is most likely secondary to depressed respiratory drive from intoxication. This patient has ventilatory insufficiency and must be monitored closely for worsening and the potential need for more aggressive ventilatory support.
- The anion gap is calculated as an increased value of 19 mmol/L, which is likely secondary to chronic kidney disease, but other unmeasured anions (such as lactate) may be contributing.
- The Δ gap can be calculated for this case.
- The deviation of the anion gap from normal is 7 mmol/L, and the deviation of the (HCO_3) from normal is 9 mmol/L.
- The difference of -2 mmol/L is not likely to represent a third acid-base process.

■ CASE 4

An 80-year-old man with hypertension, diabetes, and malnutrition is admitted to the hospital with cough, fever, and hypotension.
Chest radiograph shows a right lower lobe pneumonia.

pH	7.35
PCO_2	32 mm Hg
HCO_3^-	17 mEq/L
Na^+	132 mmol/L
K^+	4.0 mmol/L
Cl^-	103 mmol/L
PaO_2	78 mm Hg
Blood urea	20 mg/dL
Creatinine	1.4 mg/dL
Albumin	1.5 g/dL

His vital signs are:
- Heart rate 115 beats/min
- Respiratory rate 20 breaths/min (ventilator rate)
- Blood pressure 90/52 mm Hg
- Temperature 38.3° (101° F)
- Oxygen saturation on pulse oximetry 95% on oxygen supplemented at 8 L/min via nasal cannula.

Metabolic Acidosis: Diagnosis and Management

Laboratory values are as follows:
Q. 4a. Which one of the following best describes the acid-base disorder?
Ans: Acute respiratory alkalosis and metabolic acidosis.
- The pH is alkalemic and the low $PaCO_2$ indicates a respiratory process. The next step is to determine if this is an acute or chronic respiratory alkalosis. The formula for acute respiratory alkalosis is:
  - Increase in pH = $0.08 \times (40 - PaCO_2)/10$
- Using the data from this case, the expected increase in pH would be 0.2 or pH 7.6, which is higher than 7.55. The formula for chronic respiratory alkalosis is:
  - Increase in pH = $0.03 \times (40 - PaCO_2)/10$
- Applying it yields a pH increase of 0.075 or pH 7.475. These calculations suggest that there is likely to be a second acid-base disorder present.
- Calculation of the anion gap as 21 mmol/L identifies the second process of anion gap metabolic acidosis.
- The Δ gap can be also be calculated for this case.
- The deviation of the anion gap from normal is 9 mmol/L, and the deviation of the (HCO_3) from normal is 11 mmol/L.
- The difference of -2 is not likely to represent a third acid-base process.

Q. 4b. Which one of the following is a potential etiology of the acid-base disorder?
Ans: Sepsis.
- The acid-base pattern can be helpful in suggesting an etiology of a patient's condition.
- In this case, respiratory alkalosis with anion gap metabolic acidosis is the typical acid-base disorder of sepsis.
- Salicylate intoxication would also be associated with this acid-base pattern.
- Pulmonary embolism would typically result in a respiratory alkalosis, with acidosis being unlikely in a hemodynamically stable patient.
- Diuretic use would primarily result in metabolic alkalosis rather than acidosis.
- Chronic obstructive lung disease and renal failure would most likely result in a respiratory acidosis and metabolic acidosis.

■ CASE 5

A 60-year-old man with arterial vascular disease and hypertension presented to the emergency department with complaints of shortness of breath and abdominal pain.

pH	7.55
PCO_2	15 mm Hg
HCO_3^-	13 mmol/L
Na^+	135 mmol/L
K^+	3.8 mmol/L
Cl^-	101 mmol/L
PaO_2	98 mm Hg

His vital signs are:
- Heart rate 90 beats/min
- Respiratory rate 25 breaths/min (ventilator rate)
- Blood pressure 168/96 mm Hg
- Temperature 37.2° (99° F)
- Oxygen saturation on pulse oximetry 98% on oxygen supplemented at 2 L/min via nasal cannula.

Laboratory values are as follows:
Q. 5a. Which one of the following best describes the acid-base disorder?
Ans: Acute respiratory alkalosis and metabolic acidosis.
- The pH is alkalemic and the low $PaCO_2$ indicates a respiratory process. The next step is to determine if this is an acute or chronic respiratory alkalosis. The formula for acute respiratory alkalosis is:
  - *Increase in pH = 0.08 × (40 − $PaCO_2$)/10*
- Using the data from this case, the expected increase in pH would be 0.2 or pH 7.6, which is higher than 7.55. The formula for chronic respiratory alkalosis is:
  - *Increase in pH = 0.03 × (40 − $PaCO_2$)/10*
- Applying it yields a pH increase of 0.075 or pH 7.475. These calculations suggest that there is likely to be a second acid-base disorder present.
- Calculation of the anion gap as 21 mmol/L identifies the second process of anion gap metabolic acidosis.
- The Δ gap can be also be calculated for this case.
- The deviation of the anion gap from normal is 9 mmol/L, and the deviation of the (HCO_3) from normal is 11 mmol/L.
- The difference of -2 is not likely to represent a third acid-base process.

Q. 5b. Which one of the following is a potential etiology of the acid-base disorder?
Ans: Sepsis.
- The acid-base pattern can be helpful in suggesting an etiology of a patient's condition.
- In this case, respiratory alkalosis with anion gap metabolic acidosis is the typical acid-base disorder of sepsis.
- Salicylate intoxication would also be associated with this acid base pattern.
- Pulmonary embolism would typically result in a respiratory alkalosis, with acidosis being unlikely in a hemodynamically stable patient.
- Diuretic use would primarily result in metabolic alkalosis rather than acidosis.
- Chronic obstructive lung disease and renal failure would most likely result in a respiratory acidosis and metabolic acidosis

■ CASE 6

A 70-year-old woman is admitted to the ICU with syncope after several days of vomiting.

pH	7.30
PCO_2	36 mm Hg
HCO_3^-	20 mmol/L

Metabolic Acidosis: Diagnosis and Management

Na+	138 mmol/L
K+	3.0 mmol/L
Cl−	93 mmol/L
PaO₂	88 mm Hg
Glucose	90 mg/dL

Her vital signs are:
- Heart rate 140 beats/min
- Respiratory rate 24 breaths/min (ventilator rate)
- Blood pressure 80/50 mm Hg
- Temperature 37.0° (98.6° F)

Laboratory values are as follows:

Q. 6. *Which one of the following best describes the acid-base disorder?*
Ans: Anion gap metabolic acidosis and metabolic alkalosis.
- The pH is acidemic and the lower HCO_3 indicates a metabolic process. The formula for determining the expected respiratory compensation is:
  - $PaCO_2 = 1.5 \times (HCO_3) + 8 \pm 2$
- Using this, the expected $PaCO_2$ would be approximately 38 mm Hg (5.07 kPa), which is close to the $PaCO_2$ of 36 mm Hg (4.8 kPa).
- The anion gap is calculated as 25 mmol/L, which identifies the presence of an anion gap metabolic acidosis.
- The Δ gap should also be calculated for this case.
- The deviation of the anion gap from normal is 13 mmol/L, and the deviation of the (HCO_3) from normal is 4 mmol/L. The difference of 9 mmol/L suggests the presence of a metabolic alkalosis.
- The (HCO_3) did not decrease as much as expected for the degree of acidosis. The clinical scenario is also suggestive of volume depletion from vomiting, resulting in the metabolic alkalosis. An anion gap metabolic acidosis (lactic acidosis) was the result of hypotension.

■ CASE 7

A 55-year-old diabetic, hypertensive man presents with nausea, vomiting, and abdominal pain.

pH	7.45
PCO₂	34 mm Hg
HCO₃⁻	23 mmol/L
Na+	134 mmol/L
K+	3.2 mmol/L
Cl−	85 mmol/L
PaO₂	85 mm Hg
Glucose	420 mg/dL

Metabolic Acidosis: Diagnosis and Management

His vital signs are:
- Heart rate 124 beats/min
- Respiratory rate 22 breaths/min (ventilator rate)
- Blood pressure 102/50 mm Hg
- Temperature 36.4° (97.6° F)

Q. 7. Which one of the following best describes the acid-base disorder?
Ans: Respiratory alkalosis, metabolic acidosis, and metabolic alkalosis.
- The pH in this very ill patient is nearly normal, which should immediately raise the suspicion for complex acid-base disorders.
- The history is suggestive of possible diabetic ketoacidosis, so the first calculation could be the anion gap, which is increased at 26 mmol/L. Using the formula for determining the expected respiratory compensation for a metabolic acidosis:
  - $PaCO_2 = 1.5 \times (HCO_3) + 8 \pm 2$—the expected $PaCO_2$ would be approximately 42 mm Hg (5.60 kPa).
- Since the patient's $PaCO_2$ is lower at 34 mm Hg (4.53 kPa), a respiratory alkalosis is present.
- The Δ gap should definitely be calculated for this case.
- The deviation of the anion gap from normal is 14 mmol/L, and the deviation of the (HCO_3) from normal is 1 mmol/L. The difference of 13 mmol/L suggests the presence of a metabolic alkalosis.
- The (HCO_3) did not decrease as much as expected for the degree of acidosis.
- The clinical scenario is consistent with diabetic ketoacidosis with volume depletion from vomiting and a respiratory alkalosis, possibly secondary to pain.
- You could also approach the problem by identifying the pH as alkalemic. The lower $PaCO_2$ would prompt assessment of whether it is an acute or chronic respiratory process.
- Acute is more likely, so the formula for acute respiratory alkalosis would be used:
  - Increase in $pH = 0.08 \times (40 - PaCO_2)/10$.
- Based on the data from this case, the expected increase in pH would be 0.048 or pH 7.45, which is similar to the patient's value. The other acid-base processes would still be identified because the anion gap is always calculated.

CHAPTER 11

Hyponatremia

Mukesh K Sarna, Pallaavi Goel

■ INTRODUCTION

Hyponatremia is the most frequent form of electrolyte disorder. It can occur as a result of several diseases or as an isolated disease itself. It can be defined as serum sodium (Na^+) levels <135 mmol/L. The normal range of sodium is from 135 to 145 mmol/L.

Hyponatremia mostly occurs due to a relative excess of water in relation to sodium. It can either be due to marked increase in water intake or by impaired excretion of water from the body.

Total volume of water in the body is divided into two compartments—*intracellular fluid* compartment constitutes two-thirds part whereas *extracellular fluid* is the remaining one-third. Major solute of intracellular fluid is potassium, whereas major solute of extracellular fluid is sodium.

■ EPIDEMIOLOGY

Prevalence is around 25–35% in hospitalized patients; with higher incidence in ICU patients, postoperative patients, and patients with multiple comorbidities. Many studies reported a high morbidity and mortality in patients with sodium levels <125 mmol/L. Patients with coexisting liver cirrhosis have a higher risk of mortality even with low severity scores.

■ CLASSIFICATION

- **On the basis of duration:**
  - *Acute hyponatremia:* When documented duration is <48 hours.
  - *Chronic hyponatremia:* When documented duration is more than 48 hours, or when duration is undocumented and history is not suggestive of acute hyponatremia.

- **On the basis of severity:**
  - *Mild:* Na$^+$ 130–134 mmol/L
  - *Moderate:* Na$^+$ 125–129 mmol/L
  - *Profound:* Na$^+$ <125 mmol/L; (severe when with associated symptoms)
- **On the basis of volume status:**
  - *Hypovolemic hyponatremia:* Decreased total body water and sodium content, with more relative decrease in sodium.
  - *Euvolemic hyponatremia:* It implies normal sodium stores and a total body excess of free water.
  - *Hypervolemic hyponatremia:* It is characterized by a pronounced deficit of free water excretion that leads to inappropriate water retention more in comparison with the sodium concentration.
- **On the basis of plasma osmolality:**
  - *Hypotonic hyponatremia:* Excess water relative to effective osmoles in extracellular space that is caused by either a decrease in total body solute or an increase in total body water.
  - *Isotonic hyponatremia:* Pseudohyponatremia (It is defined as a state of decreased sodium levels due to an artificial reduction in sodium that is caused by elevation of the non-aqueous, non-sodium portion of plasma by proteins and lipids relative to aqueous portion with no true reduction in total sodium).
  - *Hypertonic hyponatremia:* Elevated plasma osmolality due to presence of effective osmoles and movement of water from intracellular to extracellular spaces.

ETIOLOGY

1. **Hypovolemic hyponatremia**

The key causal factor responsible is reduction in plasma volume that can be due to renal or extra renal sources.
- Nonrenal sources:
  - Urine Na$^+$ concentration <20 mmol/L
  - Gastrointestinal losses—vomiting, diarrhea
  - Insensible water loss—burns or third spacing
- Renal sources:
  - Urinary loss of Na$^+$ >20 mmol/L leading to lessening of the volume and compensatory rise in vasopressin level.
  - Mineralocorticoid deficit: Hyponatremia with hyperkalemia.
  - Salt losing nephropathies: Interstitial nephropathies, medullary cystic disease, reflux nephropathy, obstructive uropathy, and the recovery phase of acute tubular necrosis.
  - Diuretics: Thiazides, Loop diuretics
  - Excretion of osmotically active solutes that are poorly reabsorbable: Glycosuria, ketonuria, bicarbonaturia
  - Cerebral salt wasting (CSW) syndromes: Encephalitis, meningitis, traumatic brain injury, craniotomy, and subarachnoid hemorrhage.

2. **Euvolemic hyponatremia**
It is the most common type.
- Syndrome of inappropriate secretion of anti-diuretic hormone (SIADH)
- Exercise induced hyponatremia: In athletes that may develop severe hyponatremia due to excessive water intake associated with persistent ADH secretion.
- Low dietary solute intake: In beer drinkers and those who take a very poor diet. Daily solute excretion is <250 mOsmol. Daily fluid intake is >4 L/day.
- Primary polydipsia: In psychotic patients that have an overdue obsession of intake of large amount of water, hence the kidneys cannot excrete massive water load (400–600 mL/hour) that ultimately causes fatal hyponatremia even though urine is maximally dilute. There is no specific therapy except for limiting the water intake.
- Hypothyroidism
- Secondary adrenal insufficiency

3. **Hypervolemic hyponatremia**
In this case, patient develops increase in total-body water with proportionate increase in total-body Na-Cl leading to a dilutional hyponatremia.
- Renal causes: Urinary sodium concentration is >20 mEq/L and the causes are acute or chronic renal failure.
- Nonrenal causes: Urinary sodium concentration is <20 mEq/L and these includes disorders such as nephritic syndrome, congestive heart failure, and cirrhosis

PATHOGENESIS

The normal serum sodium concentration is 135–145 mmol/L. Sodium is one of the chief electrolytes that regulates serum osmolality and preserves the extracellular fluid volume. ECF sodium is upheld by the Na/K ATPase pump.

Serum osmolality can be calculated as:

Serum osmolality (mmol/kg) = $(2 \times \text{serum [Na]}) + (\text{Serum glucose}/18) + (\text{BUN}/2.8)$

Therefore, the extracellular volume and plasma osmolality need the equilibrium of sodium and water. The variations in ratio of body water and sodium occur due to abnormal water homeostasis thereby causing disorders of sodium concentration namely hyponatremia and hypernatremia. The two significant factors affecting serum osmolality are intake of water and amount of circulating vasopressin in blood faults in any of them results in sodium imbalance. Normal plasma osmolality is 275–290 mOsmol/kg. To upkeep the normal osmolality, water intake and elimination need to be balanced. Intake of water is controlled by thirst mechanisms that depend on osmoreceptors present in hypothalamus which further stimulate thirst when plasma osmolality reaches 295 mOsmol/kg. The excretion of water is regulated by antidiuretic hormone (ADH) that is produced in hypothalamus and stored in posterior pituitary. The components manipulating ADH secretion are thirst, changes in plasma osmolality, and baroreceptor stimulation. Slight contribution

to hyponatremia is by low intake of solutes. Although largely it is a consequence of abnormal water homeostasis that may be either due to:
- Increase in vasopressin concentration in blood
- Increase sensitivity of vasopressin in renal tubules
- Increase intake of free water

CLINICAL FEATURES

- Acute hyponatremia
  - Cerebral edema
  - Acute hyponatremic encephalopathy
  - Nausea, headache, and vomiting
  - Seizures, brainstem herniation
  - Coma, and finally death
  - Normocapnic or hypercapnic respiratory failure
- Chronic hyponatremia
  - Nausea, vomiting, confusion
  - Seizures
  - Gait defects with increase in falls and cognitive deficits
  - Increase in risk of fracture

Mild	Moderate	Severe
Anorexia	Personality changes	Drowsiness
Headache	Muscle cramps	Diminished reflexes
Nausea	Muscle weakness	Convulsions
Vomiting	Confusion	Coma
Lethargy	Ataxia	Death

DIAGNOSIS (FLOWCHART 1)

History and physical examination: The key aspects of the history and physical examination directed toward determining the cause of hyponatremia are as follows:
- Recent surgery
- Use of mannitol, glycerol, or intravenous immune globulin
- A history suggestive of fluid loss (vomiting, diarrhea, or diuretic therapy) that may point to hypovolemia or, on examination, signs of extracellular volume depletion, such as reduced skin turgor, a low jugular venous pressure, or orthostatic hypotension, although none of these are classical of hypovolemia
- Low protein consumption and/or high fluid consumption
- Any history suggestive of malignancy, central nervous system disease, pulmonary disease, HIV, heart failure, hepatic failure, obstructive jaundice or a plasma cell disorder.
- Signs of peripheral edema and/or ascites, which can be due to heart failure, cirrhosis, or kidney failure.
- Symptoms and signs indicating adrenal insufficiency or hypothyroidism.
- History of hyponatremia episodes

Hyponatremia

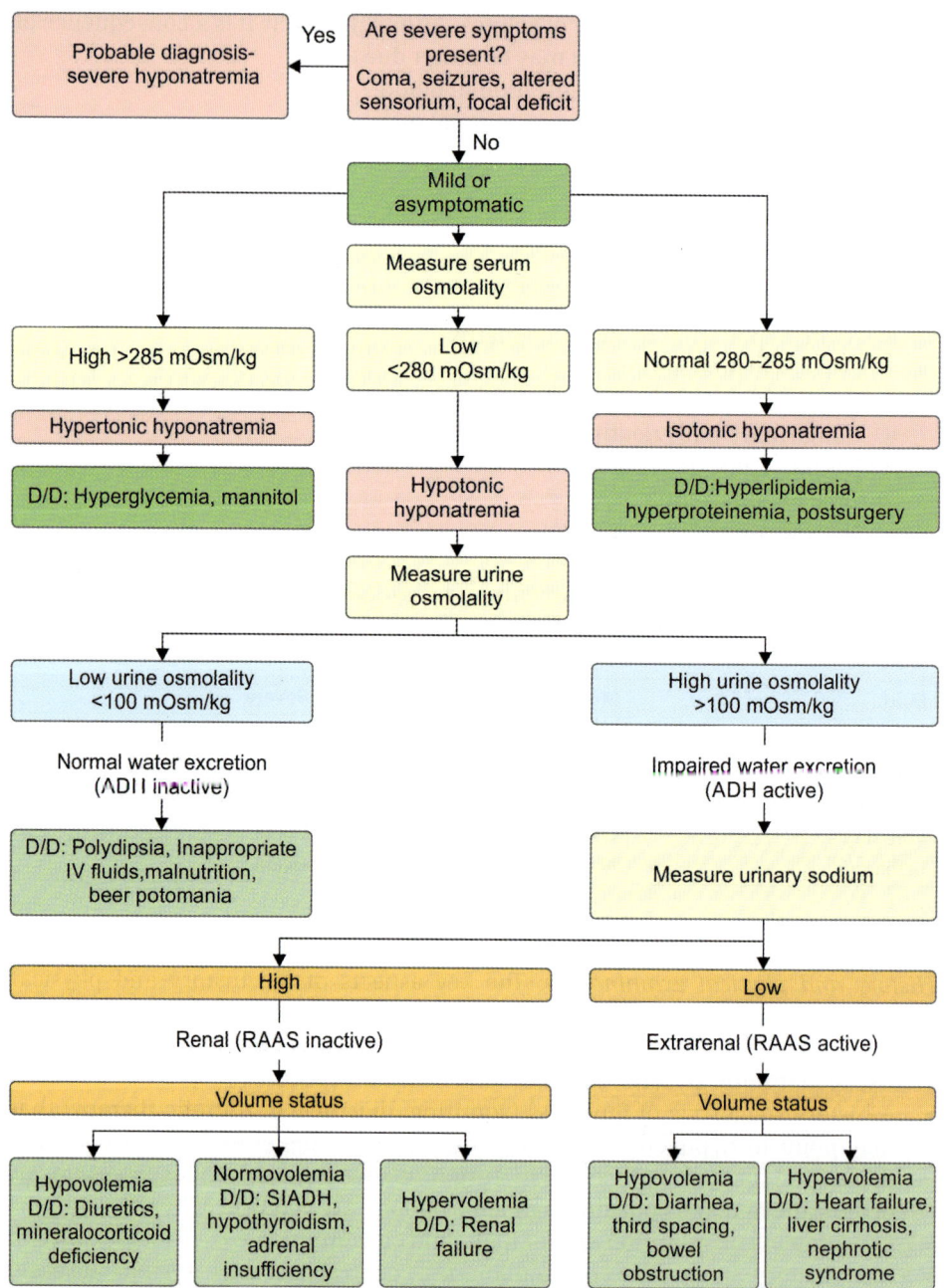

FLOWCHART 1: Approach to differential diagnosis of hyponatremia.
(D/D: differential diagnosis; RAAS: renin–angiotensin–aldosterone system)

Evaluation of the rapidity of the start of hyponatremia (if possible) and the severity of symptoms due to hyponatremia helps guide the line to therapy. Even though the history and examination offer significant clues to the cause of hyponatremia, recognition of subtle degrees of volume depletion or edema may be hard, and the history may not always reveal poor dietary protein intake or polydipsia.

Initially testing: Some laboratory tests are typically accessible at the time when hyponatremia is diagnosed, and these provide important initial information in the differential diagnosis. These include serum glucose, serum creatinine, serum potassium and bicarbonate levels. These tests are typically part of a basic metabolic panel that also comprises the serum sodium, chloride, and urea concentrations. If severe hypertriglyceridemia is present, the clinical laboratory may account the serum to be lipemic; this information suggests the likelihood of isotonic hyponatremia. When hyponatremia is first identified, results of a complete blood counts, liver function tests (alanine transaminase, aspartate aminotransferase, bilirubin, albumin), and the serum calcium may already be known. Any abnormality in these values can seldom point to an underlying illness that is causing or leading to development of hyponatremia.

When to calculate the serum osmolality: The serum osmolality, which typically ranges from 275 to 290 mOsmol/kg, is not a mandatory part of the diagnostic approach in all patients of hyponatremia; rather, it is measured in certain specific clinical scenarios.

Serum tonicity or the effective serum osmolality, is the parameter detected by osmoreceptors; serum tonicity regulates the transcellular distribution of water. Water can easily cross almost all cell membranes through aquaporin channels and shifts from an area of lower tonicity (higher water content) to an area of higher tonicity (lower water content). Tonicity is not instantly measured but is deduced from other laboratory measurements. The main difference between tonicity and osmolality is that tonicity exhibits the concentration of solutes that do not easily cross cell membranes (mostly sodium salts) and therefore affect the flow of water between cells and the extracellular fluid. By contrast, osmolality also comprises the osmotic contributions of urea and ethanol or other alcohols or glycols, which are considered "ineffective" osmoles since they can equilibrize across the cell membrane and therefore have slight effect on movement of water.

Hyperglycemia is a common cause of hypertonic hyponatremia. In patients with normal serum glucose, or in those whose serum sodium remains low after correcting for hyperglycemia, the serum osmolality should be measured if other causes of isotonic or hypertonic hyponatremia are suspected.

Ineffective osmoles: The measured serum osmolality can sometimes be misrepresentative, indicating a diagnosis of hypertonic hyponatremia or isotonic hyponatremia in a patient who instead has hypotonic hyponatremia. This most commonly occurs with:
- *Azotemia*: Patients with advanced kidney disease may develop hyponatremia because their reduced kidney function impairs their ability to excrete excess water. While the low serum sodium concentration will tend to reduce the serum osmolality, this effect is compensated to a variable degree by azotemia, which enhances the osmolality. Thus, the measured osmolality may be normal or elevated. However, despite the fact that high urea concentrations raise the osmolality, they do not change the tonicity. In contrast to sodium and glucose,

urea is an ineffective osmole since it can freely cross cell membranes and therefore does not force water movement out of cells. Hence, patients with hyponatremia and renal failure have a lesser effective serum osmolality (i.e., a low tonicity) that becomes apparent if the calculated osmolality is adjusted for the effect of urea:

$$\text{Tonicity} = \text{Measured serum osmolality} - (\text{BUN} / 2.8)$$

Dividing the blood urea nitrogen (BUN) by 2.8 converts mg/dL of urea nitrogen into mmol/L of urea, which is essential when measuring osmolality. If blood urea is measured in mmol/L, the formula is:

$$\text{Tonicity} = \text{Measured serum osmolality} - \text{Blood urea concentration}$$

- *Alcohol intoxication*: True hyponatremia is frequent in alcoholic patients. The decrease in the plasma osmolality resulting from low serum sodium concentration can be balanced in some patients by high circulating levels of ethanol. Ethanol, like urea, is an ineffective osmole since it can easily cross cell membranes and so does not force water movement out of cells. Thus, alcoholic patients with hyponatremia may have a low serum sodium concentration and a low calculated serum osmolality, but a measured osmolality that is not low. The reason for the gap between the calculated and measured serum osmolality becomes evident when the blood alcohol level is checked.

$$\text{Tonicity} = \text{Measured serum osmolality} - [\text{Ethanol}]/3.7$$

Patients who might have pseudohyponatremia. Hyperlipidemia or hyperproteinemia lowers the serum sodium concentration (and therefore the calculated serum osmolality) when it is measured with certain analyzers. Since point-of-care devices are not influenced by this laboratory artifact, a variation among the serum sodium concentration determined by a point-of-care device and the sodium concentration determined by a laboratory should imply the possibility of pseudohyponatremia.

Patients with potentially normal or elevated plasma tonicity: The majority of hyponatremic patients have hypotonic hyponatremia. However, the history, examination, and laboratory studies that are obtainable initially can designate whether a patient with hyponatremia might have pseudohyponatremia or hypertonic or isotonic hyponatremia, rather than hypotonic hyponatremia. As examples, patients with lipemic serum, obstructive jaundice, or a history of monoclonal gammopathy may have pseudohyponatremia, whereas patients with severe hyperglycemia or a history of recent surgery may have hypertonic or isotonic hyponatremia.

■ SEVEN STEPS APPROACH TO INPATIENT HYPONATREMIA

1. *Decide hyponatremia is true or pseudohyponatremia*, as in hyperlipidemia and hyperproteinemia. There is no true reduction in total sodium in pseudohyponatremia.
2. *Calculate plasma osmolality:* Normal 275–290 mOsm/kg; normal or high plasma osmolality may be because of translocational (glucose, mannitol, glycine,

maltose) or pseudohyponatremia (proteins/lipids). The low plasma osmolality is hyponatremia.
3. *Duration of hyponatremia*: Acute <48 h; chronic >48 h. This will help in deciding treatment.
4. *Is patient symptomatic?:* Moderate severe/severe hyponatremia, according to symptoms, are symptoms truly related to hyponatremia? This step will help decide rapidity of treatment.
5. *Volume status:* Get urinary spot osmolarity (<100/>100), Urinary spot sodium (<30/>30) done. This will help in diagnosis and management.
6. *Rule out hypothyroidism and adrenal insufficiency* at this level if diagnosis not achieved.
7. If SIADH: What caused the SIADH?

MANAGEMENT

I. **Start resuscitation**
   - Assess and secure the airway in a patient with severe hyponatremia who cannot maintain airway.
   - Put a peripheral line and resuscitate with suitable fluids.
   - In the hyponatremia patient, initial fluid resuscitation should be done cautiously.

II. **History and physical examination**
   - To assess severity of hyponatremia and urgency of correction.
   - Pay immediate attention to neurological symptoms such as disorientation, drowsiness, impaired consciousness, or seizures irrespective of duration of hyponatremia.
   - Other symptoms of hyponatremia are anorexia, nausea, dizziness, and lack of balance.
   - Examine previous records of serum sodium to assess chronicity.
   - Take drug history, especially for thiazide diuretics.
   - Ask for history suggestive of fluid loss such as vomiting, diarrhea, or excessive water intake.
   - Check for pedal edema, ascites, and pleural effusion.

III. **Look for the cause**
   - Assess volume status, measure serum and urine osmolality, and measure spot urine sodium
   - Calculate serum osmolality:

     $$- 2 \times [Na] + [glucose\ mg/dL]/18 + [BUN\ mg/dL]/2.8$$

   - Normal: 275–290 mOsm/kg
   - Serum osmolarity should always be measured rather than calculated to differentiate hypo-, hyper-, and iso-osmolar types of hyponatremias.
   - A patient with true hyponatremia will have low serum osmolarity.
   - Urine osmolality <100 mOsm/kg: with low serum osmolarity: suggests excess water intake.

152 Hyponatremia

- Urine osmolality >100 mOsm/kg: impaired renal excretion of water (e.g., congestive heart failure, liver cirrhosis, prerenal renal failure) or salt (e.g., salt loosing nephropathy).
- Urine osmolality may be calculated by the last two digits of urine specific gravity × 30.
- Measure spot urine sodium: Less than 20 mEq/L or more than 20 mEq/L.
- Measurement of spot urinary sodium and assessment of the volume status can help to know the etiology.

IV. Assess severity
- Mild hyponatremia: 130–135 mmol/L
- Moderate hyponatremia: 125–130 mmol/L
- Severe hyponatremia: Less than 125 mmol/L

V. Investigate further
Apart from serum osmolality, urine osmolality, and urinary sodium, send additional investigations to determine the origin and severity of hyponatremia.
- Serum K, Cl, bicarbonate
- Serum glucose, urea, creatinine, total proteins, triglycerides, uric acid
- Arterial blood gases
- Serum TSH
- Cortisol
- Urine—creatinine, uric acid
- Fractionated excretion of sodium (FE Na) = (U Na × P Cr)/(P Na × U Cr) × 100

VI. Correct sodium
- Treatment of hyponatremia must be individualized
- Factors to be considered are as follows:
  - Severity
  - Duration
  - Symptoms
- Risks of treatment (osmotic demyelination) should be balanced against benefit. Speedy correction of sodium is the most important risk factor for the development of osmotic demyelination syndrome.

VII. Fix the rate of correction
- In asymptomatic patients, the rate of correction should not be >0.5–1.00 mEq/L/h and <8 mEq over the first 24 h.
- Avoid overcorrection of serum sodium concentration.
- In symptomatic patients, sodium may be corrected at the rate of 1–2 mEq/L for an initial few hours or till seizure subsides.

VIII. To calculate sodium deficit and rate of rise of sodium

$$\text{Sodium deficit} = \text{Total body water (TBW)} \times (\text{desired serum Na} - \text{measured serum Na})$$

$$\text{TBW} = \text{Body weight (kg)} \times Y$$

The major use of this formula is in the volume depletion state and in SIADH to approximate the initial rate of administration of fluids.

Hyponatremia

For example, in a 70-kg woman with a serum sodium of 118 mEq/L with a goal of increasing sodium by 7 mEq/L in first 24 h,

$$\text{Sodium deficit} = (70 \times 0.5) \times (125-118) = 245 \text{ mEq}.$$

Hypertonic saline (3%) contains around 500 mEq of sodium per liter or 1 mEq per 2 mL. So, 480 mL (approximately 240 mEq of sodium) of hypertonic saline given over 24 h or 20 mL/h will raise serum sodium by 7 mEq (from 118 to 125 mEq/L in 24 h or 0.25 mEq/h).

This should be verified by sequential measurements of serum sodium.

$$\text{Increase in serum sodium by any fluid} = (\text{infusate sodium} - \text{serum sodium})/\text{TBW} + 1.$$

In cases when potassium is added to intravenous fluid, increase in serum sodium = [(infusate sodium + potassium) − (serum sodium)]/TBW + 1.

For example, in a 70-kg woman with a serum sodium of 112 mEq/L, if 1 L of isotonic saline (containing 154 mEq/L of sodium) is administered, the estimated rise of serum sodium will be (154 − 112)/(35+ 1) = 1.16 mEq/L.

That is, serum sodium will be 113.16 mEq/L after giving 1 L of normal saline.

Rule of thumb:
- For hypertonic (3%) saline
    Infusion rate = weight (kg) × preferred rate of correction

For example, to correct at 1 mEq/L/h in a 60-kg person,
    Infusion rate = 60 × 1 = 60 mL/h.

To correct at 0.5 mEq/L/h in a 80-kg person,
    Infusion rate = 80 × 0.5 = 40 mL/h.

- For isotonic (0.9%) saline – it corrects 1–2 mEq/L for every 1 L of NaCl

Sodium levels should always be verified by repeated sodium measurement to keep a check on the rise of sodium.

IX. **To know the underlying cause**
- **Euvolemic, hypo-osmolar, hyponatremia**
    - *Consider SIADH*
        - Clinical euvolumia
        - Urine osmolality >300 mOsm/kg
        - Urinary sodium level >40 mmol/L
        - Normal RFT, LFT
        - Normal adrenal, and thyroid function tests
        - Serum osmolality <275 mOsm/kg
        - Serum sodium <134 mEq/L
        - In severely symptomatic patients: Give 3% hypertonic saline and check serum sodium frequently
        - In asymptomatic and mildly symptomatic patients:
            - Restrict total water intake approximately to 600–1,000 mL/day (intake = 50% of output).

- Addition of salt to diet.
- Loop diuretics can be added if urine output is very low.
- Consider vasopressin antagonist (Vaptans), if available.
- Demeclocycline 600–1,200 mg/day.
  - In all cases of SIADH, correction of the underlying cause and withdrawal of any offending drug is necessary.
  - Additional causes of euvolemic, hypo-osmolar hyponatremia such as hypothyroidism, adrenal insufficiency, renal failure, and psychogenic polydipsia should be treated by water restriction, hormone replacement, and correcting the underlying disease
- **Hypervolemic, hypo-osmolar, hyponatremia**
  - Consider edematous states such as cirrhosis, nephrotic syndrome, cardiac failure, and renal failure.
  - Managed by fluid restriction, loop diuretics, treating the underlying disease, avoiding extra sodium
- **Hypovolemic, hypo-osmolar, hyponatremia**
  - Consider the volume-depleted state (renal or extrarenal).
  - Managed by volume replacement and treating the underlying disease
  - *Diuretic-induced hyponatremia*
    - May mimic SIADH, as it may be clinically euvolemic
    - Occurs mostly with thiazide diuretics, may occur within a few days of starting diuretics
    - Elderly patients with lesser body mass are more vulnerable
    - Could be associated with high water intake
    - Managed by withdrawal of diuretics, isotonic or hypertonic saline, in symptomatic cases.
    - At more risk of rapid correction after stoppage of diuretics. Therefore, watchful monitoring is required to prevent osmotic demyelination.
  - *Cerebral salt wasting*
    - It may mimic SIADH due to similar lab parameters.
    - Hyponatremia with a low plasma osmolality.
    - An inappropriately high urine osmolality (>100 mOsm/kg and often >300 mOsm/kg).
    - A urine sodium level >40 mEq/L.
    - Much less common than SIADH.
    - Occurs with acute CNS disease, mainly subarachnoid hemorrhage.
    - Clinically hypovolemic. Normal serum uric acid. Increased fractional excretion of urate.
    - Treat the underlying causes of CSW such as subarachnoid hemorrhage.
    - Insert central line to check volume status.
    - Volume replacement—match urine loss.
    - Amount of sodium required = sodium deficit × total body water

Differentiating cerebral salt wasting (CSW) versus SIADH.		
	CSW	SIADH
Plasma volume	Decreased	Normal or increased

Salt balance	Negative	Normal
Water balance	Negative	Increased or no change
Signs of dehydration	Present	Absent
Weight	Decreased	Increased or no change
CVP	Decreased	Increased or normal
HCT	Increased	Increased or normal
BUN	Increased	Normal
Total protein	Increased	Normal
Potassium	Increased or no change	Decreased or no change
Uric acid	Normal	Decreased

- **Hyperosmolar hyponatremia**
  - Consider hypertonic mannitol or other osmotic agents and hyperglycemia.
  - Stop infusion.
  - Hyperglycemia—stop or decrease glucose administration.
  - Give insulin and fluids.
  - Target a drop in glucose concentration of 75–100 mg/dL/h.
- **Iso-osmolar hyponatremia**

  Consider pseudohyponatremia (drip arm sample, hyperlipidemia, paraproteinemia); usually asymptomatic and no treatment is required.

CONCLUSION

Hyponatremia is a very common and often missed problem in clinical practice. It is associated with a high mortality and morbidity if diagnosis is missed. Immediate assessment for etiology and severity is necessary to choose appropriate treatment. Treatment mainly consists of treating underlying disorder and water restriction in some cases. Vaptans have limited role in some chronic hyponatremias, without major mortality and morbidity benefits. Early recognition improves outcome and survival.

SUGGESTED READINGS

1. Harrison's Principles of Internal Medicine 21st Edition.
2. ICU Protocols 2020. Vol 2.
3. Practical Guidelines on Fluid Therapy Pandya 2nd Ed.
4. Clinical practice guideline on diagnosis and treatment of hyponatremia. Nephrol Dial Transplant. 2014; 29 (Suppl. 2): ii1-39.
5. Diagnosis and Management of Sodium Disorders: Hyponatremia and Hypernatremia. Am Fam Physician. 2015;91(5):299-307.
6. Clinical practice guideline on diagnosis and treatment of hyponatraemia. European Journal of Endocrinology. 2014;170:G1-47.

CHAPTER 12

Rational for Antibiotics: Guidelines

Mangesh Tiwaskar, Tanuja Manohar

INTRODUCTION

Antibiotics are regarded as one of the wonder discoveries of the twentieth century. It has transformed medicine in many respects and saved countless lives. Unfortunately, the use of these wonder drugs has been accompanied by the rapid appearance of resistant strains. The overuse of antibiotics has resulted in microorganisms developing multiple mechanisms of resistance to each and every antibiotic. This resistance of microorganisms to antibiotics is a critical health issue and has advanced to become a worldwide health threat. Infections which are resistant to antibiotics manifest potentially devastating effects on public health. As a result, appropriate and conservative use of antibiotics is the need of the hour. The goal of this article is to highlight the importance of rationalizing the antibiotic usage so as to ensure the availability of this precious resource for future generations.

AN OVERVIEW OF BACTERIAL INFECTION

Bacteria, ubiquitous in nature, play an important role in maintaining the environment in which we reside. Only a small percentage of the world's bacteria cause infection and disease. Bacteria are grouped as gram positive and gram negative based on the characteristics of their cell wall, as observed under a microscope after Gram staining (developed by HC Gram in 1882). Some bacteria which cannot be classified by Gram staining, e.g., mycobacteria, requires special staining. Bacteria can also be classified as aerobes, obligate aerobes, facultative anaerobes, and obligate anaerobes, based on their need for oxygen to grow.

Clinical Manifestations of Bacterial Infections

The human body, which contains about 10^{13} cells, routinely harbors about 10^{14} bacteria called as normal microbial flora. Though all of the human organs are susceptible to bacterial infection, most often microorganisms stay in harmony with the host through mutual or commensal interactions. Each bacterial species has a predilection to infect certain organs and not others. For example, *Neisseria meningitidis* usually infects the meninges of the central nervous system causing meningitis or can infect the lungs causing pneumonia, however, it does not cause skin infection.

Infectious disease is the clinically evident illness (viz. signs and symptoms) resulting from the infection, presence and growth of pathogenic bacterial agents in an individual host organism. The list of microorganisms infecting different sites of the human body are mentioned in **Figure 1**.

ANTIBIOTICS—A BOON TO MANKIND

Infection was a major cause of morbidity and mortality, prior to the development of antibiotics. The treatment of infections faced a great challenge during those periods. Later in 1928, the discovery of penicillin, a beta-lactam antibiotic, by Alexander Fleming opened up the golden era of antibiotics. It marked a revolution in the treatment of infectious diseases and stimulated new efforts to synthesize newer antibiotics. The period between 1950s and 1970s is considered the golden era of discovery of novel antibiotic classes, with very few classes discovered since then. **Table 1** enlists the different antibiotic classes with its mode of action and target infectious microorganisms.

Antibiotics have played a vital role in achieving major advances in medicine and surgery. It has successfully prevented or treated infections that occur in patients with chronic diseases such as diabetes; end-stage renal disease or rheumatoid arthritis; complex surgeries such as organ transplants, joint replacements, or cardiac surgery; and in patients with chemotherapy treatments. Studies with antibiotics have also shown unexpected nonantibiotic effects that indicate a variety

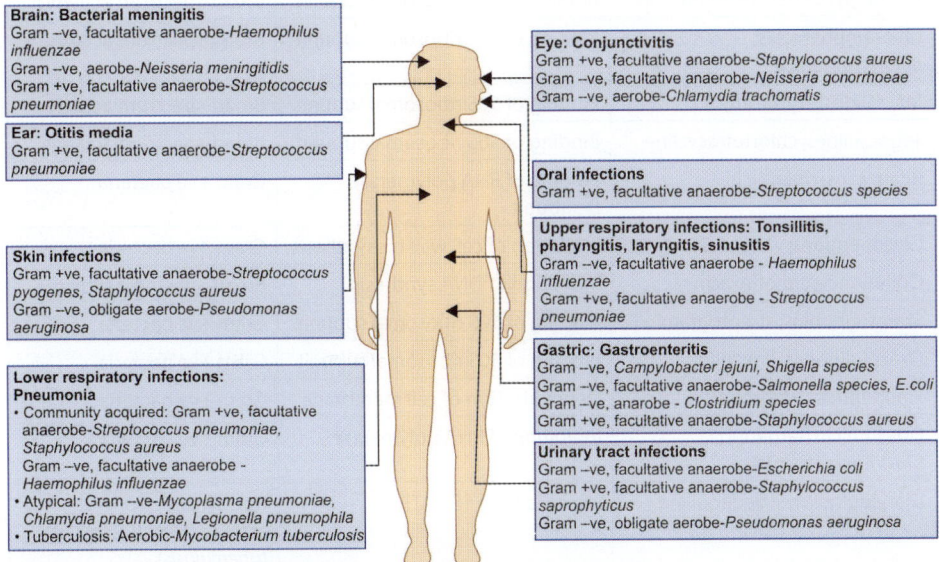

FIG. 1: Overview of bacterial infection.

(Gram -ve: gram-negative organism; Gram +ve: gram-positive organism)

of other biological activities. The results exhibited a significant number of additional therapeutic applications of "antibiotics" as antiviral, antitumor, or anticancer agents. In some cases, the alternative administrations have surpassed those of antibiotic activity in importance, such as in the treatment of cardiovascular disease or use as immunosuppressive agents. Unfortunately, the enormous requirement of these valuable drugs had a significant downside.

ANTIBIOTIC RESISTANCE—MAGIC BULLETS AND MOVING TARGETS

The successful use of any therapeutic agent is always followed by the potential development of resistance to that agent from the time it is first employed. Alexander Fleming, who won a Nobel Prize for his discovery of penicillin, had warned about the perils of antibiotic resistance. True to this prediction, resistance began to arise within 10 years of the large scale introduction of penicillin. Initially, drug-resistant strains appeared in the hospitals, where most antibiotics were being used.

Streptococcus pyogenes resistant to sulfonamide emerged in military hospitals in the 1930s while penicillin-resistant *Staphylococcus aureus* confronted London civilian hospitals shortly after the introduction of penicillin in the 1940s. Similarly,

TABLE 1: Mode of action and target of antibiotic classes.

Antibiotic class; example	Mechanism of action	Activity or target species
Sulfa drugs; prontosil	Inhibition of dihydropteroate synthetase	Gram +ve bacteria
β-lactams; penicillin	Inhibition of cell wall biosynthesis	Broad-spectrum activity
Aminoglycosides; streptomycin	Binding of 30S ribosomal subunit	Broad-spectrum activity
Chloramphenicols; chloramphenicol	Binding of 50S ribosomal subunit	Broad-spectrum activity
Macrolides; erythromycin	Binding of 50S ribosomal subunit	Broad-spectrum activity
Tetracyclines; chlortetracycline	Binding of 30S ribosomal subunit	Broad-spectrum activity
Rifamycins; rifampicin	Binding of RNA polymerase β-subunit	Gram +ve bacteria
Glycopeptides; vancomycin	Inhibition of cell wall biosynthesis	Gram +ve bacteria
Quinolones; ciprofloxacin	Inhibition of DNA synthesis	Broad-spectrum activity
Streptogramins; streptogramin B	Binding of 50S ribosomal subunit	Gram +ve bacteria
Oxazolidinones; linezolid	Binding of 50S ribosomal subunit	Gram +ve bacteria
Lipopeptides; daptomycin	Depolarization of cell membrane	Gram +ve bacteria
Fidaxomicin (targeting *Clostridium difficile*)	Inhibition of RNA polymerase	Gram +ve bacteria
Diarylquinolines; bedaquiline	Inhibition of F1F0-ATPase	Narrow-spectrum activity (*Mycobacterium tuberculosis*)

(DNA: deoxyribonucleic acid; Gram+ve: gram-positive organism; RNA: ribonucleic acid; S: Svedberg unit)

Source: Lewis K. Platforms for antibiotic discovery. Nat Rev Drug Discov. 2013;12:371-87.

TABLE 2: Modes of resistance of commonly used antibiotics.	
Antibiotic class (examples)	Mode(s) of resistance
β-Lactams (penicillins, cephalosporins, carbapenems, monobactams)	Hydrolysis, efflux, and altered target
Aminoglycosides (gentamicin, streptomycin, spectinomycin)	Phosphorylation, acetylation, nucleotidylation, efflux, and altered target
Glycopeptides (vancomycin, teicoplanin)	Reprogramming peptidoglycan biosynthesis
Tetracyclines (minocycline, tigecycline)	Monooxygenation, efflux, and altered target
Macrolides (erythromycin, azithromycin)	Hydrolysis, glycosylation, phosphorylation, efflux, and altered target
Lincosamides (clindamycin)	Nucleotidylation, efflux, and altered target
Streptogramins (synercid)	C-0 lyase (type B streptogramins), acetylation (type A streptogramins), efflux, and altered target
Oxazolidinones (linezolid)	Efflux and altered target
Phenicols (chloramphenicol)	Acetylation, efflux, and altered target
Quinolones (ciprofloxacin)	Acetylation, efflux, and altered target
Pyrimidines (trimethoprim)	Efflux and altered target
Sulfonamides (sulfamethoxazole)	Efflux and altered target
Rifamycins (rifampin)	ADP-ribosylation, efflux, and altered target
Lipopeptides (daptomycin)	Altered target
Cationic peptides (colistin)	Altered target and efflux

Source: Davies J, Davies D. Origins and Evolution of Antibiotic Resistance. Microbiol Mol Biol Rev. 2010;74(3):417-33.

streptomycin-resistant *Mycobacterium tuberculosis* appeared in the community soon after the discovery of this antibiotic. Over the years, more and more microorganisms, exposed to more and more antibiotics, eventually developed resistance to nearly all antibiotics that have been developed. **Table 2** enlists the resistance mechanisms of commonly used antibiotics. As a result, the optimism during the initial period of antibiotic discovery was tempered by the appearance of therapeutic resistant bacterial strains.

FACTORS INTENSIFYING ANTIBIOTIC RESISTANCE

Irrational use of antibiotics contributes to dramatically increasing antibiotic resistance. Irrational antibiotic use is a worldwide problem that causes significant mortality, morbidity, and increased healthcare costs. Following are some of the factors that drive antibiotic resistance:
- *Clinical overprescription and public misconceptions*: There are a plethora of ways by which humans have inadvertently escalated the evolution of resistance. Inappropriate prescriptions and over use of antibiotics contributed to the promotion of bacterial resistance. Worldwide, it has been evaluated that half of all medicines are prescribed, dispensed or sold inappropriately, and that half of all patients fail to take their medicine properly. An estimated two-thirds of global antibiotic sales occur without any prescription, while studies in Indonesia,

Pakistan, and India show that over 70% of patients are prescribed antibiotics. A vast majority—up to 90%—of injections are estimated to be administered unnecessarily. The determinants of irrational antibiotic use are mentioned below:
- *Very short consultation time*: Does not allow proper diagnosis
- *Prescription of antibiotics for nonbacterial infections*: Clinicians prescribe antibiotics to patients with nonbacterial infections, a practice that has important repercussions
- *Polypharmacy*: Too many medicines are prescribed per patient (lack of trust in or delayed laboratory results, fear of clinical failure)
- Antibiotic injections are used where oral formulations would be more appropriate
- Prolonged prophylactic therapy
- Prolonged empiric antimicrobial treatment without clear evidence of infection
- Failure to narrow antimicrobial therapy when a causative organism is identified
- Prescriptions do not follow clinical guidelines
- Patients self-medicate inappropriately
- Patients do not adhere to prescribed treatment

Antibiotic overprescribing is associated with other problems, apart from spreading resistance, *viz.,* increased medicalization of self-limiting infectious conditions, increase of more severe diseases, length of disease, risk of complications, mortality rate, healthcare costs, risk of adverse effects, and reattendance due to infectious diseases.

- *Misuse by the food industry*: The use of antibiotics in animal feed stocks has also aggravated the spread of resistance. Especially, their use for noncurative reasons such as prophylaxis, metaphylaxis and growth promotion accounted for up to 50% of all antibiotic consumption in the early 2000s.
- *Diminished pharmaceutical investment*: Antibiotic development is no longer considered to be an economically wise investment for the pharmaceutical industry as they are not as profitable as drugs that treat chronic conditions, such as diabetes, psychiatric disorders, asthma, or gastroesophageal reflux. Additionally, regulatory hurdles have also muted the interest of major pharmaceutical companies.
- *Human-independent resistance*: Though there is a pronounced human contribution to the evolution of bacterial resistance, there is also resistance that occurs in nature in the absence of human interference. Bacteria can be either intrinsically resistant to certain antibiotics or can also acquire resistance to antibiotics.

The legacy of the past decades in terms of antibiotic use and misuse has added to the development of bacterial resistance toward multiple drugs.

SUPERBUGS AND SUPER-RESISTANCE

Many of the bacterial pathogens related with the epidemics of human disease, subsequent to antibiotic use, have evolved into multidrug-resistant (MDR) forms.

The term "superbugs" refers to microorganisms with heightened morbidity and mortality due to multiple mutations conferring high levels of resistance to the antibiotic classes specifically recommended for their treatment.

- *Staphylococcus aureus (MRSA, VISA, and VRSA)*: S. aureus, a gram positive, facultative anaerobic pathogen with both hospital- and community-acquired strains, is one among the most notorious superbugs. Following the discovery of penicillin, it seemed that S. aureus infections were controllable; however, it proved to be a short-lived one. The landmark discovery and introduction of methicillin was anticipated to be a sure defense against the penicillinases, but the appearance of methicillin-resistant S. aureus (MRSA) within 3 years inexorably led to other multiantibiotic-resistant variants. MRSA is resistant to certain antibiotics, such as methicillin, dicloxacillin, oxacillin, cloxacillin, nafcillin, and closely related classes of drugs, such as cephalosporins. The use of more powerful drugs than necessary for less serious infections could be a cause of MRSA expansion. The development of resistance has led to the frequent use of vancomycin to treat MRSA infections. This greatly increased selective pressure has resulted in the emergence of MRSA isolates with reduced susceptibility to vancomycin [vancomycin-intermediate S. aureus (VISA) strains] and to the appearance of vancomycin-resistant S. aureus (VRSA) strains with high-level resistance to vancomycin.
- *Resistant Enterococci including VRE*: Resistant *Enterococci* primarily comprises of two species, E. faecalis and E. faecium, both of which are gram positive, facultative anaerobic, and opportunistic pathogens. Both E. faecalis and E. faecium have high levels of resistance rates (30–50%) against the aminoglycosides gentamicin and streptomycin.
  - *Streptococcus pneumoniae*: S. pneumoniae is a gram-positive, aerotolerant, anaerobic, and opportunistic pathogen. It has a polysaccharide capsule that makes it naturally resistant to phagocytes. About 40% of strains are no longer susceptible to penicillin, and its penicillin resistance often correlates with resistances to macrolides, sulfamides, older tetracyclines, and early generation cephalosporins. The strain is also resistant toward the third-generation antibiotics.
  - *Clostridium difficile*: C. difficile is a gram-positive, obligate anaerobic, and spore-forming opportunistic pathogen. C. difficile can be community acquired, but has a particularly high rate of acquisition in hospitals. Patients hospitalized for over 4 weeks have an approximately 50% chance of contracting C. difficile, a known causative agent for antibiotic-associated diarrhea. A study by *Pepin J et al.* showed that administration of fluoroquinolones emerged as the most important risk factor for C. difficile-associated diarrhea caused by a hypervirulent strain of C. difficile.
- *β-lactam and quinolone-resistant Enterobacter*: *Enterobacter* is a genus of gram negative, facultative anaerobic, and opportunistic pathogens. They are mainly known to exhibit antibiotic resistance through expression of an extensive variety of extended spectrum β-lactamases (ESBLs) and carbapenems including, *Klebsiella pneumoniae* carbapenemase, oxacillinases, and several metallo-β-lactamases (MBLs).

TABLE 3: Resistance mechanisms of *Pseudomonas aeruginosa*.	
Upregulation efflux pumps	Resistant to antibiotics
MexEF-OprN	Carbapenems and fluoroquinolones
MexCD-OprJ	Fluoroquinolones and some β-lactams
MexAB-OprM	Sulfonamides, β-lactams, cephalosporins, fluoroquinolones, macrolides, novobiocin, tetracycline, and chloramphenicol
MexXY-OprM	Aminoglycoside

Source: Adapted from Fair RJ, Toi Y. Antibiotics and Bacterial Resistance in the 21st Century. Perspect Medicin Chem. 2014;6:25-64.

- *MDR Pseudomonas aeruginosa*: *P. aeruginosa* is a gram-negative, facultative anaerobic, and opportunistic pathogen. It naturally has a host of siderophores (Fe^{3+} carriers) and pigments that allow it to evade the innate immune system. Furthermore, it has particularly discriminating outer membrane porins that make its outer membrane impermeable and thus naturally resistant to many antibiotics. It has a high propensity to form biofilms that can increase resistances to antibiotics by 100, to 1,000-fold. *P. aeruginosa* also has an extremely comprehensive efflux pump system. Upregulation of the efflux pumps results in resistance to an array of antibiotics **(Table 3)**.
- *Resistant Escherichia coli*: Antibiotic resistance of *E. coli* has risen rapidly due to horizontal gene transfer. ESBL positive strains in bacteraemia have shown high cross resistance to cephalosporins, fluoroquinolones, and gentamicin. *E. coli* strains in multiple continents have also acquired the New Delhi metallo-β-lactamase-1 (NDM-1) enzyme from *Klebsiella pneumoniae*, which confers a broad resistance to all β-lactams including carbapenems except for monobactam and aztreonam.

Multidrug-resistant *Acinetobacter*, MDR and Pan-drug-resistant *Klebsiella pneumoniae*, resistant *Neisseria Gonorrhoeae, and Mycobacterium tuberculosis* (MDR-TBTB and XDR-TBTB) are the other vital resistant bacteria dominating the headlines of alarming resistance.

The growing numbers of antimicrobial-resistant pathogens place a significant burden on healthcare systems and have important global economic costs. It results in high mortality and morbidity rates, increased treatment costs, diagnostic uncertainties, and lack of trust in orthodox medicine. Considering the complications associated with increasing antibiotic resistance, it is high time to promote judicious and optimized use of antibiotics worldwide.

■ GUIDELINES FOR ANTIBIOTIC STEWARDSHIP

The rise of antibiotic-resistant bacteria, which represents a serious threat to public health, can be overcome by promoting the optimized use of existing antibiotic agents and preventing transmission of drug-resistant organisms through control of infection. Rationalizing the use of antibiotics is an important patient safety and public health issue in addition to being a national priority. The following guidelines can help clinicians to ensure appropriate use of antibiotic therapy.

Evaluate the Infection by Clinical Diagnosis

The communication occurring within the consultation influences the treatment decision both for and against antibiotic prescription. Initial clinical diagnosis of an infection should always precede the clinician's decision to prescribe antibiotics. The clinician should always consider whether or not antibiotic therapy is even necessary for the patient by weighing the benefits (efficacy, rapid recovery, and comfort of patient) against the risks (antibiotic resistance and adverse effects) and costs of treatment. At the same instance, clinician should also keep in mind that many infections are self-limiting and that most of the patients just require supportive therapy to deal with the symptoms. It is of utmost importance to highlight that a clinician should never prescribe antibiotics for nonbacterial infections such as cold, flu, and sore throats. Antibiotics tackle bacteria and hence should be restricted for the treatment of bacterial infections only **(Flowchart 1)**.

Select an Appropriate Antibiotic Therapy

Following a proper clinical diagnosis, a clinician should decide whether to direct a patient to a definitive therapy or an empirical therapy or a prophylactic therapy.

Definitive Therapy

When the etiology of the infection is known, the clinician should proceed with definitive therapy. Firstly, the clinician should confirm the bacterial infection by advising for a microbiological testing (staining of secretions/fluids/exudates, culture and sensitivity, serological tests, and other tests). Microbiological testing helps to identify the specific etiologic agent and provides information about the in vitro activity of antimicrobial drugs against the microorganisms identified. It also assists the clinicians to decide whether the patient should be prescribed antibiotics, as they are often under pressure from patients who believe they need antibiotics. A negative microbiology test report can make it easier for the clinician to refuse unnecessary prescription of antibiotic. Additionally, if the patient needs treatment immediately, the test results can help in choosing the most appropriate agent.

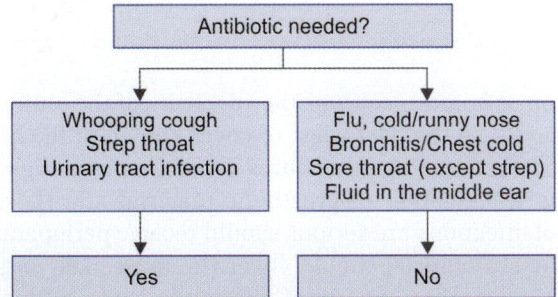

FLOWCHART 1: Common illness which requires antibiotic therapy.

Empirical Therapy

Clinician should reserve empirical therapy for critical patients, where time is inadequate for identification and isolation of the infection causing bacteria. Empiric prescribing is based on the clinician's working knowledge or experience of what is most likely to be the pathogen causing the patient's condition. For example, certain elements of the presenting illness (such as site of infection) can help the clinician to predict a broad group of pathogens such as skin and soft tissue: gram-positive cocci, urinary tract: gram-negative bacilli, intra-abdominal: gram-negative, gram-positive and anaerobic organisms. Therefore, a common approach can be prescribing a broad-spectrum antibiotic agent as initial empiric therapy with an intention to cover multiple possible pathogens commonly associated with the specific clinical syndrome.

Simultaneously, the clinician should ensure that the samples for microbiological testing are collected before starting the empirical therapy. Once microbiological results have aided in identifying the etiological agent, every attempt should be made by the clinician to narrow the spectrum of the antibiotic.

Prophylactic Therapy

Antibiotic prophylaxis should be prescribed to susceptible patients to prevent specific infections that can cause definite detrimental effects. Susceptible patients include presurgical patients, immunocompromised patients, and patients with traumatic injuries. The selection of an antibiotic for prophylaxis should be based on known or likely target pathogens, for a short duration of time. A single dose of antibiotic should be recommended for surgical prophylaxis. Long-term prophylaxis should be administered only when the benefits outweigh the risk of resistance selection or propagation.

Criteria for Choosing an Antibiotic Drug

Appropriate antibiotic selection is vital to facilitate successful treatment of infections and minimize the development of antibiotic resistance. Once the etiology of an infection is known, the clinician should recommend a most narrow spectrum antibiotic which is cost-effective and least toxic for the shortest duration possible. While prescribing an antibiotic, clinicians should consider the following treatment guidelines:

■ EFFICACY

- *Narrow spectrum or broad spectrum*: The spectrum of the antibiotic selected by the clinician should be the narrowest to cover known or likely pathogens. For instance, patients undergoing procedures associated with high infection rates, those involving implantation of prosthetic material and those in whom the consequences of infections are serious should receive perioperative antibiotics. The prophylactic antibiotic(s) should cover the most likely organisms and be present in the tissues when the initial incision is made, with adequate serum concentrations maintained during the procedure. In such situations, a single dose of a cephalosporin (such as cefazolin) administered within 1 hour before the initial incision is appropriate for most surgical procedures; this practice targets the most likely organisms (i.e., skin flora), while avoiding unnecessary broad-spectrum antimicrobial therapy.

However, in scenarios where the causative agent is not known and a delay in initiating therapy would be life-threatening or risk serious morbidity, broad-spectrum antibiotics, based on the likelihood of the pathogen(s), should be prescribed. Clinician should also make it a point to deescalate the regimen as soon as the etiological agent is known.

- *Monotherapy or combination therapy*: In order to evade antagonism between drugs and undesirable side effects of several antibiotics, it is prudent to use a single agent wherever possible in antibiotic treatment. However, there are situations when the use of an antibiotic combination is desirable. The situations are:
  - *To achieve synergistic effect against the infection*: Synergy of antimicrobial agents infers that the combined effect of the agents is greater than the sum of their independent activities when measured separately. For instance, in the treatment of serious infections for which rapid killing is essential, the combination of certain β-lactams and aminoglycosides exhibits synergistic activity against a variety of gram-positive and gram-negative bacteria (e.g., combination of penicillin and gentamicin to treat endocarditis caused by *Enterococcus* species). The addition of gentamicin to penicillin has been shown to be bactericidal, whereas penicillin alone is only bacteriostatic and gentamicin alone has no significant activity.

    Combination therapy also shortens the course of antibiotic therapy, e.g., combination of penicillin or ceftriaxone with gentamicin for 2 weeks results in more rapid clearance of the infecting microorganism as compared to penicillin or ceftriaxone alone for 4 weeks. Other combinations that act synergistically are as follows: β-lactam antibiotic + β-lactamase inhibitor, β-lactam antibiotic + glycopeptide (vancomycin/teicoplanin), and sulfamethoxazole + trimethoprim.
  - *When critically ill patients require empiric therapy before bacteriological diagnosis*: Combination therapy can be used in hospital-associated infections to ensure that at least one of the administered antibiotic agents will be active against the suspected organism(s), e.g., if a patient hospitalized for several weeks develops septic shock and the blood culture reports the growth of gram-negative bacilli, it would be appropriate to provide initial therapy with two agents that have activity against gram-negative bacilli, particularly *P. aeruginosa*, which is both a common nosocomial pathogen and frequently resistant to multiple agents. Thus in this scenario, a combination of an antipseudomonal β-lactam with a fluoroquinolone or aminoglycoside could be advisable.
  - *To extend antibiotic spectrum during polymicrobial infections*: When infections are caused by polymicrobes (more than one organism), a combination therapy can be preferred as it would extend the antimicrobial spectrum beyond that achieved by a single agent. Most intra-abdominal infections are usually caused by multiple organisms with a variety of gram-positive cocci,

gram-negative bacilli, and anaerobes. Antimicrobial combinations, such as a third-generation cephalosporin or a fluoroquinolone plus metronidazole, can be used as a potential treatment option in these cases and can sometimes be more cost-effective than a comparable single agent (e.g., a carbapenem). Bronchiectasis, peritonitis, urinary tract infections, and otitis media are the conditions considered as polymicrobial infections.
    - *To prevent the development of bacterial resistance with long-term therapy*: The development of resistant mutants in a bacterial population is the result of selective pressure from antibiotic treatment. While combining antibiotics with two different mechanisms of action, the chance of a mutant strain being resistant to both antimicrobial agents is much lower than the chance of it being resistant to either one. Additionally, use of combination therapy prevents the resistant mutant population from emerging as the dominant strain and causing therapeutic failure. This is the reason why combination therapy is considered as a standard for the treatment of infections such as tuberculosis and the human immunodeficiency virus, where treatment duration is prolonged, resistance can emerge relatively easily and therapeutic agents are limited.
- *Efficacy at the site of infection and tissue penetration*: An antibiotic which is effective at the infected site and exhibits adequate target tissue penetration should be the preferred therapy. Antimicrobial concentrations attained at some sites [namely, ocular fluid, cerebrospinal fluid (CSF), abscess cavity, prostate, and bone] are often much lower than serum levels. For example, first- and second-generation cephalosporins and macrolides are not recommended for central nervous system infections as they do not cross the blood-brain barrier. Fluoroquinolones are preferred oral agents for the treatment of prostatitis because they achieve high concentrations in the prostate. Daptomycin, an excellent bactericidal agent against gram-positive bacteria, is inactivated by the lung surfactant, hence it is not useful for the treatment of pneumonia. The tissue penetration profile of a few antibiotics are mentioned in **Table 4**.
- *Bactericidal versus bacteriostatic therapy*: An antibiotic that is able to kill an organism instead of inhibiting its growth is preferred in few clinical settings. These include infections where the site of infection is not easily penetrated, e.g., in infections such as meningitis, endocarditis, and osteomyelitis. Immunocompromised patients, in particular neutropenic patients, are also usually recommended for "cidal" therapy.

■ DOSAGE, ROUTE OF ADMINISTRATION, AND DURATION

- The clinician should consider pharmacokinetic and pharmacodynamic factors in determining the drug dose. The dosage should be high enough to ensure efficacy and minimize the risk of resistance selection, and low enough to minimize the risk of dose related toxicity.
- The clinician should ensure the most appropriate route of administration in antibiotic treatment. Oral/enteral route of administration should be preferred in patients with mild-to-moderate infections. When using oral therapy for invasive infections (such as pneumonia, pyelonephritis, or abscesses), clinicians

TABLE 4: Tissue penetration profile of few antibiotics.

Infection site	Ampicillin	Co-amoxiclav	Ceftriaxone	Aminoglycosides	Ciprofloxacin	Co-trimoxazole	Ertapenem	Meropenem	Vancomycin	Linezolid	Daptomycin
CSF	Good (in high doses)	Poor	Good (in high doses)	Poor	Good (in high doses)	Good	Poor	Good (in high doses)	Poor	Good	Poor
Lung	Good	Good	Good	Poor	Good	Good	Good	Good	Fair	Good	Poor
Soft tissue	Good	Good	Good	Fair	Good	Good	Good	Good	Poor	Good	Good
Urinary tract	Good	Fair	Good	Good (if normal GFR)	Good	Good	Good	Good	Good	Good	Good

(CSF: cerebrospinal fluid; GFR: glomerular filtration rate)

Source: Wasserman S, Boyles T, Mendelson M. (2014). A pocket guide to antibiotic prescribing for adults in South Africa. [online] Available from http://www.fidssa.co.za/Content/Documents/SAASP_Antibiotic_Guidelines_2015.pdf. [Last accessed October, 2022].

should select an agent that has excellent absorption and bioavailability (i.e., the percentage of the oral dose that is available unchanged in the serum). Examples of antibiotics with excellent bioavailability are fluoroquinolones, doxycycline, linezolid, trimethoprim-sulfamethoxazole, and metronidazole. Clinicians should reserve intravenous antibiotics for severe infection or for certain sites such as the CSF, bacteraemia, endocarditis, and bone and joint infections. New microbiological or other information (e.g., fever defervescence for at least 24 hours, marked clinical improvement; low C-reactive protein) should often permit a switch to oral antibiotic(s), or switch to an intravenous narrow spectrum alternative or cessation of antibiotics (if no infection is present).
- Antibiotic treatment should generally be continued for a maximum of 5 days or a shorter period if this is clinically appropriate; however, some specific conditions require a longer course of therapy (viz., endocarditis, osteomyelitis, etc.).

PATIENT FACTORS

The clinician should consider the age of the patient, immune status, pregnancy and lactation, associated conditions such as renal and hepatic function, epilepsy, etc., while choosing the antibacterial agent.
- *Age*: Patients at both extremes of age handle drugs differently, primarily due to differences in body size and kidney function.
- *Hepatic and renal function*: Usually, dose is reduced to prevent accumulation and toxicity in patients with reduced renal or hepatic function. However, sometimes doses might need to be increased to avoid underdosing young healthy patients with rapid renal elimination or those with rapid hepatic metabolism due to enzyme induction by concomitant use of drugs such as rifampin.
- *Pregnancy and lactation*: Human studies on safety of antibiotics in pregnancy and lactation are scarce, hence clinicians should prescribe it with utmost caution. Drugs with known toxicity or unestablished safety such as tetracyclines, quinolones, streptomycin, erythromycin, and clarithromycin are contraindicated in all trimesters while sulfa, nitrofurantoin, and chloramphenicol are contraindicated in the last trimester. Drugs with limited data on safety such as aminoglycosides, azithromycin, clindamycin, vancomycin, metronidazole, trimethoprim, rifampicin, and pyrazinamide should be used with caution when benefits overweigh the risks. Penicillins, cephalosporins, and ethambutol are safe in pregnancy. In lactating mothers, sulfa group, tetracyclines, metronidazole, nitrofurantoin, and quinolones are contraindicated.
- *Allergy or intolerance*: Clinicians should routinely obtain an evaluation of history of antibiotic allergy or intolerance.
- *Recent antibiotic use*: Eliciting a history of exposure to antimicrobial agents in the recent past (~ 3 months) can also help the clinician in selecting an antimicrobial therapy. Because the causative microorganism for a current episode of infection emerged under the selective pressure of a recently used antimicrobial agent, it is likely to be resistant to that drug and/or drug class, and an alternative agent should be used.

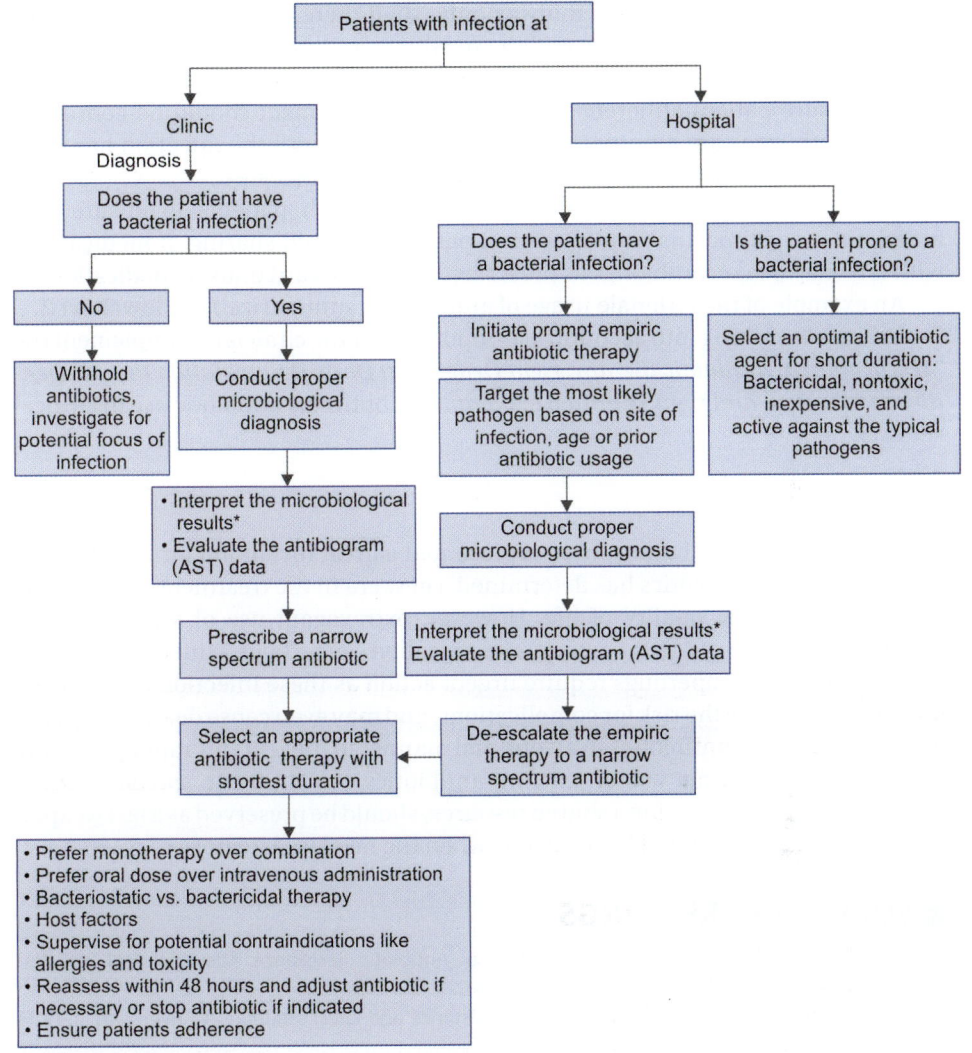

* Microbilogical testing-staining secretions/fluids/exudates, culture and sensitivity, serological tests and other tests, AST-antimicrobial susceptibility texsting

FLOWCHART 2: Summary algorithm for rational prescription of antibiotic therapy.

MONITORING RESPONSE TO THERAPY

The need for an antimicrobial therapy should be reviewed on a daily basis by reviewing laboratory evidence. Response to therapy depends on the nature and sensitivity of the agent, specificity of the drug, bioavailability, and dosage. Longer the doubling time of the organism, longer the time it takes to respond. Thus, a *Streptococcal pneumonia* can respond within 24–48 hours, but tuberculosis may take 28 weeks to respond. The clinician should wait for the adequate period before changing the drug (e.g., *Streptococcal pneumoniae* infections 24–48 hours; *E. coli* 24–48 hours; *Salmonella typhi* 4–7 days; *Mycobacterium tuberculosis* 2–8 weeks, etc.). Drugs should be changed midway only when there is absolutely no response or there is no expected response and the sensitivity report also suggests resistance. Since noncompliance is also one of the causes for treatment failure, the clinician should ensure patient adherence to the therapy. Treatment should be continued until all pathogens are eliminated from the tissues or until the infection has been sufficiently controlled for the normal host defenses to eradicate it.

Additionally, clinicians should work together with patients to ensure safe antibiotic use. Clinicians should remind patients to avoid sharing of medications with anyone, to take antibiotics as prescribed and to discard unused medication.

An example of the rationale usage of antibiotic is summarized in **Flowchart 2**.

Taking everything into account, it is important for the clinician to implement the "**4Ds** *of optimal antibiotic therapy: right* **D***rug, right* **D***ose,* **D***e-escalation to pathogen-directed therapy, and right* **D***uration of therapy*" to optimize antibiotic use in clinical settings.

CONCLUSION

Antibiotics, the magic bullets, have represented a great revolution for humankind. The discovery of antibiotics has determined a new era in the treatment of infectious diseases and in the quality of life. However, extravagant use of antibiotics has resulted in the rise of MDR bacteria, the so-called "superbugs". Infections caused by these emerging superbugs require urgent action as these infections tend to last longer, can increase the risk for complications, and may even cause death. Therefore, it is essential to use antibiotics in an optimal manner to prevent this rapidly growing issue. Only appropriate use of existing antibiotics can limit the spread of these superbugs. Antibiotics being a shared resource, should be preserved as a last weapon to treat patients and should be used only when the need is obligatory.

SUGGESTED READINGS

1. Davies J, Davies D. Origins and Evolution of Antibiotic Resistance. Microbiol Mol Biol Rev. 2010;74(3):417-33.
2. Megha MJ. Current scenario of antibiotic resistance and latest strategies to overcome it. IJCH. 2014;26(3):218-21.
3. Doron S, Gorbach SL. Bacterial infections: overview. In: Hamer D (Ed). Public Health and Infectious Diseases. United Kingdom: Elsevier Inc.; 2010. pp. 3-7.
4. Davis CP. Normal flora. In: Baron S (Ed). Medical Microbiology, 4th edition. Galveston (TX): University of Texas Medical Branch at Galveston; 1996.
5. Kumar SV, Damodar G, Ravikanth S, et al. An overview of infectious disease. Indian J Pharm Sci Res. 2012;2(2):63-74.
6. Patras K. (2013). Polymicrobial Infections: Perhaps The Rule, Not The Exception. [online] Available from http://schaechter.asmblog.org/schaechter/2013/08/polymicrobial-infections-perhaps-the-rule-not-theexception.html. [Last accessed October, 2022].
7. Pathogen Regulation Directorate. (2011). Pathogen safety data sheet-Infectious substances. [online] Available from http://www.phac-aspc.gc.ca/lab-bio/res/psds-ftss/myco-pneu-eng.php. [Last accessed October, 2022].
8. Runcie H. Infection in a pre-antibiotic era. J Anc Dis Prev Rem. 2015;3:125.
9. Centers for Disease Control and Prevention. (2016). Antibiotics: One of the Greatest Discoveries of the 20th Century. [online] Available from http://www2c.cdc.gov/podcasts/media/pdf/Antibiotics_Short.pdf. [Last accessed October, 2022].

10. Minikel E. (2015). Chemical Biology 16: Infectious Disease. [online] Available from http://www.cureffi.org/2015/11/05/chemical-biology-16/. [Last accessed October, 2022].
11. Caramia G, Ruffini E. Proper antibiotic therapy: From penicillin to pharmacogenomic. Minerva Pediatrica. 2012;64(2):225-37.
12. Aminov RI. A brief history of the antibiotic era: lessons learned and challenges for the future. Front Microbiol. 2010;1(134):1-7.
13. Lewis K. Platforms for antibiotic discovery. Nat Rev Drug Discov. 2013;12:371-87.
14. Ventola CL. The Antibiotic Resistance Crisis, Part 1: Causes and Threats. P T. 2015;40(4):277-83.
15. Bushak L. A brief history of antibiotic resistance: How a medical miracle turned into the biggest public health danger of our time. [online] Available from http://www.medicaldaily.com/antibiotic-resistancehistory-373773. [Last accessed October, 2022].
16. Rosenblatt-Farrell N. The Landscape of Antibiotic Resistance. Environ Health Perspect. 2009;117(6):A244-50.
17. Levy SB, Marshall B. Antibacterial resistance worldwide: causes, challenges and responses. Nat Med. 2004;10(2):S122-9.
18. Nanowerk. (2013). Nanotechnology solutions to combat superbugs. [online] Available from http://www.nanowerk.com/spotlight/spotid=32188.php. [Last accessed October, 2022].
19. Holloway KA. Promoting the rational use of antibiotics. Regional Health Forum 2011;15(1):122-30.
20. Fair RJ, Toi Y. Antibiotics and Bacterial Resistance in the 21st Century. Perspect Medicin Chem. 2014;6:25-64.
21. World Health Organization. (2004). The World Medicines Situation. [online] Available from http://apps.who.int/medicinedocs/en/d/Js6160e/10.html. [Last accessed October, 2022].
22. Leekha S, Terrell CL, Edson RS. General Principles of Antimicrobial Therapy. Mayo Clin Proc. 2011;86(2):156-67.
23. Ganguly NK, Arora NK, Chandy SJ, et al. Rationalizing antibiotic use to limit antibiotic resistance in India. Indian J Med Res. 2011;134(3):281-94.
24. Llor C, Bjerrum L. Antimicrobial resistance: risk associated with antibiotic overuse and initiatives to reduce the problem. Ther Adv Drug Saf. 2014;5(6):229-41.
25. Blair JMA, Webber MA, Baylay AJ, et al. Molecular mechanisms of antibiotic resistance. Nat Rev Microbiol. 2015;13:42-50.
26. Navidinia M. The clinical importance of emerging ESKAPE pathogens in nosocomial infections. J Param Sci. 2016;7(3):43-57.
27. Gardete S, Tomasz A. Mechanisms of vancomycin resistance in Staphylococcus aureus. J Clin Invest. 2014;124(7):2836-40.
28. Pépin J, Saheb N, Coulombe MA, et al. Emergence of fluoroquinolones as the predominant risk factor for Clostridium Difficile associated diarrhea: a cohort study during an epidemic in Quebec. Clin Infect Dis. 2005;41(9):1254-60.
29. Santajit S, Indrawattana N. Mechanisms of Antimicrobial Resistance in ESKAPE Pathogens. Biomed Res Int. 2016;2016:2475067.
30. Nathwani D, Sneddon J. (2013). Practical guide to antimicrobial stewardship in hospitals. [online] Available from http://bsac.org.uk/wp-content/uploads/2013/07/Stewardship-Booklet-Practical-Guide-to-AntimicrobialStewardship-in-Hospitals.pdf. [Last accessed October, 2022].
31. Centers for Disease Control and Prevention. (2013). Antibiotic Resistance Threats in the United States. [online] Available from http://www.cdc.gov/drugresistance/threat-report-2013/pdf/ar-threats-2013-508.pdf#page=6. [Last accessed October, 2022].
32. Centers for Disease Control and Prevention. Core Elements of Hospital Antibiotic Stewardship Programs. [online] Available from http://www.cdc.gov/getsmart/healthcare/implementation/core-elements.html. [Last accessed October, 2022].
33. Cabral C, Ingram J, Lucas PJ, et al. Influence of Clinical Communication on Parents' Antibiotic Expectations for Children with Respiratory Tract Infections. Ann Fam Med. 2016;14:141-7.

34. Wasserman S, Boyles T, Mendelson M. (2014). A pocket guide to antibiotic prescribing for adults in South Africa. [online] Available from http://www.fidssa.co.za/Content/Documents/SAASP_Antibiotic_Guidelines_2015.pdf. [Last accessed October, 2022].
35. Tindall WN. Modern approaches to managing bacterial infections. In: Tindall WN, Sedrak MM, Boltri JM (Eds). Patient-Centered Pharmacology: Learning System for the Conscientious Prescribe, 1st edition. Philadelphia: FA
36. Balzer D. Mayo Expert Discusses Antibiotics Overuse and Misuse. [online] Available from http://newsnetwork.mayoclinic.org/discussion/mayo-expert-discusses-antibiotics-overuse-and-misuse/. [Last accessed October, 2022].
37. Centers for Disease Control and Prevention. Antibiotics Aren't Always the Answer. [online] Available from http://www.cdc.gov/features/getsmart/. [Last accessed October, 2022].
38. Chaudhury RR, Sharma S. General principles of chemotherapy with particular reference to antimetabolites. In: Talwar GP, Hasnain SE, Sarin SK (Eds). Textbook of Biochemistry, Biotechnology, Allied and Molecular Medicine, 4th edition, New Delhi: PHI Learning Private Limited; 2016. pp. 1468-76.
39. Washington JA. Principles of diagnosis. In: Baron S (Ed). Medical Microbiology, 4th edition. Galveston (TX): University of Texas Medical Branch at Galveston; 1996.
40. Kolmos HJ, Little P. Should general practitioners perform diagnostic tests on patients before prescribing antibiotics? BMJ. 1999;318(7186):799-802.
41. Ministry of Health and Medical Services. (2011). Antibiotic Guidelines, 3rd edition. [online] Available from http://www.health.gov.fj/wp-content/uploads/2015/04/Antibiotic-Guidelines-3rdedition-2011.pdf. [Last accessed October, 2022].
42. Marcia Frellick. (2015). Clinicians and Antibiotic Prescribing: Should They Know Better? [online] Available from http://www.medscape.org/viewarticle/837039. [Last accessed October, 2022].
43. National Centre for Disease Control. (2016). National Treatment Guidelines for Antimicrobial Use in Infectious Diseases. [online] Available from http://www.ncdc.gov.in/writereaddata/linkimages/AMR_guideline7001495889.pdf [Last accessed October, 2022].
44. Jones & Bartlett Learning. General Antibiotic Prescribing Pitfalls. [online] Available from http://www.jbpub.com/physicianspress/antibioticpitfalls.htm. [Last accessed October, 2022].
45. Ernst EJ. Infectious diseases: introduction. In Richard A, Quan DJ, Herfindal ET, Gourley DR, Zeind CS, Hudson JQ, Gourley GK (Eds). Textbook of Therapeutics: Drug and Disease Management, 8th edition. Philadelphia: Lippincott Williams & Wilkins; 2006.
46. DiPiro JT. Introduction to pharmacokinetics and pharmacodynamics. In: DiPiro JT, Spruill WJ, Wade WE, Blouin RA, Pruemer JM (Eds). Concepts in Clinical Pharmacokinetics, 5th edition. Bethesda, Maryland: American Society of Health-System Pharmacists; 2010. pp. 1-18.
47. Catchpole C. 5 day Stop/Review Date Policy for Antimicrobial Prescriptions. Worcestershire: Worcestershire Acute Hospitals NHS Trust; 2013.
48. Kakkilaya BS. (2008). Rational Medicine. [online] Available from http://www.rationalmedicine.org/antibiotics.htm. [Last accessed October, 2022].
49. Kardas P. Patient compliance with antibiotic treatment for respiratory tract infections. J Antimicrob Chemother. 2002;49(6) 897-903.
50. Davey P. General principles of the treatment of infection. In: Davey P, Wilcox M, Irving W, Thwaites G (Eds). Antimicrobial Chemotherapy, 7th edition. Oxford: Oxford University Press; 2015. pp. 137-8.
51. Doron S, Davidson LE. Antimicrobial Stewardship. Mayo Clin Proc. 2011;86(11):1113–23.
52. Cascioferro S, Schillaci D. The Future of Antibiotic: From the Magic Bullet to the Smart Bullet. J Microb Biochem Technol. 2014;6:e118.

CHAPTER 13

Surgery and Diabetes: Current Concepts

BK Singh

■ INTRODUCTION

As per the American Diabetes Association (ADA), diabetes is a group of metabolic diseases characterized by hyperglycemia due to defects in insulin secretion, insulin action, or a combination of both. The current global statistics shows that 463 million people have diabetes and nearly 374 million have impaired glucose tolerance. It is predicted that between 2010 and 2030, there will be 69% increase in the number of adult diabetics in developing countries and only 20% increase in developed countries. The prevalence in India has risen from 7.1% in 2009 to 8.9% in 2019. Nearly 77 million people are suffering from diabetes and 25.2 million have impaired glucose tolerance. Due to increase in the number of diabetic patients, the number of patients going for surgery has also proportionately increased. The prevalence of hyperglycemia is 20–40% in general surgery and 80–90% in cardiac surgery. Perioperative hyperglycemia is an independent marker of poor surgical outcomes in both diabetic and nondiabetic populations.

■ METABOLIC RESPONSE AND EFFECT OF ANESTHESIA ON DIABETES

Surgical trauma, anesthesia, and illness all contribute to increase the production of stress hormones. Increased stress hormones, mainly cortisol and catecholamine, reduce insulin sensitivity, and increased sympathetic activity reduces insulin secretion and increases growth hormone and glucagon secretion. These activities lead to uncontrolled hyperglycemia, leading to increased production of proinflammatory cytokines with resultant mitochondrial injury, endothelial dysfunction, and immune deregulation. Postsurgical outcomes depend on perioperative management of hyperglycemia. The severity of hyperglycemia also depends on the type of anesthesia and surgery; longer duration of surgery with general anesthesia has higher elevation of blood glucose comparing to shorter duration of surgery with local anesthesia.

Now with introduction of newer techniques and novel agents for induction and maintenance of the desired level of anesthesia, it is very easy to control blood glucose. Local, regional, spinal, and epidural anesthesias lessen the systemic complications. General anesthesia, long surgeries, and labile diabetes increase the chance of glucose imbalance. Hypoglycemia, particularly unrecognized hypoglycemia, is dangerous during surgical procedure and leads to neurological complication if not managed appropriately. Wound healing is also delayed and poor in diabetic patients. Nearly one-third of the perioperative diabetics are first diagnosed at the time of surgery. Overall, with the use of careful glucose management strategies, the primary outcome measures of surgery are similar between diabetic and nondiabetic patients.

■ PERIOPERATIVE MANAGEMENT

Strategies for glucose management differ before, during, and after surgery **(Table 1)**. The perioperative period can be discussed under different headings:
- Screening for diabetes in preanesthetic checkup (PAC)
- Preoperative control of glucose
- Intraoperative monitoring
- Postoperative care

Screening for Diabetes in Preanesthetic Checkup

Screening for diabetes in PAC is recommended for all patients above 35 years of age and one below this age with a risk factor [obesity, hypertension, family history,

TABLE 1: Strategies for glucose management before, during, and after surgery.

Preoperative management	Intraoperative management	Postoperative management
• Verify target blood glucose concentration with frequent glucose monitoring • Use insulin therapy to maintain glycemic goals • Discontinue biguanides, alpha glucosidase inhibitors, thiazolidinediones, sulfonylureas, and GLP-1 agonists • Consider canceling nonemergency procedures if the patient presents with metabolic abnormalities (DKA, HHS, etc.) or glucose reading above 400–500 mg/dL	• Aim to maintain intraoperative glucose levels between 140 and 180 mg/dL • Physicians must take the length of surgery into account when determining an intraoperative glucose management strategy • For minor surgery, preoperative glucose protocols may be continued • IV insulin infusion is being promoted as a more efficient method of glycemic control for longer or more complex surgeries	• Target postoperative glycemic range between 140 and 180 mg/dL • In the event a patient is hypoglycemic after surgery, begin a dextrose infusion at approximately 5–10 g/h • Ensure that basal insulin levels are met, especially in type 1 diabetic patients • Postprandial insulin requirements should be tailored according to the mode in which the patient is receiving nutrition • Supplemental insulin can be used to control hyperglycemia

(DKA: diabetic ketoacidosis; GLP-1: glucagon-like peptide 1; HHS: hyperosmolar hyperglycemic state; IV: intravenous)

history of gestational diabetes mellitus (GDM), human immunodeficiency virus (HIV), and physical inactivity]. So practically, most adult patients requiring surgical intervention undergo blood glucose estimation. This screening many times makes possible the diagnosis of diabetes for the first time. If the patient is found to have impaired blood glucose, then he can be directed to lifestyle modifications, oral hypoglycemic agents, and any further investigation required. Those who are already diagnosed with diabetes will be required to do fasting followed by postprandial blood glucose with glycated hemoglobin (HbA1c) test. This test reflects the control, and any untoward effect of glucose will be minimized if it remains in the range. The desired premeal blood glucose is 90–130 mg% and postmeal is 140–180 mg%.

Preoperative Control of Blood Glucose

It is difficult to titrate oral antihyperglycemic drugs during the perioperative period due to delayed and prolonged duration of action and the risk associated with these drugs. So, the current recommendation is to withhold these drugs on the day of surgery except sodium-glucose cotransporter-2 (SGLT-2) inhibitors, which should be withheld minimum 24 hours before surgery. Dipeptidyl peptidase-4 (DPP-4) inhibitors (sitagliptin, linagliptin) do not cause hypoglycemia during the fasting state, so they can be continued. The Sita-Hospital trial clearly demonstrated that DPP-4 inhibitors are safe and efficacious in surgical patients with mild-to-moderate hyperglycemia. However, the ADA does not recommend it. Many randomized controlled trials (RCTs) are underway regarding the use of glucagon-like peptide 1 (GLP-1) agonists in a hospital setting.

Ideally, insulin should be used during operation, and modification of dose is required if the patient is on insulin therapy. If the patient is taking long-acting basal insulin either in the morning or in the evening, the dose should be reduced by 20–25%. If the patient is taking both in the morning and in the evening, both doses should be reduced by 20–25%. If the patient is taking a high dose of basal insulin or there is a high risk of hypoglycemia, then the dose should be reduced by 50–75%. For patients who are taking ultra-long-acting insulin, the dose should be reduced 3 days before surgery. Premixed insulin should be changed to long-acting insulin. If it is not possible to reduce, then the morning dose should be reduced by 50%, followed by dextrose-containing intravenous fluid. Prandial insulin should be replaced by correctional insulin during the fasting state. In critically ill patients, subcutaneous insulin should be avoided due to erratic subcutaneous absorption leading to difficulty in dose titration. Blood glucose should be checked on the day of surgery. If the blood glucose is <70 mg/dL, the patient should be treated with intravenous dextrose. If there is severe hyperglycemia, the surgery should be postponed till the blood sugar is controlled.

Intraoperative Monitoring

Blood glucose should be checked frequently during surgery, and hyperglycemia can be managed either by subcutaneous rapid-acting insulin or by intravenous insulin, depending upon the duration and type of surgery.

Postoperative Care

In the postoperative period, we should give insulin because of its merits discussed earlier. In the postoperative period, once the patient is extubated and starts taking oral diet, we can switch to subcutaneous insulin or reintroduce oral hypoglycemic agents gradually. Oral antihyperglycemic agents (OHAs), which are known to cause hypoglycemia, such as sulfonylureas, are to be avoided early in the course. It is always better to start multiple subcutaneous insulin injections, which are most physiologic and avoid chances of hypoglycemia. Doses can be titrated according to the meal and other drugs/fluids influencing blood glucose. Basal insulin is useful to control the fasting level. Its steady action decreases the chances of hyperglycemic complications too. Postoperative hyperglycemia management depends upon the condition of the patient after surgery, whether they are stable, noncritically ill, or critically ill.

Ambulatory and stable patients should be discharged with a preoperative regimen.

Noncritically ill patients should be shifted to the ward with subcutaneous insulin, and the regimen depends upon the oral intake of the patient. If the patients have poor oral intake, basal plus correctional insulin is preferred. If they have proper oral intake, then basal, prandial, and correctional regimens should be considered. Calculation of the dose of insulin should be based on the weight or prehospitalization regimen. The usual total daily insulin dose on weight basis is 0.4–0.5 U/kg/day, which can be increased or decreased according to insulin sensitivity of the patient. Blood sugar should be monitored 4–6 hourly.

Critically ill patients should be treated with regular insulin through continuous insulin infusion (CII) in an intensive care unit. Frequent blood sugar monitoring is required preferably for 1–2 hours to maintain the blood sugar in range. The NICE-SUGAR (Normoglycemia in Intensive Care Evaluation–Survival Using Glucose Algorithm Regulation) study has clearly stated that intensive glucose control, which is between 81 and 108 mg/dL, is associated with higher incidence of hypoglycemia and mortality in comparison to conventional blood glucose control (<180 mg/dL). Clinicians should be careful during the transition from CII to subcutaneous insulin dosing. Intravenous insulin has a very short half-life, and subcutaneous insulin usually takes 2–3 hours to act. So, premature discontinuation may lead to rebound hyperglycemia. The dose and type of subcutaneous insulin is as of noncritically ill patients.

Although the optimal glycemic target remains unclear, a reasonable goal in the majority of perioperative patients is to maintain blood glucose in the range of 140–180 mg/dL with the intent of avoiding both hypoglycemia (under 70 mg/dL) and severe hyperglycemia (over 180 mg/dL). Premixed insulin regimens should be avoided due to hypoglycemic risk. The use of oral or noninsulin antihyperglycemic is an area of active research and currently not recommended for glucose management in these patients.

CONCLUSION

Due to a high number of diabetic patients, the rate of those going to surgery is nearly 10%. There is no definite consensus guideline for the perioperative treatment of diabetes. Many societies have given different views, but careful planning considering the type of surgery, duration of surgery, comorbidities of patients, and expected complication is very important. Proper coordination between the physician, surgeon, diabetologist, anesthesiologist, nurses, and diabetic educator is essential for the optimal perioperative management of diabetic patients. The treatment plan should be made according to the needs of the patient. Proper communication between different specialties is essential to improve clinical outcomes.

SUGGESTED READINGS

1. Shaw JE, Sicree RA, Zimmet PZ. Global estimates of the prevalence of diabetes for 2010 and 2030. Diabetes Res Clin Pract. 2010;87(1):4-14.
2. Kotagal M, Symons RG, Hirsch IB, et al. Perioperative hyperglycemia and risk of adverse events among patients with and without diabetes. Ann Surg. 2015;261(1):97-103.
3. Palermo NE, Gianchandani RY, McDonnell ME, et al. Stress hyperglycemia during surgery and anesthesia: pathogenesis and clinical implications. Curr Diab Rep. 2016;16(3):33.
4. Pasquel FJ, Gianchandani R, Rubin DJ, et al. Efficacy of sitagliptin for the hospital management of general medicine and surgery patients with type 2 diabetes (Sita-Hospital): a multicenter, prospective, open-label, noninferiority randomized trial. Lancet Diabetes Endocrinol. 2017;5(2):125-33.
5. Hulst AH, Plummer MP, Hollmann MW, et al. Systematic review of incretin therapy during perioperative and intensive care. Crit Care. 2018;22(1):299.
6. Demma LJ, Carlson KT, Duggan EW, et al. Effect of basal insulin dosage on blood glucose concentration in ambulatory surgery patients with type 2 diabetes. J Clin Anesth. 2017;36:184-8.
7. Jacobi J, Bircher N, Krinsley J, et al. Guidelines for the use of an insulin infusion for the management of hyperglycemia in critically ill patients. Crit Care Med. 2012;40(12):3251-76.
8. Umpierrez GE, Smiley D, Hermayer K, et al. Randomized study comparing a basal-bolus with a basal plus correction insulin regimen for the hospital management of medical and surgical patients with type 2 diabetes: basal plus trial. Diabetes Care. 2013;36(8):2169-74.
9. NICE-SUGAR Study Investigators, Finfer S, Chittock DR, Su SY, et al. Intensive versus conventional glucose control in critically ill patients. N Engl J Med. 2009;360(13):1283-97.
10. American Diabetes Association. 14. Diabetes care in the hospital: standards of medical care in diabetes-2018. Diabetes Care. 2018;41(Suppl 1):S144-51.

CHAPTER 14

How Often Estimation of Urinary Albumin to Creatinine Ratio do Help to Identify Early DM Nephropathy?

Dipankar prakas Bhaumik, M Roy, Soma Saha

■ OVERVIEW

Diabetic nephropathy (DN) is in the top of common causes of end-stage renal disease (ESRD) worldwide. Urinary albumin excretion is one of the early signs of development of nephropathy in Diabetes. Glomerular filtration rate (GFR) represents actual renal function. Serum creatinine is crude to indicate GFR. Modification of diet in renal disease (MDRD) equation is considered as the standard method of estimation of GFR (eGFR). Many normoalbuminurics may have reduced eGFR. Presence of albuminuria was found highly variable in different studies, depending upon methodology. Type 2 diabetes mellitus (T2DM) patients may have albuminuria even at diagnosis and prevalence of albuminuria is significant. It has been similar in a study done in Tripura, a state of North East India. Combining urinary albumin to creatinine ratio (UrACR) and eGFR, in regular manner, progression to ESRD of a patient having diabetes can be better predicted.

Case 1

About 3 years back, Mr Chakraborty, a 58-year-old gentleman, diabetic, and hypertensive for 8 years, came to me with complaints of fatigue and leg cramp for 6 months. His previous documents were suggestive of irregular medication, poorly controlled sugar and BP but recent blood sugar and BP reports were in normal range. He was taking vitamins beside sulfonylurea, metformin, amlodipine, and nebivolol. On work-up, creatinine was 2.1 mg/dL, UrACR was 1,000 mg/gCr, and eGFR was 36 mL/min/1.73 m^2.

Case 2

In few days interval, Mr Debnath, a 63-year-old gentleman with diabetes mellitus (DM) for 13 years, hypertension (HTN) for 12 years, postpercutaneous transluminal coronary angioplasty (PTCA) to left anterior descending artery (LAD) 3 years back, presented with tingling sensation of both lower limb for 3 months. His history revealed dyslipidemia, acute coronary syndrome (ACS) though diabetes, and HTN was managed satisfactorily to great extent. On work up, creatinine was 1.8 mg/dL, urinary ACR was 124 mg/gCr, and eGFR was 42 mL/min/1.73 m².

Mr Chakraborty landed to ESRD in next 8 months. Renal replacement therapy (hemodialysis) was initiated. In next 6 months of renal replacement therapy (RRT) initiation, he had acute NSTEMI and demised next day. Presently, Mr Debnath is having creatinine 2.72 mg/dL, urinary ACR 324 mg/gCr, and eGFR 25 mL/min/1.73 m² Ur. He has been primed for possible RRT in future and access construction has been advised.

INTRODUCTION

Diabetes mellitus remains the most common cause of end-stage renal disease (ESRD) in the developed world and diabetic nephropathy is the leading specific primary renal diagnosis for patients commencing renal replacement therapy (RRT) in the UK. The development of microalbuminuria has been considered as one of the first clinical signs in diabetic nephropathy eventually leading to ESRD. Albuminuria is pervasive and seen to increase with age and depends upon body mass, blood pressure, sugar, lipid, alcohol intake, glomerulonephropathies and inversely related to birthweight.

Kidney disease in T2DM is more heterogeneous. The UK Prospective Diabetes Study even demonstrated that 51% of patients who progressed to chronic renal failure had no preceding albuminuria. However, the proportions of patients with low GFR among type 2 diabetic patients with normoalbuminuria, microalbuminuria or macroalbuminuria remain uncertain. Serum creatinine reflects GFR poorly, but direct measures of GFR in routine clinical practice is not feasible. The National Kidney Disease Education Program and the National Kidney Foundation recommend use of the abbreviated Modification of Diet in Renal Disease (MDRD) equation to estimate GFR in adults utilizing age, sex, and ethnicity as surrogates for muscle mass. This is now recommended as the best validated means for transforming serum creatinine measurements into eGFR.

Hyperfiltration and albuminuria may occur independently of each other in early stages of diabetes, but decline in eGFR and albuminuria follow a parallel course later, suggesting there may be common pathophysiological mechanisms or they may be causally linked. Albuminuria, diabetes, and hypertension (not smoking dyslipidemia, and obesity) were markers for increased risk of natural and cardiovascular death. Relative risk associated with albuminuria was independent of diabetes and hypertension. Albuminuria was more common than either diabetes or hypertension and represents a target for intervention to reduce not only progression to renal disease, but also overall mortality. Rising ACR level is predictive of microalbuminuria, independent of HbA1c, beside poor glycemic control is involved in pathogenesis of diabetic nephropathy and early intervention with to reduce fall in GFR may be beneficial even before onset of microalbuminuria.

Type 2 diabetes mellitus is a leading cause of ESRD worldwide, it is important to determine the magnitude of renal disease and risk of ESRD. As normoalbuminuric T2DM patients could have low GFR, measurement of both UAE and eGFR in combination may improve prediction of ESRD and thereby improving the outcome. Factors associated with albuminuria and low GFR may be common but could be independent. Most of the studies have used development of microalbuminuria as primary endpoint, with data on GFR being limited.

■ REVIEW OF LITERATURE

Diabetic nephropathy is defined as the appearance of persistent clinical albuminuria in a diabetic (in absence of urinary tract infection, renal disease, and heart failure) for >5 years and concomitant retinopathy. The earliest clinical evidence of nephropathy is albuminuria ≥30 mg/day, referred as microalbuminuria. Many methods for the screening of microalbuminuria can be performed but the albumin to creatinine ratio is found easiest, convenient, accurate, and correlate well with 24-hour samples.

In a study, it was seen that though there may be higher GFR in people having subtle albuminuria but with further increase in albuminuria, there is augmented reduction of GFR with individual variation. Other factors significantly influence GFR reduction include cholesterol, HTN, and blood sugar beside few others. Those patients had baseline microalbuminuria with eGFR ≥60 mL/min/1.73 m^2 found to have 5.0-fold risk of developing endpoint renal outcome (95% CI 2.8–8.8; $p < 0.001$) in a prospective study. During an average 10.7 years follow-up, mortality rates increased with greater albuminuria and with lower levels of eGFR. Within categories of eGFR, mortality increased with higher albuminuria; within albuminuria categories mortality increased with decreasing eGFR. Participants with eGFR 15–29 mL/min/1.73 m^2 with macroalbuminuria, had mortality rate 7.1 times higher to those having eGFR 90–119 mL/min/1.73 m^2 with normoalbuminuria. A proportional hazards model, included albuminuria and eGFR, provided significantly better prediction of mortality than either albuminuria ($p = 2.0 \times 10^{-7}$) or eGFR ($p = 1.2 \times 10^{-7}$).

The natural history of nephropathy in T2DM is not unlike that of T1DM, with some notable exceptions. At diagnosis, UAE may be raised. In cross-sectional studies in established diabetes, prevalence of microalbuminuria is 10–42%, depending on population selection. Without specific interventions, about 80% of subjects with type 1 diabetes mellitus, having microalbuminuria, UrACR increase at a rate of ~10–20% yearly to the stage of overt nephropathy (≥300 mg/24 h) over a period of 10–15 years. A higher proportion of individuals with T2DM have microalbuminuria and overt nephropathy at diagnosis, because diabetes is actually present for many years before diagnosis. The overall sequence is similar in T2DM patients, but uncertainties may exist because of inaccurate dating of diabetes onset. The decline is more variable in T2DM patients and progression rate to ESRD may be as low as 20% over 20 years. Among 1,425 (876 males and 549 females) South Indian T2DM patients overall prevalence of microalbuminuria was 36.3% (32.1% males and 39.9% females). Multivariate regression analysis revealed age, diastolic blood pressure, HbA1c, FPG, and DM duration is associated with microalbuminuria. UK Prospective Diabetes Study (UKPDS) revealed that over a median of 15 years' follow-up, risk factors for development of albuminuria were male sex, TG, LDL-C, A1c, smoking and retinopathy and those for renal insufficiency were female sex, age, and neuropathy. The UKPDS demonstrated that 51% of patients progressing to chronic renal failure had no albuminuria.

National Institute for Clinical Excellence (NICE) guidelines (September, 2008) recommends annual assessment of eGFR and UrACR. US National Kidney Foundation Kidney Disease Outcomes Quality Initiative guidelines (NKF-KDOQI) and the American Diabetes Association (ADA) guidelines, both also recommend annual testing of eGFR regardless of their degree of urine albumin excretion to aid early detection and prevention of progression in patients with early kidney disease.

Merlin C Thomas et al. examined the frequency and predictors of nonalbuminuric renal impairment (eGFR 60 mL/min/1.73 m^2) in a nationally representative cohort of 3,893 patients with T2DM. Out of 23.1% subject having eGFR 60 mL/min/1.73 m^2, 55% had UrACR in normal range and concluded that nonalbuminuric renal impairment may not be more common but albuminuria is having greater impact. Hiroki Yokoyama et al. explored prevalence of normoalbuminuric type 2 diabetic patients having renal insufficiency (RI). 15.3% of subjects had renal insufficiency (low eGFR), of those 11.4% had normoalbuminuria, 14.9% had microalbuminuria, and 47.3% had macroalbuminuria. Study finding revealed that a significant proportion of T2DM patients have RI with normoalbuminuria. Richard J Macisaac et al., in a cross-sectional survey, examined 301 outpatients, using plasma disappearance of isotopic ^{99m}Tc-diethylene-triamine-penta-acetic acid to measure GFR and urinary albumin excretion rate over 24 hours to determine albuminuria. A total of 109 patients (36%) had a low GFR. Among this 109 subjects, 43 (39%) had normoalbuminuria, 38 (35%) had microalbuminuria, and 28 (26%) macroalbuminuria. The rates of decline in GFR were not significantly different for level of albuminuria. Stein I Hallan et al. [Nord-Trondelag Health (HUNT 2) Study, 1995–1997, $n = 65,589$)] found 124 patients progressed to ESRD after 10.3 years of follow-up. In multivariable survival analysis, eGFR and albuminuria were independently and strongly associated with progression to ESRD. Time-dependent receiver operating characteristic analyses showed that considering both UrACR and eGFR substantially improved diagnostic accuracy. This large population-based sample identified the combination of eGFR and albuminuria as a powerful predictor of progression to ESRD.

In our study in NE state Tripura (Bhaumik DP, Roy M, unpublished) ($n = 544$), 45.55% patients had albuminuria (microalbuminuria in 35% and macroalbuminuria in 10.84%). Subjects with albuminuria were having eGFR reduced in comparison to those who were not having significant albuminuria (i.e., UrACR <30 mg/gCr). Those who were having overt proteinuria (i.e., >300 mg/gCr) were having mean of eGFR very low (male 43.275 mL/min/1.73 m^2 and female 44.515 mL/min/1.73 m^2) **(Table 1)**.

TABLE 1: UrACR and eGFR in a study of diabetics of a state in North East.

Urinary ACR Mg/gCr	Mean of eGFR by MDRD equation (mL/min/1.73 m²)		No. of patients	Total
0–30	Male	84.651	138	294
	Female	65.523	156	
31–300	Male	75.285	101	191
	Female	61.996	90	
>300	Male	43.275	34	59
	Female	44.515	25	
	Male: 273, Female: 271			544

(ACR: albumin to creatinine ratio; eGFR: estimation of glomerular filtration rate; MDRD: modification of diet in renal disease; UrACR: urinary albumin to creatinine ratio)

CONCLUSION

It is clearly evident, even though many of the diabetics may progress to ESRD without having significant albuminuria, higher albumin excretion is associated with higher risk of rapid progression of nephropathy. When UrACR and eGFR are combined together to stratify risk of progression to terminal renal condition, it helps to identify subjects in higher risk group and can prompt active focused management. Higher UrACR is also increased risk of having cardiac events. Different studies, including our study, show high prevalence of albuminuria among T2DM patients. So estimation of ACR periodically along with serum creatinine and eGFR will help primary care providers to identify high-risk patients early. That will prompt us to take aggressive measures to slow down progress of nephropathy and by that we may be able to defer cardiac events also.

SUGGESTED READINGS

1. Ansell D, Tomson CR. UK Renal Registry 11th Annual Report (December2008): Chapter 2 Introduction to the 2008 UK Renal Registry Report. Nephron Clin Pract. 2009;111:c3-12.
2. Mogensen CE, Christensen CK, Vittinghus E. The stages in diabetic renal disease. With emphasis on the stage of incipient diabetic nephropathy. Diabetes. 1983;32(Suppl 2):64-78.
3. Hoy WE. Renal disease in Australian Aborigines. Nephrol Dial Transplant. 2000;15:1293-7.
4. Retnakaran R, Cull CA, Thorne KI, et al. UKPDS Study Group. Risk factors for renal dysfunction in type 2 diabetes: U.K. Prospective Diabetes Study 74. Diabetes. 2006;55:1832-9.
5. Levey AS, Bosch JP, Lewis JB, et al. A more accurate method to estimate glomerular filtration rate from serum creatinine: a new prediction equation. Modification of Diet in Renal Disease Study Group. Ann Intern Med. 1999;130:461-70.
6. Magri CJ, Fava S. Albuminuria and glomerular filtration rate in type 2 diabetes mellitus. Minerva Urol Nefrol. 2011;63(4):273-80.
7. McDonald S, Wang Z, Hoy WE. Physical and biochemical predictors of death in an Australian Aboriginal cohort. Clin Exp Pharmacol Physiol. 1999;26:618-21.
8. Amin R, Turner C, van Aken S, et al. The relationship between microalbuminuria and glomerular filtration rate in young type 1 diabetic subjects: The Oxford Regional Prospective Study. Kidney Int. 2005;68(4):1740-9.

9. Caramori ML, Fioretto P, Mauer M. The need for early predictors of diabetic nephropathy risk: is albumin excretion rate sufficient? Diabetes. 2000;49:1399-408.
10. Thomas S, Carlo Viberti G. Diabetic nephropathy. Medicine. 2006;34:83-6.
11. American Diabetes Association. Diabetic nephropathy. Diabetes Care. 2002;25:S85-S89.
12. Hoy WE, Wang Z, Vanbuynder P, et al. The natural history of renal disease in Australian Aborigines. Part 1. Changes in albuminuria and glomerular filtration rate over time. MATHEWS Kidney Int. 2001;60:243-8.
13. Tanaka N, Babazono T, Takagi M, et al. Albuminuria and reduced glomerular filtration rate for predicting the renal outcomes in type 2 diabetic patients. Nephrology (Carlton). 2015;20(8):531-8.
14. Berhane AM, Jennifer Weil E, Knowler WC, et al. Albuminuria and Estimated Glomerular Filtration Rate as Predictors of Diabetic End-Stage Renal Disease and Death. Clin J Am Soc Nephrol. 2011;6(10):2444-51.
15. Allawi J, Rao PV, Gilbert P, et al. Microalbuminuria in non-insulin-dependent diabetes: its prevalence in Indian compared with Europid patients. Br Med J. 1988;296:462-4.
16. Gall MA, Rossing P, Skott P, et al. Prevalence of micro and macroalbuminuria, arterial hypertension, retinopathy and large vessel disease in European type II (non-insulin dependent) diabetic patients. Diabetologia. 1991;34:655-61.
17. Collins VR, Dowse GK, Finch CF, et al. Prevalence and risk factors for micro- and macroalbuminuria in diabetic subjects and entire population of Nauru. Diabetes. 1989;38:1602-10.
18. Nelson RG, Knowler WC, Pettitt DJ, et al. Incidence and determinants of elevated urinary albumin excretion in Pima Indians with NIDDM. Diabetes Care. 1995;18:182-7.
19. Unnikrishnan RI, Rema M, Pradeepa R, et al. Prevalence and risk factors of diabetic nephropathy in an urban South Indian population: the Chennai Urban Rural Epidemiology Study (CURES 45). Diabetes Care. 2007;30:2019-24.
20. American Diabetes Association. Standards of medical care for patients with diabetes mellitus. Diabetes Care. 2002;25(S1):S33-49.
21. Varghese A, Deepa R, Rema R, et al. Prevalence of microalbuminuria in type 2 diabetes mellitus at a diabetes centre in southern India. Postgrad Med. 2001;77:399-402.
22. National Kidney Foundation. K/DOQI clinical practice guidelines for chronic kidney disease: evaluation, classification, and stratification. Am J Kidney Dis. 2002;39:S1-S266.
23. American Diabetes Association. Clinical Practice Recommendations 2007. Diabetes Care. 2007;30.
24. Thomas MC, Macisaac RJ, Jerums G, et al. Nonalbuminuric Renal Impairment in Type 2 Diabetic Patients and in the General Population (National Evaluation of the Frequency of Renal Impairment co existing with NIDDM [NEFRON] 11). Diabetes Care 2009; 32:1497–1502 .
25. Yokoyama H, Sone H, Oishi M, et al. Prevalence of albuminuria and renal insufficiency and associated clinical factors in type 2 diabetes: the Japan Diabetes Clinical Data Management study (JDDM15). Nephrol Dial Transplant. 2009;24:1212-9.
26. Macisaac RJ, Tsalamandris C, Panagiotopoulos S,et al. Nonalbuminuric Renal Insufficiency in Type 2 Diabetes. Diabetes Care. 2004;27:195-200.
27. Hallan SI, Ritz E, Lydersen S, et al. Combining GFR and Albuminuria to Classify CKD Improves Prediction of ESRD. J Am Soc Nephrol. 2009;20:1069-77.

CHAPTER 15

Difficult Case Scenarios in Diabetes Mellitus Management

Anil Kumar Virmani

■ INTRODUCTION

Type 2 diabetes mellitus (T2DM) is a heterogenous disease with various phenotypes and different presentations. Thus, the treatment becomes very challenging and requires a detailed clinical history and a high index of suspicion for the unusual presentations. The following series of five case presentations highlight the same.

■ CASE 1

A 52-year-old woman, history of diabetes mellitus since 10 years; obese with history of weight gain in the last 2 years after she started insulin; and tiredness in the afternoons, started on antidepressants.

Issues

- Poorly controlled diabetes mellitus
- High insulin dose contributing to weight gain
- Recurrent hypoglycemia with fear leading to snacking
- Similarity of symptoms with depression

The perception and fear of hypoglycemia is a major problem for individuals treated with insulin, and it is often unrecognized by healthcare providers.

Uncontrolled blood sugar leads to increased insulin dose and calorie restriction leads to weight gain and hypoglycemic episodes (snacking).

With caloric restriction, if insulin doses are not lowered a vicious cycle sets in of hypoglycemia with overeating, further hyperglycemia, and increased insulin requirements with subsequent weight gain → this may mimic or exacerbate depression.

Learning Points

Caloric restriction in obese, insulin-treated patients should always be accompanied by decrease in insulin doses at the same time.

Insulin-treated patients with diabetes mellitus and obesity should be assessed for symptoms of hypoglycemia and overeating.

Metformin in optimum doses can help decrease insulin requirements and assist with weight loss.

Addition of sodium–glucose cotransporter-2 inhibitors (SGLT2i)/basal insulin + glucagon-like peptide-1 receptor agonist (GLP-1 RA) can further reduce insulin dose and reduce weight.

Treating hyperglycemia can alleviate symptoms of depression.

CASE 2

A 35-year-old male with history of diabetes mellitus since 2 years, on tablet metformin 2 g and tablet glimepiride 4 mg daily. Weight loss of about 8 kg in the last 2 years; body mass index (BMI) 20 kg/m^2.

Fasting blood sugar (FBS)—180 mg%, postprandial blood sugar (PPBS)—260 mg%, glycated hemoglobin (HbA1c)—9.3%.

Serum C-peptide was low (0.34 ng/mL); glutamic acid decarboxylase 65-kilodalton isoform (GAD65 Ab) was absent; but islet antigen 2 (IA-2) was strongly positive: 3.4 U/mL (normal <0.8 U/mL).

Latent autoimmune diabetes mellitus in adults (LADA): Started on insulin glargine and Novorapid. Oral hypoglycemic agent (OHA) stopped.

After 2 months: FBS—110 mg%, PPBS—150 mg%, HbA1c—6.9%

According to the Immunology of Diabetes Society (IDS), there are three criteria to define LADA:
1. Age usually ≥30 years
2. *Any one of the following autoantibodies should be positive*: Islet cell autoantibody (ICA), GAD autoantibody, tyrosine phosphatase-related IA-2, and insulin autoantibodies (IAA)
3. Did not require insulin within the first 6 months after diagnosis

Why this Patient has Latent Autoimmune Diabetes Mellitus in Adults?

- Fits the proposed IDS criteria for diagnosing LADA
- Age >30 years
- Although he was GAD-negative, his IA-2 was positive in high titers. At least one antibody was positive.
- He did not require insulin treatment in the initial 6 months after diagnosis.
- C-peptide levels were low.
- Besides these criteria, his clinical course was that of a typical misdiagnosed LADA patient initially treated with oral medications, as would be a patient with T2DM.

- Despite adherence, these medications failed to achieve glycemic lowering, and he had an A1c of 9.3% by the time he was first seen at the clinic.
- Similar to a patient with type 1 diabetes mellitus (T1DM), he also continued to lose weight.

Management

In a patient with LADA, besides insulin, other drugs that can be used are dipeptidyl peptidase 4 inhibitors (DPP-4i), GLP-1 RA, and thiazolidinediones that can preserve β-cell function.

Sulfonylureas (SU) should be avoided since they increase the rate of deterioration of C-peptide secretion and further deplete insulin levels.

CASE 3

A 40-year-old female, diabetic since 5 years. Well controlled (FBS—110 mg%, PPBS—150 mg%, HbA1c—6.8%) on tablet metformin 1 g BD and tablet glimepiride 4 mg OD.

Developed autoimmune hemolytic anemia, was treated with tablet prednisolone 60 mg/day.

After 6 months of steroid therapy, presented with FBS—140 mg%, PPBS—270 mg%, HbA1c—8.0%.

How to Manage?

Steroid-induced diabetes mellitus (SIDM) is defined as an abnormal increase in blood glucose levels, in patients on glucocorticoids who may or may not have a prior history of diabetes mellitus.

Pathogenesis: Glucocorticoid effects on glyceroneogenesis in adipose tissue and liver are that phosphoenolpyruvate carboxykinase (PEPCK) is reciprocally upregulated in liver and downregulated in adipose, thus leading to increase of free fatty acid (FFA) ultimately resulting in insulin resistance and increased gluconeogenesis.

Treatment: Different management strategy than nonsteroid-induced diabetes mellitus since postprandial hyperglycemia (PPHG) is the dominant feature.

Basal-bolus insulin therapy is the most flexible option for patients along with a supplemental correction factor insulin.

The timing of glucocorticoids, to a mid-day or an evening meal with concomitant administration of intermediate-acting insulin, would be the ideal situation.

Metformin may cause nausea/vomiting, hypoxia, and liver or kidney disease, and hence is not recommended.

Sulfonylureas do not specifically control PPHG, and thus long-acting agents may be associated with hypoglycemia. However, SU used once daily in the morning may best manage the glucose excursion associated with a once-daily oral steroid.

However, in patients with mild hyperglycemia, short-acting secretagogues such as glinides taken before meals could be considered.

Key messages: Glucocorticoids are generally used to treat inflammatory diseases and to prevent organ transplant rejection, but unfortunately they lead to hyperglycemia and diabetes mellitus.

Glucocorticoid-induced hyperglycemia is due to a direct action via glucocorticoid signaling in metabolic organs and tissues (liver, adipose tissue, muscle, bone, and pancreatic β-cells) and indirectly via interorgan hormone and metabolite flux.

There is no consensus regarding optimal screening of patients on glucocorticoids for hyperglycemia, because of various context-dependent factors, but measurement of postprandial glucose is recommended.

Insulin sensitizers and insulin provide satisfactory glucose control and have to be adjusted according to the dose and type of glucocorticoid used.

It is very difficult to develop selective glucocorticoid modulators that will dissociate the diabetogenic from the anti-inflammatory effects of glucocorticoids; however, new pharmacological targets that prevent diabetogenic effects are being developed.

CASE 4

A 44-year-old, previously healthy woman presented with polyuria and polydipsia for 6 weeks, along with progressive worsening of dry mouth; no family history of diabetes mellitus; she gave history of losing 7 kg weight over the past 3 months.

FBS—190 mg%; PPBS—340 mg%; HbA1c—2.5%; BMI of 23.2 kg/m^2; urine positive for ketones (>7.8 mmol/L)

She was treated with intensive insulin therapy and intravenous (IV) fluids.

After 2 weeks, her insulin requirements started coming down and due to recurrent hypoglycemia, her insulin was stopped after 2 months.

Two months after stopping all medications → FBS—100 mg%; PPBS—148 mg%; HbA1c—6.4%; serum C-peptide—695 pmol/L (normal: 364–1,655 pmol/L); anti-GAD antibody and anti-islet cell antibody negative.

What is the Diagnosis?

Atypical or Ketosis-prone T2DM (Flatbush Diabetes Mellitus)

The patient had polyuria, polydipsia, and weight loss with unprovoked diabetic ketoacidosis (DKA).

Majority of patients will undergo spontaneous remission with discontinuation of insulin therapy within a few weeks; however, an estimated 60–70% of patients relapse within 2 years and require either oral hypoglycemic agents or insulin. Hence, close follow-up is needed.

These patients characteristically do not have markers of autoimmune β-cell failure, including the various autoantibodies.

As shown by various studies, there is a transient secretory defect of β cells during the acute phase, with 60–80% improvement in insulin-secreting capacity during remission. There is also a concomitant severe reduction in insulin sensitivity during the acute hyperglycemia phase, which improves by 200% upon restoration of normoglycemia.

Clinical Pearls
- All patients who present with DKA may not require lifelong insulin.
- In the early stages, these patients often behave as T1DM, but a rapidly falling requirement for insulin over the first few weeks is a strong indicator of the possibility of this diagnosis.
- Markers of autoimmune β-cell failure are usually not seen in patients with atypical diabetes mellitus.

■ CASE 5

A 48-year-old cachectic male with history of chronic alcohol abuse and recurrent pancreatitis was admitted with dehydration, excess thirst, fatigue, and blurred vision. He had history of abdominal pain, intermittent diarrhea/steatorrhea, and poor appetite.

Fasting blood sugar—250 mg%, HbA1c—7.1%; low levels of vitamin 25(OH) D and B, negative anti-GAD antibody.

Diagnosis → type 3c diabetes mellitus (T3cDM) (pancreatogenic or pancreatic diabetes mellitus).

Challenging Issues in Management
- Malnutrition leads to low glycogen stores making counter-regulation difficult, and this leads to a high risk of undernutrition and hypoglycemia.
- Normal HbA1c due to long-standing poor nutrient absorption
- Severe fluctuations of glucose levels ("brittle diabetes mellitus")
- Exaggerated response to smaller doses of insulin
- Choice of OHA

Prevalence: About 8%

Etiology: Chronic pancreatitis/cystic fibrosis/hemochromatosis/pancreatectomy/pancreatic cancer

Pathophysiology:
- Unlike T1DM where pancreatic inflammation causes only β-cell destruction, in these patients there is also a loss of glucagon and pancreatic polypeptide (PP) from the islet α cells and PP cells besides the loss of insulin from the islet β cells.
- Incretin secretion is also impaired due to nutrient maldigestion and malabsorption.
- The circulating insulin levels are low, and there is a compensatory increase in peripheral insulin sensitivity, but there is also a decrease in hepatic insulin sensitivity with unsuppressed hepatic glucose production, which aggravates hyperglycemia and is associated with the reduction in pancreatic PP secretion.

Diagnosis
- *Major criteria*:
  - Pancreatic exocrine insufficiency

- Pathological pancreatic imaging
  - Absence of T1DM-associated autoantibodies
- *Minor criteria*:
  - Absent PP secretion
  - Impaired incretin secretion
  - Absence of excessive insulin resistance
  - Impaired β-cell function
  - Low serum levels of fat-soluble vitamins

Principles of management: The goals are to prevent hypoglycemia and hyperglycemia, exacerbation of malnutrition and malabsorption, comorbidities associated with diabetes mellitus (e.g., retinopathy, renal disease).

Management strategies: Starchy carbohydrates with regular small, frequent meals/cut down on high sugar and high glycemic foods/measurement of glucose levels frequently/avoid alcohol/smoking cessation/adequate pancreatic enzyme replacement therapy (PERT)/maintaining a diary to record diet, glucose levels, PERT, exercise, at least until acceptable glucose control is maintained/routine dietitian assessment/monitoring.

Clinical Pearls

- Insulin will be required in the majority to control rampant hyperglycemia, and its anabolic effects will be beneficial in those with undernutrition.
- In patients with mild hyperglycemia and concomitant insulin resistance, metformin could be used if not contraindicated.
- Continuous glucose monitoring (CGM) may have an important role to play in patients with brittle diabetes mellitus.

CONCLUSION

Five unusual presentations and challenges in diagnosis and treatment have been presented. Over-insulinasation in obese patients, Latent Auto-immune Diabetes of Adults (LADA), Steroid-induced diabetes, Atypical or Ketosis-prone diabetes and pancreatogenic diabetes have been discussed. These cases highlight some of the challenges in the treatment of T2DM.

SUGGESTED READINGS

1. Naik RG, Brooks-Worrell BM, Palmer JP. Latent autoimmune diabetes in adults. J Clin Endocrinol Metab. 2009;94:4635-44.
2. Pipi E, Marketou M, Tsirogianni A. Distinct clinical and laboratory characteristics of latent autoimmune diabetes in adults in relation to type 1 and type 2 diabetes mellitus. World J Diabetes. 2014;5:505-10.
3. Brophy S, Davies H, Mannan S, et al. Interventions for latent autoimmune diabetes (LADA) in adults. Cochrane Database Syst Rev. 2011;9:CD006165.
4. Cadoudal T, Leroyer S, Reis AF, et al. Proposed involvement of adipocyte glyceroneogenesis and phosphoenolpyruvate carboxykinase in the metabolic syndrome. Biochimie. 2005;87:27-32.
5. Oyer DS, Shah A, Bettenhausen S. How to manage steroid diabetes in the patient with cancer. J Support Oncol. 2006;4(9):472-82.

6. Hwang JL, Weiss RE. Steroid-induced diabetes: a clinical and molecular approach to understanding and treatment. Diabetes Metab Res Rev. 2014;30(2):96-102.
7. Mauvais-Jarvis F, Sobongwi E, Porcher R, et al. Ketosis-prone type 2 diabetes in patients of sub-Saharan African origin; clinical pathophysiology and natural history of beta-cell dysfunction and insulin resistance. Diabetes. 2004;53(3):645-53.
8. Cui Y, Andersen DK. Pancreatogenic diabetes: special considerations for management. Pancreatology. 2011;11(3):279-94.
9. Ewald N, Hardt PD. Diagnosis and treatment of diabetes mellitus in chronic pancreatitis. World J Gastroenterol. 2013;19(42):7276-81.
10. Duggan SN, Ewald N, Kelleher L, et al. The nutritional management of type 3c (pancreatogenic) diabetes in chronic pancreatitis. Eur J Clin Nutr. 2017;71(1):3-8.
11. Cadoudal T, Leroyer S, Reis AF, et al. Proposed involvement of adipocyte g;hyperemesis phosphoenolpyruvate carboxykinase in the metabolic syndrome. Biochinie. 2005;87:27–32.

CHAPTER 16

Type 2 Diabetes Mellitus: Asian Indian Phenotype

GD Ramchandani, Sugandha Sharma, Rahul Ramchandani, Divyansh Mathur

■ INTRODUCTION

Currently, India is global hub for chronic metabolic conditions such as type 2 diabetes mellitus (T2DM) and dyslipidemia. There are certain factors such as genetic predisposing factors, diet factors, and socioeconomic factors are involved for development of this. There is a need to have appropriate multidisciplinary approach to restrict development of this condition.

India is one of the epicenters of the global diabetes epidemic having large population of T2DM. In early 70's, diabetes prevalence was ~2–3%, but recent update shows that it has increased to nearly 20% and 10% in urban and rural part of India, respectively. Studies mentioned that South Asians (SA), specifically Indians are more prone to develop early onset of T2DM because of adoption of western lifestyle and some extent due to genetic predisposition of higher rate of insulin resistance. In SA population, cut off body mass index (BMI) rate is low but high waist circumference hip ratio indicating a greater degree of central body obesity, which contributes for higher insulin levels along with insulin resistance, and leads increment in new onset of diabetes in SA population. Insulin resistance and hyperinsulinemia are a challenge in SA population since adolescence and at some extent since birth, which is much matter of discussion. In this issue, Bakker et al. find abnormality of mitochondrial fatty acid oxidation in SA population, leading to increased visceral fat deposition and consequent development of insulin resistance. In his study, he found that following hyperinsulinemic-euglycemic clamp, insulin levels rose only in SA compared to caucasians, indicating lower levels of insulin sensitivity in this group.

As per available studies, two major pathological mechanisms are predominant in SA population. Likewise, higher rate of impaired nonoxidative glucose disposal (NOGD) and the second one is the nutrient-sensing mammalian target of rapamycin (mTOR) pathway, activation of which could conceivably impair mitochondrial beta oxidation of fatty acids and lead to ectopic deposition of fat in the peripheral tissues.

In SA populations, there are multiple reasons for increasing diabetes and obesity, like wise; economic growth, excess intake of junk food, lack of physical activities, occupational stress and because of these reasons; since last many years, elevation of diabetes cases has been observed in rural population more than urban. It has been observed that over the last two decades, consumption of saturated fat and oil is increased in India. Though overall fat consumption is <15% of diet in Indian population; it is more likely that the high intake of refined carbohydrates (e.g., polished white rice or other refined cereals) and the consequent high glycemic load is contributing to the increased insulin resistance and T2DM and metabolic syndrome in this population. SA population has adversely accepted "WESTERN DIET" along with rich carbohydrate consumption, but still there is no significant mechanism is established to show higher propensity of insulin resistance and T2DM in respective class of people. Raising awareness among the population regarding the deleterious effects of a high-fat, high-carbohydrate, high-calorie diet, and encouraging them to continue the more healthy traditional foods could help individuals make healthy dietary choices, helping to reduce the risk of not only T2DM but of cardiovascular disease as well.

CONCLUSION

Insulin resistance and T2DM are now highly prevalent conditions across the globe, but it more aggressive and develops at very young age in SA populations, which is a major concern. Appropriate spread of awareness and education about this disease, certainly going to be helpful to curtail its spread further.

SUGGESTED READINGS

1. Unwin N, Whiting D, Guariguata L, et al. Diabetes Atlas, 5th edition. Brussels, Belgium: International Diabetes Federation; 2011. pp. 11-74.
2. Ahuja MMS. Epidemiological studies on diabetes mellitus in India. In: Ahuja MMS (ed). Epidemiological studies on diabetes mellitus in India. Epidemiology of Diabetes in Developing Countries. New Delhi: Interprint; 1979; pp. 29-38.
3. Anjana RM, Ali MK, Pradeepa R, et al. The need for obtaining accurate nationwide estimates of diabetes prevalence in India—rationale for a national study on diabetes. Indian J Med Res. 2011;133:369-80.
4. Anjana RM, Pradeepa R, Deepa M, et al.; ICMR–INDIAB Collaborative Study Group. Prevalence of diabetes and prediabetes (impaired fasting glucose and/or impaired glucose tolerance) in urban and rural India: phase I results of the Indian Council of Medical Research-INdiaDIABetes (ICMR-INDIAB) study. Diabetologia. 2011;54:3022-7.
5. Ramachandran A, Snehalatha C, Viswanathan V, et al. Risk of noninsulin dependent diabetes mellitus conferred by obesity and central adiposity in different ethnic groups: a comparative analysis between Asian Indians, Mexican Americans and Whites. Diabetes Res Clin Pract. 1997;36:121-5.
6. Mohan V, Sharp PS, Cloke HR, et al. Serum immunoreactive insulin responses to a glucose load in Asian Indian and European type 2 (non-insulin-dependent) diabetic patients and control subjects. Diabetologia. 1986;29:235-7.
7. Sharp PS, Mohan V, Levy JC, et al. Insulin resistance in patients of Asian Indian and European origin with non-insulin dependent diabetes. Horm Metab Res. 1987;19:84-5.
8. McKeigue PM, Shah B, Marmot MG. Relation of central obesity and insulin resistance with high diabetes prevalence and cardiovascular risk in South Asians. Lancet. 1991;337:382-6.

9. Misra A, Vikram NK, Arya S, et al. High prevalence of insulin resistance in postpubertal Asian Indian children is associated with adverse truncal body fat patterning, abdominal adiposity and excess body fat. Int J Obes Relat Metab Disord. 2004;28:1217-26.
10. Yajnik CS, Lubree HG, Rege SS, et al. Adiposity and hyperinsulinemia in Indians are present at birth. J Clin Endocrinol Metab. 2002;87:5575-80.
11. Bakker LEH, van Schinkel LD, Guigas B, et al. A 5-day high-fat, high calorie diet impairs insulin sensitivity in healthy, young South Asian men but not in Caucasian men. Diabetes. 2014;63: 248-58.
12. Shulman GI, Rothman DL, Jue T, et al. Quantitation of muscle glycogen synthesis in normal subjects and subjects with non-insulin-dependent diabetes by 13C nuclear magnetic resonance spectroscopy. N Engl J Med. 1990;322:223-8.
13. Nair KS, Bigelow ML, Asmann YW, et al. Asian Indians have enhanced skeletal muscle mitochondrial capacity to produce ATP in association with severe insulin resistance. Diabetes. 2008;57:1166-75.
14. Radhika G, Sathya RM, Ganesan A, et al. Dietary profile of urban adult population in South India in the context of chronic disease epidemiology (CURES-68). Public Health Nutr. 2011;14:591-8.
15. Ministry of Statistics and Programme Implementation, Government of India. National Sample Survey Organisation. Nutritional Intake in India. 66thRound NSS Consumer Expenditure Survey. New Delhi, India: Ministry of Statistics and Programme Implementation; 2012.
16. National Family Health Survey (NFHS-3). (2007). International Institute for Population Sciences (IIPS) and Macro International. National Family Health Survey (NFHS-3), 2005–06: India, Vol I.Mumbai, IIPS. [online] Available from . https://dhsprogram.com/pubs/pdf/frind3/frind3-vol1andvol2.pdf [Last accessed October, 2022].
17. Mohan V, Radhika G, Sathya RM, et al. Dietary carbohydrates, glycaemic load, food groups and newly detected type 2diabetes among urban Asian Indian population in Chennai, India (Chennai Urban Rural Epidemiology Study 59). Br J Nutr. 2009;102:1498-506.
18. Radhika G, Van Dam RM, Sudha V, et al. Refined grain consumption and the metabolic syndrome in urban Asian Indians (Chennai Urban Rural Epidemiology Study 57). Metabolism 2009;58: 675-81.
19. Sun Q, Spiegelman D, van Dam RM, et al. White rice, brown rice, and risk of type 2 diabetes in US men and women. Arch Intern Med. 2010;170:961-9.

CHAPTER 17

Interpretation of Urine of a Diabetic Patient

Prabhat Agrawal, Mudit Khurana, Nikhil Pursnani, Kanika Agarwal, Ashish Gautam

■ INTRODUCTION

With the increasing prevalence of diabetes mellitus, there is a substantial increase in its microvascular as well as macrovascular complications.

Diabetes is the most common cause of chronic kidney disease or end-stage renal disease (ESRD) due to multiple mechanisms such as glomerular hyperfiltration, oxidative stress due to advanced glycation products (AGE), increased vascular proliferation mediated by increase in VEGF, interstitial fibrosis, and atrophy of tubules with advancement of the disease leading to decrease in estimated glomerular filtration rate (eGFR). However, it is almost impossible to clearly predict the prevalence of diabetic kidney disease as it is a diagnosis of biopsy which being an invasive procedure is infrequently performed. Therefore, the diagnosis of diabetic kidney disease is presumed to have based on the clinical history and laboratory evaluation. Although diabetic patients mostly experience diabetic nephropathy, they might also present with other renal disorders, pathologically unrelated to diabetes known as nondiabetic kidney disease (NDKD).

■ DIABETIC NEPHROPATHY

Diabetic nephropathy is characterized pathologically by thickening of glomerular basement membrane, endothelial damage, mesangial expansion, nodule formation, and podocyte loss. But the term "diabetic kidney disease (DKD)" is clinically defined as the presence of a persistently high urine albumin-to-creatinine ratio (UACR) ≥30 mg/g and/or the sustained reduction in eGFR below 60 mL/min/1.73 m^2. DKD is further divided into stages which are elaborated in **Figure 1**.

■ SCREENING FOR KIDNEY DISEASE IN DIABETIC PATIENTS

Increasing prevalence of kidney disease in diabetic patients necessitates early diagnosis and expeditious management. Ergo, urinalysis serves to be one of the

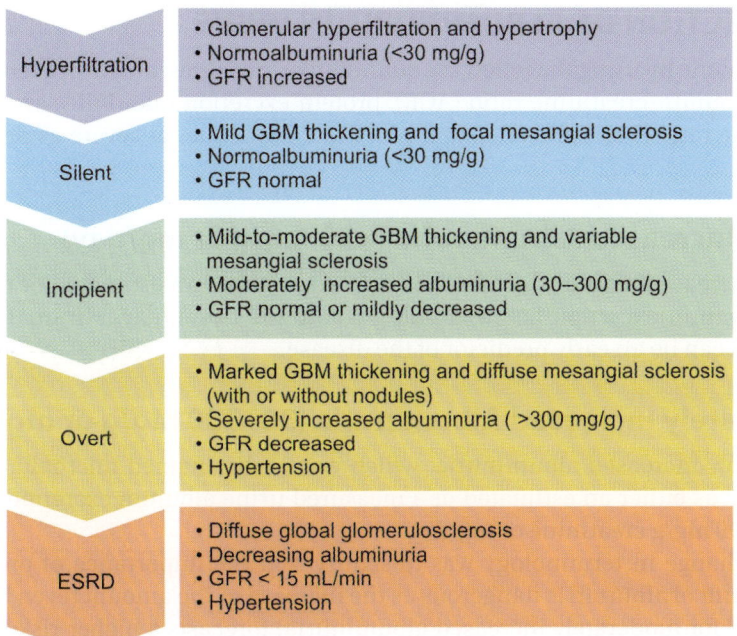

FIG. 1: Stages of diabetic kidney disease.
(ESRD: end-stage renal disease; GBM: glomerular basement membrane; GFR: glomerular filtration rate)

most important investigations to diagnose DKD early as well as to assess the disease severity and it also helps to differentiate from nondiabetic causes of kidney disease in diabetic patients that might be mistaken for diabetic nephropathy. Urinalysis is an easy-to-conduct, noninvasive method for early identification of the disease which helps to prevent the further progression of the disease as regardless of etiology. Chronic kidney disease is classified according to the combined measures of albuminuria and eGFR to indicate prognosis for acute kidney injury, progressive kidney disease, renal failure, cardiovascular mortality, and all-cause mortality. In patients at high cardiovascular risk, the incidence of cardiovascular events is approximately 2.5 times higher for every 10-fold increase in urine albumin excretion and approximately twofold higher for every halving of eGFR. Early institution of therapy will help reverse the albumin loss at the level of glomerulus and improve eGFR decreasing the incidence of cardiovascular mortality and further complications.

■ URINALYSIS IN DIABETIC PATIENTS

Urinalysis should be done annually in all the patients with type 2 diabetes mellitus (T2DM) from the point of diagnosis and in type 1 diabetes mellitus (T1DM) patients beginning 5 years after the diagnosis unless the patient has hypertension, which if present, then urinalysis should be done earlier.

Routine screening in diabetic patients includes albuminuria detection in urine (spot UACR, 24-hour urinary protein), complete urine analysis, and estimated GFR.

DETECTION OF ALBUMINURIA IN URINE

It can be done by using the following quantitative measures: albumin excretion rate (AER), albumin/creatinine ratio (ACR), protein excretion rate (PER), and protein/creatinine ratio (PCR) and staging it into mild, moderate, or severe as depicted in **Table 1**.

Mildly Increased Albuminuria (<30 mg/g or mg/day)

Mildly increased albumin excretion is defined as either an estimated or measured urine albumin excretion below 30 mg/g creatinine or mg/day. Minimal albumin excretion can be an early predictor of the disease.

Moderately Increased Albuminuria (30–300 mg/g or mg/day)

Moderately increased albuminuria, which was earlier named microalbuminuria, is defined as either an estimated or a measured urine albumin excretion between 30 and 300 mg/g creatinine or mg/day.

The change in terminology was to signify that the importance of presence of any amount of albumin is dangerous as the increase in the amount (even below the threshold for moderately increased albuminuria) forecasts a higher risk for future kidney and cardiovascular disease.

Severely Increased Albuminuria (>300 mg/g or mg/day)

Previously termed macroalbuminuria, it is described as either an estimated or a measured urine albumin excretion > 300 mg/g or mg/day.

It provides forecast for the increased severity of disease with worsening in GFR, or development of ESRD. Severely increased albuminuria may also provide a clue to the presence of other kidney pathology instead of DKD and therefore warrants further evaluation.

A better way to assess for albuminuria is 24-hour urinary protein measurement but spot urine albumin creatinine ratio (UACR) has similar outcomes and therefore can be used instead.

TABLE 1: Various parameters used to quantify proteinuria.

	Categories for albuminuria and proteinuria		
	Normal to mildly increased	Moderately increased	Severely increased
AER (mg/day)	<30	30–300	>300
ACR (mg/g)	<30	30–300	>300
PER (mg/day)	<150	150–500	>500
PCR (mg/g)	<150	150–500	>500
Protein dipstick	Negative to trace	Trace to 1+	>1+

(AER: albumin excretion rate; ACR: albumin/creatinine ratio; PCR: protein/creatinine ratio; PER: protein excretion rate)

COMPONENTS OF ROUTINE URINALYSIS

The first early morning urine sample is more concentrated and therefore has better chances of detection of sediments but due to chronic stasis there is also an increased risk of lysis of cells.

Due to the same reason, mid-stream of second urine sample in morning is preferred in all the patients. A mid-stream sample also decreases the contamination with vaginal secretions in females. The urine sample should be examined within 2 hours of collection, otherwise cell lysis ensues. If required, the sample can be preserved at 2–4°C up to 24 hours.

Complete urinalysis consists of the following three components as listed in **Box 1**:
1. Gross assessment of the urine
2. Urine dipstick analysis
3. Urine sediments (microscopy)

DIFFERENTIATING FEATURES BETWEEN DKD AND NDKD USING URINALYSIS

The prevalence of NDKD ranges in diabetic patients ranges from 10 to 85% in different literature. As per the study performed at the Columbia University, approximately 24% of all the native kidney biopsies were taken from diabetic patients, 37% of which had DKD alone, 36% had NDKD alone, and 27% had both DKD with NDKD. In the DKD with NDKD group, the most common finding was acute tubular injury whereas in the group with NDKD ALONE the most frequent diagnosis came out to be focal segmental glomerulosclerosis:

Microscopic hematuria and active urinary sediments: Urine sediment in diabetic nephropathy is usually bland, but microscopic hematuria can occur. In a report from Japan, glomerular hematuria was observed in 17% patients of diabetes mellitus and almost half of these had NDKD, but hematuria was also observed

---

BOX 1: Three components of complete urinalysis.

1. Gross assessment of urine:
   - Urine color
   - Turbidity
   - Urine odor
2. Dipstick analysis:
   - Specific gravity
   - pH
   - protein
   - glucose
   - ketone
   - Blood (heme)
   - Urobilinogen
   - Nitrite
   - Leukocyte esterase
3. Urine sediments:
   - Cells:
     - Red blood cells (RBC)
     - White blood cells (WBC)
     - Epithelial cells
   - Casts:
     - RBC cast
     - WBC cast
     - Granular cast/waxy cast
     - Renal tubular epithelial cells
   - Crystals and microorganisms

TABLE 2: Difference between glomerular and nonglomerular hematuria.

	Glomerular hematuria	Nonglomerular hematuria
Urine color	Dark red, cola-colored, smoky	Bright red
Presence of clots	Absent	Present
Proteinuria (>1 g)	Present	Absent
RBC morphology	Dysmorphic (especially acanthocytes)	Isomorphic
Blood pressure	Increased	Mostly normal
Pedal edema	Present	Absent
Urinary voiding symptoms	Absent	Present
Renal function	Decreased	Initially normal, later reduced
Trauma	Absent	Present

in a minority of DKD patients. More severe diabetic nephropathic changes were observed on renal biopsy if hematuria was present. Although sensitivity and specificity of microscopic hematuria for detecting NDKD is poor, the presence of dysmorphic RBC in the urine is highly specific (94%) for NDKD. Evaluation of spun urine on a high-power microscope reveals dysmorphic RBCs varying in size, shape, and hemoglobin content, thereby revealing glomerular hematuria whereas isomorphic RBCs reflect nonglomerular bleed (from lesions such as calculi, papilloma, and carcinoma). Glomerular versus nonglomerular hematuria can further be differentiated on the basis of clinical features, examination, and laboratory criteria as discussed in **Table 2**.

- *Onset of proteinuria*: The onset of proteinuria within 5 years from documented onset of diabetes mellitus is suspicious of NDKD, since the latent period of overt diabetic nephropathy is usually 10-15 years. However, the time of onset is difficult to ascertain in patients of T2DM.
- *Heavy proteinuria*: An average healthy adult does not excrete more than 150 mg of total protein per day, consisting of 20-30 mg of albumin, 10-20 mg of low molecular weight protein that has undergone glomerular filtration, and 40-60 mg of proteins secreted by the distal tubules such as Tamm–Horsfall protein. Proteinuria can be detected by a reagent strip test which is based on the effect of albumin on a buffer, causing a change in pH proportional to the concentration of albumin itself. Color changes can help in the semiquantitative analysis of albuminuria. Heavy proteinuria may be an indication of NDKD and therefore warrant further investigations including biopsy.
- *Rapid progression of disease*: Diabetic nephropathy is a slowly progressive disorder and rapid deterioration suggests NDKD.
- *Morphology of RBC*: Presence of dysmorphic RBC in the urine is highly specific (94%) for NDKD.
- *Sudden increase in proteinuria*: A sudden increase in albuminuria of >5-10-fold or eGFR decline of >5 mL/min/1.73 m^2/year.
- *Discrepancy between total urinary protein and dipstick albumin*: Dipstick test detects only albumin in the urine; therefore, presence of other proteins such as free light chain may be missed and therefore increased total protein in the urine helps in the diagnosis.

- *Pyuria*: Diabetes mellitus is an immunocompromised state exposing the patient to the threat of recurrent infection; therefore, urinary tract infection is common in diabetic patients. On routine urine examination, it can be easily revealed as the presence of pus cells. Pyuria is defined as the presence of:
    - 10 or more WBC per mm^3 in an unspun specimen of urine
    - 3 or more WBC per mm^3 of spun specimen of urine
    - Urinary dipstick analysis that turns out to be positive for leukocyte esterase

    Usually, culture of such urinary specimens reveals a causative organism but sometimes there might be *Sterile Pyuria* which can be defined as the persistent presence of WBC in the urine with the absence of bacteria, as determined by the means of aerobic laboratory techniques. Sterile pyuria can be due to infective or noninfective causes. The most common cause of sterile pyuria is prior antibiotic use and therefore cultures should always be sent before the initiation of antibiotics. Other infective causes can be prostatitis, balanitis, urethritis, genitourinary tuberculosis, fungal infection. WBC can also be present due to inflammation without any infection such as in interstitial nephritis, nephrolithiasis, urothelial tumors, and polycystic kidneys.
- *Other features*: Proteinuria in the absence of retinopathy (especially in T1DM) and neuropathy as usually retinopathy precedes the presence of nephropathy.

    Such atypical findings on urinalysis warrant further investigations such as ultrasound, kidney function test (KFT), and if indicated renal biopsy which is discussed further.

CLINICAL INDICATIONS FOR KIDNEY BIOPSY IN DIABETIC PATIENTS

Kidney biopsy remains to be the gold standard investigation for diagnosis, treatment decisions, and prediction of outcome in patients with kidney disease. But as currently there are no standard guidelines for indications of biopsy, it is mainly based on the personal opinion of the physician. It is mostly done for patients where it is difficult to differentiate between DKD and NDKD, that is, patients presenting with atypical features such as:
- Nephrotic range proteinuria or kidney failure with duration of diabetes <5 years
- Presence of nephrotic range proteinuria in patients with normal kidney function
- Nephrotic range proteinuria or kidney failure in the absence of diabetic retinopathy
- Acute kidney injury or presence of unexplained microscopic hematuria
- Rapid worsening of kidney function in patients with previously stable kidney function

CONCLUSION

Early evaluation of urine in diabetic patients is a simple, noninvasive, and cost-effective method for diagnosis of kidney disease and to initiate proper management as soon as possible. Albuminuria can be decreased and eGFR can be improved significantly if therapy is started early in the course of the disease. Urinalysis also helps to differentiate patients having kidney disease due to nondiabetic causes which might be mistaken for DKD. Presence of atypical features in urine warrants further investigation, such as biopsy to identify the cause. Therefore, urinalysis in diabetic patients is a first and basic investigation which should be done to identify the cause of kidney disease in diabetic patients.

SUGGESTED READINGS

1. Chen TK, Knicely DH, Grams ME. Chronic kidney disease diagnosis and management: a review. JAMA. 2019;322(13):1294-304.
2. Helal I, Fick-Brosnahan GM, Reed-Gitomer B, Schrier RW. Glomerular hyperfiltration: definitions, mechanisms and clinical implications. Nat Rev Nephrol. 2012;8(5):293-300.
3. National Kidney Foundation. KDOQI Clinical Practice Guideline for Diabetes and CKD: 2012 Update. Am J Kidney Dis. 2012;60(5):850-86. [Erratum in Am J Kidney Dis. 2013;61(6):1049].
4. Ninomiya T, Perkovic V, de Galan BE, et al; ADVANCE Collaborative Group. Albuminuria and kidney function independently predict cardiovascular and renal outcomes in diabetes. J Am Soc Nephrol. 2009;20(8):1813-21.
5. Zimmet PZ, Magliano DJ, Herman WH, et al. Diabetes: a 21st century challenge. Lancet Diabetes Endocrinol. 2014;2(1):56-64.
6. Summary of Recommendation Statements. Kidney Int Suppl (2011). 2013;3(1):5-14.
7. Zhuo L, Ren W, Li W, et al. Evaluation of renal biopsies in type 2 diabetic patients with kidney disease: a clinicopathological study of 216 cases. Int Urol Nephrol. 2013;45(1):173-9.
8. Sharma SG, Bomback AS, Radhakrishnan J, et al. The modern spectrum of renal biopsy findings in patients with diabetes. Clin J Am Soc Nephrol. 2013;8(10):1718-24.
9. Levin A, Stevens PE, Bilous RW, et al. Kidney disease: Improving global outcomes (KDIGO) CKD work group. KDIGO 2012 clinical practice guideline for the evaluation and management of chronic kidney disease. Kidney Int Suppl. 2013;3(1):1-150.
10. Hogan JJ, Mocanu M, Berns JS. The native kidney biopsy: Update and evidence for best practice. Clin J Am Soc Nephrol. 2016;11(2):354-62.
11. Gonzalez Suarez ML, Thomas DB, Barisoni L, et al. Diabetic nephropathy: Is it time yet for routine kidney biopsy? World J Diabetes. 2013;4(6):245-55.

CHAPTER
18

Sulfonylureas in 2022: Are They Still Relevant?

Abhishek Kumar, Sudhir Kumar, Niharika Sinha

■ INTRODUCTION

Blood glucose control is the cornerstone of diabetes management. Metformin and lifestyle changes are the first-line management of newly diagnosed type 2 diabetes mellitus (T2DM). Sulfonylureas (SUs) are one of the most potent oral antidiabetic drugs (OADs) among at least 12 classes of currently available medicines for the management of T2DM and it gives a robust glycated hemoglobin (HbA1c) reduction of about 1.5%. SUs are popular among masses because of their long-established track record on several endpoints like efficacy, treatment adherence, tolerability over time, and affordability. But after the availability of newer agents, the international guidelines differ regarding its position in treatment hierarchy mainly due to concerns about its cardiovascular safety. The controversy about SUs safety emerged during University Group Diabetes Program (UGDP) study that suggested that tolbutamide therapy was no more effective than diet alone, and an increase in all-cause and cardiovascular mortality compared with other treatment groups. However, over the time the major trails like ADVANCE (Action in Diabetes and Vascular Disease: Preterax and Diamicron Modified Release Controlled Evaluation), CAROLINA (Cardiovascular Outcome Study of Linagliptin versus Glimepiride in Patients with Type 2 Diabetes), and TOSCA.IT (Thiazolidinediones Or Sulfonylureas and Cardiovascular Accidents Intervention Trial) has proven its cardiovascular (CV) safety beyond doubt.

■ A CASE SCENARIO

A 44-year-old gentleman presented to OPD with history of polydipsia, frequent urination and weakness from past 6 months. On evaluation, he was normotensive, BMI 26.5, fasting sugar 264, postprandial 445, HbA1c 11.6, low-density lipoprotein (LDL) 110, triglyceride (TG) 156, serum glutamic pyruvic transaminase (SGPT) 42, thyroid-stimulating hormone (TSH) 2.13, creatinine 0.6, and urine albumin-creatinine ratio (UACR 20). His parents were diabetic and mother was on insulin.

He was from a lower middle-class family taking care of family including parents and younger brother. The fellow had just gained a private job in a firm almost 250 km away from the city. The working conditions and the local environment of workplace are not exactly known. He was put on metformin and lifestyle modifications. After 6 months fasting sugar 184, postprandial 226, and HbA1c 9.2. Thus, the patient is newly diagnosed symptomatic T2DM from low economic class on metformin and lifestyle modifications, living away from family (expecting slow/poor lifestyle changes), with expected poor follow-up. Then the question arises; what will be the second line OAD?

■ CLASSIFICATION OF SULFONYLUREAS

Sulfonylureas can be classified by two ways: Based on duration of action and by hierarchy of its development **(Table 1)**.

It is worth to note here that the modern SUs differ in its mechanism of action with their predecessors which makes it more CV safe.

■ MECHANISM OF ACTION OF SULFONYLUREAS

In brief, SUs bind to sulfonylurea receptor (SUR) on the beta cells of the pancreatic islets and stimulate the release of insulin via closure of the adenosine triphosphate (ATP) sensitive potassium (K_{ATP}) channel. The conventional SUs bind strongly with the SUR and cause a continuous release of insulin from the β-cells causing hypoglycemia and weight gain. However, the modern SUs like glimepiride bind to a distinct 65-kD protein site on K_{ATP} channel and have high association/dissociation rate at the SUR. Thus, only the required amount of insulin is released rapidly and not continuously. Hence, modern SU has several benefits compared to conventional causing low risk of hypoglycemia, preservation of beta-cell functions, less secondary failure and less weight gain. Apart from pancreatic beta cells, the K_{ATP} channels are also found in other cells like muscles (skeletal, cardiac, and smooth) and neurons. These extrapancreatic K_{ATP} channels respond to different SU classes based on their SUR affinities. The older SUs like tolbutamide inhibit the mitochondrial K_{ATP} channels on cardiac myocytes more avidly, which may cause impairment of ischemic preconditioning. However; modern SUs do not bind to

TABLE 1: Classification of sulfonylureas.	
Classification based on duration of action	
Short acting	Tolbutamide
Intermediate acting	Gliclazide and glipizide
Long acting	Glibenclamide, glimepiride, gliclazide modified-release (MR), and glipizide MR
Classification based on hierarchy of development	
Conventional	Tolbutamide, glibenclamide, and glipizide
Modern/second generation	Glimepiride, gliclazide, gliclazide MR, and glipizide MR

cardiac SUR in such manner thus, they do not inhibit ischemic preconditioning of cardiac myocytes giving cardiovascular safety.

EFFICACY AND SAFETY

The addition of modern SUs (glimepiride and gliclazide modified release) as second-line agents in patients who have not achieved predecided glycemic target are effective and safe. Compared to metformin up-titration beyond half-maximal dose, the addition of SU to metformin demonstrates better glucose-lowering efficacy and tolerability than pioglitazone, a dipeptidyl peptidase 4 (DPP-4) inhibitors, and comparable glucose-lowering efficacy with sodium-glucose cotransporter-2 (SGLT-2) inhibitors. SUs show similar glycemic efficacy, with acceptable safety at lower cost if compared to glucagon-like peptide 1 receptor agonists (GLP-1-RA).

The ADVANCE trail proved that tighter and longer duration (5 years) glycemic control (HbA1c 6.5) in T2DM patients can be achieved using a SU-based regimen, which gives about 14% reduction in microvascular events. Its observational follow-up study (5 years post-trial), ADVANCE-ON, also shows a significant cumulative benefit (up to 46%) in end-stage kidney disease (ESKD), suggesting that renal protection persisted even longer. This trail did not give any mortality benefit but it was considered safe and practical regarding use of modern SUs in patients of wide CV risk strata. CAROLINA is the only DPP-4 inhibitor CVOT study with an active comparator. It demonstrated that compared to glimepiride, linagliptin poses noninferior risk for major adverse cardiovascular events (3P MACE). The safety profile of SUs appeared to be worse than that of DPP-4 inhibitors prior to this study. In CAROLINA, death from any cause was comparable for the groups, however, glimepiride group had modest weight gain (up to 1.54 kg) and more hypoglycemia. The safety and efficacy of gliclazide modified-release (MR) versus sitagliptin in postmetformin monotherapy patients were retrospectively compared by Zaccardi and colleagues in the UK CPRD observational study. In this study, gliclazide MR was found to be superior over sitagliptin in terms of rapid achievement of target (HbA1c 7.0%) just within 3 months. Thus, the results of ADVANCE and CAROLINA trials, as well as CPRD observational study, largely secured the place of newer-generation SUs, gliclazide MR, and glimepiride in particular in modern T2DM management. The TOSCA.IT assessed the CVOT in >3,000 T2DM patients with mild-to-moderate CV risk randomly assigned to receive either pioglitazone or a SU (gliclazide, glimepiride, or glibenclamide) for a follow-up period of almost 5 years. According to the results, the pioglitazone and SU groups did not differ significantly neither in fatal or nonfatal cardiovascular events, nor in all-cause mortality. These findings reinforced the use of SUs as additional therapies to metformin given their long-term safety profiles.

SPECIAL CONSIDERATIONS

Sulfonylureas and Ramadan

Fasting during Ramadan can lead to excessive gluconeogenesis in people with diabetes, thereby increasing the risk of dehydration, diabetic ketoacidosis, both hypoglycemia and hyperglycemia, and thrombosis. Modern SUs may be used in combination with other drugs during Ramadan, with appropriate counseling and proper dose modifications. In long-standing diabetes, the safety profile of gliclazide makes it the SU of choice during Ramadan.

In Elderly
Risk of hypoglycemia is higher among the elderly with SU therapy. However, modern SUs alone or in combinations can be used in elderly patients because of low risk of hypoglycemia.

In Comorbidities
There is insufficient evidence to suggest that modern SUs increase CV risk. Appropriate dose modifications in hepatic and chronic renal comorbidities are recommended.

Weight Gain
Sulfonylurea use is associated with weight gain, a secondary effect that also occurs with agents like insulin, TZD, and glinides. It may be due to improved utilization of consumed glucose. Modern SUs such as glimepiride and gliclazide MR cause less weight gain if it up-titrated slowly.

Cost Consideration
Cost of medications plays an important role in the management of any chronic disease in underdeveloped and developing countries. Patients without any medical insurance and below the poverty line encounter numerous challenges if costly medicines are prescribed and it affects the compliance. However, SUs are associated with a significantly lower cost per quality-adjusted life-years (QALYs) and result in the longest time to insulin dependence.

■ SULFONYLUREAS AS STANDARD OF CARE
In low- and middle-income countries (LMICs) of Asia and Africa, SUs are the main OAD alone or in combination with metformin. The South Asian Federation of Endocrine Societies (SAFES) recommends glimepiride and gliclazide MR to be preferred over conventional SUs due to its better CV outcomes, reduced mortality and renal protection. The Dutch and Italian guidelines prefer gliclazide because of its lower CV risk, lesser hypoglycemic episodes, relative weight neutrality, and established microvascular benefits. European Association for the Study of Diabetes/American Diabetes Association (EASD/ADA) consensus report says the second-generation SUs (glimepiride, gliclazide, and glipizide) are the last but reasonable choice in people with T2DM with established atherosclerotic cardiovascular disease (ASCVD) or chronic kidney disease (CKD) and/or heart failure (HF) in recourse limited settings. The Research Society for the Study of Diabetes in India (RSSDI) recommends newer SUs, such as gliclazide MR and glimepiride in people with T2DM due to less CV adverse events as add on therapy to metformin. Practically

in countries like India, SUs are the backbone of management of T2DM, as the combination of SUs and metformin is prescribed in about 80% of patients across the age, duration of diabetes, BMI, or disease complications. Also, about 65% of elderly diabetes are on modern SU and/or combinations, endorsing its safety.

CONCLUSION

The efficacy, safety, tolerability, access, and treatment cost are the pillars of management of diabetes. Wherever accessibility and treatment cost permit, the newer agents like SGLT-2 inhibitor, GLP-1 RA has a role in management of T2DM. It is also appropriate as add-on therapy in patients at higher CV risks. Since the second-generation SUs have demonstrated efficient glycemic control, benefits in microvascular and macrovascular outcomes, cardiovascular safety and less hypoglycemia thus, in regions like our country where resources are limited, the SU remains an accessible and affordable treatment option as an add on therapy when metformin alone is inadequate to achieve glucose targets. Thus, the SUs are relevant today and will remain relevant in future supported by their robust and long-standing evidence base.

SUGGESTED READINGS

1. Al-Saleh Y, Sabico S, Al-Furqani A, et al. Sulfonylureas in the Current Practice of Type 2 Diabetes Management: Are They All the Same? Consensus from the Gulf Cooperation Council (GCC) Countries Advisory Board on Sulfonylureas. Diabetes Ther. 2021;12:2115-32.
2. Scheen AJ. Cardiovascular safety of DPP-4 inhibitors compared with sulphonylureas: results of randomized controlled trials and observational studies. Diabetes Metab. 2018;44(5):386-92.
3. Zaccardi F, Jacquot E, Cortese V, et al. Comparative effectiveness of gliclazide modified release versus sitagliptin as second- line treatment after metformin monotherapy in patients with uncontrolled type 2 diabetes. Diabetes Obes Metab. 2020;22(12):2417-26.
4. Kalra S, Bahendeka S, Sahay R, et al. Consensus recommendations on sulfonylurea and sulfonylurea combinations in the management of type 2 diabetes mellitus—International Task Force. Indian J Endocrinol Metab. 2018;22:132-57.
5. Zhang Y, McCoy RG, Mason JE, et al. Second-line agents for glycemic control for type 2 diabetes: Are newer agents better? Diabetes Care 2014;37:1338-45.
6. Kalra S, Aamir A, Das A, et al. Place of sulfonylureas in the management of type 2 diabetes mellitus in South Asia: a consensus statement. Indian J Endocrinol Metab. 2015;19:577.
7. Mohan V, Saboo B, Khader J, et al. Position of sulfonylureas in the current ERA: Review of National and International Guidelines. Clinical Medicine Insights: Endocrinol Diabetes. 2022;15:1-8.

CHAPTER 19

Remission and Reversal in Diabetes

Navneet Agrawal

■ INTRODUCTION

Type 2 diabetes mellitus (T2DM) is a complicated, multifaceted metabolic disorder which is culminated as a result of increase in consumption of unhealthy food and chronic overeating, modern lifestyle and sedentary habits in addition to genetic constitution of the individual. Worldwide prevalence of T2DM was found to be more than 530 million in 2019. With the realization that overall high calorie dietary patterns of processed food rich in sugar content and saturated fat, and concurrent reduction in healthy dietary components including natural fibers, green leafy vegetable and fresh organic foods, has led to a steep rise in development of T2DM. This condition calls for action toward a remedy for reversal, which could aid the staggering healthcare systems and societies across the world. This chapter reviews the current knowledge regarding the possible reversibility of T2DM.

■ TREATMENT OF T2DM FOR REVERSAL

Previous perception of T2DM as a chronic and nonreversible condition has been questioned and recent studies and reports have raised the hope of reversing the condition and facilitate remission of the disease. Reversal of the T2DM in patients has been defined as the maintenance of acceptable blood glucose level for a period of at least 3 months without the need for any antidiabetic medications.

Surgical Reversal for T2DM Remission

Bariatric surgery is believed to reverse T2DM and result in favorable outcomes. Bariatric surgery was associated with postoperative improvement in sugar control, improvement in sensitivity of insulin, better homeostasis of various GI hormones and dramatic improvement in GI microflora from obesogenic to lean profile. In a long-term study, patients with T2DM who underwent bariatric surgery had reversal rate of over 51% at 12 years with an average concurrent weight loss of 35 kg. Factors contributing toward the long-term outcomes of bariatric surgery include the type of surgery, presence of comorbidities, efforts to practice a healthier lifestyle. The Second Diabetes Surgery Summit recommended the use of bariatric surgery in T2DM adults with body mass index >40, or >35 kg/m^2 in those with obesity-related comorbidities. The remission rate in obese adolescents with T2DM were 99%, >5 years and 85% at 5 years. However, there exists a small risk of associated complications in bariatric surgery such as high rates of reoperations and various nutritional deficiencies. The prospective Swedish Obese Subjects study reported remission rates of T2DM at 2, 10 and 15 years of follow-up as 72.3%, 38.1% and 30.4%, respectively. With the results mirrored in a retrospective cohort study with average remission time after bypass being 8.3 years, with 35.1% suffering from T2DM relapse by 5th year. Recently "pill balloons" which are part of the obesity management bridge the gap between the challenges in implementing rigorous lifestyle modifications and remain a nonsurgical alternative to bariatric surgery. However, large scale longitudinal studies are being pursued to evaluate their real-world application. Further mechanistic research and larger prospective randomized studies would be needed to identify the optimal treatment strategies for post-bariatric weight regain and relapse of T2DM with residual or recurrent metabolic disease.

■ PHARMACOTHERAPY FOR T2DM REMISSION AND REVERSAL

Pharmacotherapy aimed to reverse T2DM remains a more feasible option compared to surgical modality. However, taking into account that T2DM is multifactorial disorder, drug therapy by itself may not be successful making remission unlikely with high a chances of relapse. The evidence of desired benefits is observed only in 16% of patients treated with antidiabetics. Pharmacological remission is used as a first-line option for management. In a meta-analysis, short-term intensive insulin therapy was found to significantly improve islet function and induce remission in 46% of patients at 12 months, and 42% at 24 months. Beta-cell redifferentiation was considered as an important underlying mechanism for the treatment effect, providing another treatment strategy for modifying T2DM. In addition, the triple regimen of metformin, pioglitazone and repaglinide, initially used at their maximum tolerated dosage have been shown to be a potential regimen to reverse the newly diagnosed T2DM, followed by dose corrections.

A combination of metformin, pioglitazone with gliclazide was found to be efficacious for the reversal of the disease within couple of years. Even for T2DM patients who have had the disease for a period of 5 years and progressed to insulin without comorbidities, add-on combination drug therapy resulted in lack of need for insulin in 43% of patients within a period of 6 months.

Lack of reversal of T2DM using conventional pharmacotherapy could be because it targets the levels of blood glucose without taking into accounts the involvement of visceral fat. A major study in USA observed only a 0.23% remission rate even with the best practice standard of care despite a staggering increase in expenditure. This highlighted the lack of effectiveness of conventional pharmacotherapy in T2DM reversal. Interventions that can mimic energy deficit can drive similar beneficial effects on T2DM as bariatric surgery. Orlistat, an antiobesity drug, considered to be a calorie restriction mimetic (CRM) was found to be effective.

A study in Japanese patients found the alpha-glucosidase inhibitors effective for reversal in obese T2DM, with miglitol being the most effective. Phase 3 trials with high dose glucagon-like peptide-1 (GLP-1) analogs (like semaglutide) or GLP-1/GIP dual analogs (like tirzepatide) have improved treatment and seem to be promising game-changers in reversing T2DM. In the SURPASS-1 study of tirzepatide, efficacy and treatment regimens were evaluated for three tirzepatide doses (5 mg, 10 mg and 15 mg) compared to placebo for 40 weeks. 51.7% of participants assigned the highest dose achieved a nondiabetic HbA1c value of 5.7% with average weight loss at 9.5 kg. Participants in the tirzepatide treatment arms had a mean diabetes duration of 4.7 years and baseline HbA1c with no severe hypoglycemia or severe hyperglycemia. Treatment discontinuation rates due to adverse events were <7% in each tirzepatide treatment arm.

In a 68-week study of the therapeutic effect of semaglutide in T2DM, subjects on a high dose of the drug (2.4 mg) lost an average of 6.2% more of their body weight in comparison to placebo. Common side effects of high dose semaglutide included nausea, vomiting, diarrhea, and constipation, which 88% of participants reported. The average reduction in body weight with high dose semaglutide was 10 kg. These results indicate the potential of semaglutide in the possible reversal of T2DM. At the end of the trial, participants on the high dose had an average prediabetic range in HbA1c of 6.4%, in comparison to placebo, 7.8% which falls into diabetic range.

Very Low Energy Diets

Very low energy diets (VLEDs) are diets containing energy levels below 800 kcal per day while meeting the nutritional requirements. A retrospective cohort study of T2DM patients receiving standard American Diabetes Association (ADA) care (including dietary advice) found a 7-year cumulative remission rate of just 0.14%. As DiRECT study demonstrated that 50% of the participants who had VLED had long-term reversal with a weight loss of 10 kg, and 90% with 15 kg provided that this was achieved within 6 years of their diagnosis translating a remission of 46% and 36% at 1 and 2 years follow-up respectively. Another long-term study, over 3-year period with 5,000 participants, has indicated a remission rate of 61% in 12 months, strengthened by replications in different studies with different populations.

Low Carbohydrate Diets

Low carbohydrate diets (LCDs) are based broadly on restricting carbohydrate intake between 20–130 g of carbohydrates per day. The classification of LCDs by Feinman et al. has become the most popular definition among dietetic practitioners, as summarized in **Table 1**.

Much evidence has been published on restricting carbohydrate intake including sugar, grains and starchy vegetables in improvement of T2DM. The greatest reductions in HbA1c and diabetic medication use were seen when carbohydrates were restricted to <10% of calorie intake. In a 2-year ad libitum low-carbohydrate T2DM trial, included patients with a longer duration of diabetes (8.4 years on average) and which did not exclude any patients on insulin. With 75% of the patients completing the study, normoglycemia (off medications other than metformin) was

TABLE 1: Definition of low carbohydrate diets (LCDs).		
Definition	Carbohydrate (g/day)	Carbohydrate (% of energy)
Very low carbohydrate diet	20–50 g	6–10%
Low carbohydrate diet	<130 g	<26%
Moderate carbohydrate diet	130–225 g	26–45%
High carbohydrate diet	>225 g	>45%

achieved in 54% out of 75% of participants, suggesting higher retention. Typically, weight loss of 10% was recorded despite no calorie restriction.

LCDs may also have an advantage for long-term weight maintenance. Participants assigned to a low carbohydrate diet after losing weight had significantly higher energy expenditure with a linear trend of 52 kcal per day for every 10% decrease in the calorific contribution of carbohydrate to total energy intake and lower levels of ghrelin than those assigned to a high carbohydrate diet, despite genetic and epigenetic factors driving weight gain.

A major limitation of the LCD literature base is that there are few studies of LCDs showing T2DM remission without also reporting weight loss. It is difficult to attribute pure causality to the LCD as a result. A lack of long-term studies is partly attributed to difficulties in maintaining pure LCD for the long term.

Exercise

The Nutrition Practice Guideline (NPG) sets out an individualized exercise plan for diabetes which suggests aiming for >150 min/week of moderate-intensity aerobic physical activity, divided between 3 days per week, and with no gap of >2 consecutive days without exercise.

There is evidence that neuromuscular electrical stimulation (NMES) can play an important role in controlling T2DM. The average improvement in HbA1c of 0.8 ± 0.7% with NMES therapy is clinically significant and compares well with lifestyle intervention studies where an exercise effect of 0.62% improvement can be expected. Further, another study proposed the benefits of targeting type 2b muscle fibers in exercise for T2DM, as it uses oxidative metabolism with carbohydrate as substrate. Research on elucidating the basic metabolic mechanisms on exercise can help optimize exercise prescription with NMES therapy for T2DM.

■ DURABLE REMISSION FOR BETTER LONG-TERM OUTCOMES IN T2DM PATIENTS

In order to improve reversal of T2DM, it is important to address how to convert reversal into a durable remission, and whether long-term remission can translate into the prevention of any (further) macrovascular, and more importantly, microvascular damage caused by the T2DM. Certain factors have been identified as predictors of remission following bariatric surgery which include diabetes duration, degree of medication use, glycemic control, BMI, manifestation and severity of comorbidities, C-peptide levels and age. Hence, focus and study into understanding the heterogeneity of predictors can help optimize and personalize treatment for T2DM and provide a framework for targeting and personalizing effective support for remission to take place in addition to making it more durable.

CONCLUSION

Multiple, disparate therapeutic interventions confirm that T2DM patients can become normoglycemic again, and early results suggest that this reversal could be maintained long term. Remission should be a treatment goal for those who are still prediabetic, newly diagnosed T2DM, and T2DM diagnosed <6 years ago. Combination therapy will be the key feature of successful reversal and remission due to its multifactorial nature. The pathophysiological complexity seems to boil down to metabolic interventions. Further studies can shed light into understanding the major factors that could contribute to strong remission and perhaps reversal of T2DM.

SUGGESTED READINGS

1. Magkos F, Hjorth MF, Astrup A. Diet and exercise in the prevention and treatment of type 2 diabetes mellitus. Nat Rev Endocrinol. 2020;16(10):545-55.
2. International Diabetes Federation. IDF Diabetes Atlas. [online] Available from: https://diabetesatlas.org/. [Last Accessed October, 2022].
3. Hallberg SJ, Gershuni VM, Hazbun TL, et al. Reversing Type 2 Diabetes: A Narrative Review of the Evidence. Nutrients. 2019;11(4):766.
4. Riddle MC, Cefalu WT, Evans PH, et al. Consensus Report: Definition and Interpretation of Remission in Type 2 Diabetes. Diabetes Care. 2021;44(10):2438-44.
5. Taylor R. Reversing the irreversible: T2DM and you. England: Newcastle University; 2014.
6. Federico A, Dallio M, Tolone S, et al. Gastrointestinal hormones, intestinal microbiota and metabolic homeostasis in obese patients: effect of bariatric surgery. In vivo. 2016;30:321-30.
7. Medina DA, Pedreros JP, Turiel D, et al. Distinct patterns in the gut microbiota after surgical or medical therapy in obese patients. Peer J. 2017;5:e3443.
8. Buchwald H, Estok R, Fahrbach K, et al. Weight and type 2 diabetes after bariatric surgery: systematic review and meta-analysis. Am J Med. 2009;122(3):248-56.
9. Buchwald H, Avidor Y, Braunwald E, et al. Bariatric surgery. A systematic review and metaanalysis. JAMA. 2004;292(14):1724-37.
10. Pories WJ, MacDonald KG, Morgan EJ, et al. Surgical treatment of obesity and its effect on diabetes: 10-y follow-up. Am J Clin Nutr. 1992;55(2 Suppl):582S-85S.
11. Taylor R. Type 2 diabetes: etiology and reversibility. Diabetes Care. 2013;36(4):1047-55.
12. Rubino F, Nathan D, Eckel RH, et al. Delegates of the 2nd Diabetes Surgery Summit. Metabolic surgery in the treatment algorithm for T2DM: a joint statement by International Diabetes Organizations. Diabetes Care. 2016;39:861-77.
13. Qi L, Guo Y, Liu CQ, et al. Effects of bariatric surgery on glycemic and lipid metabolism, surgical complication and quality of life in adolescents with obesity: a systematic review and meta-analysis. Surg Obes Relat Dis. 2017;13(12):2037-55.
14. Ruiz-Cota P, Bacardí-Gascón M, Jiménez-Cruz A. Long-term outcomes of metabolic and bariatric surgery in adolescents with severe obesity with a follow-up of at least 5 years: a systematic review. Surg Obes Relat Dis. 2018;15:S1550.
15. Inge TH, Courcoulas AP, Jenkins TM, et al. Five-year outcomes of gastric bypass in adolescents as compared with adults. N Engl J Med. 2019;380(22):2136-45.
16. Olbers T, Beamish AJ, Gronowitz E, et al. Laparoscopic Roux-en-Y gastric bypass in adolescents with severe obesity (AMOS): a prospective, 5-year, Swedish nationwide study. Lancet Diabetes Endocrinol. 2017;5(3):174-83.

17. Adams TD. In teens with severe obesity, can bariatric surgery wait until adulthood? N Engl J Med. 2019;380(22):2175-7.
18. Sjöström L, Peltonen M, Jacobson P, et al. Association of bariatric surgery with long-term remission of type 2 diabetes and with microvascular and macrovascular complications. JAMA. 2014;311(22):2297-304.
19. Arterburn DE, Bogart A, Sherwood NE, et al. A multisite study of long-term remission and relapse of T2DM mellitus following gastric bypass. Obes Surg. 2013;23:93-102.
20. Ienca R, Al Jarallah M, Caballero A, et al. The procedureless elipse gastric balloon program: multicenter experience in 1770 consecutive patients. Obes Surg. 2020;30(9):3354-62.
21. Daigle CR, Chaudhry R, Boules M, et al. Revisional bariatric surgery can improve refractory metabolic disease. Surg Obes Relat Dis. 2016;12(2):392-7.
22. Wieseler B, McGauran N, Kaiser T. New drugs: where did we go wrong and what can we do better? BMJ. 2019;366:l4340.
23. Weng J, Li Y, Xu W, et al. Effect of intensive insulin therapy on beta-cell function and glycaemic control in patients with newly diagnosed type 2 diabetes: a multicentre randomised parallel-group trial. Lancet. 2008;371(9626):1753-60.
24. Chen A, Huang Z, Wan X, et al. Attitudes toward diabetes affect maintenance of drug-free remission in patients with newly diagnosed type 2 diabetes after short-term continuous subcutaneous insulin infusion treatment. Diabetes Care. 2012;35(3):474-81.
25. Kramer CK, Zinman B, Retnakaran R. Short-term intensive insulin therapy in type 2 diabetes mellitus: a systematic review and meta-analysis. Lancet Diabetes Endocrinol. 2013;1(1):28-34.
26. Wang H, Kuang J, Xu M, et al. Predictors of long-term glycemic remission after 2-week intensive insulin treatment in newly diagnosed type 2 diabetes. J Clin Endocrinol Metab. 2019;104(6):2153-62.
27. McInnes N, Hall S, Sultan F, et al. Remission of type 2 diabetes following a short-term intervention with insulin glargine, metformin, and dapagliflozin. J Clin Endocrinol Metab. 2020;105(8):dgaa248.
28. Kramer CK, Zinman B, Choi H, et al. Predictors of sustained drug-free diabetes remission over 48 weeks following short-term intensive insulin therapy in early type 2 diabetes. BMJ Open Diabetes Res Care. 2016;4(1):e000270.
29. Jennings AS, Lovett AJ, George TM, et al. Getting to goal in newly diagnosed type 2 diabetes using combination drug "subtraction therapy". Metabolism. 2015;64(9):1005-12.
30. Panikar V, Chandalia HB, Joshi SR, et al. Beneficial effects of triple drug combination of pioglitazone with glibenclamide and metformin in type 2 diabetes mellitus patients on insulin therapy. J Assoc Physicians India. 2003;51:1061-4.
31. Prasad V. Rosiglitazone, medical reversal, and back to basics for diabetes. Am Fam Physician. 2014;90(6):368-70.
32. Shibib L, Al-Qaisi M, Ahmed A, et al. Reversal and Remission of T2DM: An Update for Practitioners. Vasc Health Risk Manag. 2022;18:417-43.
33. Karter AJ, Nundy S, Parker MM, et al. Incidence of remission in adults with T2DM: the diabetes and aging study. Diabetes Care. 2014;37:3188-95.
34. Kalra S, Jacob JJ, Gupta Y. Newer antidiabetic drugs and calorie restriction mimicry. Indian J Endocrinol Metab. 2016;20(1):142-6.
35. Sugihara H, Nagao M, Harada T, et al. Comparison of three α-glucosidase inhibitors for glycemic control and bodyweight reduction in Japanese patients with obese type 2 diabetes. J Diabetes Investig. 2014;5(2):206-12.
36. Rosenstock J, Wysham C, Frías JP, et al. Efficacy and safety of a novel dual GIP and GLP-1 receptor agonist tirzepatide in patients with type 2 diabetes (SURPASS-1): a double-blind, randomised, phase 3 trial. Lancet. 2021;398(10295):143-55.
37. Davies M, Færch L, Jeppesen OK, et al; STEP 2 Study Group. Semaglutide 2.4 mg once a week in adults with overweight or obesity, and type 2 diabetes (STEP 2): a randomised, double-blind, double-dummy, placebo-controlled, phase 3 trial. Lancet. 2021;397(10278):971-84.

38. Mustajoki P, Pekkarinen T. Very low energy diets in the treatment of obesity. Obesity Rev. 2001;2(1):61-72.
39. Lean MEJ, Leslie WS, Barnes AC, et al. Durability of a primary care-led weight-management intervention for remission of T2DM: 2-year results of the DiRECT open-label, cluster-randomised trial. Lancet Diabetes Endocrinol. 2019;7(5):344-55.
40. Feinmann J. Low calorie and low carb diets for weight loss in primary care. BMJ. 2018;360:k1122.
41. Nicholas AP, Soto-Mota A, Lambert H, et al. Restricting carbohydrates and calories in the treatment of type 2 diabetes: a systematic review of the effectiveness of 'low-carbohydrate' interventions with differing energy levels. J Nutr Sci. 2021;10:e76.
42. Feinman RD, Pogozelski WK, Astrup A, et al. Dietary carbohydrate restriction as the first approach in diabetes management: critical review and evidence base. Nutrition. 2015;31(1):1-13.
43. Saslow LR, Daubenmier JJ, Moskowitz JT, et al. Twelve-month outcomes of a randomized trial of a moderate-carbohydrate versus very low-carbohydrate diet in overweight adults with T2DM mellitus or prediabetes. Nutr Diabetes. 2017;7:304.
44. Leonetti F, Campanile FC, Coccia F, et al. Very low-carbohydrate ketogenic diet before bariatric surgery: prospective evaluation of a sequential diet. Obes Surg. 2015;25:64-71.
45. Wolever TM, Gibbs AL, Mehling C, et al. The Canadian trial of carbohydrates in diabetes (CCD), a 1-yr controlled of low-glycemic index dietary carbohydrate in T2DM: no effect on glycated hemoglobin but reduction in C-reactive protein. Am J Clin Nutr. 2008;87:114-25.
46. Yamada Y, Uchida J, Izumi H, et al. A non-calorie-restricted low-carbohydrate diet is effective as an alternative therapy for patients with T2DM. Int Med. 2014;53:13-9.
47. Tay J, Thompson CH, Luscombe-Marsh ND, et al. Effects of an energy-restricted low-carbohydrate, high unsaturated fat/low saturated fat diet versus a high-carbohydrate, low-fat diet in T2DM: a 2-year randomized clinical trial. Diabetes Obes Metab. 2018;20:858-71.
48. Hallberg SJ, McKenzie AL, Williams PT, et al. Effectiveness and safety of a novel care model for the management of T2DM at 1 year: an open-label, non randomized, controlled study. Diabetes Ther. 2018;9:583-612.
49. Athinarayanan SJ, Adams RN, Hallberg SJ, et al. Long-term effects of a novel continuous remote care intervention including nutritional ketosis for the management of T2DM: a 2-year non-randomized clinical trial. Front Endocrinol. 2019;10:348.
50. Kaska L, Sledzinski T, Chomiczewska A, et al. Improved glucose metabolism following bariatric surgery is associated with increased circulating bile acid concentrations and remodeling of the gut microbiome. World J Gastroenterol. 2016;22:8698-719.
51. Shai I, Schwarzfuchs D, Henkin Y, et al. Weight loss with a low-carbohydrate, Mediterranean, or low-fat diet. N Engl J Med. 2008;359:229-41.
52. Ebbeling CB, Feldman HA, Klein GL, et al. Effects of a low carbohydrate diet on energy expenditure during weight loss maintenance: randomized trial. BMJ. 2018;363:k4583.
53. Franz MJ, MacLeod J, Evert A, et al. Academy of nutrition and dietetics nutrition practice guideline for type 1 and type 2 diabetes in adults: systematic review of evidence for medical nutrition therapy effectiveness and recommendations for integration into the nutrition care process. J Acad Nutr Diet. 2017;117:1659-79.
54. Jabbour G, Belliveau L, Probizanski D, et al. Effect of low frequency neuromuscular electrical stimulation on glucose profile of persons with T2DM: a pilot study. Diabetes Metab J. 2015;39(3):264-7.
55. Thomas DE, Elliott EJ, Naughton GA. Exercise for T2DM mellitus. Cochrane Database Syst Rev. 2006;(3):CD002968.
56. Miyamoto T, Slone J, Song X, et al. A fructose receptor functions as a nutrient sensor in the Drosophila brain. Cell. 2012;151(5):1113-25.
57. Min T, Barry JD, Stephens JW. Predicting the resolution of T2DM after bariatric surgical procedures: a concise review. J Diabetes Metab. 2015;6:617.

CHAPTER 20

Protecting the Diabetic Target Organs: Kidneys/Heart/Retina and the Liver

Daya Kishore Hazra, Padmamalika Khanna nee Hazra, Gaurav Ashish Khanna, Srishta Hazra

INTRODUCTION

Preventing the effects of diabetes on the target organs constitutes tertiary prevention, but in fact saving these organs starts with primordial prevention, commencing with the diabetes family, which we consider as the primary focus of prevention, and at Agra we have a miniregistry of diabetic families under APIDS (the Agra Preventive Intervention Diabetes Study): families with more than one diabetic and especially the offspring of biconjugal diabetic couples. Protection thus needs to start at birth! Dysglycemia passes through the stages of impaired fasting glucose (IFG) and impaired glucose tolerance (IGT), or both before diabetes supervenes. However, we can pick up abnormalities in nondysglycemic members of diabetic families, such as in MUGA studies! Family members, who have witnessed target organ complications in other members, are all the more receptive to advice!

Since the pathophysiology of diabetic complications is to a large extent common to the various target organs, many of the preventive measures are common to the various target organs, and in fact these are useful even in retarding ageing and reducing diseases such as cancer and Alzheimer's. Alzheimer's is sometimes called type 3 diabetes mellitus! Many also may retard the other forms of Reaven's metabolic syndrome (which we have renamed as "Ravanna syndrome" because of multiple manifestations). *Today inflammation, free radicals, reactive oxygen species, pollutants, and lack of exercise—physical and mental—are incriminated as causal mechanisms in all of these.*

Professor Gyan P Elhence, beloved teacher to Dr Hazra, and countless others always made it a point to emphasize ancillary factors, and would say that an apparent case of Kimmelstiel Wilson syndrome may not be suffering from diabetic nephropathy and may be salvaged by focusing on other factors damaging the kidney, including renal tuberculosis, obstruction, etc.

We have therefore considered ancillary causes of target organ damage when describing target organ protection!

It is therefore essential to avoid ancillary pathogenetic triggers such as free sugars, alcohol, nonsteroidal anti-inflammatory drugs (NSAIDs), obesity, tobacco in its various forms—smoking, chews, snuff, and *dentifrices*, many of which contain tobacco even without labeling! Tobacco no doubt numbs dental pain, but proper dental hygiene and treatment is a much better alternative. Keeping the teeth and gums healthy also eliminates a common source of inflammation!

Preventing obesity by discouraging sweet tooth habits (sugary foods, sweets, sugar in the milk) in infancy, and avoiding excess fat in the food, and encouraging physical activity through games/running and trekking need to be established right from childhood.

Controlling the blood sugar is the sine qua non in protecting the target organs, and apart from self-monitoring of the blood sugar, various equivalents such as glycosylated hemoglobin and fructosamine are in common use. Since fructosamine is dependent on sugar over the last 3 weeks, we find it more useful in assessing recent control, more so than glycosylated hemoglobin. Continuous glucose monitoring is now gaining popularity because it can assess not only the time in the physiological range but also the extent of variability which is considered to be a predictor of complications independent of the mean sugar. Microangiopathy and macroangiopathy manifestations show differences in relation to glycemic control, as evidenced in long-term the United Kingdom Prospective Diabetes Study (UKPDS).

Adequate education, literacy, and group activities prevent depression, physical and mental inertia, and so do meditation, Yoga, and participation in Satsangs and the like.

ORGAN-SPECIFIC PROTECTION

We will now list specific protective measures for the target organs.

Kidneys

Nephrotoxic agents such as NSAIDs and aminoglycoside antibiotics should be avoided unless absolutely unavoidable.

Blood Pressure Control

Since hypertension damages the kidneys, blood pressure should be monitored and controlled.

Restriction of sodium intake and avoiding fluid overload need to be remembered.

Agents such as renin–angiotensin system (RAS) inhibitors/angiotensin receptor blocker (ARB)/beta blockers/mineralocorticoid antagonists have now been supplemented by the sodium–glucose co-transporter 2 (SGLT-2) inhibitors as preferred agents for reducing the BP while protecting the kidneys. Earlier calcium channel blockers cause fluid retention, but nifedipine is renoprotective.

Other agents have been recently reviewed (Sonkar and Verma, 2022).

The LEADER trial showed benefits from liraglutide. SUSTAIN 1-7 trials suggested benefits from semaglutide. Dipeptidyl peptidase-4 (DPP-4) inhibitors such as linagliptin and sitagliptin are being studied. Both SGLT-2 inhibitors and DPP-4 inhibitors have been claimed to reduce fibrosis in the kidney!

Other Agents for Reducing Renal Fibrosis

Antifibrotic drugs, such as pirfenidone, and pentoxifylline and finerenone a new mineralocorticoid antagonist, are in phase 3 trials for diabetic kidney disease.

The anti-AGE (advanced glycation end-product) drug pyridoxamine derived from vitamin B6 and the JAK STAT inhibitor baricitinib have been studied for reducing free radicals and the inflammatory cascade, respectively.

Infections

Urinary tract infection (UTI), pyelonephritis, and tuberculosis of the kidneys sometimes complicate diabetic nephropathy and diabetic kidney disease.

Controlling UTI is important for protecting the kidneys, and one needs to stress that apart from diabetes other mechanisms damaging the kidneys need attention.

The urine needs to be examined for microalbuminuria and pus cells more than 5 per high power field warrant culture and sensitivity.

Diagnosing UTI and eliminating obstructions such as due to the prostrate are important. Avoidable catheterization can introduce infection, and should not be routinely done.

Nonproteinuric Diabetic Kidney Disease and Biomarkers

Nonproteinuric diabetic kidney disease is being increasingly recognized. Biomarkers attracting attention are cystatin C, kidney injury molecule-1 (KIM1), tumor necrosis factor 1 and 2, and MMP-9/NGAL (matrix metalloproteinase-9/neutrophil gelatinase-associated lipocalin), etc.

These can supplement periodic monitoring of the serum creatinine and the estimated glomerular filtration rate (e-GFR).

Since some diabetic families show a predilection for early kidney involvement diabetics in such families need close attention.

Diet

Switching to a plant-based vegetarian diet instead of nonvegetarian proteins is probably beneficial, as well as using a low-protein diet.

Salt restriction helps prevent hypertension.

Retina

There are some instances where what is beneficial for a particular target organ is possibly harmful in another. Vascular endothelial growth factor (VEGF) inhibition is an accepted mode of treatment for diabetic retinopathy, where new blood vessels are undesirable, but in coronary artery disease one mode of therapy is creating and stimulating new blood vessels to feed the myocardium! Similarly hyperbaric oxygen helps diabetic foot ulcers but may promote free radical formation!

The routine use of retinal photography, coupled with use of artificial intelligence analysis, is making it far easier to detect retinopathy. It is exciting that using laser photocoagulation and VEGF antagonist injections one can prevent the progress of retinopathy, and a patient guide for watching retinal health is summarized below. The main anti-VEGF therapies in current use are bevacizumab (Avastin), ranibizumab (Lucentis), and aflibercept (Eylea). In addition Rho kinase inhibitors are of interest. Rho kinase inhibitors work to treat diabetic retinopathy by decreasing the adhesion of leukocytes and by slowing leukocyte-induced damage. Used as an intravitreal injection, the Rho kinase inhibitor slows the synthesis of various downstream proteins in the Rho pathway as well as intercellular adhesion molecule 1 (ICAM-1). Ruboxistaurin and other inhibitors of protein kinase C are not in common use.

Some of the points in the patient guide that are logical for the early detection of diabetic retinopathy are listed here:
- Routine eye checks, starting at 40 years, and then at least every 2 years, including indirect ophthalmoscopy retinal examination. This must be done to supplement direct retinal examination.
- Proper nutrients: Vitamin A/C/lutein/zeaxanthin/fatty acids
- Minimizing screen time: Computer breaks with eye moistener drops
- Eliminating tobacco
- Avoid stress, that raises BP and blood sugar
- Wearing eye protection: Glasses with 100% UV protection/screens eliminating blue light
- Pay attention to vision changes: Increases in muscae volitantes/field defects/blurred vision
- Monitor retina during diabetes checkups by simple fundus photography

Rho kinase inhibitors, taurodeoxycholic acid, dexamethasone implants, and glibenclamide are being evaluated in experimental models.

Heart

This target organ can be affected not only by coronary artery atherosclerosis but also by cardiomyopathy, and both can lead to heart failure, diastolic or systolic, without or with reduction of the ejection fraction, which is an important cause of morbidity and mortality in diabetes. EKG and echocardiography are simple tools for monitoring the heart.

The earliest detection of coronary artery disease is, in terms of clinical symptoms, suggestive of myocardial ischemia, but in diabetes because of concurrent autonomic neuropathy silent involvement is common, and therefore early detection of cardiac involvement can be problematic.

Periodic clinical assessment can be supplemented by Tc MIBI perfusion scanning and magnetic resonance imaging cardiac assessment, so that interventions can be considered before cardiac muscle is lost. Fractional flow measurements easily supplements angiography to indicate the functional importance of a visualized coronary artery narrowing.

It is wise to combine nitrates with agents that enhance the myocardium utilization of available blood: trimetazidine and ranolazine are extensively used and clinically rewarding, especially in small vessel disease, where stenting or coronary artery bypass graft (CABG) is not feasible.

In addition to the general preventive measures, heart protection focusses on controlling hypertension and blood lipids.

Lowering serum cholesterol, especially low-density lipoprotein cholesterol (LDL-C), is easily achieved by high intensity statins supplemented by ezetimibe. These respectively reduce endogenous and ingested sources of cholesterol. The advantages of a vegetarian, or better still vegan diet have been already mentioned. It is best to combine statins with coenzyme Q supplementation.

In high-risk cases modulation of the LDL receptors can be achieved by antibodies or by mRNA modification, albeit these are currently expensive.

Lowering triglycerides is also important, and saroglitazar is an extremely effective agent for this. Furthermore unlike the fibrates there are no overlapping toxicities with the statins.

In patients with episodic symptoms a Holter monitor for 1-7 days can pick up transient arrhythmias and particularly paroxysmal atrial fibrillation. These can be efficiently managed by drugs or devices.

Pacemakers can if necessary be supplemented by implanted cardiac defibrillators (ICD)!

Psychiatric or family physician counseling to the patient and the family can often help eliminate psychological stresses that precipitate angina and/or arrhythmias.

As regards blood sugar very tight control and achieving this too rapidly has been shown to enhance cardiovascular mortality! The HbA1c goal has to be adjusted according to age and cardiovascular risk. *Hypoglycemia has to be avoided*! Many of the newer antidiabetics help protect the heart.

Cardiac failure—diastolic or systolic is easily diagnosed by echocardiography and this can be supplemented by myocardial magnetic resonance imaging. For ischemia, CT angiography and CT calcium scoring can avoid invasive angiography. Myocardial perfusion scanning with Tc MIBI should precede invasive angiography.

Cardiac failure is treated by the four-pronged approach: beta blockers, angiotensin-converting enzyme (ACE)/ARB, mineralocorticoid antagonists such as eplerenone or finerenone, and angiotensin receptor neprilysin inhibitor (ARNI) (sacubitril–valsartan combinations) with significant benefit both clinical and by echocardiographic assessment. Again sodium restriction and stress reduction should not be forgotten! Cardiac chamber synchronization is sometimes useful in left bundle branch block. Left ventricular assist surgery and as an ultimate option heart transplant may need to be remembered!

The newer hyperglycemia therapies such as SGLT-2 inhibitors switch myocardial metabolism from glucose to ketones and this has long-term benefits not only to the heart but also to the kidneys and the liver, as shown in various studies. Cardiovascular outcomes trial (CVOT) studies are now mandatory by the Food and Drug Administration (FDA) for all new antidiabetic agents!

The fears of ketoacidosis are now being challenged by the advocacy of ketogenic diets, and at Agra we encourage a vegan/vegetarian Agra Diet that is mildly ketogenic!

Liver

This is probably the least understood, as compared to heart, kidney, and retina protection. This is despite the almost ubiquitous demonstration of fatty livers in our diabetics.

Exercise, sugar and fat dietary restriction, vitamin E, and saroglitazar have been advocated. Methyl donors such as S-Adenosyl methionine may be useful, and also glutathione.

Thiazolidinediones (TZDs) though touted, are not used by us because of their deleterious effects on the heart (in North India swelling of the feet is regarded as a harbinger of approaching death!).

It is important to eliminate other hepatotoxic agents such as alcohol/heavy metals (in well water or in Ayurvedic tonics), amoebiasis, and drinking water in copper vessels which is widespread in our subcontinent.

Liver protective foods in common use include radishes, turnips, sprouts, and turmeric.

Hyperhomocystinemia is common, and diagnosing this protects the heart too using B6/folate/B12 supplements at very low cost!

CONCLUSION

Prevention is possible and far cheaper than dealing with the consequences of target organ damage. We have outlines both systemic and organ-wise approaches. Deo Gratia, the results are rewarding!

SUGGESTED READINGS

1. Hazra D, Gupta A, Jain V, et al. Comparison of MUGA assessment with ANU photorheography for assessment of early cardiac dysfunction in prediabetics and diabetics. J Nucl Med. 2008;40(Supplement 1):199P.
2. Sonkar SK, Verma J. Diabetic nephropathy. In: Shyam Sundar (Ed). Medicine Update 2022, volume 32. Evangel; 2022. pp. 976-84.
3. Behar-Cohen F, Loewenstein A. Current and Future Treatments for Diabetic Retinopathy. Pharmaceutics. 2022;14:812.
4. Hazra DK, Padmamalika K. The Agra Diet Poster Presentation at Diabetes India Meet, Jaipur; 2015.

CHAPTER
21

Gestational Diabetes Mellitus: A Window of Opportunity for Noncommunicable Disease Prevention

Saurabh Srivastava

■ INTRODUCTION

High prevalence and immense potential for diabetes prevention makes gestational diabetes mellitus (GDM) a public health priority in our country. Diabetes in pregnancy, has been well recognized as a significant contributor to the epidemic of type 2 diabetes mellitus (T2DM) in the country. Taking into consideration the above contribution, the pregnant women has been the focus of attention, as a critical target for diabetes prevention strategies.

During pregnancy physical, hormonal, and humoral changes take place in woman's body to supply the necessary nutrients and for the development of fetus. This biological phenomenon is considered as a window for the future health of both offspring and mother. Fetal origin of adult metabolic disorder is the concept introduced by Dr D Barker which stated that the adverse uterine environment during pregnancy can lead to metabolic disorders in fetal life.

Gestational diabetes mellitus is defined as hyperglycemia or glucose intolerance which is first recognized during pregnancy. As per the estimates of International Diabetes Federation GDM accounts for 14% of the pregnancies worldwide representing around 18.4 million births annually. Indian women have a relatively high prevalence of GDM (7.2%) as well as several times higher risk of developing T2DM within 3–5 years following the pregnancy during which GDM was experienced.

One in four pregnancies is affected by hyperglycemia in pregnancy, in the Southeast Asian region, which has the highest prevalence in the world. GDM occurs at a lower body mass index (BMI), and T2DM at a younger age in Asians. Urbanization is the major contributor for the growing epidemic of GDM. Prevalence of GDM ranges from 3.8 to 21% in different parts of India. There are >200,000 cases of GDM annually, as around 7% of pregnancies are complicated by GDM. As compared to Caucasian women, Indian woman are at 11-fold increased risk of developing glucose intolerance during pregnancy.

METABOLIC ADAPTATIONS DURING PREGNANCY

During pregnancy mother's body undergoes various physiological changes to support the growing demand of fetus. These physiological changes include various adaptations of cardiovascular, hematologic, renal, respiratory, and adds metabolic systems. The most important metabolic adaptation is insulin sensitivity. In early pregnancy, there is increase in insulin sensitivity which promotes uptake of glucose into adipose stores, to be used in the later part of pregnancy. With advancement of pregnancy, there is surge of local and placental hormones such as estrogen, progesterone, cortisol, placental lactogen, and placental growth hormone which promotes insulin resistance. As a result of this insulin resistance, glucose levels are elevated, and glucose is transported across the placenta for the growth of fetus. In order to maintain homeostasis, there is hypertrophy and hyperplasia pancreatic beta cells leading to hyperinsulinemia. However, the maternal insulin sensitivity returns to prepregnancy levels within few days of delivery.

METABOLIC ADAPTATIONS DURING GESTATIONAL DIABETES MELLITUS (FLOWCHART 1)

Normal pregnancy is characterized by declining maternal insurance sensitivity from mid-gestation onward to supply the nutrients to the fetus. There is chronic defect in beta-cell function, in women developing GDM, caused due to maternal hyperglycemia. The beta cells, in these patients are not able to compensate for the challenge of insulin resistance posed by late pregnancy. GDM may represent a transient "unmasking" of preexisting latent metabolic disturbances. Maternal

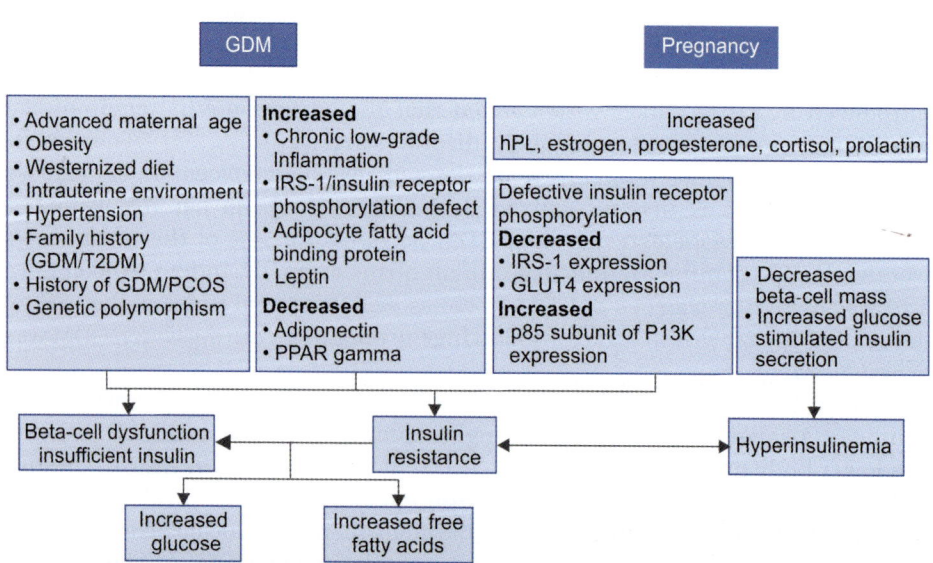

FLOWCHART 1: Metabolic adaptations in gestational diabetes mellitus (GDM).

(IRS: insulin receptor substrate; PPAR: peroxisome proliferator-activated receptor; T2DM: type 2 diabetes mellitus)

genetic predisposition coupled with environmental and fetoplacental factors initiates a chain of events affecting mother and fetus in both the short and long term.

RISK FACTORS FOR GESTATIONAL DIABETES MELLITUS

Risk factors for GDM are indirectly or directly related to impaired beta-cell function and/or insulin sensitivity. Important factors include obesity, overweight, advanced maternal age, hypertension, westernized diet, intrauterine environment, ethnicity, family history of GDM or T2DM, and personal history of GDM or polycystic ovarian syndrome. Other factors responsible are increased insulin receptor substrate 1 (IRS-1) phosphorylation, insulin receptor phosphorylation defects, chronic low-grade inflammation, hyperleptinemia, decreased adiponectin and peroxisome proliferator-activated receptor gamma (PPARγ), and increased adipocyte fatty acid-binding protein.

WHY IS GESTATIONAL DIABETES IMPORTANT?

There are well-documented clinical issues that follow GDM in pregnancy. GDM plays an important role in increasing the prevalence of obesity, metabolic syndrome, and diabetes, hence, it has been considered as a major public health issue. In the evolution of (T2DM), GDM is considered to be an intermediate stage.

Immediate Implications

Fetal hyperglycemia which is a consequence of maternal hyperglycemia stimulates fetal insulin secretion. Fetal hyperinsulinemia promotes excessive growth due to anabolic effects of insulin. This overgrowth can contribute to a host of adverse neonatal outcomes like prematurity, perinatal mortality, birth injury, macrosomia, shoulder dystocia, and need for cesarean section.

The hyperglycemia and adverse pregnancy outcomes (HAPO) study showed a continuous association of maternal glycemia with adverse outcomes and clinical consequences of maternal glycemia—namely fetal overgrowth and fetal hyperinsulinemia.

Future Implications (Flowchart 2)

Gestational diabetes mellitus has long term implications for mother and child. The offspring born out of GDM pregnancy has an increased prevalence of overweight/obesity, metabolic syndrome dyslipidemia, and dysglycemia, in childhood. There is a high risk of development of T2DM later in the life (21 vs. 4%) in the children born of GDM mothers as compared to non GDM mothers. Glucose intolerance develops before the age of 17 years in about one-third of children born of diabetes pregnancies.

Metabolic dysfunction linking mother and child may be the consequence of several elements including: (1) The home environment and associated lifestyle, (2) Fetal exposure to the altered intrauterine environment of the GDM pregnancy, and (3) Shared genetic factors, which may program adverse developmental pathways as per the Developmental Origins of Health and Disease (DOHaD) paradigm.

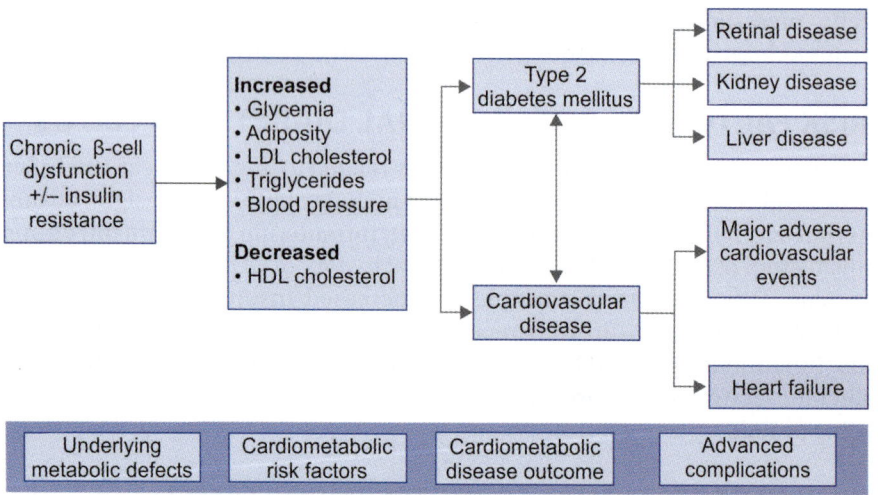

FLOWCHART 2: Future implications of gestational diabetes mellitus.
(HDL: high-density lipoprotein; LDL: low-density lipoprotein)

The hyperglycemia associated with GDM results in fetal overnutrition and a higher risk of obesity and diabetes in the offspring through various mechanisms including epigenetic changes. Postnatal overnutrition in the above scenario leads to higher incidence of early onset adult T2DM along with childhood and adolescent obesity. This in turn increases the prevalence of GDM and sets off a vicious cycle of GDM and T2DM in the community. Metabolic disease susceptibility is increased lifelong, following epigenetic changes in various genes and, thus, the likelihood for a new generation of mothers with GDM and/or obesity.

Women, diagnosed with GDM, during pregnancy are at high risk of future development of T2DM. Pregnancy with GDM is considered as index pregnancy and it is estimated that ~10% of women with GDM have diabetes mellitus soon after delivery. Of the remaining, 20–60% develop diabetes within 5–10 years. Factors that are responsible for early development of diabetes mellitus after pregnancy include markers of severe decompensation, in the form of marked insulin resistance, high glucose levels, and poor beta cell function. There is also an increased frequency of cardiovascular risk factors and cardiovascular events in patients with history of GDM.

■ CAN THE RISK OF GDM REDUCED?

Antenatal and perinatal outcomes as well as long term outcome of both mother and child can be prevented by the control of hyperglycemia during the pregnancy.

Antenatal and Perinatal Outcomes

Two randomized control trials, viz., Australian Carbohydrate Intolerance Study in Pregnant Women (ACHOIS) and Maternal Fetal Medical Units Network in the USA, reveal a consistent pattern. There are various studies which state that relative risk of maternal hypertensive disorders, fetal overgrowth, and shoulder dystocia is lowered by diagnosing and treating GDM either by nutritional advice, glucose self-monitoring, or if required, exogenous insulin. However, this benefit is evident in only a small fraction of pregnancies, as most pregnancies do not have adverse perinatal outcomes in the absence of treatment.

Long-term Maternal Outcomes

There are direct evidence showing the benefits of interventions during GDM, in the prevention of future T2DM. Lifestyle intervention during postpartum period prevents the occurrence of T2DM and cardiovascular disease among the women with GDM. Use of metformin and intensive lifestyle intervention is highly effective in delaying or preventing diabetes in women with impaired glucose tolerance (IGT) and a history of GDM. As GDM is recognized as a chronic cardiometabolic disorder there is a potential opportunity that early risk-modifying intervention can be aimed at primary prevention of cardiovascular disease (CVD) and T2DM. However, there are clinical challenges and hurdles that need to be overcome for this approach.

Long-term Fetal Outcomes (Fig. 1)

Preventive measures for T2DM should be started during intrauterine period and have to be continued throughout life. Several observational studies have shown that breastfeeding as compared to bottle feeding, has been associated with a reduced long-term risk of obesity and diabetes mellitus. The pregnant mother with diabetes is highly motivated and can serve as a very effective starting point for a diabetes prevention strategy as she can deliver the message to the family, effectively. Recently a subanalysis of HAPO follow-up on 4,832 mothers with untreated GDM as well as their 10-14 years old children, confirmed that BMI and glycemia, measured during mid-pregnancy, serve as joint predictors of childhood adiposity outcomes. The original HAPO study demonstrated that the combination of maternal obesity and untreated GDM was associated with higher odds for new-born body fat, birth

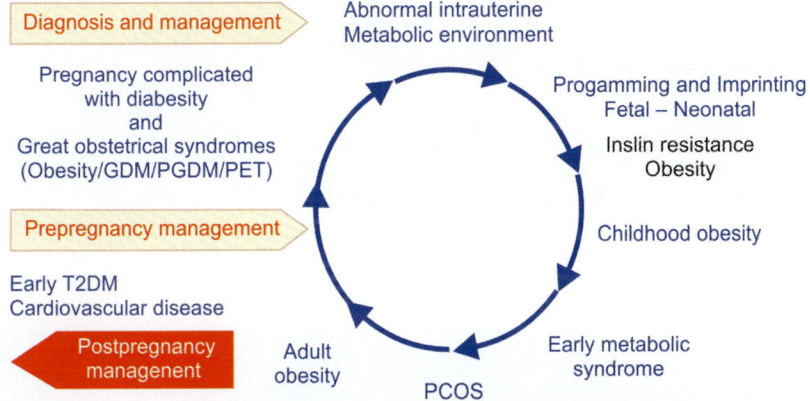

FIG. 1: Fetal outcome in GDM pregnancy.

(GDM: gestational diabetes mellitus; PGDM: pregestational diabetes; PET: pre-eclampsia/toxemia; T2DM: type 2 diabetes mellitus)

weight, and cord C-peptide >90th percentile, compared with the odds for either GDM or obesity separately. This suggests that there is more than additive association of obesity and GDM with neonatal outcomes.

CONCLUSION

Changes in carbohydrate and lipid metabolism occur during pregnancy to ensure a continuous supply of nutrients to the growing fetus despite intermittent maternal food intake. These metabolic changes are progressive and may be accentuated in women who develop GDM. However, in the woman's life, this biological phenomenon is considered as a window on the future health of both mother and offspring. Instituting preconception care and effective postdelivery follow-up, especially for those who had GDM, can provide windows of opportunity for promoting long-term health.

SUGGESTED READINGS

1. Zeng Z, Liu F, Li S. Metabolic Adaptations in Pregnancy: A Review. Ann Nutr Metab 2017;70(1):59-65.
2. Buchanan TA, Xiang AH, Page KA. Gestational Diabetes Mellitus: Risks and Management during and after Pregnancy. Nat Rev Endocrinol. 2012;8(11):639-49.
3. Berberoglu Z. Pathophysiology of Gestational Diabetes Mellitus. EMJ Diabet. 2019;7(1):97-106.
4. Fu J, Retnakaran R. The life course perspective of gestational diabetes: An opportunity for the prevention of diabetes and heart disease in women. E Clinical Medicine. 2022;45:101294.
5. Madhu SV. Diabetes in pregnancy–A critical window of opportunity. Int J Diabetes Dev Ctries. 2018;38(1):1-3.
6. Chen LW, Soh SE, Tint MT, et al. Combined analysis of gestational diabetes and maternal weight status from pre-pregnancy through post-delivery in future development of type 2 diabetes. Sci Rep. 2021;11(1):5021.

CHAPTER 22

Diabetes and Vaccination: The Need and Guideline

Puneet Saxena, Aradhana Sharma, Suresh Kumar Yadav

INTRODUCTION

Diabetes mellitus is a chronic metabolic disorder that share the phenotype of hyperglycemia. Diabetes is one of the rapidly spreading health problem across the low-and-middle income countries like India. It is predicted that by 2025 the number of cases with diabetes in India would be 69.9 million with majority of undiagnosed cases. Diabetic patient both type 1 diabetes mellitus (T1DM) as well as type 2 diabetes mellitus (T2DM) are at higher risk for certain vaccine preventable disease, which would lend up to hospitalization and sometime even die. Diabetic people are more at risk of disease because it makes immune system weaker to fight against infection, even in well controlled blood sugar. This could be prevented up to some extent by vaccination against infections.

INFECTION IN DIABETES

- *Pneumococcal infection*: It's mortality rate average 10–20% while may it may exceed 50% in high-risk group, according to World Health Organization (WHO). It is found that diabetic people are almost three times at higher risk of death by pneumonia related complications.
- *Influenza infection*: The people with diabetes are six times more hospitalized than those without diabetes during an influenza epidemic and mortality also varying between 5 and 15%.
- *Hepatitis B infection*: Diabetic people are at a 2.1 times increased risk of infection than nondiabetics by the hepatitis B infection (HBV).

PATHOPHYSIOLOGY OF INFECTION IN DIABETES

Adults with diabetes are more prone to infections because of hyperglycemic condition and complications that reduces T-cell response, neutrophil function, disorders of humoral immunity, antioxidant system depression, and low secretion of inflammatory cytokines.

RECOMMENDED ADULT IMMUNIZATION SCHEDULE (TABLE 1)

- Recommended vaccination for adults who meet age requirement, lack documentation of vaccination, or lack evidence of past infection.
- Recommended vaccination for adults with an additional risk factor or another indication.
- Recommended vaccination based on shared clinical decision-making.
- No recommendation/not applicable.

Pneumococcal Vaccine

Two types of pneumococcal vaccine are recommended in diabetic patients.
1. *Pneumovax 23 (PPSV23)*: All 19–64 years age group persons vaccinate with one dose of Pneumovax vaccine and age >65 years received second dose of Pneumovax at least 5 years after from first dose of pneumovax vaccine.
2. *PCV13*: Adults age >19 years with an immunocompromising conditions like chronic renal failure (CRF), etc., vaccinate with PSV13 single dose.

TABLE 1: Vaccination in diabetic patient based on age and special population.

Group	19–26 Years	27–49 years	50–64 years	>65 years	Pregnant women	HIV and immunocompromised
Pneumococcal	A	A	A	A	B	C
COVID-19	Above 12 years-A	A	A	A	A	A
Hepatitis B	A	A	B	B	A	A
Influenza IIV4/RIV4	A	A	A	A	A	A
Influenza LAIV4	C	C	D	D	D	D
HPV	A	C	D	D	D	D
Herpes zoster	B	B	A	A	D	A
Tdap diphtheria pertussis tetanus	A	A	A	A	A	A
MMR	B	B	B	D	D	D
Hepatitis A	B	B	B	B	C	C
Meningococcal	B	B	B	B	C	D
Haemophilus influenza B (HIB)	C	C	C	C	D	C

(HIV: human immunodeficiency virus; HPV: human papillomavirus; IIV4: influenza inactivated; LAIV4: influenza live attenuated; MMR: measles, mumps, and rubella; RIV4: influenza recombinant; Tdap: tetanus, diphtheria, and pertussis)

Contraindications

Pneumococcal vaccine is contraindicated if there is a severe allergic reaction (e.g., anaphylaxis) after a previous dose or to a vaccine component, and also with any diphtheria–toxoid-containing vaccine or to its component.

Precautions

Moderate or severe acute illness with or without fever.

COVID-19

All the people with diabetes are recommended to get series of COVID-19 vaccine (Covaxin, Covishield, Pfizer-BioNTech, etc.) plus booster dose whenever eligible.

Contraindications

History of a severe allergic reaction (e.g., anaphylaxis) after a previous dose or to a component of the COVID-19 vaccine.

Precautions

- History of anaphylaxis after any vaccine other than COVID-19 vaccine or after any injectable therapy.
- History of a nonsevere, immediate allergic reaction with onset <4 hours after a dose of one type of COVID-19 vaccine.
- History of an allergy-related contraindication to one type of COVID-19 vaccine should have a precaution to the other types of COVID-19 vaccines.

Hepatitis B

All the people with age <60 years are recommended to complete a 2- or 3-series of hepatitis B vaccine. If a person is 60 years or older than that, then the vaccination may be decided based on the patient's likelihood of acquiring hepatitis B infection.

Contraindications

History of severe allergic reaction (e.g., anaphylaxis) after a previous dose or to a vaccine component.

Precautions

- In case of pregnancy for Heplisav-B only.
- Moderate or severe acute illness with or without fever.

Influenza Vaccine

One dose of influenza vaccine (quadrivalent inactivated influenza vaccine) is recommended annually for all diabetic patients who lack of evidence of past infection. It advises not to use live attenuated influenza vaccine in diabetic patients.

Special Situations

- *Egg allergy, hives only*: Any influenza vaccine appropriate for age and health status annually.
- *Egg allergy—any symptom other than hives*, e.g., angioedema and respiratory distress) or required epinephrine or another emergency medical intervention.
- *Severe allergic reaction* (e.g., anaphylaxis) to a vaccine component or a previous dose of any influenza vaccine.
- *History of Guillain-Barré syndrome* within 6 weeks after previous dose of influenza vaccine.

Human Papillomavirus

Two or three doses of human papillomavirus vaccine are recommended through 26 years depending on age of initial vaccination or condition.

Contraindications

History of severe allergic reaction (e.g., anaphylaxis) after a previous dose or to a vaccine component

Precautions

Moderate or severe acute illness with or without fever.

Herpes Zoster

Series of two dose is recommended in age 19 yeas or older and have weak immune system or are age 50 years or older.

Contraindications

History of severe allergic reaction (e.g., anaphylaxis) after a previous dose or to a vaccine component.

Precautions

- Moderate or severe acute illness with or without fever.
- History of current herpes zoster infection.

Tetanus, Diphtheria, and Whooping Cough (Pertussis)

One dose tetanus, diphtheria, and pertussis (Tdap), then Td or Tdap booster every 10 years. Tdap need to get if person have not received at or after age 11 years. After that need Tdap or Td booster ever 10 years.

Contraindications

- History of severe allergic reaction.
- For Tdap only, encephalopathy, not attributable to another cause within 7 days of administration of previous dose of DTP, DtaP, or Tdap.

Precautions
- Guillain–Barré syndrome (GBS) within 6 weeks after a previous dose of tetanus–toxoid-containing vaccine.
- History of Arthus-type hypersensitivity reactions after a previous dose of diphtheria–toxoid-containing or tetanus–toxoid-containing vaccine; defer vaccination until at least 10 years have elapsed since the last tetanus–toxoid-containing vaccine.
- Moderate or severe acute illness with or without fever.
- *For Tdap only*: Progressive or unstable neurological disorder, uncontrolled seizures, or progressive encephalopathy until a treatment regimen has been established and the condition has stabilized.

Additional vaccines protection against Hepatitis A, *Haemophilus influenza* type B (HIB), meningococcal, varicella, measles, mumps, and rubella (MMR) may be recommended for adult with diabetes depending on vaccination history, comorbidities, and risk of exposure.

CONCLUSION

Diabetes is a chronic disease and persons with diabetes are prone to infections. Hence, apart from considering for microvascular and macrovascular complications, infections can also be prevented to some extent by vaccine preventable diseases. Vaccination strategies in diabetic cases should be involved as part of routine care.

SUGGESTED READINGS

1. Misra A, Gopalan H, Jayawardena R, et al. Diabetes in developing countries. J Diabetes. 2019;11(7):522-39.
2. World Health Organization. (2004). Diabetes. [online] Available from https://www.who.int/health-topics/diabetes#tab=tab_1 [Last accessed October, 2022].
3. World Health Organization. (2004). Pneumococcal vaccine. [online] Available from http://www.who.int/vaccines/en/pneumococcus.shtml [Last accessed October, 2022].
4. Akbar DH. Bacterial pneumonia: Comparison between diabetics and non-diabetics. Acta Diabetol. 2001;38(2):77-82.
5. Smith SA, Poland GA. Use of influenza and pneumococcal vaccines in people with diabetes. Diabetes Care. 2000;23(1):95-108.
6. Warren-Gash C, Smeeth L, Hayward AC. Influenza as a trigger for acute myocardial infarction or death from cardiovascular disease: A systematic review. Lancet Infect Dis. 2009;9(10):601-10.
7. Reilly ML, Poissant T, Vonderwahl CW, et al. (2011). Incidence of acute hepatitis B among adults with and without diabetes, 2009-2010. [online] Available from https://idsa.confex.com/idsa/2011/webprogram/Paper31404.html [Last accessed October, 2022].
8. U.S. Food and Drug Administration. (2022). Vaccines Licensed for Use in the United States. [online] Available from https:/www.fda.gov/vaccines-blood-biologics/approved-products/vaccines-licensed-use-united-states [Last accessed October, 2022].
9. Centers for Disease Control and Prevention. (2022). Contraindications and Precautions. [online] Available from https://www.cdc.gov/vaccines/hcp/aicp-recs/general-recs/contraindications.html [Last accessed October, 2022].
10. Centers for Disease Control and Prevention. (2022). Use of COVID-19 Vaccines in the United States. [online] Available from https/www.cdc.gov/vaccines/covid-19/clinical-considerations/covid-19-vaccine-us.html [Last accessed October, 2022].

CHAPTER 23

Prediabetes

Vijay Garg, Himanshu Jain, Vimlesh Patidar, Sukrati Maheshwari

INTRODUCTION

Prediabetes, a metabolic disorder, is considered as a precursor for diabetes mellitus. There is a rapid increase in the prevalence of diabetes in India. Prediabetes is characterized by impaired fasting glucose or impaired glucose tolerance.

Prediabetes is a widely understood term for individuals whose glucose levels are below threshold cutoffs for a diagnosis of diabetes but are elevated beyond what is considered normal "diabetes and prediabetes" represent a significant healthcare burden and increasing challenge for clinicians. The absolute numbers of individuals with prediabetes are projected to increase by approximately one-third by the middle of this century. It is estimated that there will be >470 million people with prediabetes in 2030. According to the National Urban Diabetes Survey, the estimated prevalence of prediabetes is 15% in India. Prediabetes is not benign. It is necessary to start early and adequate intervention in order to prevent the development of complications and progression to overt diabetes.

WHAT IS PREDIABETES?

- A metabolic disorder.
- Precursor for diabetes mellitus.
- Characterized by impaired fasting glucose or impaired glucose tolerance.
- Blood sugar levels are consistently higher than normal, but not high enough to cause symptoms or to be diagnosed as diabetes.
- Although it is still possible at this stage to prevent the slide into full-blown diabetes, but risk of developing type 2 diabetes mellitus (T2DM) is greatly increased.
- Prediabetes is not benign, hence, it is necessary to start early intervention to prevent progression to overt diabetes and development of complications.

Prediabetes

■ MAGNITUDE OF PROBLEM
- The prevalence of prediabetes is increasing worldwide (around 15% in India).
- According to the Centers for Disease Control and Prevention, about 84 million adults in the US have prediabetes in 2015 and 70% of them will develop diabetes in the long term.
- It is projected that over 470 million people will have prediabetes by 2030.
- 5–10% of people with prediabetes progress to diabetes every year, while the same proportion converts back to normal blood sugar levels.

■ INDIAN SCENARIO
- The Chennai Urban Population Study (CUPS) epidemiological study
- In a report published in 2008 (J Assoc Physicians India) the researchers, led by Dr V Mohan, informed that the rate of prediabetes was 13.1 per 1,000 person-years.
- Mohan et al. reported that 40.5% of prediabetes participants converted to T2DM within 8 years of follow-up.
- Chennai Urban Rural Epidemiology Study (CURES) found the rate to be a whopping 29.5 per 1,000 person-years.
- It documented a high prevalence of prediabetes as compared to T2DM (24.7% vs. 7.3%).
- The high rate of prediabetes, compared to T2DM, signals that prediabetes, too, is at an epidemic trend in India.
- Moreover, it signifies that the diabetes epidemic is far from over.

■ TYPES OF PREDIABETES
There are two types of prediabetes:
1. *Impaired fasting glucose (IFG)*: IFG is present if the glucose level is 100–125 mg/dL (126 mg/dL is diagnostic for diabetes) after an overnight fasting of at least 8 hours.
2. *Impaired glucose tolerance (IGT)*: IGT is present if people have a blood glucose of 140–199 mg/dL after consuming 75 g of glucose during a 2-hour oral glucose tolerance test (OGTT).

■ DIAGNOSIS OF PREDIABETES
Prediabetes broadly refers to an intermediate stage between completely normal glucose levels and the clinical entity of T2DM, encompassing both impaired fasting glucose and impaired glucose tolerance. Prediabetes is defined by different organizations accordingly **(Table 1)**.

Diagnosis impacts prognosis, because patients diagnosed with both IFG and IGT develop diabetes approximately twice as often as individuals with either isolated IFG or isolated IGT. In addition, cardiovascular risk is greater in those with IGT or diabetes based on the 2 hours PG.

Upon presentation, an OGTT should be considered to definitively diagnose whether the patient has prediabetes or has unrecognized T2DM.

TABLE 1: Definitions of prediabetes by different organizations.			
	American Diabetes Association	**American Association of Endocrinology**	**World Health Organization**
Fasting blood glucose	100–125 mg/dL (5.6–7.0 mmol/L)	≥100–125 mg/dL (5.6–7.0 mmol/L)	110 mg/dL
2 h plasma glucose during 75 g—OGTT	140–199 mg/dL (7.8–11.1 mmol/L)	≥140–199 mg/dL (7.8–11.1 mmol/L)	140–199 mg/dL
HbA1c	5.7–6.4%	5.5–6.4%	ND

WHAT IS THE CRITERIA FOR DIABETES OR PREDIABETES TESTING IN ASYMPTOMATIC ADULTS?

Testing should be considered in adults who are overweight or obese BMI ≥25 kg/m^2 Asian-Americans having one or more following risk factors:
- First-degree relative with diabetes
- History of cardiovascular disease
- Hypertension with blood pressure >140/90 mm Hg or taking medication for hypertension
- HDL cholesterol level 35 mg/dL and/or a triglyceride level 250 mg/dL
- Physical inactivity
- Other clinical conditions associated with insulin resistance (e.g., severe obesity, and acanthosis)
- HIV

NATURAL HISTORY OF DIABETES AND PREDIABETES

Approximately all patients with T2DM spend an extensive phase in prediabetes stage of nearly 10 years duration. Prediabetes is linked with abnormalities in the form of insulin resistance and beta-cell dysfunction. The conversion rate of prediabetes to diabetes is around 5–10%.

Prediabetes should not be considered as a clinical entity, in fact, prediabetes poses an increased risk for diabetes and CVD.

Baseline HbA1c is a stronger predictor of diabetes as well as cardiovascular events. Several prospective studies have demonstrated a strong connection between HbA1c and diabetes development subsequently. Systematic reviews from 16 cohort studies which included 44,203 reviews individuals with HbA1c ranging between 5.5 and 6 exhibited a substantially increased risk of diabetes.

Pathophysiologic Defects in Prediabetes
- Beta-cell volume loss
- Insulin action and secretion defects
- Endothelial dysfunction
- Arterial stiffness
- Increased lipolysis

- Decreased incretin levels
- Increased glucose production in liver
- Impaired glucagon levels
- Dysregulated cytokines

WHAT IS THE NATURAL COURSE OF UNTREATED PREDIABETES?

The progression from prediabetes to T2DM occurs over many years before the development of overt hyperglycemia seen in diabetes. The risk of progressing to diabetes is greater in individuals with both IFG and IGT compared with isolated IFG or isolated IGT alone.

The risk of progressing to diabetes depends on the degree of insulin resistance and deficiency of insulin secretion as well as other diabetes risk factors, such as age, family history, overweight/obesity, or history of gestational diabetes or polycystic ovary syndrome.

PROGRESSION FROM PREDIABETES TO DIABETES (FIG. 1)

Complications of Prediabetes (Fig. 2)

The most obvious sequela of prediabetes is the risk of development of T2DM. In addition to the progression to T2DM, the prediabetes state is associated with a spectrum of microvascular and macrovascular complications including:

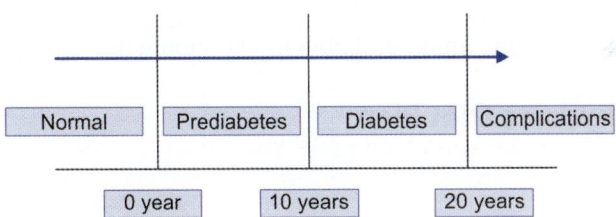

FIG. 1: Progression from prediabetes to diabetes.

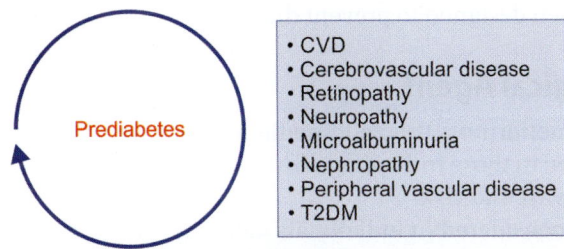

FIG. 2: Complication of prediabetes.

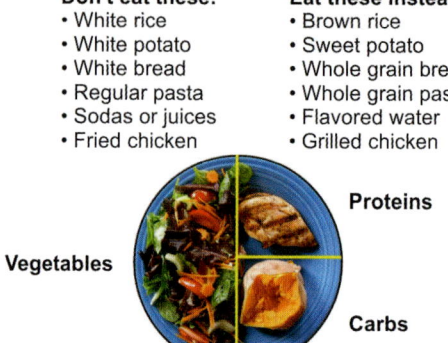

FIG. 3: Dietary approaches to stop hypertension.

MANAGEMENT OF PREDIABETES

- *Lifestyle modification* including—an amalgamation of diet and exercise, weight loss—for every 1 kg decrease in weight, the risk of developing diabetes in future was reduced by 16%. In the DPP, lifestyle intervention with a goal of at least 7% weight loss and at least 150 min of physical activity per week appeared to have greater impact on older persons and those with a lower BMI.

    With a BMI goal of <22 kg/m^2 in the intensive lifestyle group compared with <24 kg/m^2 in the standard group, a Japanese study in males with IGT resulted in a 67.4% risk reduction in diabetes over 4 years.
- *Nutrition*: Total fat intake should <30% of energy intake, saturated-fat intake should be <10% energy intake and fiber intake should be 15 g/1,000 kcal.

Low-carbohydrate Diet Plan
Refer **Figure 3**.

Physical Activity (Figs. 4A and B)
Moderate-intensity physical activity improves insulin sensitivity. Moderate-intensity physical activity (150 min/week), such as brisk walking has shown beneficial effects in those with prediabetes. Resistance training can also be included in exercise regimen designed to prevent diabetes.

Pharmacological Agent
Drugs such as metformin, thiazolidinediones, and alpha-glucosidase inhibitors may be considered in those individuals with high risk of progression to diabetes and increased cardiovascular risk.
- *Metformin* is considered in individuals <60 years of age, individuals with a BMI of at least 35 kg/m^2, and individuals with increased risk such as family history of diabetes in first-degree relatives, BMI ≥35 kg/m^2, aged 60 years, and women with

Being Active

Being active will:
- Lower blood sugar levels.
- Decrease your risk of diabetes.
- Help you lose weight by burning calories.
- Help your balance and lowers your risk of falls.
- Reduce your stress.
- Increase your feeling of wellbeing.
- Help you control your blood pressure.
- Help you increase your good cholesterol.

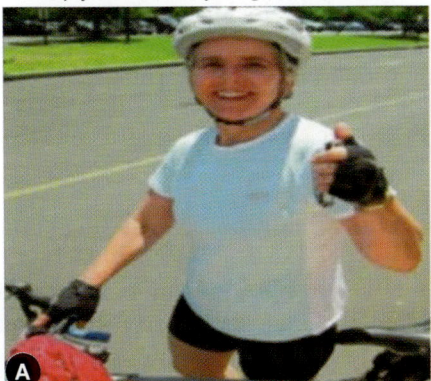
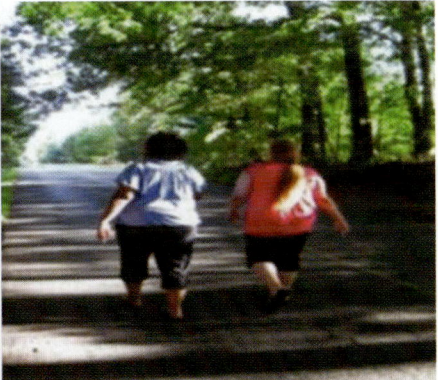

Tips to Increase Activity

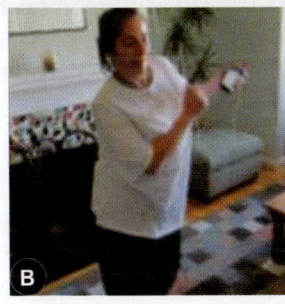
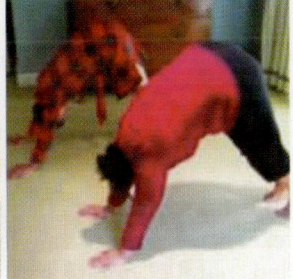
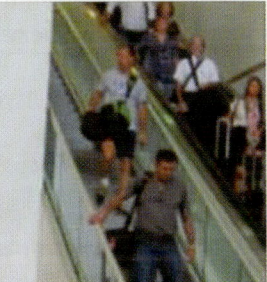

Make increased activity a habit that you will enjoy.
- Try dancing, walking, swimming, or riding a bicycle.
- Exercise with a friend. This will help you to stay motivated.
- Park farther away from stores or work. You will walk more.
- Take the stairs instead of the elevator or escalator.

Get Started!
- Be active 10 minutes a day, 3 days a week.
- Try to move up to 5 days a week.
- Slowly increase your activity to 30 minutes a day.

Activity I will do this week:

FIGS. 4A AND B: Tips of being active and to increase activity.

prior history of GDM, elevated triglycerides, reduced HDL-C, hypertension, or HbA1c >6.0%.
- *Acarbose* was associated with a 25% reduction in progression from IGT to diabetes after 3 years in the STOP-NIDDM (Study to Prevent Non-Insulin Dependent Diabetes Mellitus) trial. This effect disappeared with discontinuation of the acarbose, suggesting that acarbose may have masked the progression to diabetes.
- *Rosiglitazone*: In the DREAM study (Diabetes Reduction Assessment with Ramipril and Rosiglitazone Medication), *rosiglitazone* increased the regression of IFG or IGT to normoglycemia and reduced the incidence of the composite outcome of diabetes or death by 60% over 3 years. Rosiglitazone also reduced the risk of renal disease, suggesting that maintenance of normoglycemia may impact development of microvascular disease.

Others

- Weight loss therapies may be considered in morbidly obese including bariatric surgery
- Multifactorial risk factor management which includes smoking cessation, management of hypertension, dyslipidemia, nonalcoholic fatty liver disease, polycystic ovarian syndrome
- Prevention program to achieve and maintain 7% loss of initial body weight. Moderate-intensity physical activity (such as brisk walking) should be increased to minimum 150 min/week.
- The Diabetes Prevention Program (DPP) demonstrated that lifestyle modification and metformin interventions can delay or prevent the development of T2DM by 11 and 3 years, respectively, and reduce the absolute incidence of diabetes by 20% and 8%, respectively.

PRE-D TRIAL

It was designed to assess the on-treatment effects on glycemic variability of dapagliflozin, metformin or exercise for 6 weeks as well as 13 weeks. The Pre-D trial was a randomized, controlled, parallel, multi-arm, open-label, and nonblinded trial. It was performed at Steno Diabetes Center, Denmark. About 120 participants of the 404 screened with BMI ≥25 kg/m^2 in the age group of 30–70 years, and having prediabetes with an HbA1c of 5.7–6.4% were randomized 1:1:1:1 to dapagliflozin (10 mg once daily), metformin (1,700 mg daily), interval-based exercise or habitual lifestyle. There were minor improvements in glucometabolic outcomes with all treatment modalities. In addition. exercise was associated with additional cardiometabolic benefits.

CONCLUSION

Prediabetes, a common metabolic condition is etiologically related to obesity (especially abdominal or visceral obesity), and associated with an increased risk of T2DM, CVD, and all-cause mortality.

Lifestyle intervention would delay the onset of diabetes by 11.1 years, and metformin would delay the onset of diabetes by 3.4 years. Lifestyle intervention would increase life expectancy by 0.5 years and reduce the incidence of blindness by 39%, end-stage renal disease by 38%, amputation by 35%, stroke by 9%, and coronary heart disease by 8%. HbA1c by itself lacks sufficient sensitivity to diagnose diabetes. However, HbA1c correlates well with long-term complications and is a good indicator of chronic glycemic control.

With trends toward increased prevalence, but effective therapeutic interventions available, it is very important to increase efforts to identify and effectively manage prediabetes as early as possible so that we may avoid the impending global epidemic of diabetes. T2DM prevention and prediabetes "reversal" should be principal goals in diabetes care.

TAKE HOME MESSAGE

- Prediabetes, a metabolic disorder, is a precursor of diabetes.
- The estimated prevalence in India is around 14%.
- It is etiologically related to obesity.
- The micro- and macrovascular complications are similar to diabetes.
- Prediabetes reversal must be a principal goal in diabetes care.
- Mainstay of management is lifestyle modification and drug such as "metformin".

SUGGESTED READINGS

1. American Diabetes Association. Economic costs of diabetes in the U.S. in 2007. Diabetes Care. 2008;31:596-615.
2. https://drmohans.com/what-is-prediabetes-and-how-to-control/
3. Tuso P. Prediabetes and lifestyle modification: time to prevent a preventable disease. Perm J. 2014;18(3):88-93.
4. https://www.hopkinsmedicine.org/news/articles/a-holistic-prediabetes-clinical-approach

CHAPTER 24

Insulin: Initiation, Intensification, and Barriers

Arvind Gupta, Rajeev Gupta, NK Singh

■ INTRODUCTION

Early insulin therapy is indicated in type 2 diabetes patients mellitus (T2DM) to provide insulin replacement to preserve the ongoing destruction of Beta cells. The deleterious effects of Insulin resistance and poor glycemic control ultimately lead to exhaustion of beta-cell activity. Early initiation of insulin therapy in patients with relevant clinical indications can address this vicious cycle and help preserve beta cell function, improve glycemic control and reduce complications.

■ HISTORY OF INSULIN: DIABETES HAS BEEN KNOWN SINCE ITS ANTIQUITY

A turning point in the history of diabetes mellitus took place in 1889 after the experiments of Minkowski and von Mering. In 20th Century comes Dr Banting's Miracle Drug changing career for Frederick Banting from study of ministry 27 to medical officer in Canadian hospital in England. The relation of the Islets of Langerhans to diabetes and anatomy of diabetes was well established. Banting came with the big idea for diabetes—ligate pancreatic ducts of dog. Keep dogs alive till acini degenerate leaving islets. Try to isolate the internal secretion of these to relieve glycosuria. Banting sold the idea to Macleod and there was a cool reception between the two to take the extraction of insulin to next level.

Dr August Krogh visited Toronto for a conference and impressed by insulin extracts as his wife had type 1 diabetes mellitus (T1DM) and wanted to take this idea to Europe and initiated the Nordisk Insulin Laboratories.

Insulin is an anabolic hormone secreted from the β-cells in the islet of Langerhans in the pancreas. Active insulin protein consists of two chains of amino acids linked by two disulphide bonds chain contains 21 amino acids and B-chain contains 30 amino acids. The anti-inflammatory, antiapoptotic, cardioprotective and neuroprotective effects of insulin have been demonstrated in humans and animal models. The vasodilatory reactive oxygen species (ROS)-suppressive, antiplatelet, antithrombotic and profibrinolytic effects have been demonstrated in humans.

INSULIN REGIMENS

Basal only (in combination with oral antidiabetic drugs)—one dose of basal insulin at bedtime.

Basal plus: One dose of basal insulin at bedtime and one dose of bolus insulin with major meal.
- Basal-bolus therapy: Basal-bolus therapy is closest to physiologic insulin profile. One dose of basal insulin at bed time and 3 dose of short-acting insulin before each major meal. It is recommended to calculate the total insulin dose as 0.3–0.5 U/kg body weight. 40% of the total dose to be given as basal insulins as a single dose at bedtime and 60% of the total dose to be given as prandial insulin as 3 doses just before each meal or just after the meal. It is recommended to titrate the dose once in a week based on PPG and modify dose based on the lowest/mean value of the three most recent PPG values. A lower starting dose, slower titration, and higher targets may be recommended for those patients at higher risk of hypoglycemia.
- Premixed therapy/Co-formulation therapy: It is a ready mixture of short acting and prolonged acting insulin in a fixed ratio to reduce the mixing and dosing errors by the patient. When twice daily premix/co-formulation is necessary, it is recommended to start at 6U BD at prebreakfast and predinner. The recommended target for titration is premeal value of 80–130 mg/dL, prebreakfast dose to be modified, if titrated based on predinner values and vice versa.

Insulin Initiation and Intensification

Insulin initiation and titration can be challenging for many primary care providers who are involved in the treatment of patients with T2DM. Despite the introduction of advanced insulin analogues and improvements in insulin delivery devices, many patients with T2DM continue to experience suboptimal glycemic control. With an increasing number of treatment options available, T2DM management is moving away from a "one size-fits-all" approach and toward individualized treatment regimens based on patient needs. Given this, nurse practitioners, physician assistants, pharmacists, and certified diabetes educators are becoming increasingly valuable resources in busy primary care practices.

CURRENT GUIDELINES FOR INSULIN INITIATION AND TITRATION

The American Diabetes Association (ADA) recommends initiation of basal insulin at 10 units/day or 0.1–0.2 units/kg/day, adjusted by 10–15% or 2–4 units once or twice weekly to reach a target fasting plasma glucose (FPG) in patients whose HbA1c remains uncontrolled after >3 months of triple combination therapy, whose HbA1c is >10%, whose blood glucose is >300 mg/dL, or who are symptomatic of hyperglycemia. Treatment intensification recommendations for patients whose

HbA1c remains uncontrolled after basal insulin initiation and titration. Three regimen options should be considered:
- Regimen 1: Administer one rapid acting insulin injection before the meal with the greatest carbohydrate content; if the glycemic target is not met, progress to two or more rapid-acting insulin injections before meals (basal-bolus regimen).
- Regimen 2: Add a GLP-1 receptor agonist. If target HbA1c remains unmet or the regimen is not tolerated, patients may discontinue the GLP-1 receptor agonist and switch to regimen 1 or 3.
- Regimen 3: Replace basal insulin with premixed insulin at a 75/25, 70/30, or 50/50 mix twice (usually before breakfast or dinner) or thrice daily (before breakfast, lunch, and dinner). Basal insulin and GLP-1 receptor agonists should be discontinued before initiating premixed insulin.

Switching to Newer Generation Basal Insulins

- From OD/BID basal insulin therapy or basal component of prior basal-bolus regimen/premix insulin: Unit-to-unit switch.
- A total of 20% dose reduction to be considered when switching from a BID insulin to newer generation insulins such as insulin degludec.
- Glar U100–U300: Dose reduction to be done by 20%.
- Glar U300–U100: Unit-to-unit basis, but a higher Toujeo dose (~10–18%) may be needed to achieve target ranges for plasma glucose levels.

Switching to Newer Generation Co-formulations

- Switch from human premixes: Unit-to-unit switch.
- Unit-to-unit switch when switching from basal/premix OD/BID to newer generation co-formulations.
- Switching from basal-bolus to newer co-formulations is done on individual basis according to patient's requirements.

■ BARRIERS TO INSULIN INITIATION

Patient and clinician factors contribute to delays in adding insulin to treatment regimens or in transitioning from oral antidiabetic agents (OADs) to insulin. Patient barriers are numerous and include the inconvenience of insulin regimens, a need for more frequent self-monitoring of blood glucose (SMBG), fear of hypoglycemia, weight gain, and injection pain. Many patients lack confidence in their ability to self-manage their diabetes, with emotional factors such as an unwarranted sense of failure, guilt, and shame representing some of the most significant barriers to insulin use. In the DAWN (Diabetes Attitudes, Wishes, and Needs) study, 48% of patients initiating insulin believed they had failed to manage their diabetes correctly, 52% were worried about initiating insulin, and only 23% believed insulin would help manage their diabetes. Additionally, nonscientific beliefs such as the notion that insulin causes limb loss or kidney failure, lack of awareness of improved insulin delivery devices, and concerns about treatment costs are important factors that influence insulin adherence. Among primary care physicians (PCPs), there is often resonance with patients regarding fear of hypoglycemia, as well as a lack of confidence in patients' ability to manage insulin therapy. Factors such as a patient's presumed unwillingness or inability to inject contribute to the reluctance of PCPs to initiate insulin. Importantly, a lack of awareness of patient fears, beliefs, and expectations may affect the quality of PCP-patient relationships and create further barriers to achieving glycemic control. Provider or clinician factors, including a lack of integrated care, uncertainty regarding insulin type, complexity of titration algorithms, and concerns that the complexity of insulin therapy is too great to be managed in primary care often led PCPs to delay insulin initiation.

CONCLUSION

Insulin therapy is the corner stone of treatment in T2DM patients. It leads to an improvement in glycaemic control, helps in the preservation of beta-cell function and improves the quality of life. Early introduction to the insulin therapy has shown a significant reduction in the micro and macrovascular complications in T2DM patients. There is an unmet need for early initiation and intensification of insulin therapy. Various barriers based at the level of both patients and healthcare providers need to be addressed to overcome and alleviate the symptoms of T2DM.

SUGGESTED READINGS

1. Owens DR. Clinical evidence for the earlier initiation of insulin therapy in type 2 diabetes. Diabetes technology and therapeutics. 2013;15(9):776-85.
2. Albers JW, Herman WH, Pop-Busui R, Feldman EL, Martin CL, Cleary PA, Waberski BH, Lachin JM, DCCT/EDIC Research Group. Effect of prior intensive insulin treatment during the Diabetes Control and Complications Trial (DCCT) on peripheral neuropathy in type 1 diabetes during the Epidemiology of Diabetes Interventions and Complications (EDIC) Study. Diabetes care. 2010;33(5):1090-6.
3. Inzucchi SE, Bergenstal RM, Buse JB, Diamant M, Ferrannini E, Nauck M, et al. Management of hyperglycemia in type 2 diabetes: a patient-centered approach: position statement of the American Diabetes Association (ADA) and the European Association for the Study of Diabetes (EASD). Diabetes care. 2012;35(6):1364-79.
4. American Diabetes Association. 7. Diabetes technology: standards of medical care in diabetes—2020. Diabetes Care. 2020;43(Supp 1):S77-88.
5. Polonsky WH, Arsenault J, Fisher L, Kushner P, Miller EM, Pearson TL, Tracz M, Harris S, Hermanns N, Scholz BM, Pollom RK. Initiating insulin: how to help people with type 2 diabetes start and continue insulin successfully. International Journal of Clinical Practice. 2017;71(8).
6. Swinnen SG, Hoekstra JB, DeVries JH. Insulin therapy for type 2 diabetes. Diabetes care. 2009;32(Suppl 2): S253-9.

CHAPTER
25

Technology Transforming Diabetes Care

Ajay Kumar

■ INTRODUCTION

Technological innovations have enormously empowered every stakeholder in diabetes management. Keeping pace with these innovations is a daunting task for each of them. However, empowered with technology we can positively impact clinical outcomes in diabetes in a big way. It is imperative that these innovations are understood properly by each stakeholder and applied in clinical practice with prudence. This alone should ensure long-term benefits in terms of reduced mortality, decreased microvascular and macrovascular complications, and provide better quality of life.

■ PHYSICIAN'S EMPOWERMENT BY TECHNOLOGICAL INNOVATION

Physicians are at the center of entire disease management strategy. Majority of diabetes clinics today are technologically savvy with respect to appointments, patient's data collection, digital prescriptions, effective communication, and data analysis for research projects. It not only enables a better decision-making process but also ensures transparency in the delivery of diabetes care.

Scope of technology encompasses measurement, documentation, education, and treatment facilitation. Home blood glucose monitoring popularly known as self-monitoring of blood glucose (SMBG) is now widely performed and has become integral part of diabetes management. Patients can easily transfer the data to log books and share the information with treating physicians, who in turn can make considered treatment decision in a seamless, comprehensive, and scientific manner. Furthermore continuous glucose monitoring systems (CGMS) with or without hypoglycemia alarm have completely revolutionized glucose measurement.

Patient's education is pivotal to diabetes management. Technology now enables physicians and other stakeholders to facilitate education and training with respect to diet, exercise, carbohydrate counting, and social support measures. Desired notifications, insulin dose adjustments, and hypoglycemia alarms further enhance patient's empowerment. Better glucose sensing and insulin delivery devices help manage diabetes efficiently and reduce the cost of treatment by reducing the incidences of hospitalizations.

Information technology-enabled diabetes management (ITDM) enables synthesis of information and delivery of knowledge. It also improves the efficiency of communication and allows for coordination of care along delivery teams. Diabetes registries have shown enormous potential in improving outcomes and reducing cost.

ELECTRONIC HEALTH RECORDS

Documentation of clinical data has become an integral part of diabetes care. Such data can be easily accessed for treatment decisions and at the same time can be shared within the clinic or with other experts for scientific discussions. However, there are several ethical concerns related with electronic health records (EHRs). These include privacy and confidentiality of data, availability, and data integrity. Digital prescriptions can obviate issues pertaining to legibility of handwritten prescriptions and can save lives by avoiding treatment error (famous Daonil vs. Diavol story).

Recent advancements in technology in healthcare delivery include:
- Telemedicine
- M-health
- Smartphone application
- Machine learning technology
- Artificial intelligence

TELEMEDICINE

Medical consultation provided remotely through audiovisual technology is called telemedicine. Notwithstanding logistics and legal issues around the use of telemedicine, it is slowly being accepted as an effective and convenient method of diabetes management. In coronavirus disease (COVID-19) times, particularly it has saved several lives.

Digital health technology called *Digiceuticals* has been approved by the Food and Drug Administration (FDA). Cloud-based data collection systems with data security features are now available in various countries. *Tidepool* is a nonprofit organization for patients and healthcare providers. The web-based system is compatible with various devices. *Glooko* is a data management platform and integrates data from different devices. It has a standard uploader and enables data transfer to applications on android or apple smartphones through Bluetooth technology.

Blockchain technology has enormous potential by creating blocks of individual patient's data that can be shared among people, devices, and electronic medical systems. Through this technology the patient can give access to their healthcare providers, insurers, and other approved agencies.

EVIDENCE OF BENEFIT OF TECHNOLOGY IN DIABETES CARE

Number of studies have unequivocally shown improved clinical outcomes by using digital technology. In a 6-month, randomized, open label, parallel group, and multicenter study significant improvement in glycated hemoglobin (HbA1c) was demonstrated in poorly controlled type 1 diabetic subjects using individualized insulin dose adjustment combined with telemedicine. A meta-analysis of 35 randomized controlled trials (RCTs) of telemedicine (video, phone, and email) from China [involving a pooled population (3,514) over 3–6 months] demonstrated HbA1c reduction by 0.35% (p-value <0.001). In a Cochrane review of 21 RCTs; use of telemedicine demonstrated 0.31% reduction in HbA1c (p-value <0.001). In another systematic review of 46 studies in subjects both with type 1 diabetes mellitus (T1DM) and type 2 diabetes mellitus (T2DM) showed HbA1c reductions (0.12–0.86 in T1DM and 0.01 to 1.13% in T2DM).

A snapshot of technological innovations transforming diabetes care includes:
- Smart weighing scales
- Smart watches
- Smart socks
- Smart electrocardiogram (ECG)
- Smart blood pressure (BP) machines
- Smart contact lenses
- Insulin pumps
- CGMS devices
- Mobile apps
- Artificial pancreas
- Smart drugs

Smart weighing scales not only provide body weight measurement but also the body mass index (BMI), body fat percentage and pulse wave velocity. *Smart socks* can sense temperature, detect infection and inflammation, and in turn help prevent amputations. *Smart watches* provide deep insight into physical activity, sleep pattern, heart rate, glucose levels, and geolocation facilitating smart management. Arrhythmias can be picked up by watches and certainly with *smart ECG* machines. *Smart dugs* can demonstrate physiological response to treatment, body temperature, and drug regimen compliance.

INSULIN DELIVERY DEVICES

Vials and syringes have stood the test of time for insulin administration. However, they are complicated, time consuming, and error prone. Modern delivery devices such as pre-filled and durable pens have completely changed the level of acceptance on account of ease of use, accuracy, discreetness, and improved convenience. Switching from vials and syringes to smart pens has vastly improved adherence to insulin treatment. Modern needles are shorter and thinner and cause less pain and anxiety. They are easily attached and detached providing convenience. Connected pre-filled and durable pen containing both basal and prandial insulins is another gem among technological marvels.

MOBILE APPS IN DIABETES MANAGEMENT

Varieties of health apps in management of diabetes have empowered subjects with diabetes on an unimaginable scale. These apps include:
- Nutrition apps
- Physical activity apps
- Glucose monitoring apps
- Insulin dose adjustment apps
- Insulin delivery apps

Diabetes Buddy app, LogFrog DB app, and WaveSense Diabetes Manager app are few examples. From calorie count to step count, medication reminder, and blood glucose tracker; all have made life convenient for diabetic subjects.

INSULIN PUMP

Continuous subcutaneous insulin infusion (CSII) pumps have a remarkable journey since their first discovery in 1960s. Modern CSII devices are smaller and more user friendly as compared with early devices of the size of a back pack. It has been an evolutionary continuum from open-loop (SAP) to hybrid closed-loop and finally to fully closed-loop systems. While the open-loop system requires manual input in terms of basal and bolus dose adjustments, hybrid closed-loop systems set bolus for meals and inform the system about exercise. In a fully closed-loop system, no manual input is required for normal operation. Insulin delivery based on CGM requires manual adjustments in open-loop systems. In hybrid modes, it is automatic but requires manual food and correctional boluses. However, fully closed-loop systems are fully automated. Artificial pancreas today is a reality.

Patch pumps are now available which directly attach to the skin and do not require a line of plastic tubing to deliver insulin to the cannula. The Omnipod and The Omnipod DASH are few such examples. Finally *bionic pancreas* discovered in 2015 has a closed-loop system consisting of two infusion pumps (separately for insulin and glucagon) and are connected to a CGM via a smart phone app. In this system, automated dosing assessments of insulin and glucagon are made every 5 minutes based on appraised CGM data.

GLUCOSE MONITORING

Glucose test strips for SMBG have become a household name. Smart meters have such tantalizing features such as storage for strips, no battery requirement, easy integration with mobile phone, and easy sharing of data. They are bound to enhance positive outcomes in diabetes management. Current developments in glucose monitoring include instruments which can be attached on the body like flash glucose monitoring (FGM) or Dexcom CGM or implantable devices including Eversense and GlySens.

Continuous glucose monitoring system can provide 288 glucose measurements in 24 hours. CGM data can be real-time helping quick adjustment of treatment or can be accessed retrospectively. Most popular in use today in India is Abbott's FreeStyle Libre [flash monitoring of glucose (FMG)] which was approved by the FDA in 2017. One sensor lasts for up to 14 days and no calibration with finger pricks is needed. It is cheaper than CGM and is extremely useful. Other FDA approved FGM/CGM devices include Eversense, FreeStyle Libre 2, Dexcom G6, and MiniMed 670G. Eversense can be worn for 180 days and provides real-time measurements. Dexcom G6 is a single use sensor and can provide data for 10 days. MiniMed 670G is a hybrid system that measures glucose and automatically adjusts insulin dose.

Continuous glucose monitoring system has enabled the scientific fraternity to develop newer metrics of blood glucose control such as *time in range (TIR), time below range (TBR), and time above range (TAR)*. Many other calculations provide great insight to target blood glucose anomalies smartly and provide better clinical outcomes. TIR obviates many of the limitations of widely used metrics HbA1c. TIR and HbA1c used together could be a game changer in diabetes management and is slowly become common practice. Numerous RCTs have started measuring TIR in the process of new drug development.

Noninvasive glucose monitoring is the holy grail. Wearable and noninvasive devices are bound to increase compliance and in turn provide better glucose control. Biological fluids other than blood such as tears and sweat can be used to measure glucose. Optical measurement might become a reality soon through smart lenses.

Diabetic temporary tattoos are another remarkable innovation in the field of glucose monitoring. Precisely patterned electrodes are printed on the temporary tattoo paper. This in turn is applied to the skin and a mild electrical current is set. Tiny sensors collect and provide glucose data.

SCOPE OF DIGITAL TECHNOLOGY

- Advance diagnostics and screening
- Precision medicine
- Patient remote monitoring
- Drug development and research
- Clinical decision support
- Population health analytics

Many of the modern insulins and glucagon-like peptide 1 (GLP-1) based therapies are the result of smart molecular engineering and have provided safer and efficacious molecules addressing issues of compliance, hypoglycemia, and patient acceptability. Oral semaglutide is one of the best examples of this great innovation. Ultra-long-acting basal insulins are now widely available. Weekly administrable basal insulins are on the horizon completing phase 3 clinical trials. Glucose-responsive "smart" insulin called i-insulin consists of analog insulin attached with glucose transporter (GLUT) inhibitor. Built-in sensitivity in this insulin will obviate the risk of hypoglycemia by automatic switch on and switch off depending upon glucose levels.

CONCLUSION

Technological advancements are revolutionizing diabetes therapy. New technology effectively ensures individualization of treatment which is pillar of modern diabetes management. Advancements in technology from syringes and pens to pumps and do it yourself artificial pancreas aim to accomplish 100% TIR and 0%

hypoglycemia. Technology has the potential to enormously empower subjects with diabetes in terms of self-management skills, behavioral changes, and smart communication with other stakeholders in the management. It is important that healthcare providers embrace this change and become more professional rather than becoming dinosaurs of our age. However technological advancements cannot replace the need for physicians in patient care. While artificial intelligence can improve and aid the triage of diagnosis, reduce cost, increase access, and reduce medical errors and administrative burden; it cannot be completely free from data issues, substitute years of on ground experience and certainly cannot empathize with patient situations.

▍SUGGESTED READINGS

1. Ashrafzadeh S, Hamdy O. Patient-Driven Diabetes Care of the Future in the Technology Era. Cell metab. 2019;29(3):564-75.
2. Unnikrishnan R, Sharma M, Mohan V, et al. Technology in the management of diabetes mellitus. J Diabetol. 2018;9(1):3-11.
3. Bailey TS, Walsh J, Stone JY. Emerging technologies for diabetes care. Diabetes Technol Ther. 2018;20(S2):1-7.
4. Zhai YK, Zhu WJ, Cai YL, et al. Clinical and Cost effectiveness of Telemedicine in type 2 diabetes mellitus; a systematic review and meta-analysis. Medicine (Baltimore). 2014;93(28):e312.
5. Fiodgren G, Rachas A, Farmer AJ, et al. Interactive Telemedicine: Effect on professional practice and health care outcomes. Cochrane Database Syst Rev. 2015;9:CD002098.
6. Timpel P, Oswald S, Scwarz PE. Mapping the Evidence on the Effectiveness of Telemedicine Interventions in Diabetes, Dyslipidemia, and Hypertension: An Umbrella Review of Systematic Reviews and Meta-Analyses. J Med Internet Res. 2020;22(3):e16791.
7. Cobelli C, Renard E, Kovatchev BP. Artificial pancreas: past, present, future. Diabetes. 2011;60: 2672-82.
8. Bergenstal RM, Tamborlane WV, Ahmann A, et al.; STAR 3 Study Group. Effectiveness of sensor-augmented insulin-pump therapy in type 1 diabetes. N Engl J Med. 2010;363:311-20.
9. Ly TT, Nicolas JA, Retterath A, et al. Effect of Sensor-Augmented Insulin Pump Therapy and Automated Insulin Suspension vs Standard Insulin Pump Therapy on Hypoglycemia in Patients With Type 1 Diabetes: A Randomized Clinical Trial. JAMA. 2013;310:1240-7.
10. www.animascorp.co.uk/insulin-pumps/vibe-insulin-pump
11. Medtronic. www.medtronicdiabetes.com.
12. Beta Bionics. www.betabionics.org/publications.
13. Kesavadev J, Saboo B, Krishna MB, et al. Evolution of Insulin Delivery Devices: From Syringes, Pens, and Pumps to DIY Artificial Pancreas. Diabetes Ther. 2020;11:1251-69.
14. Heinemann L, Freckmann G. CGM versus FGM; or, continuous glucose monitoring is not flash glucose monitoring. J Diabetes Sci Technol. 2015;9:947-50.
15. Bailey T, Bode BW, Christiensen MP, et al. The performance and usability of a continuous glucose monitoring system. Diabetes Technol Ther. 2015;17:787-94.
16. Abbott. www.freestylelibre.co.uk.
17. Kovatchev B, Covelli C. Glucose Variability: Timing, Risk Analysis, and Relationship to Hypoglycemia in Diabetes. Care. 2016;39(4):502-10.
18. Jiang F, Jiang Y, Zhi H, et al. Artificial intelligence in healthcare: past, present and future. Stroke Vasc Neurol. 2017;2(4):230-43.
19. Lau J, Bloch P, Schaffer L, et al. Discovery of the once-weekly glucagon-like peptide-1 (GLP-1) analogue semaglutide. J Med chem. 2015;58:7370-80.

20. Kapitza C, Nosek L, Jensen L, et al. Semaglutide, a once-weekly human GLP-1 analog, does not reduce the bioavailability of the combined oral contraceptive, ethinylestradiol/levonorgestrel. J Clin Pharmacol. 2015;55:497-504.
21. Marbury TC, Flint A, Jacobsen JB, et al. Pharmacokinetics and Tolerability of a Single Dose of Semaglutide, a Human Glucagon-Like Peptide-1 Analog, in Subjects With and Without Renal Impairment. Clin Pharmacokinet. 2017;56:1381-90.
22. Rosenstock J, Bajaj HS, Janež A, et al. Once-Weekly Insulin for Type 2 Diabetes without Previous Insulin Treatment. N Eng J Med. 2020;383(22):2107-16.
23. Wang J, Yu J, Gu Z, et al. Glucose transporter inhibitor-conjugated insulin mitigates hypoglycaemia. Proc Natl Acad Sci. 2019;116(22):10744-8.
24. Danne T, Heinemann L, Bolinder J. New insulins, biosimilars, and insulin therapy. Diabetes Technol Ther. 2017;19(S1):S42-58.

CHAPTER 26

Selection of Footwear in Patient with Diabetic Foot

Vaibhav Saxena, Rajnish Saxena, SS Dariya

INTRODUCTION

Diabetic foot ulcers (DFUs) are the most common non-traumatic cause of lower limb amputation. Management of DFU mainly depends upon proper achievement of offloading of foot with glycemic control with control of infection and maintenance of circulation. Causative factors of foot ulceration include presence of triad of neuropathy, vasculopathy, and alteration of biomechanics of foot.

Dr Paul Brand stated in the year 1954 that "there is hope of saving the neuropathic foot, only when it is recognized that the real problem is due to biomechanical abnormalities," means there is strong relation between abnormal plantar pressure and foot ulceration.

Footwear selection after healing of wound after stage I is very important to protect the foot and recurrence of ulceration. As you know diabetic patients already have insensitive foot due to diabetic neuropathy.

Offloading of diabetic foot—redistribution of foot pressure is essential aspect of diabetic foot care. Foot pressure, shock, and shear force be reduced by using appropriate footwear, insoles, and socks. Total non-weight bearing allows wound to be at rest, so it heals very quickly. If suitable footwear is not worn by patient then other problems such as postural instability, infection, ischemia, deep ulcer, and gait deformity like ataxic gait can develop.

Foot examination is very important before selecting appropriate foot appliance. Examination begins with inspection of foot, both plantar, and dorsal aspect with palpation of pedal pulsation. Examination of footwear is also important giving ideas regarding altered plantar pressure area of feet. Protective sensation examination is done by Semmes–Weinstein monofilament. Biothesiometer (VPT) and ABI are also important tools to assess neuropathy and ischemia. Examine strength of intrinsic muscles by paper grip test. Plantar pressure assessment is done with Harris mat and computer assessment (Podia scan).

CHARACTERISTICS OF IDEAL OR PREVENTIVE DIABETIC FOOTWEAR

Footwear should have tough wide tough toe box, rigid sole, extra width, and total heal counter with shoe closure system, i.e., Velcro. Depth of diabetic footwear should be ½ to 5/8" to 3/16 inch deeper than standard oxford shoes, heal <2 cm with widest point at 1st MTP joint. Length <1.25 cm than length of foot and weight should be <700 g per pair.

Always avoid anything with toe straps, nails, stitches, metal eyelets, and projections or waves like shapes are not recommended. Hunter type or long leather shoes extending above the ankle should be avoided.

Sandals with heal counter and adequate width are more economical, more open (allow free airflow) and cannot hold moisture in comparison to shoes.

Footwear should have extra depth to accommodate dorsal deformity and dressings. It should have removable soft insole material such as microcellular rubber (MCR), microcellular polymer (MCR) or plastazote or evazote. Ankle high leather shoe prevents excessive pronation and supination; stabilizes and controls rotation at ankle. Two feet are not identical in diabetic patients so shoes are manufactured accordingly.

HOW FREQUENTLY SHOULD FOOTWEAR BE CHANGED?

Assessment of footwear must be advised after every follow-up visit of patient. If insole shows bottoming out then change immediately. Also check for heal wear and tear, if excessively skewed change it. Normally we advise to change the insole after every 6 months.

If patient's neuropathy status or biomechanics changed, change the footwear to adjust or accommodate deformity and redistribute the planter pressure evenly.

Selection of Therapeutic Footwear

- *Risk category 1 (normal foot or low risk patients)*: Diabetes patients who have no neuropathy or vasculopathy, i.e., with normal sensation and muscle strength, no deformity or skin changes with normal response to monofilament and normal ABI and normal plantar pressure on foot scanning. More than 85% of diabetic patients are at low risk for developing ulceration, according to natural history of diabetic foot stage I included in this category.
  Footwear prescription: We recommend preventive footwear including sandals or closed shoes with insole of MCR, MCP or ethylene vinyl acetate (EVA) of 8–19 mm thickness for low risk patients.
- *Risk category 2 (the high risk feet)*: Patients with loss of protective sensation included in this group. Foot is at the risk of developing ulcer. This group includes:
  - Patients with neuropathy and/or vasculopathy.
  - Mobile foot deformity such as high or low arches.
  - Altered biomechanics of foot lesions such as callus, corns, healed scar mark, and partially healed plantar ulcers.
  - Patients with intrinsic muscle paralysis and foot deformities.

Footwear prescription: MCR sandal with add-ons is advised to these patients. Footwear selection depends upon mobile deformity mainly arch of foot weather low or high arch foot.
- In case of normal arch MCR "Y" strap sandals are prescribed. MCR above 150 shores is advised for both preventing ulcers and recurrence of ulceration.
- Correct fitted sport shoe for neuropathic foot is better choice.
- Molded shoes
- Customized or bespoke shoe—if the shape of feet is abnormal and cannot be fitted with routine footwear.
- Temporary readymade shoes for ulcerated foot to accommodate the dressings.

  Insoles are advised for redistribute the abnormal plantar pressure even. Extra cushioning under MT head is achieved with fibro fatty padding.

  Regular podiatrist consultation and debridement of callus with nail care is very important for reducing high pressure from vulnerable sites.

- *Risk category 3 (ulcerated foot)*: Patient with insensate feet and foot deformity and non-infected neuropathic ulcers is included in this category. In neuropathic ulcer, total contact cast (TCC) is gold standard for achieving total offloading. If patient is not accepting TCC then temporary readymade shoe with cushioning insole is prescribed.

In neuropathic foot aim is to save vulnerable margins of foot.
- In case of partially healed plantar ulcer, OrthoWedge shoes with site of wedge depending upon the site of ulcer. A smaller ulcer can be managed with insole wing pad to relive pressure on the ulcer bearing area is prescribed.
- In case of diabetic with foot deformity molded total contact cradle (TCC) insoles are used **(Fig. 1)**. TCC insole is made up from different materials such as polyethylene, Plastazote and cork rubber and fitted inside the shoes with wide toe box, extra depth, and rocker bottom with complete heel counter.

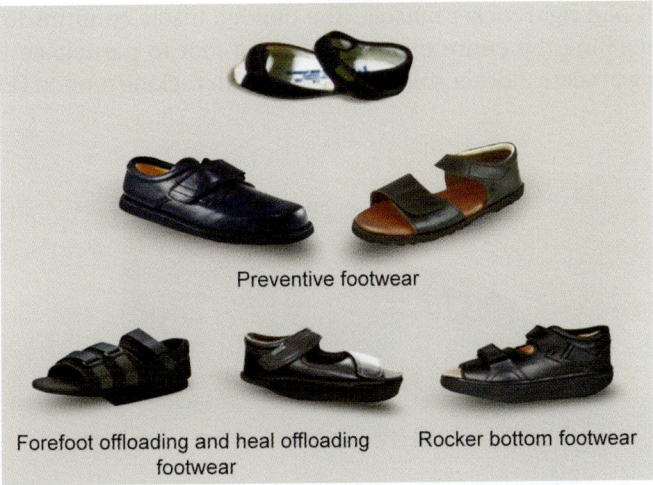

FIG. 1: Preventive and offloading footwear.
Courtesy: SDCC, Ajmer.

In case of low arched foot there will be no bulging in inside part of footwear but heel should be turned inside. Additional changes in different conditions are done as mentioned below:
- Low arch foot without scarring or no pressure lesion—tarsal cradle or medial heel wedge is also advised.
- Low arch with pressure lesion—if lesion at MT heads than tarsal cradle and MT pad cut out and if lesion at heel, then elephant pad is applied.
- Low arch foot with excessive forefoot scarring—tarsal cradle with anterior rocker is advised.

If foot is with high arch deformity increased bulging of inside part of footwear is done with heel turned out with additional changes in different conditioned as mentioned below:
- High arch foot without scarring or no pressure lesion—tarsal platform or lateral heel wedge is advised.
- High arch foot with pressure lesion—if lesion at metatarsal leads, then MT should be filled with pad without cut and if lesion at heel then heal meniscus is applied.
- High arch foot with excessive forefoot scarring—tarsal platform with anterior rocker is advised **(Fig. 2)**.

If foot is partially amputated then amputated portion space should be filled with soft material in the shoe (shoe filler).

Footwear prescription is better decided by podiatrist or diabetic foot specialist, but in day-to-day practice a physician can prescribe easily if ulcer at forefoot then front offloading footwear, if ulcer at heal then heal offloading, if at mid foot then mid foot offloading footwear is prescribed.

These patients are with loss of protective sensation, intrinsic muscle paralysis, fixed deformities, severe scars, and high plantar pressure areas. Footwear prescription for these patients includes shoes and braces.

If foot is rigid with <50% weight bearing area lost due to scarring then molded shoes are prescribed. Molded shoes consist of two parts molded insoles and rigid rocker outsole. The molded insole confirms to the shape of foot enabling the entire plantar surface of foot to participate in the weight bearing process. Rocker sole provides smooth rocking motion **(Fig. 3)**.

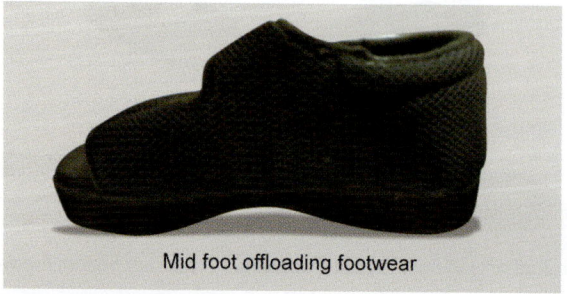

Mid foot offloading footwear

FIG. 2: Mid foot offloading footwear.
Courtesy: SDCC, Ajmer.

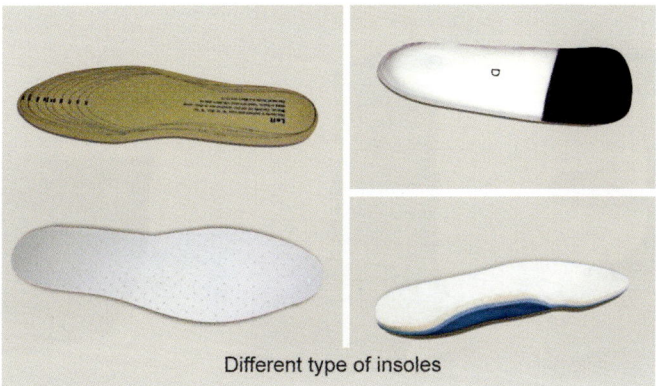

FIG. 3: Different types of insoles.
Courtesy: SDCC, Ajmer.

- *Risk category 4 and 5 (stage of cellulitic and necrotic foot)*: Patient with insensate foot with or without structural deformities or Charcot foot and previous history of ulceration and ischemia.
  Footwear prescription—custom-molded or extra depth footwear with 2–3 layered insoles with internal and external modification may be added depending on the biomechanical deformity of foot. Patient with extensive cellulites should not walk. Advise bed rest and increase use of crutches, Zimmer frames or wheelchair for movement of day-to-day activity.
  In neuroischemic feet non-weight bearing is advised until wound is not healed. Patient should wear Scotchcast boot in bed to protect heal.

OTHER METHODS FOR OFFLOADING

Mandakini offloading, S K offloading, and Samadhan offloading device are very economical techniques for achieving offloading.

If unstable ankle joint or Charcot's deformity is present then fixed ankle brace (FAB) also known as ankle foot orthosis (AFO) is prescribed. It restricts all the joint movements. So reduce stress and protect the joint **(Fig. 4)**.

If foot is rigid, unstable with <30% weight bearing surface then patellar tendon bearing (PTB) brace or orthosis is advised.

Temporary shoes such as Drushoe has two removable Plastazote insole and OrthoWedge such as rocker bottom shoes OrthoWedge surgical shoes or half-shoes to offload pressure from forefoot, i.e., MTH and toes.

CONCLUSION

For healing of diabetic foot ulcers proper offloading is mandatory, it can be achieved by advising suitable footwear along with metabolic, microbiological and wound control with education of patient.

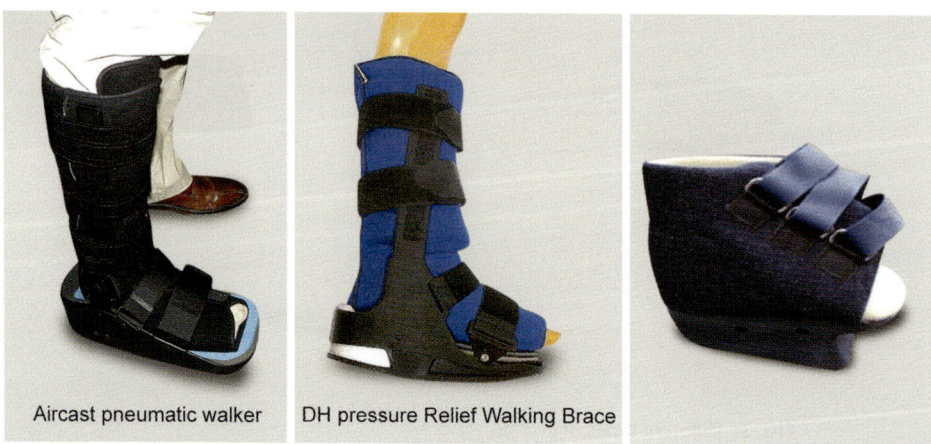

FIG. 4: Different methods of offloading.
Courtesy: IPA workbook.

SUGGESTED READINGS

1. IDF Atlas. https://diabetesatlas.org/upload/resources/previous/files/8/IDF_DA_8e-EN-final.pdf
2. Edmonds ME, Foster AVM. Managing the Diabetic Foot; 2002 Chapter 1 & 8. pp. 2-24,115-21.
3. Boulton AJ. The diabetic foot: grand overview, epidemiology and pathogenesis. Diabetes Metab Res Rev. 2008;24 (Suppl 1).S3-S6.
4. Armstrong DG, Boulton AJ, Bus SA. Diabetic foot ulcers and their recurrence. N Engl J Med. 2017;376(24):2367-75.
5. Tripathi K, Saboo B. Sadikot's International Textbook of Diabetes. 1st edition. New Delhi: Jaypee Brothers Medical Publishers; 2019. pp. 638-44, 655.
6. Edmonds ME, New treatment for diabetic foot ulcers, In: Boulton AJM, Coor H, Cavanagh PR (Eds). The Foot in Diabetes. Wiley & Sons; 2000. pp.1551-59.

CHAPTER 27

Interplay between T2DM, Dyslipidemia and NASH

Anuj Maheshwari, Naman Shukla, Ajoy Tewari

INTRODUCTION

Globally, diabetes is rising rapidly. In India, every year 2 million people with diabetes are being added. Major determinant in India is *insulin resistance (IR)*. In India, prevalence of IR is around 35% in young age even if they are not having diabetes. The major cause of mortality remains death due to cardiovascular diseases (CVDs). This is because majority of patients with diabetes are suffering from comorbidities such as lipid abnormalities (dyslipidemia) and hypertension. Insulin resistance is a common link for these metabolic conditions such as hypertension, dyslipidemia, and nonalcoholic fatty liver disease (NAFLD). In India, every 9 out of 10 diabetic patients suffer from dyslipidemia. According to INTERHEART study, dyslipidemia is one of the major risk factors associated with acute myocardial infarction. In India, we see different pattern of diabetic dyslipidemia compared to Caucasian counterpart which is "high triglycerides (TG) and low high-density lipoprotein (L-HDL)". It is more prevalent form of dyslipidemia in type 2 diabetes mellitus (T2DM) and is associated with 44% higher risk of CVDs. Such lipid pattern is associated with increased proportion of small dense low-density lipoprotein (sdLDL) particles which, is considered as more atherogenic in nature. Hence, diabetic dyslipidemia is also termed as "atherogenic diabetic dyslipidemia (a triad of high TG, low HDL and increased sdLDL)". Triglyceride is strongly associated with NAFLD among markers of hyperlipidemia and T2DM. TG to HDL ratio works as a surrogate marker for NAFLD. Gradually, it is taking a shape of neglected epidemic with 25% fatty liver without inflammation or hepatocyte ballooning across the world ending in steatohepatitis (NASH) and cirrhosis. Overall prevalence of NAFLD in India is up to 32%. In obesity, it is 80%, ranging between 70 and 80% in T2DM. Almost half of them progress to advanced fibrosis. Odds ratio for NASH between patients with T2DM and without is 1.76 while it is for cirrhosis is 2.57. Polycystic ovarian disease is one of the common comorbidities occurring with NAFLD. So NAFLD is rising fast in population with T2DM and obesity but there is a huge diagnosis gap.

EVALUATION AND MANAGEMENT OF NAFLD IN PATIENTS WITH T2DM: A CALL TO ACTION

Around 17% of patients with T2DM may have significant fibrosis when assessed by noninvasive imaging tools. American Diabetes Association (ADA) recommends NASH and fibrosis screening in persons with T2DM or prediabetes and elevated ALT or fatty liver. If liver ultrasonography is found abnormal it is an indication for assessment of fibrosis which can be done with MR elastography, Transient elastography and fibrosis biomarker panel. Long-standing T2DM (>10 years), evidence of steatosis, high HbA1c ≥8.5%, triglycerides >250 mg/dL and genetically prone are considered as high risk for NAFLD followed by NASH. They all should be candidates for periodic evaluation even if they keep their ALT >30 IU/L in male and >19 IU/L in females. Liver enzymes may be normal in up to 80% of NAFLD patients, not so much sensitive even for NASH, poorly correlating to histology. Liver biopsy is the confirmatory.

TREATMENT: PHARMACOLOGICAL OR NONPHARMACOLOGICAL?

Lifestyle management is the key approach. More than or 10% weight loss can cause fibrosis regression in 45% patients and 7% loss in weight brings resolution of NASH in 64–90% individuals. On sustaining weight loss for 1 year can further do fibrosis regression 10% and 18% resolution of NASH. Even 3% weight loss can cause steatosis improvement in 33–100% individuals or if it can be made up to 5% weight loss or more it reduces inflammation and ballooning of fat cells in 41–100% people which can further reduce 30% if it could sustain weight loss up to 1 year.

Role of Statin or Other Available Options

As far as pharmacological options are concerned, most of them are used as off-label medications may it be metformin, vitamin E, PPAR-γ agonists, PUFA, pentoxifylline, GLP-1a, UDCA, obeticholic acid, silymarin and statins. Statins are good to control the diabetic dyslipidemia along with lifestyle therapy and proper glycemic control. Guidelines aggressively recommend statin therapy (moderate-to-high intensive statin) in almost all diabetic patients, unless contraindicated. Although not enough evidences are there, proving beneficial in reducing NAFLD. Others medications also have insufficient evidences to be used. It is estimated that statin therapy may reduce the risk of CV events by 20–30%. Residual risk still stays there.

Role for Upcoming Molecules?

A dual PPAR α/γ agonist, saroglitazar is known for its impact on atherogenic diabetic dyslipidemia together with statin but also effective against NAFLD and NASH. It is recommended in addition to statin which is supposed to reduce the risk of CV events by 20–30%. Various other uncontrolled risk factors (such as high TG, low HDL, uncontrolled obesity, high blood pressure, smoking and bad dietary habits) might be contributing to the residual CV risk. Various latest large observational studies have established the positive association between uncontrolled TG and

CV risk. Results from the Strong Heart Study (published recently in Diabetes Care 2017) showed that people with diabetes having high TG (>150 mg/dL) and low HDL (<40 mg/dL in male and <50 mg/dL in female) carry 54% significantly higher risk of CHD and more than two times higher risk of stroke compared to people with diabetes having normal TG and HDL values. The subgroup analysis from ACCORD and FIELD studies (in patients with baseline TG >203 mg/dL and HDL <34 mg/dL) showed that TG lowering therapy may reduce the CV events significantly compared to placebo therapy. After statin therapy, currently available options for controlling TG levels are fibrates, saroglitazar, and omega-3-fatty acids. Treatment with fibrate therapy may have some limitations as they might increase the risk of muscle related side effects, particularly in patients with diabetes, renal diseases, elder patients, or patients who are on statin therapy. Fibrates may also cause reversible increase in serum creatinine.

Saroglitazar reduces TG by 45–62%, non-HDL 21–36%, sdLDL 20.3%, HbA1c reduction 0.7–1.6% and improvement in ALT by 28–67%. Biopsy Driven P-III Study from India has proven effectiveness of PPAR agonists saroglitazar in nonalcoholic steatohepatitis. It decreased NAFLD activity score (NAS) ≥2 was observed in 52.3% of patients without worsening of fibrosis at week 52 together with liver and lipid parameters. Study concluded that Saroglitazar leads to significant improvement in transaminases, LSM, and CAP in NAFLD patients with DD. It has shown significant reduction in NAFLD score (NAS) in 52.3% patients and 30% reduction in liver fat content in 40.7% patients. Saroglitazar also caused 45.8% reduction in liver enzymes beyond baseline. It also has positive impact on insulin sensitivity and has been approved to use in patients of NAFLD and NASH. According to the recent study, saroglitazar may also reduce sdLDL levels. Omega-3-fatty acids can also be an option for treatment of high TG in diabetic patients. The major limitations of omega-3-fatty acids are its poor tolerability and multiple daily doses.

Saroglitazar is a dual PPAR α/γ agonist, approved and available in India for the treatment of hypertriglyceridemia in T2DM not controlled with statin alone. Along with significant TG lowering action, saroglitazar also improves insulin sensitivity (through PPAR-γ agonistic action) in patients with diabetic dyslipidemia.

CONCLUSION

Indian patients with T2DM are different in perspective of atherogenic dyslipidemia conspicuous of hypertriglyceridemia and low HDL. Currently, Indians are getting T2DM about two decades earlier in their life time compared to Caucasian counterparts. Poor physical activity together with carbohydrate predominant dietary habits makes Indians more vulnerable to this interplay among T2DM, dyslipidemia and NAFLD or NASH. Hypertriglyceridemia remains a common factor in all three serving as surrogate marker of this interplay.

SUGGESTED READINGS

1. Van der Aa MP, Fazeli Farsani S, Knibbe CAJ, et al. Population-Based Studies on the Epidemiology of Insulin Resistance in Children. J Diab Res. 2015:362375.
2. Chandalia M, Abate N, Garg A, et al. Relationship between generalized and upper body obesity to insulin resistance in Asian Indian men. J Clin Endocrinol Metab. 1999;84(7):2329-35.

3. Krishnamurthy V, Kerekoppa, AR. (2019). Cross-sectional study of pattern of Dyslipidemia and Prevalence of Atherogenic Diabetic Dyslipidemia in newly detected Diabetic patients. Asian J Med Sci. 2019;10(6):45-9.
4. Yusuf S, Hawken S, Ounpuu S, et al; INTERHEART Study Investigators. Effect of potentially modifiable risk factors associated with myocardial infarction in 52 countries (the INTERHEART study): case-control study. Lancet. 2004;364(9438):937-52.
5. Dhamija E, Paul SB, Kedia S. Non-alcoholic fatty liver disease associated with hepatocellular carcinoma: An increasing concern. Indian J Med Res. 2019;149(1):9-17.
6. Kruk B, Liebe R, Milkiewicz M, et al. PNPLA3 p.I148M and TM6SF2 p.E167K variants do not predispose to liver injury in cholestatic liver diseases: a prospective analysis of 178 patients with PSC. PLoS One. 2018;13(8):e0202942.
7. Vilar-Gomez E, Martinez-Perez Y, Calzadilla-Bertot L, et al. Weight Loss Through Lifestyle Modification Significantly Reduces Features of Nonalcoholic Steatohepatitis. Gastroenterology. 2015;149(2):367-78.e5.
8. Leoni S, Tovoli F, Napoli L, et al. Current guidelines for the management of non-alcoholic fatty liver disease: a systematic review with comparative analysis. World J Gastroenterol. 2018;24(30): 3361-73.
9. Kaul U, Parmar D, Manjunath K, et al. New dual peroxisome proliferator activated receptor agonist-Saroglitazar in diabetic dyslipidemia and non-alcoholic fatty liver disease: integrated analysis of the real world evidence. Cardiovasc Diabetol. 2019;18(1):80.
10. Gawrieh S, Noureddin M, Loo N, et al. Saroglitazar, a PPAR-α/γ Agonist, for Treatment of NAFLD: A Randomized Controlled Double-Blind Phase 2 Trial. Hepatology. 2021;74(4):1809-24.
11. Chauhan S, Kodali H, Noor J, et al. Role of Omega-3 Fatty Acids on Lipid Profile in Diabetic Dyslipidaemia: Single Blind, Randomised Clinical Trial. J Clin Diagn Res. 2017;11(3):OC13-16.

CHAPTER 28

Early Detections and Therapeutic Interventions in Diabetes Kidney Disease

SK Sharma, Niharikaa Sharma

INTRODUCTION

Diabetic kidney disease (DKD) represents the most common cause of end-stage renal disease (ESRD) that accounts for the high mortality rate in patients with diabetes. It contributes to about 30% of ESRD. DKD occurs in ~20–30% of people with type 1 diabetes mellitus (T1DM) and 25–40% of people with type 2 diabetes mellitus (T2DM).

Patients with T2DM often develop other renal diseases, pathologically unrelated to diabetes and known as nondiabetic renal disease (NDRD). Diabetic nephropathy is diagnosis of exclusion. Exclusion of other causes of renal involvement in diabetic patients is very important. Absence of diabetic retinopathy, shorter duration of diabetes mellitus (<5 years), lower glycated hemoglobin (HbA1c), and lower blood pressure (BP), presence of active urinary sediments (hematuria, pyuria, and casts), grossly elevated lipids, history, or clinical features of primary renal disease preceding onset of diabetes may help to distinguish NDRD from DKD in patients with diabetes.

DEFINITION OF DIABETIC KIDNEY DISEASE

Diabetic kidney disease is defined by characteristic structural and functional changes. The pathophysiological interactions of DKD consists of persistent (>3 months) albuminuria [urinary albumin-to-creatinine ratio (UACR) >30 (μg/min)] and/or estimated glomerular filtration rate (eGFR) <60 mL/min/1.73 m^2 in a patient with diabetes, usually in the presence of retinopathy and often associated with hypertension and progressive decline in renal function. Glomerular filtration rate (eGFR) should be estimated by Modification of Diet in Renal Disease (MDRD) formula at initial screening.

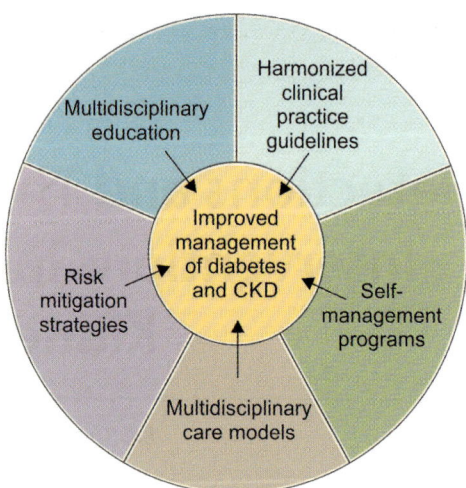

FIG. 1: Steps in care of diabetic kidney disease management.

Overcoming barriers to management of chronic kidney disease (CKD) such as low CKD awareness, high complexity of care, difficulties with adhering to increasingly complex treatment regimens, and low recognition and application of guideline-directed management all contribute to suboptimal management of patients with diabetes and CKD. Implement multidisciplinary models of care, structured risk mitigation strategies, and education [Kidney disease. Improving Global Outcomes (KDIGO) Diabetes Work Group 2022].

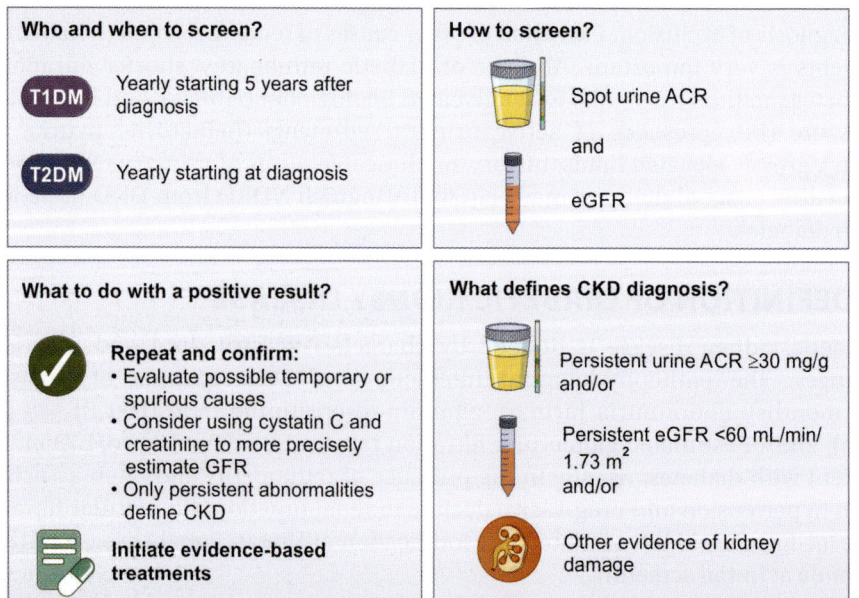

FIG. 2: Holistic approach in patients with diabetes and CKD.

CHRONIC KIDNEY DISEASE CLASSIFICATION BASED ON GLOMERULAR FILTRATION RATE AND ALBUMINURIA

Chronic kidney disease is defined as abnormalities of kidney structure or function, present for >3 months, with implications for health. CKD is classified based on cause, GFR category (G1–G5), and albuminuria category (A1–A3), abbreviated as CGA.

CKD is classified based on:
- **Cause (C)**
- **GFR (G)**
- **Albuminuria (A)**

GFR categories (mL/min/1.73 m^2) Description and range			Albuminuria categories description and range: A1 Normal to mildly increased <30 mg/g <3 mg/mmol	A2 Moderately increased 30–299 mg/g 3–29 mg/mmol	A3 Severely increased ≥300 mg/g ≥30 mg/mmol
G1	Normal or high	≥90	Screen 1	Treat 1	Treat and refer 3
G2	Mildly decreased	60–89	Screen 1	Treat 1	Treat and refer 3
G3a	Mildly to moderately decreased	45–59	Treat 1	Treat 2	Treat and refer 3
G3b	Moderately to severely decreased	30–44	Treat 2	Treat and refer 3	Treat and refer 3
G4	Severely decreased	15–29	Treat and refer 3	Treat and refer 3	Treat and refer 4+
G5	Kidney failure	<15	Treat and refer 4+	Treat and refer 4+	Treat and refer 4+

- Low risk (if no other markers of kidney disease, no CKD)
- Moderately increased risk
- High risk
- Very high risk

FIG. 3: Risk of CKD progression, frequency of visits, and referral to nephrology according to GFR and albuminuria.

STRATEGIES FOR RISK MITIGATION AND PREVENTION OF DIABETIC KIDNEY DISEASE

High morbidity and mortality with DKD suggest primary prevention of its development and secondary prevention to retard its progression once it is established. In most cases, DKD remains silent before the first signs of kidney damage are evident and thus go unrecognized to both patients and physicians.

Clinical predictors for CKD, based on the patient's history, should be assessed for every patient of T2DM at the time of diagnosis, and at subsequent visits as appropriate. These include the presence of hypertension, presence of dyslipidemia, history of smoking, poor glycemic control, family history of DKD, and presence of other vascular complications. Albuminuria and eGFR both have independent diagnostic and therapeutic implications. Measurement of eGFR is a must, as mere serum creatinine assessment, may mislead interpretation. Albuminuria, serum creatinine, and eGFR must be assessed at the time of diagnosis of T2DM and followed-up at-least-once annually. A positive albuminuria finding should be confirmed by two additional assessments, each being at least 1–3 months apart.

TREATMENT

Multifactorial multidisciplinary approach management for prevention and halting progression of DKD is important. In DKD patients, multiple risk factor control which included HbA1c of <7%, BP of <140/90 mm Hg, total cholesterol <185 mg/dL and no smoking was associated with a significantly lower risk of all-cause and cardiovascular (CV) mortality and lower risk of adverse CV events such as coronary heart disease and stroke.

Lifestyle Modifications

Recognizing the potential benefits and known risks associated with various levels of dietary protein, recommended dietary allowance (RDA) 0.8 g protein/kg/day is recommended by the American Diabetes Association (ADA) (~10% of daily calories). Kidney Disease: Improving Global Outcomes (KDIGO) and the National Kidney Foundation (NKF) suggest a target dietary protein intake of 0.8 g/kg/day for people with or without diabetes mellitus and eGFR <30 mL/min/1.73 m^2 accompanied with nutrition education and close monitoring of clinical and biochemical parameters. Protein restriction helps in reducing hyperfiltration and intraglomerular pressure.

Indian diet is low in protein and is mainly of vegetarian origin; hence, protein restriction is often not needed in Indian patients. When albumin excretion rate is still normal avoid high protein intake, particularly high protein intake from animal sources. Keep protein intake within 10–20% of total energy intake. When albumin excretion rate is raised and diabetic nephropathy suspected than reduce protein intake to target of 0.8 g/kg body weight/day (not below 0.6 g/kg body weight/day).

Diabetic kidney disease patients with raised blood pressure (>130/80 mm Hg), reduce salt intake to target of 5 g/day.

If serum cholesterol is elevated [Cho >185 mg/dL or low-density lipoprotein (LDL) >115 mg/dL], restrict intakes of saturated fatty acid (SFA) and trans FA (<10% of total energy) and dietary cholesterol intake (<300 mg/day).

Physical activity has been associated with improved physical fitness, BP, lipid profile, insulin sensitivity, and CV outcomes in patients with diabetes. However, few clinical studies have examined the effects of physical activity on DKD.

Avoid Smoking

The impact of smoking exposure on CV morbidity and mortality has been well documented in the population with CKD, both before and in that undergoing dialysis. However, most studies included both patients with and without diabetes. Guidelines recommend providing smoking cessation counseling as an integral part of CKD treatment, regardless of the etiology.

Management of Hyperglycemia in DKD

Inadequate glycemic control is considered as an independent predictor of development of albuminuria and/or ESRD. Trials, namely DCCT and UKPDS, highlighted intensive glycemic control has long-lasting favorable effect on the risk of DKD. Intensive glycemic control carries a "legacy effect" (metabolic memory) and prevents or retard DKD. Strict control of blood glucose and blood pressure significantly lowered the development and progression of DKD in both T1DM and T2DM. Glycemic control to A1c <7% reduces the appearance of DKD.

In DCCT, 35–45% lower risk for development of microalbuminuria in tight glycemic control group. In UKPDS, 25–30% reduction for development of microalbuminuria in the intensive glycemic treatment group. In KUMAMOTO study with primary prevention cohort, there is 62% reduction for development of microalbuminuria in the intensive treatment group. In secondary prevention cohort 52% risk reduction in risk of progression of albuminuria in intensive control group was achieved (KDIGO 2022 Clinical Practice Guideline for Diabetes Management in Chronic Kidney Disease. Kidney Int. 2022).

Antidiabetic Therapy in Diabetic Kidney Disease

- *Biguanides* are contraindicated if eGFR <30; reduce dose if eGFR is between 30 and 45
- *Sulfonylureas* are best avoided; shorter acting agents like glipizide and gliclazide may be used in mild to moderate renal insufficiency.
- *Repaglinide* is safe in kidney failure.
- *Glitazones* and *acarbose* are best avoided.
- *Gliptins* (sitagliptin, saxagliptin, and vildagliptin) can be given with dose adjustment and linagliptin can be used without dose adjustment.
- *Insulin* is the antidiabetic agent of choice; regular insulin and rapid-acting analogs are preferred.

According to the ADA guidelines, a patient-centered approach should be used to guide the choice of pharmacologic agents. Considerations include CV comorbidities, hypoglycemia risk, impact on weight, cost, the risk for side effects, and patient preferences. Strict glycemic control decreases development of diabetic nephropathy in both T1DM and T2DM patients.

Intensive insulin therapy partially reverses the glomerular hypertrophy and hyperfiltration, delays the development of microalbuminuria, reduce the onset or progression of diabetic nephropathy.

Among T2DM patients with established atherosclerotic CV disease or indicators of high risk, established kidney disease, or heart failure, a sodium-glucose cotransporter 2 (SGLT2) inhibitor or glucagon-like peptide 1 receptor agonist (GLP-1RA) with demonstrated CV disease benefit is recommended as part of the glucose-lowering regimen independent of HbA1c and in consideration of patient-specific factors.

	Progression of CKD	ASCVD	Heart failure	Glucose-lowering efficacy	Hypoglycemia risk	Weight effects	Cost
Metformin	Neutral	Potential benefit	Potential benefit	High	Low	Neutral	Low
SGLT-2 inhibitors	Benefit[a]	Benefit[c]	Benefit	Intermediate	Low	Loss	High
GLP-1 receptor agonists	Benefit[b]	Benefit[c]	Potential benefit	High	Low	Loss	High
DPP-4 inhibitors	Neutral	Neutral	Potential risk[c] (saxagliptin)	Intermediate	Low	Neutral	High
Insulin	Neutral	Neutral	Neutral	Highest	High	Gain	High (analogs) / Low (human)
Sulfonylureas	Neutral	Neutral	Neutral	High	High	Gain	Low
Thiazolidinediones	Neutral	Potential benefit (pioglitazone)	Increased risk	High	Low	Gain	Low
α-Glucosidase inhibitors	Neutral	Neutral	Neutral	Intermediate	Low	Neutral	Low

Legend:
- Neutral
- Potential benefit or intermediate glucose-lowering efficacy
- Benefit (organ protection, high efficacy, low hypoglycemia risk, weight loss, or low cost)
- Potential risk or high cost to patient
- Increased risk for adverse effects

FIG. 4: Selecting glucose lowering agents in patients with T2DM and DKD.

[a] Benefit supported by primary and secondary outcome data.
[b] Benefit supported by secondary outcome data.
[c] Benefit or risk is agent specific.

(ASCVD: atherosclerotic cardiovascular disease; CKD: chronic kidney disease; DKD: diabetes kidney disease; DPP-4: dipeptidyl peptidase 4; GLP-1: glucagon-like peptide 1; SGLT-2: sodium-glucose cotransporter-2)

Early Detections and Therapeutic Interventions in Diabetes Kidney Disease

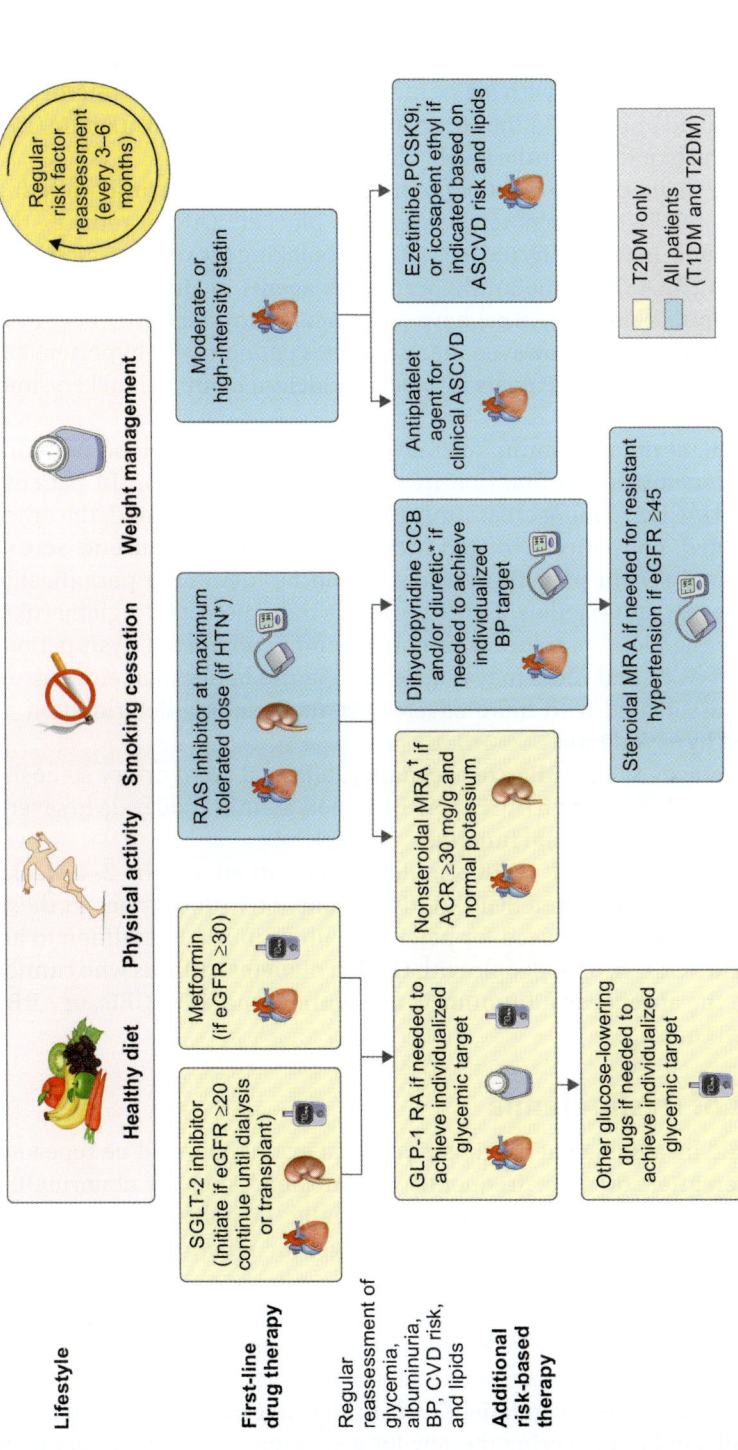

FIG. 5: Holistic approach for improving outcomes in patients with diabetes and CKD.

*ACE inhibitors or ARB should be first-line therapy for hypertension when albuminuria is present, otherwise dihydropyridine CCB or diuretic can also be considered; all three classes often needed to attain BP targets.

†Finerenone is currently the only nonsteroidal MRA with proven clinical kidney and cardiovascular benefits.

(ACE: angiotensin-converting enzyme; ACR: albumin-creatinine ratio; ARB: angiotensin receptor blocker; ASCVD: atherosclerotic cardiovascular disease; BP: blood pressure; CCB: calcium channel blocker; CGM: continuous glucose monitoring; eGFR: estimated glomerular filtration rate; GLP-1 RA: glucagon-like peptide-1 receptor agonist; HbA1c: glycated hemoglobin; HTN: hypertension; LDL-C: low-density lipoprotein cholesterol; MRA: mineralocorticoid receptor antagonist; PCSK9i: proprotein convertase subtilisin/kexin type 9 inhibitor; SGLT-2: sodium-glucose cotransporter-2; T1DM: type 1 diabetes mellitus; T2DM: type 2 diabetes mellitus;; TG: triglycerides)

Management of Hypertension in Diabetic Kidney Disease

Hypertension is also an important risk factor for DKD. Each 10 mm Hg increase in mean systolic BP was associated with a 15% increase in the risk of both micro- and macroalbuminuria and impaired kidney function defined as eGFR <60 mL/min/1.73 m^2 or doubling of the blood creatinine level.

Blood pressure reduction to <130/80 mm Hg with angiotensin-converting enzyme inhibitors (ACEIs) or angiotensin receptor blockers (ARBs) reduces the appearance of diabetic nephropathy in T2DM. Drugs blocking the renin angiotensin aldosterone system (RAAS) are the antihypertensive agents of choice. ACEIs and angiotensin II receptor blockers (ARBs) have additional renoprotective effect over and beyond their effects on BP. However, many diabetes patients with hypertension need additional drugs to reach BP goals (β-blocker, calcium channel blockers, and diuretics).

An ACEI or ARB, at the maximum, tolerated dose indicated for blood pressure treatment, is the recommended first-line treatment for hypertension in patients with diabetes and UACR ≥30 mg/g creatinine. If one class is not tolerated, the other should be substituted. For patients treated with an ACEI, ARB, or diuretic, serum creatinine/eGFR, and serum potassium levels should be monitored periodically. Mechanism of renoprotective action of ACEIs involves reduction of intraglomerular pressure and systemic blood pressure with correction of endothelial dysfunction. The combination of ACEI and ARBs may reduce proteinuria better than either drug alone, but is also associated with more adverse events including deterioration of renal function and hyperkalemia.

Contraindications to ACEI/ARBs are pregnancy, bilateral renal artery stenosis, intolerance, particularly dry cough (ACEI > ARB), hyperkalemia, moderate to severe aortic stenosis, and worsening renal function.

Serum potassium levels and eGFR should be monitored within 2-4 weeks after initiating an ACEI, an ARB, a SGLT-2i, finerenone, or with changes in these medications. Finerenone can be used for persistent albuminuria in addition to an ACEI or an ARB and SGLT-2i, or in people with CKD in diabetes mellitus who cannot take a SGLT-2i. In the absence of albuminuria and with normal BP, ACEIs, or ARBs do not prevent DKD onset.

Management of Dyslipidemia

Lipid profile should be assessed at diagnosis or initial evaluation, and be repeated every 5 years thereafter, or more frequently if indicated. After an abnormality is detected, lipid profile should be assessed annually. Low-density lipoprotein cholesterol (LDL-C) is the primary therapeutic target for atherosclerotic cardio-vascular disease (ASCVD) risk management.

The KDIGO and KDOQI clinical guidelines recommend using LDL-C lowering medicines, such as statins or statin/ezetimibe combination, to reduce the risk of major atherosclerotic events in patients with DKD (including those who have received a kidney transplant). The recommendations were based largely on post hoc analyses that reported results of lipid-lowering therapy for a subpopulation of patients with CKD and diabetes mellitus compared with placebo. Owing to the lack of mortality benefit, statin therapy may not be started in patients treated with dialysis; however, the risks and benefits of reducing nonfatal CV events need to be considered.

Early Detections and Therapeutic Interventions in Diabetes Kidney Disease 267

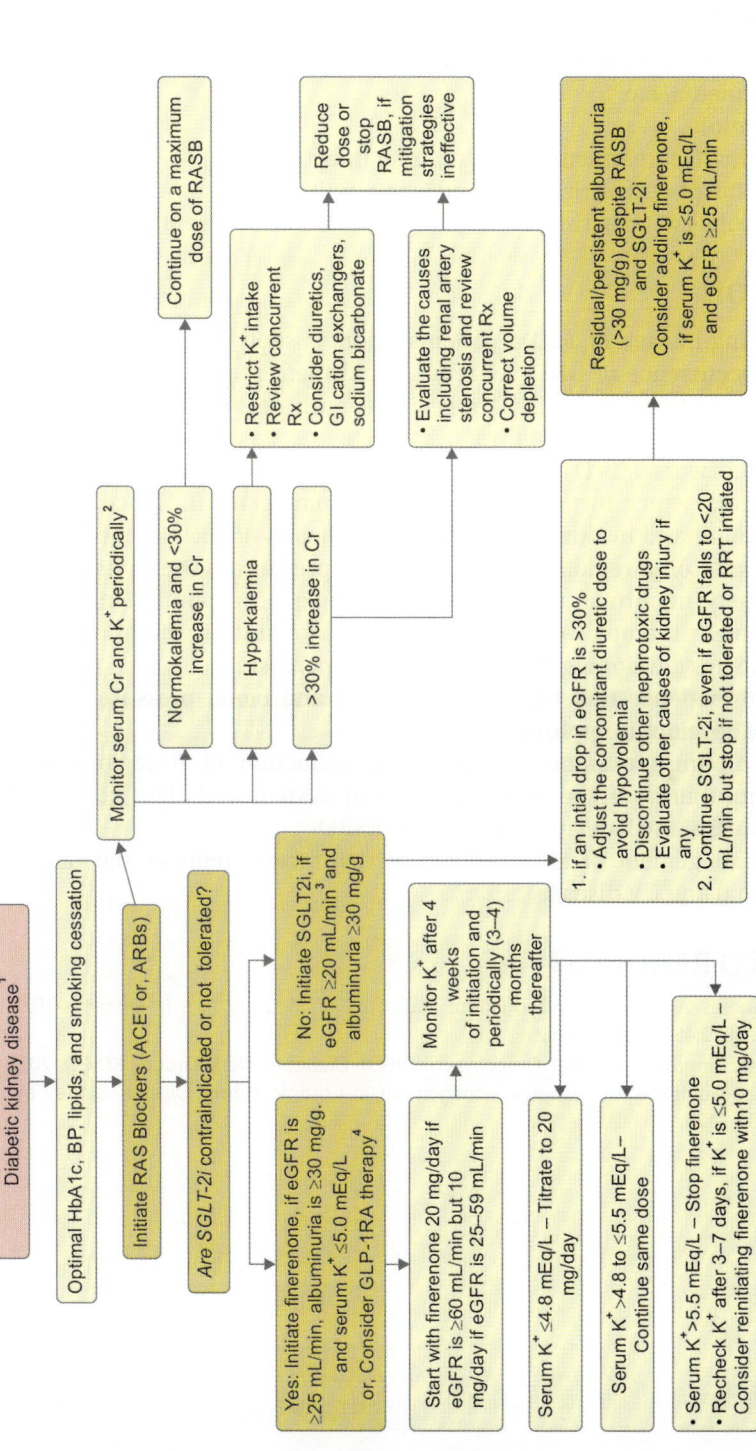

FLOWCHART 1: Positioning of RASB, SGLT-2 inhibitors, and finerenone in treatment of diabetic kidney disease.

[1] Diabetic kidney disease is defined as albuminuria >30 mg/g and or reduction in eGFR.
[2] KDIGO 2022 and AACE/ACE 2022 guidelines recommend monitoring serum potassium every 2–4 weeks.
[3] Indications and eGFR threshold may vary by region.
[4] GLP-1RA are another class of agent that is recommended in DKD if SGLT-2i are contraindicated or not tolerated and also as an addon agent after SGLT-2i if further HbA1c lowering is required.

(AACE: American Association of Clinical Endocrinology; ACE: angiotensin-converting enzyme; ARBs: angiotensin II receptor blockers; CKD: chronic kidney disease; Cr: creatinine; eGFR: estimated glomerular filtration rate; GI: gastrointestinal; GLP-1RA: glucagon-like peptide-1 receptor agonists; HbA1c: glycated hemoglobin; BP: Blood pressure; K^+: potassium; KDIGO: Kidney Disease Improving Global Outcome; RASB: renin-angiotensin system blockers; Rx: treatment; SGLT-2i: sodium-glucose cotransporter-2 inhibitors)

Other Measures
- Avoid nephrotoxic substances—nonsteroidal anti-inflammatory drug (NSAID), radiocontrast media, etc.
- Avoid dehydration
- Early and aggressive treatment of urinary tract infection (UTI)
- Sodium and phosphate restriction as and when indicated
- Refer to nephrologist if creatinine rises or hyperkalemia is present.

CONCLUSION

With the increasing burden of T2DM patients, India is soon going to witness an increase in the occurrence of DKD. As renal impairment remain subclinical for many years before the first signs of DKD are evident, early detection is often missed by both patients and physicians.

To make matters worse, CVD is frequently associated with DKD, and both share common risk factors, which further complicates the management. Hence, regular follow-up assessment and evaluation of clinical predictors of DKD at the time of T2DM diagnosis and on a regular basis is crucial to prevent DKD and its further progression. Diabetic nephropathy is currently the single most common indication for renal replacement therapy worldwide, and in most countries the numbers of patients with diabetes developing ESRD continues to increase.

There is good evidence that tight blood glucose and blood pressure control reduce the risk of developing nephropathy.

Once urine albumin excretion is increased, reduction of intraglomerular pressure using inhibitors of the renin-angiotensin system and tight control of systemic blood pressure will delay progression to ESRD.

Aggressive management of all classical CV risk factors reduces the rate of progression of renal and CV disease.

SUGGESTED READINGS

1. American Diabetes Association. Introduction: Standards of Medical Care in Diabetes-2022. Diabetes Care. 2022;45(Suppl 1):S1-S2.
2. Kidney Disease: Improving Global Outcomes (KDIGO) Diabetes Work Group. KDIGO 2022 Clinical Practice Guideline for Diabetes Management in Chronic Kidney Disease. Kidney Int. 2022;102(4S):S1-S123.

CHAPTER 29

Diabetes in Young: Current Concepts

BK Singh

◼ INTRODUCTION

Diabetes in young has been classically defined as onset of diabetes <35 years of age. But according to Indian Council of Medical Research (ICMR), age ≤25 years were considered in the Registry of People with Diabetes with Young Age at Onset (YDR). Here is controversy regarding the age, in western population age of onset of diabetes is higher so the upper limit of age of young diabetics are also higher around <40 years. According to International Diabetes Association, cut-off age of 40 years was chosen to define young onset diabetes because patients of diabetes were stratified as 20–39, 40–59, and 60–79 years for estimating the prevalence of diabetes in the world.

◼ EPIDEMIOLOGY

The prevalence of young diabetes is increasing worldwide because of increasing obesity, more sedentary habits, lack of exercise, increased level of stress, intake of high fat, and refined carbohydrate in diet and epigenetic factors. Nearly 65% of population of India is young. The SEARCH study indicated that there has been overall increase by 21.1% of type 1 diabetes mellitus (T1DM) and 30.5% of type 2 diabetes mellitus (T2DM) between 2001 and 2009. The highest rate of progression from prediabetes to T2DM in India is 14–18%. As per observation of Sahoo et al. the prevalence of T2DM and T1DM in young in India is almost same nearly 40%.

◼ TYPE OF DIABETES IN YOUNG

According to ADA 2020, epidemiology, pathophysiology, developmental consideration, and recommended care as well as response to treatment, and treatment outcome are different for pediatric onset diabetes and adult diabetes, so different tools are needed to classify diabetes in this group.

As per observation of Sahoo et al. the most common etiologies for diabetes mellitus (DM) in young are:
- T2DM (40%)
- T1DM (40%)
- Fibrocalculous pancreatic diabetes (FCPD, 15%)
- Maturity-onset diabetes of the young (MODY) (2%)
- Flatbush diabetes (2%)
- Mitochondrial diabetes (1%)

CLASSIFICATION (ICMR YDR DATA): YOUNG ONSET DIABETES (<25 YEARS)
- T1DM (63.9%)
- T2DM (25.3%)
- Gestational diabetes (3.9%)
- Maturity-onset diabetes of the young (3.1%)
- Chronic pancreatitis (1.3%)
- Secondary diabetes (1.0%)
- Latent autoimmune diabetes in adults (LADA) (1.0%)
- Drug-induced diabetes (0.3%)
- Malnutrition-modulated diabetes (0.1%)
- Congenital and neonatal diabetes (rare)

APPROACH TO PATIENT

If the age of patient in < 6 months, molecular diagnosis/genetic diagnosis is important to rule out congenital and neonatal forms (NDM). More recent studies show that monogenic forms of NDM may still occur up to 12 months of age, although with reduced frequency.

If the age is > 6 months to 10 years, T1DM and monogenic diabetes are considered most. So c-peptide test and pancreatic autoantibodies test is required to rule out T1DM.

In other group when age > 10 years up to age of 25 years, this represents the majority of young diabetes group, a complete work up including of urine ketones, serum glucose, c-peptide, plasma insulin, autoantibodies, and a pancreatic ultrasound should be performed. Other routine investigation like lipid assessment, renal function, liver function, and funduscopic examination must be done. Genetic testing in this group is also indicated when there is clinical and laboratory suspicion of MODY a form of monogenic diabetes.

SALIENT FEATURES OF DIFFERENT TYPES OF YOUNG DIABETES
- *Neonatal diabetes mellitus (NDM)* is a monogenic form of diabetes, a rare disease (one to 100,000–500,000 live births). It can occur in the first 6 months of life but may be found up to 12 months. Infants with NDM do not produce enough insulin, leading to increase blood glucose. There are two types:

i. *Transient NDM*—observed in both term and preterm babies, but more common in preterm caused by immaturity of islet B-cells due to chromosome 6q24 imprinting abnormalities and *K ATP* channel genes. Polyuria and dehydration are prominent, but baby looks well and suck vigorously treatment is insulin. Disappears in 4–6 weeks.

ii. *Permanent NDM*—a familial form of diabetes that appears shortly after birth and continues for life. The usual genetic and immunologic markers of T1DM are absent although insulin requiring, but ketosis resistant. There is mutation in ATP sensitive K channel subunit (KCNJ11 and ABCCB8) and insulin genes and these cases can be treated with high-dose sulfonylurea. It is often associated with other congenital anomalies and syndromes, e.g., Wolcott-Rallison syndrome and DNED syndrome (developmental delay, epilepsy and diabetes).

- *T1DM*—characterized by absolute insulin deficiency. There are two forms—autoimmune and idiopathic. There is pancreatic beta-cell destruction resulting in total deficit of circulating insulin. These patients are prone to ketosis. In autoimmune form, there is presence of autoantibodies (85%) which are absent in idiopathic type. Younger age of onset, absent C-peptide, presence, or absent of antibodies points toward T1DM. Treatment is lifestyle modification and insulin. From 9 months to 10 years almost all diabetes is caused by islet autoimmunity. Diabetic ketoacidosis (DKA) may be the clinical presentation. Measurements of autoantibodies—GAD65, IA-2, ZnT8, C-peptides, and genetic testing may be required, commonly associated genes are *HLA-DR4-DQ8* and *DR3-DQ2*.

- *T2DM in young*—T2DM is a disease normally seen to appear after 40 years of age but the age of onset of T2DM is falling globally. There is a shift of age of onset toward younger age groups. T2DM in childhood and adolescence is a new disease that has emerged in last two to three decades. Insulin resistance especially during puberty and childhood obesity is major risk factor for causing childhood diabetes. Asian populations are prone to have T2DM. Youth diagnosed with T2DM are more prone to develop comorbid complications such as hypertension, hyperlipidemia, and other diabetic complications at earlier age.

The pathophysiology of early-onset T2DM subjects is like those above 40 years, i.e., insulin resistance and B-cell impairment or abnormal insulin secretion but with some unique features. The earliest abnormality observed is insulin resistance which is at peak of puberty (due to pubertal hormones) leading to progressive β-cell failure leading to diabetes. In fact, adolescents with T2DM have approximately 50% lower insulin sensitivity and approximately 75% lower first-phase insulin secretion when compared with nondiabetic adolescents matched for similar BMI as well as abdominal adiposity. There is sharp decline in B-cell function 15% per year as compared to 6% per year as seen in older type.

The most common type of diabetes affecting these group nearly >40% of total DM. Features favoring a diagnosis of T2DM are overweight or obesity, age > 10 years, sign of insulin resistance, strong family history, normal c-peptides, and absence of autoantibodies.

It is very difficult to achieve glycemic target due to physiological and psychological factors. Treatment is lifestyle modification, medical nutrition therapy, metformin, and insulin. The TODAY (Treatment Options for type 2 Diabetes in Adolescents and Youth) study is the largest clinical trial of 10-17 years age group. Participants were randomized to metformin alone, metformin with lifestyle modification and metformin with rosiglitazone. Loss of glycemic control occurs in metformin and metformin plus lifestyle modification group but those receiving rosiglitazone with metformin had superior outcome, but safety is doubtful. The TODAY study also focused on standardized diabetes education program. But in young adult treatment is same as that of adult and selection of medication depend on the clinical judgment of treating clinician.

- *Gestational diabetes mellitus (GDM)*: Glucose intolerance developing during second and third-trimester during pregnancy is called gestational diabetes. Most of GDM reverts to normal in postpartum period but with a 35-60% risk of future development of T2DM. Glucose intolerance detected in first trimester is called preexisting pregestational diabetes by American Diabetes Association. Diabetes mellitus in pregnancy differs from GDM, in the former hyperglycemia is more severe and does not resolve after pregnancy as it does with GDM. Treatment is lifestyle modification, medical nutrition therapy and insulin. Oral drugs like metformin and glyburide are used in pregnancy but they are second line and cross placenta (neonatal hypoglycemia) and lack long-term safety data.

- *Maturity onset diabetes of young*—MODY is misdiagnosed as both T1DM and T2DM and only molecular diagnosis can make a correct diagnosis. But in practice it is often delayed for many years. It is a monogenic form of diabetes which runs in families because of a change in a single gene which is passed on by affected parents to their children.

    Though it is not as common as Scandinavian people, limited source of genetic testing may be the reason for underdiagnoses. Number of MODYs has increased significantly in recent years from 6 to more than 14 different specific genes. It is now well known that many patients with MODY may present de novo with the absence of strong family history of diabetes.

    When to suspect MODY—if patient is normal weight, no sign of insulin resistance, normal c-peptides, and no autoantibodies. Correct clinical diagnosis is important to predict clinical outcome.
    Targeting treatment to the genetic etiology:
    - GCK MODY—no treatment required
    - HNF-1A and HNF-4A MODY—SU sensitivity, CV risk with HNF-1A statins if >40 years
    - KCNJ11/ABCC8 NDM—insulin not required. High dose SU
    - Management of pregnancy
    - GCK MODY—BW depends on fatal/maternal genotype
    - HNF-4A MODY—macrosomia and hyperinsulinemic hypoglycemia

- *Fibrocalculous pancreatic diabetes*—tropical calcific pancreatitis, better known as FCPD. It is predominantly limited to tropics characterized by pancreatic intraductal calcifications, ketosis-resistant lean diabetes, progressive and irreversible destruction of pancreatic parenchyma, good initial response to oral diabetes medications, and high-risk of carcinoma pancreas in the long run. Etiopathogenesis remains unknown. Poor nutrition or malnutrition has been implicated as possible factor. Dietary toxin such as cyanogens (found in cassava) intake and micronutrient deficiencies may be possible factors. Serine protease inhibitor *Kazal type 1 (SPINK1)* gene variations is associated with FCPD. FCPD contributes significantly to the burden of diabetes in young in this part of the world. Further studies with regard to the burden of FCPD in young are needed from other parts of India, especially West Bengal, Kerala, and Tamil Nadu.

OTHER TYPES OF DIABETES

Another form of diabetes, which is unique to South Asia, is the Flatbush diabetes. These patients present with very high blood glucose values, varying degree of ketosis, have one of more features of insulin resistance, initially respond poorly to oral antidiabetic medications, and are well managed with insulin in the acute setting. Once glycemic control is achieved in a few weeks, insulin can be commonly stopped in these patients and they do well with oral antidiabetic medications for long periods of time similar to T2DM.

Mitochondrial diabetes is caused by poor functioning of beta-cell and/or by the emergence of insulin resistance due to mitochondrial disorder. Mutation of mtDNA or nuclear DNA can cause mitochondrial disorder. Symptoms are similar to those of T1DM or T2DM. It is diagnosed by genetic testing. In comparison to MODY2, it is progressive disorder. Treatment is difficult particularly in children and needs regular monitoring to adjust treatment to their changing needs.

Drug induced diabetes—many drugs like corticosteroids, antipsychotics can produce hyperglycemia in susceptible individual and young are not an exception. Diabetogenic drugs can impair insulin secretion or action and result in diabetes which may be transient or sometimes permanent.

Secondary diabetes—it develops as consequence of other diseases. Many endocrine disease may cause secondary diabetes such as Cushing's syndrome and glucagonoma.

CONCLUSION

Incidence and prevalence of diabetes in young are increasing not only in India but globally. Early detection and differentiation are necessary to plan treatment. Childhood obesity is increasing day-by-day due to unhealthy lifestyle like high calorie junk food and sedentary behavior. Management is really challenging in this group due to physical, social, and emotional growth. Future research is needed to halt or reverse the diabetes or its complications.

SUGGESTED READINGS

1. Thanabalasingham G, Pal A, Selwood MP, et al. Systematic assessment of etiology in adults with a clinical diagnosis of young-onset type 2 diabetes is a successful strategy for identifying maturity-onset diabetes of the young. Diabetes Care. 2012;35:1206-12.
2. ICMR- YDR. Executive Summary: ICMR-YDR Registry (Phase-1) Report2. [online] Available from https://main.icmr.nic.in/sites/default/files/reports/Executive%20summary.pdf [Last accessed October, 2022].
3. Sahoo SK, Zaidi G, Vipin VP, et al. Heterogeneity in the etiology of diabetes mellitus in young adults: A prospective study from north India. Indian J Med Res. 2019;149:479-88.

4. Pradeep A. Praveen, Sri venkata madhu, Viswanathan mohan et al. Registry of youth onset diabetes in India (YDR). J Diabetes Sci Technol. 2016;10(5):1034-41.
5. Arslanian S, Bacha F, Grey M, et al. Evaluation and management of youth-onset type 2 diabetes: a position statement by the American Diabetes Association. Diabetes Care. 2018;41:2648-67.
6. Indian Ministry of Health and Family Welfare. National guideline for Diagnosis and management of gestational Diabetes Mellitus. New Delhi: Indian Ministry of Health and Family Welfare; 2018.
7. Kolly A, Shivaprasad C, Pulikkal AA, et al. High prevalence of serine protease inhibitor *Kazal type 1* gene variations detected by whole gene sequencing in patients with fibrocalculous pancreatic diabetes. Indian J Endocrinol Metab. 2017;21:510-4.
8. Jha S, Waghdhare S, Siddiqui S, et al. First identification of Flatbush diabetes in patients of Indian origin. Diabetes Care. 2015;38:e164-5.
9. Pandit MK, Burke J, Gustafson AB, et al. Drug-induced disorders of glucose tolerance. Ann Intern Med. 1993;118:529-39.

CHAPTER 30

Prediabetes: A Synopsis

Sarita Bajaj

INTRODUCTION

Diabetes mellitus represents a significant healthcare burden and increasing challenge for clinicians. The prevalence of elevated glycemic levels in both developed and developing countries is rising quickly. The absolute numbers of individuals with prediabetes are projected to increase by approximately one-third by the middle of this century. It is estimated that there will be more than 470 million people with prediabetes in 2030. According to the National Urban Diabetes Survey, the estimated prevalence of prediabetes is 14% in India.

Prediabetes is not a benign state as one thinks. Early and adequate intervention is needed to prevent the development of complications and progression to overt diabetes mellitus.

Prediabetes is now a widely understood term for individuals whose glucose levels are below threshold cutoffs for a diagnosis of diabetes mellitus but are elevated beyond what is considered "normal."

DIAGNOSIS OF PREDIABETES

Patients with prediabetes are defined by the presence of impaired fasting glucose (IFG) and/or impaired glucose tolerance (IGT) and/or A1c 5.7–6.4% **(Table 1)**.

TABLE 1: Criteria defining prediabetes.			
	ADA	**AACE**	**WHO**
FPG	100–125 mg/dL (IFG)	≥100–125 mg/dL (IFG)	110 mg/dL
2-hour PG during 75-g OGTT	140–199 mg/dL (IGT)	≥140–199 mg/dL (IGT)	140–199 mg/dL
HbA1c	5.7–6.4%	5.5–6.4%	ND

(AACE: American Association of Endocrinology; ADA: American Diabetes Association; FPG: fasting plasma glucose; HbA1c: glycated hemoglobin; ND: not defined; OGTT: oral glucose tolerance test; PG: plasma glucose; WHO: World Health Organization)

CRITERIA FOR TESTING FOR DIABETES MELLITUS OR PREDIABETES IN ASYMPTOMATIC ADULTS

- Testing should be considered in adults with overweight or obesity [body mass index (BMI) ≥25 kg/m² or 23 kg/m² in Asian Americans] who have one or more of the following risk factors:
    - First-degree relative with diabetes mellitus
    - High-risk race/ethnicity (e.g., African American, Latino, Native American, Asian American, Pacific Islander)
    - History of cardiovascular disease (CVD)
    - Hypertension (≥140/90 mm Hg or on therapy for hypertension)
    - High-density lipoprotein (HDL) cholesterol level <35 mg/dL (0.90 mmol/L) and/or a triglyceride level >250 mg/dL (2.82 mmol/L)
    - Women with polycystic ovary syndrome
    - Physical inactivity
    - Other clinical conditions associated with insulin resistance (e.g., severe obesity, acanthosis nigricans)
- Patients with prediabetes (A1c ≥5.7%, IGT, or IFG) should be tested yearly.
- Women who were diagnosed with gestational diabetes mellitus (GDM) should have lifelong testing at least every 3 years.
- For all other patients, testing should begin at age 45 years.
- If results are normal, testing should be repeated at a minimum of 3-year intervals, with consideration of more frequent testing depending on initial results and risk status.
- Human immunodeficiency virus (HIV)

NATURAL HISTORY OF DIABETES MELLITUS AND PREDIABETES

Nearly all patients with type 2 diabetes mellitus (T2DM) pass through an extensive phase of prediabetes (average duration of nearly 10 years) **(Fig. 1)**.

Prediabetes is linked with the abnormalities in the form of insulin resistance and β-cell dysfunction. The conversion rate of prediabetes to diabetes mellitus is around 5–10%. Prediabetes should not be viewed as a clinical entity but as an increased risk for diabetes mellitus and CVD. Baseline A1c is a stronger predictor of subsequent diabetes mellitus and cardiovascular events. Several prospective

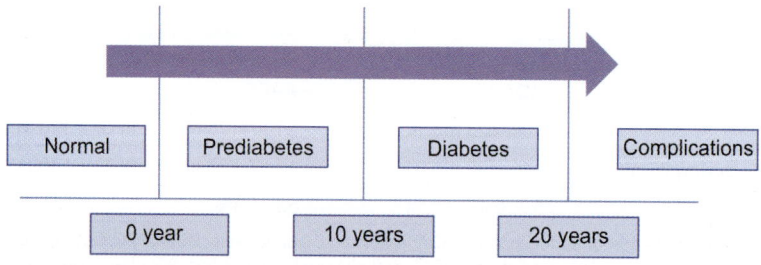

FIG. 1: Progression from prediabetes to diabetes mellitus.

studies have demonstrated a strong, continuous association between A1c and subsequent diabetes mellitus. In a systematic review of 44,203 individuals from 16 cohort studies with A1c between 5.5 and 6.0% with a follow-up interval averaging 5.6 years (range 2.8–12 years), there was a substantially increased risk of diabetes mellitus (5-year incidence from 9 to 25%). Those with an A1c range of 6.0–6.5% (42–48 mmol/mol) had a 5-year risk of developing diabetes mellitus between 25 and 50% and a relative risk 20 times higher compared with A1c of 5.0% (31 mmol/mol).

PATHOPHYSIOLOGIC DEFECTS IN PREDIABETES

- Loss of β-cell volume
- Defects in insulin action and secretion
- Endothelial dysfunction
- Arterial stiffness
- Increased lipolysis
- Reduced incretin levels
- Increased hepatic glucose production
- Impaired glucagon levels
- Dysregulated cytokines

COMPLICATIONS OF PREDIABETES

The most obvious sequela of prediabetes is the risk of development of T2DM. In addition to the progression to T2DM, the prediabetes state is associated with a spectrum of microvascular and macrovascular complications **(Fig. 2)**.

Microvascular Complications

The three classical microvascular complications in people with prediabetes are retinopathy, neuropathy, and nephropathy. In the Diabetes Prevention Program (DPP), 8% of the subjects with IGT had retinopathy. This was similar to the prevalence of retinopathy observed among individuals with prediabetes in the Gutenberg Health Study in Germany, 8.1%. In another study, the estimated prevalence of microalbuminuria among subjects with prediabetes was 15.5%.

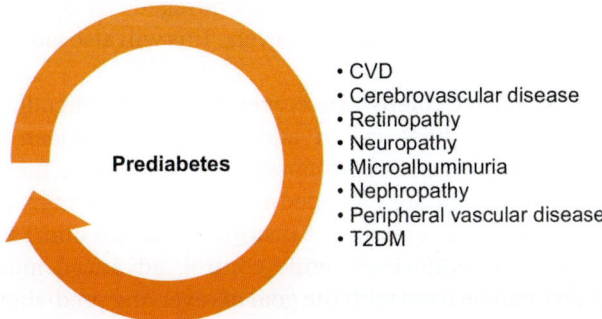

FIG. 2: Complications of prediabetes.

(CVD: cardiovascular disease; T2DM: type 2 diabetes mellitus)

Macrovascular Complications of Prediabetes

Prediabetes state is a significant risk factor for macrovascular disease. Although some of the risk may be due to the progression to overt diabetes mellitus, individual risk factors still exist in people who have not yet progressed to diabetes mellitus. A meta-analysis of 38 prospective studies in which CVD or mortality was the end point concluded that increasing glucose levels displayed a linear relationship with CVD risk.

The macrovascular disorders associated with prediabetes include CVD, stroke, and peripheral vascular disease. This depicts that although these disorders are established in patients with T2DM, their initiation and progression are well recognized to occur during the prediabetes stage. In fact, the traditional CVD risk factors (dyslipidemia, obesity, hypertension) are quite prevalent among individuals with prediabetes.

■ MANAGEMENT OF PREDIABETES

Lifestyle intervention is a cost-effective approach to the prevention of diabetes mellitus. It reduces the relative risk reduction for the future development of T2DM by 40–70%. If proper glycemic control is not achieved with lifestyle modification, several medications are prescribed to prevent diabetes mellitus among people with prediabetes.

- *Lifestyle modifications*: The combination of diet and exercise is the single most important factor that could halt the progression towards T2DM in patients with prediabetes.
- *Nutrition*: A variety of eating patterns such as the Mediterranean-style and low-carbohydrate eating plans may be appropriate for patients with prediabetes. Observational studies have also shown that vegetarian, plant-based (may include some animal products), and dietary approaches to stop hypertension (DASH) eating patterns are associated with a lower risk of developing T2DM.
- *Physical activity*: Moderate-intensity physical activity has been shown to improve insulin sensitivity and reduce abdominal fat in children and young adults. 150 min/week of moderate-intensity physical activity, such as brisk walking, has shown beneficial effects in those with prediabetes. Resistance training can also be included in exercise regimen designed to prevent diabetes mellitus. Breaking up prolonged sedentary time may be encouraged, as it is associated with moderately lower postprandial glucose levels. This will also aid in the prevention of GDM.
- *Pharmacological agent*: There are currently four medications for treating the prediabetes subpopulation. In addition, the American Association of Endocrinology (AACE) has also proposed two weight loss therapies—orlistat, and phentermine/topiramate extended-release (ER)—to manage obesity with the goal of halting the progression of insulin resistance and T2DM. If medical management fails to achieve glycemic control, advanced measures such as bariatric surgery can be used with the goal of reversing prediabetes and helping obese patients lose weight **(Flowchart 1)**. All surgical procedures are complex processes that require mental preparedness on the part of the patient and an in-

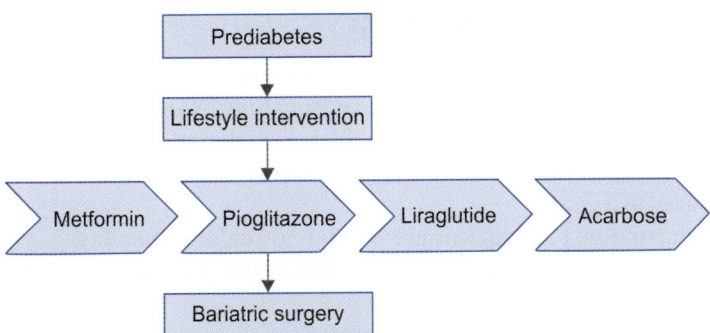

FLOWCHART 1: Lifestyle interventions in prediabetes adapted from the American Association of Clinical Endocrinologists guidelines.

depth understanding of how it will impact their lifestyle. Hence, surgery should be reserved for those who are resistant to other forms of treatment.

As per the American Diabetes Association (ADA) 2021, metformin therapy for the prevention of T2DM should be considered in those with prediabetes, especially for those with BMI ≥35 kg/m², those aged <60 years, and women with prior GDM.

The ADA also recommends that patients with prediabetes should be referred to an intensive lifestyle behavior change program modeled on the DPP to achieve and maintain 7% loss of initial body weight and increase moderate-intensity physical activity (such as brisk walking) to at least 150 min/week.

The DPP demonstrated that lifestyle modification and metformin interventions can delay or prevent the development of T2DM by 11 and 3 years, respectively, and reduce the absolute incidence of diabetes mellitus by 20% and 8%, respectively. However, evidence is lacking in individuals with IFG or prediabetes assessed by glycated hemoglobin (HbA1c).

PRE-D Trial

The PRE-D trial was designed to investigate on-treatment effects of dapagliflozin, metformin, or exercise on glycemic variability for 6 weeks as well as 13 weeks. It was a randomized, controlled, parallel, multiarm, open-label, nonblinded trial performed at the Steno Diabetes Center Copenhagen, Gentofte, Denmark. 120 participants of the 404 screened with BMI ≥25 kg/m², 30–70 years of age, and prediabetes [HbA1c 39–47 mmol/mol (5.7–6.4%)] were randomized 1:1:1:1 to dapagliflozin (10 mg once daily), metformin (1,700 mg daily), interval-based exercise (5 days/week, 30 min/session), or control (habitual lifestyle), $n = 30$ in each group.

All treatments were associated with small improvements in glucometabolic outcomes. However, exercise was associated with additional cardiometabolic benefits.

REVERSAL OF PREDIABETES

Intensive lifestyle changes support prediabetes remission and lower a person's risk for developing T2DM. This was seen in a recent study, which included 158 African-Americans and European-Americans with prediabetes and parental history of T2DM. The study assessed the effects of six intensive lifestyle modification therapies over the course of 5 years:

1. *Calorie restriction*: Participants ate 1,200–1,500 calories per day.
2. 3 hours of physical activity per week. Most participants chose brisk walking as their physical activity.
3. A personal weight loss goal of 10% or more
4. *Increased face-to-face visits with a healthcare professional*: Monthly sessions for the first 6 months, followed by quarterly visits for the rest of the time
5. *Meal replacement*: Two shakes and two protein bars for two meals per day for participants who had not met their weight goals, 6–12 months after the start of the study
6. Increased self-monitoring through logging of daily calorie intake and physical activity

Only 6.5% of the participants were diagnosed with T2DM over 10 years. 43.5% of the people in the study achieved prediabetes remission within 10 years. Prediabetes remission was defined as "restoration of normal glucose regulation," or fasting plasma glucose (FPG) <100 mg/dL and 2-hour plasma glucose (PG) <140 mg/dL.

CONCLUSION

Prediabetes is a common metabolic condition etiologically related to obesity (especially abdominal or visceral obesity), and associated with increased risk of T2DM, CVD, and all-cause mortality.

With trends toward increased prevalence, but effective therapeutic interventions available, it is very important to increase efforts to identify and effectively manage prediabetes as early as possible so that we may avoid the impending global epidemic of diabetes mellitus.

Type 2 diabetes mellitus prevention and prediabetes "reversal" are achievable with lifestyle modification, and both should be the primary goals in diabetes mellitus care. Each person's diabetes mellitus journey is different; making small steps toward achievable goals is a great place to start.

SUGGESTED READINGS

1. Standards of medical care in diabetes—2021. Diabetes Care. 2021;44(Suppl 1):S1-2.
2. Kumar S, Anand A, Nagarathna R, et al. Prevalence of prediabetes, and diabetes in Chandigarh and Panchkula region based on glycated hemoglobin and Indian diabetes risk score. Endocrinol Diabetes Metab. 2021;4(1):e00162.
3. Jose J, Thomas N. How should one tackle prediabetes in India? Indian J Med Res. 2018;148(6):675.
4. Garber AJ. Combined pharmacologic/nonpharmacologic intervention in individuals at high risk of developing type 2 diabetes. Diabetes Care. 2009;32(Suppl 2):S184-8.
5. Handelsman Y, Bloomgarden ZT, Grunberger G, et al. American Association of Clinical Endocrinologists and American College of Endocrinology clinical practice guidelines for developing a diabetes mellitus comprehensive care plan. Endocr Pract. 2015;21(Suppl 1):1-87.

6. Khetan AK, Rajagopalan S. Prediabetes. Canadian J Cardiol. 2018;34(5):615-23.
7. Brannick B, Dagogo-Jack S. Prediabetes and cardiovascular disease: pathophysiology and interventions for prevention and risk reduction. Endocrinol Metab Clin North Am. 2018;47(1):33-50.
8. Brannick B, Wynn A, Dagogo-Jack S. Prediabetes as a toxic environment for the initiation of microvascular and macrovascular complications. Exp Biol Med (Maywood). 2016;241(12):1323-31.
9. Zand A, Ibrahim K, Patham B. Prediabetes: why should we care? Methodist DeBakey Cardiovasc J. 2018;14(4):289.
10. Herman WH, Hoerger TJ, Brandle M, et al. The cost-effectiveness of lifestyle modification or metformin in preventing type 2 diabetes in adults with impaired glucose tolerance. Ann Intern Med. 2005;142(5):323-32.
11. Færch K, Blond MB, Bruhn L, et al. The effects of dapagliflozin, metformin, or exercise on glycemic variability in overweight or obese individuals with prediabetes (the PRE-D trial): a multi-arm, randomized, controlled trial. Diabetologia. 2021;64(1):42-55.
12. Cardillo C. (2021). "Reversing" prediabetes may be possible with intensive lifestyle changes. [online] Available from https://diatribe.org/reversing-prediabetes-with-intensive-lifestyle-changes. [Last accessed October, 2022].
13. Rett K, Gottwald-Hostalek U. Understanding prediabetes: definition, prevalence, burden and treatment options for an emerging disease. Curr Med Res Opin. 2019;35(9):1529-34.

CHAPTER 31

Addison Disease, Clinical Challenges, and Treatment

Gursaran K Sidhu

■ INTRODUCTION

Addison's disease also known as adrenal insufficiency is an endocrine disorder characterized by inadequate production of steroid hormones-cortisol, aldosterone, and androgen by the adrenal glands. Adrenal glands also called suprarenals are two in number located one each on top of both the kidneys. The paired adrenal glands are triangular shaped measuring approximately 5 cm by 2 cm and weighing 4 to 5 g each. The adrenal glands play vital role in the body's fight or flight response. They generate stress hormones that activate physiological adaptation to counter act changes in external environment, and significant role in regulating the body's immune system, body metabolism and salt and water balance.

History

Addison's disease is named after Thomas Addison, the British physician who first described the condition in "On the Constitutional and Local Effects of Disease of the Suprarenal Capsules" in 1855.

The condition was initially considered a form of anemia associated with the adrenal glands. Tuberculosis used to be a major cause of Addison's disease and acute adrenal failure worldwide. It remains a leading cause in developing countries today.

Epidemiology

This incidence is estimated at 1 in 100,000 human population. Addison's disease can affect persons of any age, sex, or ethnicity, but it typically presents in adults between 30 and 50 years of age. About 70% of Addison's disease occurs due to autoimmune reactions, which cause damage to the adrenal cortex.

The adrenal glands is composed of two distinct tissues: The outer cortex and the inner medulla. The adrenal cortex is yellowish and much larger than smaller medulla. It is composed of three distinct zones.

Zona glomerulosa (outer layer) produces aldosterone, play important role in electrolyte balance and regulation of blood pressure.

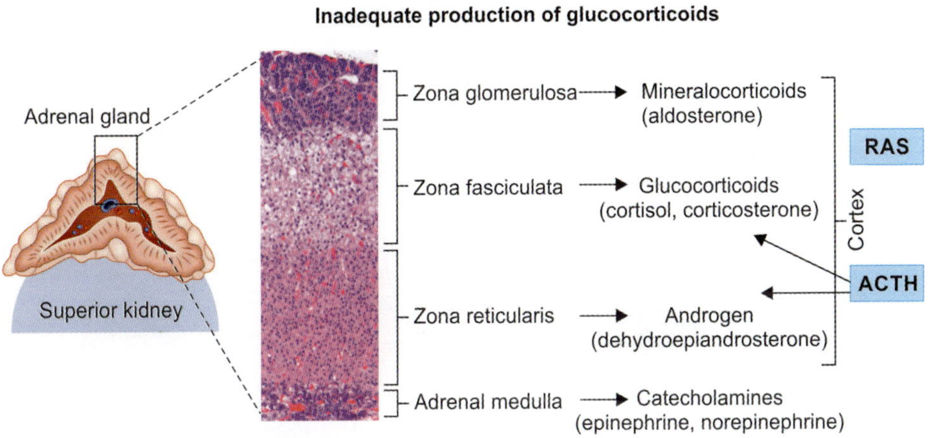

Inadequate production of glucocorticoids

FIG. 1: Adrenal gland structure and function.

Zona fasciculata (middle layer) produces glucocorticoids (cortisol) playing role in regulation of blood sugar, modulating immune system and metabolism of fat protein and carbohydrate.

Zona reticularis (inner zone) produces androgens dehydroepiandrosterone (DHEA) and plays a role in development of secondary sexual characteristics. DHEA is the precursor for synthesis of other hormones such as progesterone, estrogen, cortisol and testosterone.

The function of these three zones can be remembered by the mnemonic "Salt, Sugar, Sex" as to correlate the function of the hormones produced in each layer of adrenal cortex.

Adrenal medulla synthesizes catecholamines (epinephrine and nonepinephrine).

The hypothalamus produces corticotropin-releasing hormones (CRH) that stimulates the pituitary gland to secrete adrenocorticotropic hormone (ACTH). ACTH than stimulates the adrenal glands to make and release cortisol hormones into the blood. The glucocorticoids (cortisol) and androgens are regulated by pituitary adrenocorticotropic hormone (ACTH).

Mineralocorticoids (aldosterone) are regulated by kidneys through the renin-angiotensin–aldosterone system (RAAS).

Adrenal insufficiency is of two types:
1. Primary
2. Secondary

Primary adrenal insufficiency also called Addison's disease is the disorder in which the adrenal gland produces insufficient amount of hormones.

Secondary adrenal insufficiency is due to disorder in anterior pituitary and hypothalamus and results in low cortisol and adrenal androgens.

Common Causes of Adrenal Insufficiency

In developed countries the etiology of Addison's diseases is often attributed to idiopathic damage by body's own immune system and in developing countries most

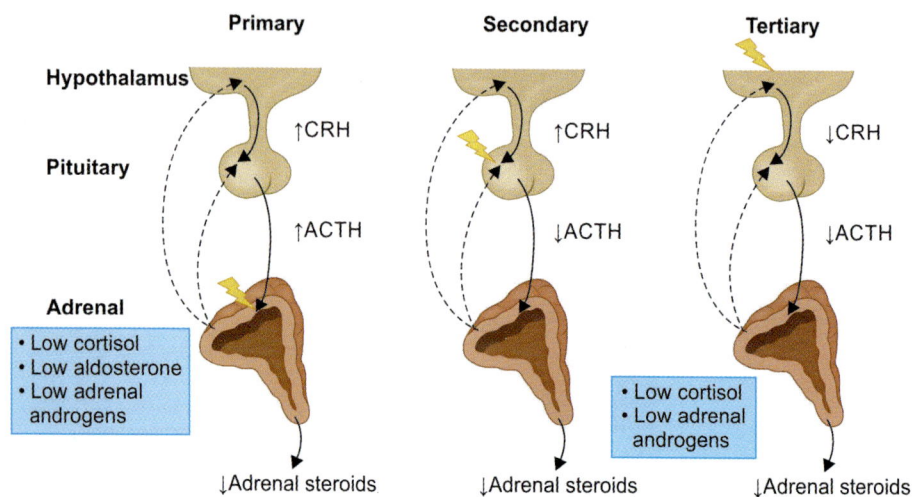

FIG. 2: Regulation of adrenal hormone secretion.

often due to tuberculosis. Other causes include septicemia, hemorrhage, infarction, tumors, metastasis, surgical B/L adrenalectomy, and certain medications.

Etiology of Different Types of Adrenal Insufficiency

Primary AI	Secondary AI	Tertiary AI
• Autoimmune • Infection • Infiltrative disorders • Infarction and hemorrhage • Tumors and metastasis • Bilateral adrenalectomy • Genetic—CAH, adrenoleukodystrophy	• Congenital hypopituitarism • Pituitary tumors • Hypophysitis • Trauma, surgery, radiation • Infarction • Infection • Infiltrative disorders • Drugs—immune check-point inhibitors	• Exogenous glucocorticoids (>5 mg prednisolone for >3–4 weeks) • Opioids • Hypothalamic tumors

(AI: adrenal insufficiency; CAH: congenital adrenal hyperplasia)

Causes of Primary Adrenal Insufficiency

- *Autoimmune adrenalitis*: Isolated (30–40%) or as part of autoimmune Polyglandular syndrome (APS) 60–70%
- *APS*: It is of two types:
  i. *APS 1*: Also called as autoimmune polyendocrinopathy ectodermal dystrophy (APECED). It includes hypoparathyroidism, Addison's disease, and chronic mucocutaneous candidiasis. APS 1 is caused by mutation in autoimmune regulator gene *AIRE*.
  ii. *APS 2:* It has polygenic inheritance, associated with human leukocyte antigen (HLA)-DR3. It includes thyroid disorders, type 1 diabetes mellitus, pernicious anemia, and Addison's disease.

- *X-linked adrenoleukodystrophy*: There is mutation of peroxisomal membrane transporter protein ABCD-1. This results in accumulation of long chain fatty acids.
- *Destruction of gland*:
  - Infection: Tuberculosis is the frequent cause in developing countries.
  - Hemorrhage: Water house Friderichsen syndrome
    Antiphospholipid antibodies (APLAs) may cause vascular thrombi and hemorrhagic infarction in antiphospholipid syndrome resulting in primary adrenal insufficiency.
  - *Infiltration*: Metastasis, lymphomas, amyloidosis, and hemochromatosis
- *Drug induced*: Mitotane, ketoconazole, INF-alpha, ribavirin
- *Triple A syndrome*: It includes alacrima, achalasia-cardia, and Addison's disease are caused by mutation in *AAAS* gene.
- Congenital adrenal hyperplasia (CAH)

Causes of Secondary Adrenal Insufficiency
- Pituitary tumors
- Craniopharyngioma, meningioma, ependymoma
- Pituitary irradiation
- Autoimmune hypophysitis
- *Pituitary hemorrhage*: Sheehan's syndrome, surgery, pregnancy
- *Pituitary infiltration*: Tuberculosis, actinomycosis, sarcoidosis, and metastasis
- Combined pituitary hormone deficiency (CPHD)

Tertiary Adrenal Insufficiency
The most common cause of tertiary adrenal insufficiency is sudden stoppage corticosteroids after taking them for a long time.

This is treated by glucocorticoid (e.g., hydrocortisone replacement) and not mineralocorticoid or androgen replacement.

Signs and symptoms of Adrenal Insufficiency
It should be suspected as it is potentially life-threatening.

Signs and symptoms caused by mineralocorticoids deficiency:
- Abdominal pain, nausea, and vomiting
- Dizziness, hyponatremia, salt craving, and hyperkalemia
- Postural hypotension and muscle cramps

Signs and symptoms caused by GC deficiency:
- Fatigue, lack of energy, weight loss
- Joint pain, fever, hypoglycemia or unexplained reduction in antidiabetic doses
- Low blood pressure (BP), postural hypotension
- Hyponatremia [due to loss of feedback inhibition of arginine vasopressin (AVP) release]

- Hyperpigmentation on extensor surfaces, elbows, knuckles, and lips is seen only in primary adrenal insufficiency.

Signs and symptoms caused by androgen deficiency:
- Lack of energy, dry and itchy skin
- Loss of libido, loss of axillary and pubic hair
- These signs and symptoms are mostly seen in females.

Symptoms of Secondary Adrenal Insufficiency
- Other pituitary hormone deficits present
- Usually no aldosterone deficiency so less electrolyte disturbances
- Hyponatremia may still occur due to reduced water clearance

ACUTE ADRENAL INSUFFICIENCY
- It is also called adrenal crisis. Most frequently seen in patients with primary adrenal insufficiency due to both GC and mineralocorticoid deficiency.
- It may mimic acute abdomen with abdominal pain, tenderness, nausea, vomiting, and fever.
- Postural hypotension may progress to hypovolemic shock.
- Acute metabolic disturbances and altered sensorium

Definition	Other symptoms	Causes
Major impairment of general health with at least two of the following signs/symptoms: • Hypotension (systolic blood pressure <100 mm Hg) • Nausea or vomiting • Severe fatigue • Fever • Somnolence • Hyponatremia (<132 mmol/L) or hyperkalemia • Hypoglycemia	• Fatigue, lack of energy, weight loss • Hypovolemia to hypovolemic shock • Cardiomyopathy • Anorexia, abdominal pain (peritonitis) • Skin abnormalities (PAI hyperpigmentation vs. SAI alabaster-like paleness) • Prerenal failure, normochromic anemia, lymphocytosis, eosinophilia	• Infections (gastroenteritis) • Surgery • Pain • Strenuous exercise • Severe emotional stress • Accidents • Unsuitable dose adjustments • No clear cause
		Grading: Grade 1: Outpatient care only Grade 2: Hospital care Grade 3: Admission to ICU Grade 4: Death from adrenal crisis

(ICU: intensive care unit; PAI: primary adrenal insufficiency; SAI: secondary adrenal insufficiency)

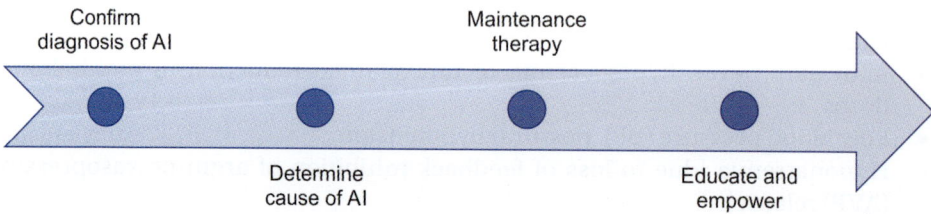

FIG. 3: Clinical presentation and symptomatology.

Addison Disease, Clinical Challenges, and Treatment

When to suspect: Suspect a lean built, young female/male presenting with dehydration, drowsy, hypotension, or shock with mild abdominal tenderness.

Confirmation of diagnosis: Complete blood count (CBC), serum electrolytes, renal functional test, thyroid profile test, cortisol level, and ACTH levels.

Diagnosis and Evaluation

Serum cortisol concentrations determined at 8 hours of <3 μg/dL (80 nmol/L) are strongly suggestive of adrenal insufficiency.
- Normal basal cortisol: 3–10 μg/dL (<100 nmol/L).
- Less than 3 μg/dL strongly suggestive,
- More than 10 μg/dL unlikely
- Plasma ACTH: More than two to three times of upper normal limit confirms—primary AI.

Adrenocorticotropic hormone stimulation test: It involves administration of cosyntropin (it contains ACTH 1-24 AA) 0.25 mg intramuscular (IM)/intravenous (IV) followed by collection of blood sample at 0, 30, and 60 minutes.

Normal response is defined as cortisol level >50–20 μg/dL in 30–60 minutes after cosyntropin administration.
- *Plasma renin and aldosterone*: Elevated renin and low aldosterone in primary adrenal insufficiency.
- If the basal and stimulated cortisol levels are abnormal, the diagnosis of adrenal insufficiency is suspected. Exclude the concurrent and recent use of exogenous use of steroids. Measure the ACTH levels.

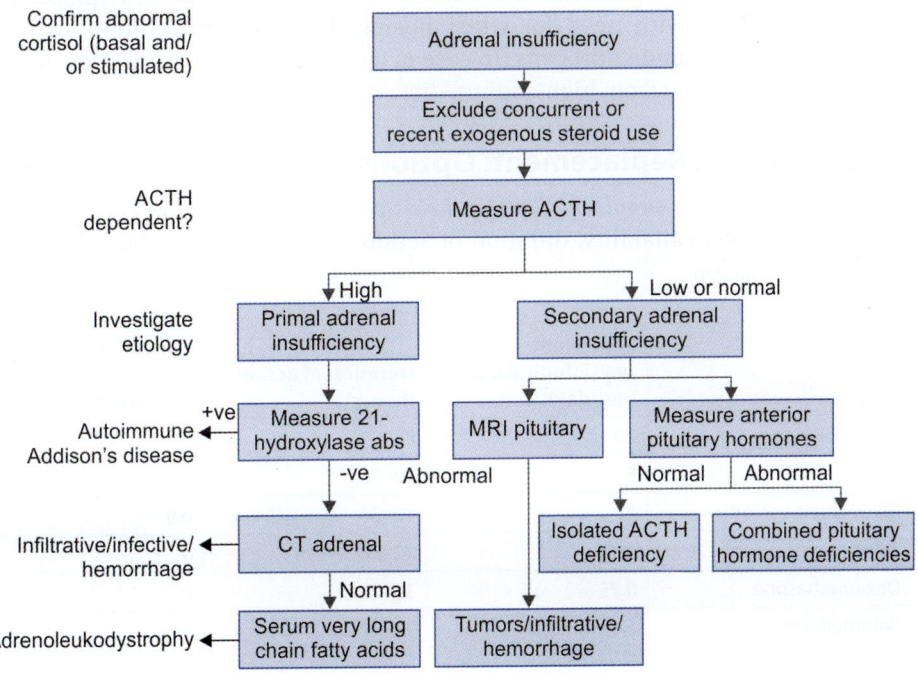

FLOWCHART 1: Diagnosis and evaluation.

- If high investigate as primary AI. Causes may be autoimmune, infiltrative/infective/hemorrhage in adrenal glands
- If low investigate as secondary AI. Then causes may be pituitary hormone deficiency

Treatment and Management

On suspicion of acute adrenal insufficiency, draw sample for cortisol and ACTH and initiate treatment without waiting for results.
- *Fluid resuscitation*: 1 L 0.9% saline (20–30 mL/kg) in first hour, 500 mL in second hour, followed by maintenance fluid—125–250 mL/h. Monitor vitals, BP, electrolytes with continous cardiac monitoring.
- *Glucocorticoid replacement*: Drug of choice is hydrocortisone 100 mg IV/IM bolus, 200 mg/24 hours, then taper down.

Avoid—dexamethasone as it has no mineralocorticoid effect.
- *Treat precipitating factor*:
  - Infection
  - Surgical stress and trauma

Start fludrocortisone 50–100 µg/day in primary adrenal insufficiency.
Blood pressure and sensorium will start improving in next 2 hours.

Subsequently by day-3 patient can be shifted to oral hydrocortisone 100 mg along with tablet fludrocortisone 100 mg/day.

■ CHRONIC TREATMENT IN ADRENAL INSUFFICIENCY

Goal is to provide symptomatic relief and prevent adverse effects. Replacement therapy is lifelong with need for stress dosing. Replacement is done for GCs, mineralocorticoids, and androgens (in case of female). Those with low-aldosterone levels may also benefit from high-sodium diet.

Glucocorticoid Replacement: Options

Structural changes in steroid nucleus and side chains determine PK/PD properties: Differences in bioavailability, duration of action, relative potency, MR effect, and genomic modulation.

Glucocorticoids	Equivalent physiological doses (mg/day)	Duration of action (hours)	Mineralocorticoid activity relative to hydrocortisone
Hydrocortisone	20	8–12	1
Prednisone	5	12–36	0.8
Methylprednisolone	4	12–36	0.5
Triamcinolone	4	12–36	0
Dexamethasone	0.75	36–72	0
Betamethasone	0.6	36–72	0

Addison Disease, Clinical Challenges, and Treatment

- *Mimic endogenous cortisol secretion:* Endogenous cortisol production is 6–8 mg/m² BSA circadian rhythm
- *Drug of choice*: Hydrocortisone alternative—prednisolone
- *Avoid*: Dexamethasone, betamethasone, deflazacort

Glucocorticoid Replacement: ES Guidelines

- Hydrocortisone or cortisone acetate

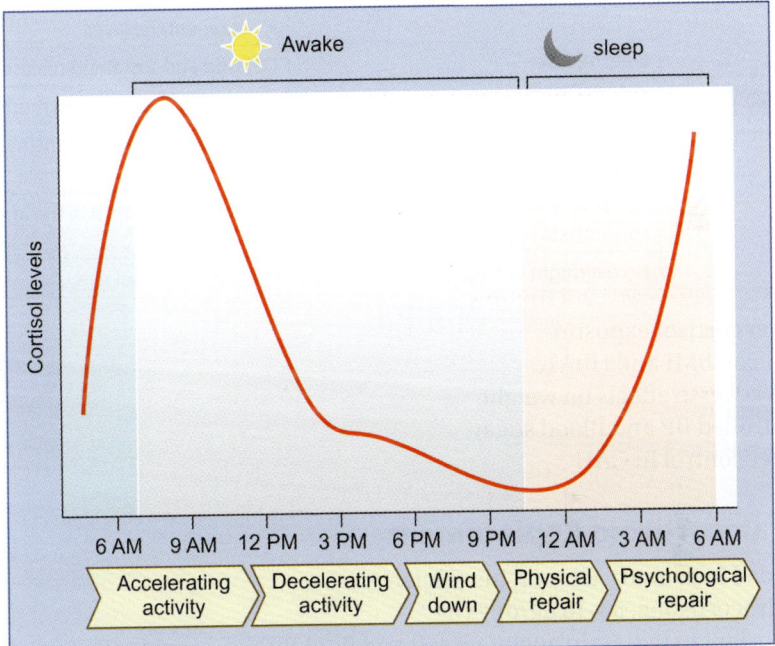

- Hydrocortisone 15–255 mg/day (>25 mg rarely needed) in two to three divided doses
- First dose on awakening, second in late afternoon (e.g., 7 AM, 3 PM)
- First dose on awakening, second in early afternoon, third 4–6 hours before bedtime (e.g., 7 AM, 12 noon, 5 PM)

Prednisolone: 3–5 mg once daily

How to monitor GC replacement?
- *Under treatment will cause symptoms like:* Anorexia, weight loss, vomiting, fatigue, increasing pigmentation
- *Overtreatment will produce:* Weight gain, Cushingoid habitus, disturbed sleep, glucose intolerance, hypertension, decreased bone mineral density (BMD)
- *Biochemical monitoring:* There are no reliable biochemical parameters of dose adequacy—cortisol, ACTH, 24-hour urinary free cortisol (UFC) are not good indicators of tissue exposure to cortisol.

There is a strong need for stress doses in acute medical or surgical stress.
    Treating EMO's and patient himself/herself should be educated and empowered with this knowledge.

Recent Advances in Glucocorticoid Replacement
- Continuous subcutaneous hydrocortisone infusion
- Modified release hydrocortisone

	Plenadren®	Multiparticulate Chronocort®
Composition	Immediate-release hydrocortisone outer-layer coating extended-release core	• Inert core coated with a hydrocortisone layer, coated with polymeric layers • Outer enteric layer
	Dual release	Delayed and sustained release
Dose regimen	Once daily, morning	Twice daily (evening and morning)
Distribution profile	Higher morning cortisol concentrations	Early peak of cortisol in the morning
	Lower evening cortisol concentrations	Early peak of cortisol in the afternoon
	No overnight cortisol rise	Overnight cortisol rise

- Lower cortisol exposure
- Reduced BMI and HbA1c
- Less adverse effects on weight
- Controlled BP and Blood sugar
- Better control in CAH

Mineralocorticoid Replacement
- Needed in primary adrenal insufficiency
- Fludrocortisone: 50–10 µg/day OD
- Important to maintain adequate salt and fluid intake—avoid salt restriction
- Inadequate MC replacement and/or salt intake can cause recurrent adrenal crisis and compensatory GC over replacement.
- It should be monitored clinically as well as biochemically.
- *Clinical* symptoms of insufficient dose are lightheadedness, fainting, salt craving, postural hypotension.
- Overdose can cause edema and new onset hypertension.
- *Biochemical*—maintain electrolytes in normal range. And maintain the plasma rennin (or PRA) in upper reference range or slightly higher.

Practical Aspects in Mineralocorticoids Replacement
Higher doses are required in children, young adults, and pregnant ladies also increase the doses of salt and fluid intake in hot and humid climate and during exercise.

In case of hypertension, carefully reduce dose of fludrocortisone, but do not stop it. And avoid diuretics and aldosterone receptor blockers. If required, start antihypertensives—RAS blockers, CCB. Patients need to be counseled properly regarding medication, adequate salt, and fluid intake. Patients may not feel unwell if few doses are omitted, but there is a very high risk of adrenal crisis which needs to be avoided.

Dehydroepiandrosterone Replacement: When and How?

Low libido, reduced well-being, and impaired quality of life (QoL) in women. DHEA replacement in premenopausal women will help improve mood and well-being, reduce depression, and anxiety scores. Improve sexual interest and satisfaction and improvement in body composition and BMD.

Give a trial of 6 months (25–50 mg DHEA), if women have persistent reduced well-being, if symptoms do not improve discontinue medication.

Long-term Risks of Overtreatment
- Infections
- Weight gain, adiposity
- Hypertension and dyslipidemia
- Glucose intolerance and diabetes mellitus
- Increased cardiovascular (CV) risk and increased mortality
- Osteoporosis, fracture risk

Secondary Adrenal Insufficiency

The causes could be:
- Pituitary macroadenoma
    - Nonfunctional
- Combined anterior pituitary hormone deficits produce
    - Secondary adrenal insufficiency, secondary hypothyroidism, and secondary hypogonadism

Management: Replace the deficits, these patients do not require mineralocorticoids replacement. Most important dictum to remember is steroid replacement before thyroid replacement

■ CONCLUSION

The clinician must have a high index of suspicion to diagnose adrenal insufficiency. Patients need hormone replacement therapy to balance the levels of steroid hormones in their body. Therefore, they need to take medicines on the daily basis, and continuous treatment require.

Educate to Prevent Crisis: To decrease the risk of adrenal crisis, patient education, and empowerment is key.

Equip patients with:
- Supply of hydrocortisone and fludrocortisone to account for sick days
- Leaflets about stress dosing
- Medical alert card with diagnosis, medical information, and contact details of endocrine team
- Emergency injection kit

SUGGESTED READINGS

1. National Organization for Rare Disorders. 2020. Addison's disease. [online] Available from https://rarediseases.org/rare-diseases/addisons-disease/ [Last accessed October, 2022].
2. Pazderska A, Pearce SHs. Adrenal insufficiency - recognition and management. Clin Med (Lond). 2017;17(3):258-62.
3. Nowotny H, Ahmed SF, Bensing S, et al. Therapy options for adrenal insufficiency and recommendations for the management of adrenal crisis. Endocrine. 2021;71(3):586-94.
4. Pelewicz K, Miśkiewicz P. Glucocorticoid withdrawal-An overview on when and how to diagnose adrenal insufficiency in clinical practice. Diagnostics (Basel). 2021;11(4):728.
5. Bornstein SR, Allolio B, Arlt W, et al. Diagnosis and treatment of primary adrenal insufficiency: An Endocrine Society Clinical Practice Guideline. J Clin Endocrinol Metab. 2016;101(2):364-89.
6. Ruiz-Babot G, Hadjidemetriou I, King PJ, et al. New directions for the treatment of adrenal insufficiency. Front Endocrinol (Lausanne). 2015;6:70.
7. Irina B, Hahner S, Tomlinson J, et al. Diagnosis and management of adrenal insufficiency. Lancet Diabetes Endocrinol. 2015;3(3):216-26.
8. Oprea A, Bonnet NCG, Pollé O, et al. Novel insights into glucocorticoid replacement therapy for pediatric and adult adrenal insufficiency.Ther Adv Endocrinol Metab. 2019;10: 2042018818821294.
9. Younes N, Bourdeau I, Lacroix A, et al. Latent adrenal insufficiency: From concept to diagnosis. Front Endocrinol (Lausanne). 2021;12:720769.
10. Bovenberg SA, van Uum SHM, Hermus ARMM, et al. Dehydroepiandrosterone administration in humans: evidence based? Neth J Med. 2005;63(8):300-4.
11. Gurnell EM, Hunt PJ, Curran SE, et al. Long-term DHEA replacement in primary adrenal insufficiency: a randomized, controlled trial. J Clin Endocrinol Metab. 2008;93(2):400-9.
12. Prete A, Bancos I. Glucocorticoid induced adrenal insufficiency. BMJ. 2021;374:n1380.

CHAPTER 32

Treatment Issues in Hypothyroidism

Rahin Mahata, Partha Pratim Chakraborty

■ INTRODUCTION

Hypothyroidism, a clinical state of deficient thyroid hormone (TH) action in peripheral tissues, is broadly classified into three groups: (i) primary hypothyroidism, (ii) secondary or central hypothyroidism (CH), and (iii) peripheral hypothyroidism. Primary hypothyroidism results from disorders of the thyroid gland itself, and accounts for about 99% of all cases of hypothyroidism. CH develops due to deficiency of thyrotropin-releasing hormone (TRH) and/or thyroid-stimulating hormone (TSH), as encountered in a variety of hypothalamic or pituitary diseases. Peripheral hypothyroidism is the rarest form of hypothyroidism in which TH secretion is normal or increased but TH action is impaired due to peripheral tissue resistance or increased degradation of active THs. Primary hypothyroidism is further divided into overt hypothyroidism (OH) [low serum concentrations of total thyroxine (T4) or free T4 (FT4)] and subclinical hypothyroidism (SCH), also termed as "mild thyroid failure" in which serum TSH level is high but serum FT4 values remain within the population specific reference range.

■ TREATMENT OF OVERT HYPOTHYROIDISM

Levothyroxine sodium (LT4) is widely accepted as the treatment of choice for all forms of hypothyroidism. Absorption after oral administration in fasting state is acceptable (around 70–80%), and the half-life of about a week allows once daily dosing. Administered LT4 is converted to active triiodothyronine (T3) by deiodination in peripheral tissues and relatively stable serum concentrations of both T4 and T3 are achieved. Patients with hypothyroidism have higher circulatory T4/T3 ratio compared to euthyroid subjects to maintain normal TSH. Though serum TSH actually reflects pituitary effect of T3, in clinical practice, TSH is used as surrogate marker of TH action at the peripheral tissues.

Objectives of treatment in OH are:
- Alleviate symptoms of hypothyroidism
- Normalize serum TSH
- Avoidance of iatrogenic thyrotoxicosis

Initiation of LT4 Therapy

Starting dose of LT4 depends on underlying etiology of primary hypothyroidism (congenital, autoimmune, postsurgery or postradioiodine ablation), underlying age, and degree of residual thyroid gland function (decline in FT4 and elevation of TSH). In adults with minimal/no residual thyroid function, as seen in post-total thyroidectomy or post-radioiodine ablation, and no underlying cardiovascular disease LT4 therapy is initiated at full dose (1.6–1.8 µg/kg/day). Elderly patients, those with coronary artery disease and untreated severe, long-standing hypothyroidism, should initially be put on low dose of LT4 (25 µg/day). In neonates with congenital hypothyroidism (CH) the starting dose of LT4 is 10–15 µg/kg/day. Children, particularly those between 8 and 12 years of age, with profound primary hypothyroidism are at risk of developing pseudotumor cerebri after initiation of treatment with conventional doses. Thus, treatment is initiated with one-third to one-half of the usual dose of LT4 in this age group. In children, the magnitude of the height deficit is proportional to the duration of hypothyroidism, which can be estimated as the difference between the chronological age and bone age. When these children are treated with conventional doses of LT4, accelerated skeletal maturation is observed, with the skeletal age advancing disproportionately faster than gain in height. Thus, predicted height falls, and genetic growth potential may not be achieved. A small proportion of patients with primary autoimmune hypothyroidism may have coexistent primary adrenal insufficiency (PAI) as components of autoimmune polyglandular syndrome (APS). Glucocorticoid replacement should always be started before or concurrently with LT4 therapy to prevent life-threatening adrenal crisis.

The time interval between treatment initiation and effect(s) depends on the dose of LT4 and severity of hypothyroidism. An early clinical response in moderate to severe hypothyroidism is diuresis with a weight loss of around 2–4 kg. Serum sodium level increases quite early in those with hyponatremia. This is often followed by increase in pulse rate and pulse pressure, improvement in appetite and constipation, if present. Improvement in psychomotor activity and delayed relaxation of deep tendon reflexes then becomes apparent. Changes in skin and hairs persist for several months.

If patients forget to take their schedule LT4 dosage on a particular day, little decrement in FT4 concentrations, if any, would be expected because of the long half-life of LT4. The omitted dose can be taken as soon as the lapse is recognized.

Monitoring and Adjustment of LT4 Therapy

Serum TSH is the best indicator available to monitor LT4 therapy. Serum TSH indicates TH effect on pituitary tissue and a normal serum TSH may not necessarily indicate euthyroidism in all tissues and organs of the body. This is the reason why a subset of patients with biochemical euthyroidism continue to experience persistent symptoms of hypothyroidism.

LT4 dosage is often adjusted based on serum TSH concentration and repeat testing should be performed after 6–8 weeks of therapy initiation or dose modification. Target TSH depends on a number of factors that include age of the patient, underlying comorbidities, pregnancy, and etiology of primary hypothyroidism (like surgery in thyroid malignancy). In majority of patients with primary hypothyroidism, the target TSH is between 0.5 and 2.5 µIU/mL. If TSH is above the target range but <10 µIU/mL, or subnormal but not undetectable, an increase or decrease of 12.5 µg, respectively, may suffice to normalize the TSH concentration. More deranged TSH values may require more substantial dosage changes. However, individual sensitivity to any dose of LT4 varies markedly; hence dose titration should be based on individual patient's response. Some patients may be under-replaced or over-replaced with the lowest available doses (12.5 µg) and may require fine tuning of dosage such as alternate use of different available doses, omitting the dose or doubling the dose on a particular day of the week. However, complex replacement regimens should be avoided if possible.

Once the TSH goal is achieved, serum TSH should be repeated every 3 to 6 months and then every 6–12 months to ensure continued adherence therapy and euthyroidism. Restoration of euthyroidism increases the metabolic clearance of LT4; a dose that was adequate to normalize TSH during the early phase of therapy may not be sufficient when the patient is rendered metabolically euthyroid owing to accelerated TH clearance. In addition, patients with chronic lymphocytic thyroiditis who are being treated with relatively small LT4 doses may require progressive increment of LT4 doses during follow-up, as remaining thyroid function gradually declines.

Some clinicians routinely perform FT4 along with TSH during follow-up of primary hypothyroid patients treated with LT4. FT4 as a monitoring tool is particularly important in patients with Graves' disease (GD), CH, and in those with questionable compliance. In patients with GD who have undergone total thyroidectomy or radioactive iodine (I-131) ablation TSH often remains suppressed for a considerable period even if those individuals are clinically and biochemically hypothyroidism (low FT4). These patients should be treated with full LT4 replacement therapy and monitored not with TSH, but with FT4 and total T3, particularly during the initial months. Serum FT4 levels to be kept in the mid-normal to high-normal reference range. In CH, the characteristic "inverse log-linear relationship" between FT4 and TSH may not be apparent due to altered set point; hence, dose adjustment should be based on both FT4 and TSH concentrations.

TSH concentration is much less influenced by the timing of phlebotomy than is FT4 level, and increment in serum FT4 of about 15% from baseline may be encountered approximately 3.5 hours after LT4 administration. FT4 value in LT4-treated patients need to be interpreted keeping in mind the time of LT4 administration. Sampling for FT4 should preferably be done before the morning dose of LT4.

Fluctuating Thyroid-stimulating Hormone

Unexpected fluctuations in serum TSH in LT4-treated patients with previously "normal" TSH are not uncommon in clinical practice. The most common etiology of persistently elevated TSH or intermittently elevated TSH, particularly in those having large dosage of LT4, is noncompliance. Variable adherence may falsely suggest the need for an increased LT4 dose. The prevalence of nonadherence between 22–52% in different studies. Combination of a high TSH and a high-normal/normal FT4 is consistent with recent resumption of LT4 intake in a noncompliant patient prior to a scheduled blood test. It may be necessary to choose a schedule of medication administration that is practical, even if absorption is affected, if this ensures that doses are not omitted. If repeated efforts to encourage regular daily consumption of LT4 are unsuccessful, options include observed therapy, including twice weekly or weekly dosing of LT4. Weekly dosing of LT4 should be done very cautiously in older patients or those with known cardiac disease.

The next important factor is to ensure adequate absorption of the administered LT4 dose. A number of medications and factors interfere with LT4 absorption and have been listed in **Table 1**. LT4 should be administered at empty stomach every day and nothing is allowed (except water) for at least 30 minutes (preferably 60 minutes) after the LT4 dosage to ensure satisfactory and consistent absorption. The metabolism of LT4 may also be altered by different drugs. Drugs that have been shown to increase hepatic metabolism of T4 and T3 are phenobarbital, phenytoin, carbamazepine, rifampicin, sertraline, and imatinib. Drugs accelerating the conversion of T3 to reverse T3 (inactive metabolites) are imatinib, sorafenib, masitinib, and sunitinib. Patients may also require an increased dose of LT4 to maintain a normal serum TSH when amiodarone is initiated. The effects of amiodarone (type III antiarrhythmic, having high iodine content, 37% iodine by weight) include transient suppression of T4 release, inhibition of deiodinase, and decrease binding of T3 to its receptor.

TABLE 1: Factors affecting LT4 absorption.				
	Drugs	Foods and beverages	Patient's condition	Timing of LT4 intake
Decrease LT4 absorption	• Calcium carbonate • Phosphate binders • Antacids • Ferrous sulfate • Cholestyramine • Colesevelam • Sucralfate • Raloxifene • PPI/H2 blockers • Orlistat	• Meals • Fiber • Soy products • Coffee • Milk	• Atrophic gastritis • Celiac disease • Lactose intolerance • Severe obesity • Bariatric surgery • Aging	Order from best to most impaired LT4 absorption are as follows: • 60 minutes BBF • Bedtime • 30 minutes BBF • With breakfast
Increase LT4 absorption	Vitamin C		Bariatric surgery	

(BBF: before breakfast; H2 blockers: histamine-2 blockers; LT4: levothyroxine sodium; PPI: proton pump inhibitors)

A change from one product to another (tablet from one brand to another brand, brand to generic tablet), significant weight change, or intervening pregnancy may also be associated with fluctuation in TSH. Different brands of LT4 tablets have different bioavailability due to different excipients (color agents and filters); hence a switch between brands is to be discouraged.

Once factors related to compliance, LT4 formulation, absorption, metabolism, and plasma protein binding (mainly with thyroid binding globulin) have been confidently ruled out in patients with fluctuating TSH, potential interferences by macro TSH or heterophile antibodies (human anti-mouse antibodies) should be sought for (especially in asymptomatic patients) by measuring TSH in a different platforms, or in serial dilution. Changing patterns of TSH receptor antibody (between neutral, blocking, and stimulating) need to be considered when there is unexpected fluctuation of serum TSH (high to suppressed) in a patient who was previously biochemically euthyroid on a stable LT4 dose. Ingestion of high doses of biotin may cause spurious low TSH values in immunometric assays that utilize a streptavidin-biotin immobilization technique.

On rare occasions, patients with autoimmune hypothyroidism have coexistent atrophic gastritis that might alter LT4 absorption. Thr92Ala polymorphism of the deiodinase also necessitates higher LT4 dosage.

Adverse Effects of LT4 Therapy

Avoidance of long-term iatrogenic thyrotoxicosis is desirable in patients treated with LT4. Iatrogenic thyrotoxicosis is particularly of concern in those above 65 years of age, and in patients with comorbidities. Overtreatment with LT4 increases the risk of atrial fibrillation, causes accelerated bone loss, particularly in the elderly. On rare occasions, patients may develop an allergy to one of the components (excipients) of the LT4 tablets. Switching the brand might be helpful in these patients.

■ TREATMENT OF SUBCLINICAL HYPOTHYROIDISM

SCH (early thyroid failure/mild hypothyroidism/preclinical hypothyroidism) is a biochemical diagnosis, defined as an elevated serum TSH in combination with serum FT4 within the population-specific reference range. The incidence of SCH varies between populations and ranges from 3 to 15% depending upon gender, age, thyroid autoimmunity, and iodine status. Due to the inverse log-linear relationship between serum TSH and FT4, a relatively small decrease in FT4 even within the reference range, can result in relatively large increase of serum TSH, putting TSH outside the reference range. The risk of progression to OH is about 2-6% per year, with highest risks in those with higher TSH elevations, positive antithyroid antibodies, and those with low-normal FT4 levels. The association of SCH with an increase risk for atherosclerotic heart disease has been shown in some studies. The impact of LT4 therapy to reduce the risk of atherosclerotic heart disease, however, is not clear. Heterophile antibodies or macro TSH, recovery phase of nonthyroidal illness (sick euthyroid syndrome), recovery phase of thyroiditis, and medication use often give rise to the biochemical picture of SCH. So, mildly elevated TSH concentrations should be confirmed after 3-6 months before treatment is initiated. It has been seen that in SCH, high TSH normalizes in about 62% individuals on subsequent remeasurement without any intervention.

Indications of LT4 Treatment for Subclinical Hypothyroidism

- Patient is symptomatic (put them on therapeutic trial. LT4 therapy may be stopped if no clinical improvement after 3–6 months normalization of TSH)
- TSH ≥10 µIU/mL
- Rising TSH on subsequent measurement
- Positive antithyroid antibodies
- Presence of goiter
- Menstrual abnormality
- Women with infertility
- Pregnant women
- Patients aged 70 years or below with cardiovascular disease or associated risk factors

Dose of LT4 in Subclinical Hypothyroidism

Due to residual thyroid function in patients with SCH, the LT dose required to normalize TSH is usually lower than in OH. A daily dose of 25–75 µg LT4 is usually sufficient, depending on the degree of TSH elevation.

Target TSH in Subclinical Hypothyroidism

Thyroid-stimulating hormone should be kept within the euthyroid reference range; patients aged 70 years or less should have their TSH between 0.5 and 2.5 µIU/mL. Target TSH in older patients is around 1–5 µIU/mL. In pregnant women, TSH should be kept at lower half of the trimester-specific range (if available) or <2.5 µIU/mL.

▍TREATMENT OF CENTRAL HYPOTHYROIDISM

CH coexists with multiple pituitary hormone deficiencies (MPHDs). The hypothyroid state is mild to moderate in most CH patients, as some TH secretion occurs by constitutive activity of the TSH receptors. In addition, manifestations can be masked by symptoms of MPHDs. The diagnosis is usually made biochemically with low serum FT4 and low/normal/inappropriately elevated TSH.

Central hypothyroidism is treated with daily administration of LT4 dose (final dose about 1.4–1.7 µg/kg). Concomitant central adrenal insufficiency must always be excluded before starting LT4 therapy, to avoid the risk of precipitating adrenal crisis. Treatment is monitored by serum FT4 which should be kept at upper half of the laboratory reference range. Measurement of serum FT4 should be done from samples collected before the morning dose of LT4. Reassessment of the dose of LT4 should be done whenever additional replacement with other pituitary hormones (recombinant human growth hormone) is started.

CONCLUSION

LT4 therapy alone is the current standard of care in patients with all forms of hypothyroidism. Decision on LT4 initiation and starting dose of LT4 depend on multiple factors. The target TSH in majority of patients with primary hypothyroidism is 0.5–2.5 µIU/mL; however, it must be individualized. Those with central hypothyroidism should be followed up with FT4 and not with TSH. Patients having coexistent adrenal insufficiency should be prescribed glucocorticoids before initiating LT4. A significant number of LT4-treated patients are either undertreated or overtreated. Maintaining TSH value within the target range is challenging in some patients. Out of range TSH values in such patients may be due to multiple factors starting from noncompliance to concurrent medications, changing antibody pattern or assay-specific interferences.

SUGGESTED READINGS

1. Melmed S, Auchus RJ, Goldfine AB, et al. (Eds). Williams Textbook of Endocrinology, 14th edition. Philadelphia, PA: Elsevier; 2020.
2. Braverman LE, Cooper DS, Koop PA (Eds). Werner & Ingbar's The Thyroid, 11th edition. Wolters Kluwer; 2020.
3. Sperling MA (Ed). Pediatric Endocrinology, 5th edition.
4. Peeters RP. Subclinical hypothyroidism. N Engl J Med. 2017;377(14):1404.

CHAPTER 33

Subclinical Hypothyroidism

AK Gupta, Ajit Singh Chahar, Ashutosh Kumar

▪ INTRODUCTION

Subclinical hypothyroidism (SCH) is defined as a state of increased thyroid-stimulating hormone (TSH) levels with circulating thyroxine (T4) and triiodothyronine (T3) concentration within the normal range.

The word SCH appears to be misnomer by endocrinologists. Subclinical word is right in those circumstances where there is no clinical symptoms or sign and the values are detected on routine investigations. However at times, the thyroid profile is done on some clinical suspicion and increased TSH with normal T3 and T4 values are found. Since the investigation was advised on some clinical ground, the word subclinical seems unjustified.

Yet conventionally increased TSH with normal T3 and T4 comes in the category of SCH and here we will discuss the same.

Subclinical hypothyroidism is akin to impaired glucose tolerance in many ways. Though diagnosis on biochemical basis is well defined yet the initiation of treatment is uncertain. Certain group of persons stress for starting the therapy, while others opine that they should be watched and followed periodically.

▪ EPIDEMIOLOGY

In population-based studies, the prevalence of SCH ranges from 4 to 15%. The prevalence rises with age and is higher in females than males.

▪ ETIOLOGY

The causes of SCH are the same as of overt hypothyroidism.

Most patient have chronic autoimmune (Hashimoto's) thyroiditis with high serum concentrations of anti-thyroid peroxidase (anti-TPO, formerly called antithyroid microsomal) antibodies. Other major causes include prior ablative or antithyroid drug therapy for hyperthyroidism caused by Graves' disease;

prior partial thyroidectomy; external radiation therapy in patients with Hodgkin lymphoma, leukemia, or brain tumors; inadequate T4 (levothyroxine) replacement therapy for overt hypothyroidism; and drugs impairing thyroid function.

CLINICAL FINDINGS

Most patients with SCH have serum TSH level <10 mU/L and are asymptomatic. However, some of them on questioning explain vague complaints mainly drier skin, poorer memory, slower thinking, greater tiredness, and more constipation.

Some older patients also have vague similar complaints but on investigations are found euthyroid. Most of the times attempts to identify patients clinically have not been successful.

DIAGNOSIS

The diagnosis of SCH is based upon biochemical testing alone.
Subclinical hypothyroidism is defined as:
- Normal serum free T4
- Elevated TSH

It may occur in the presence or absence of mild symptoms of hypothyroidism.

In most circumstances, the initial screening test for thyroid disease is the serum TSH. If the serum TSH concentration is elevated, the TSH measurement should be repeated along with a serum free T4 before making the diagnosis of SCH. Because the serum TSH concentration can be transiently elevated, a serum TSH measurement should be repeated preferably after 2–3 months interval to confirm the diagnosis.

PREGNANCY AND SUBCLINICAL HYPOTHYROIDISM

If we understand little physiology of pregnancy, it will be easier to understand the values of TSH during pregnancy. In pregnancy, thyroid-binding globulin is raised (↑TBG) and therefore total T3 and T4 values go up but free T3 and T4 values are normal. Secondly, human chorionic gonadotropin (hCG) values are rising in the pregnancy. hCG has got a thyroid-stimulating effect like TSH, therefore T3 and T4 values are raised and consequently TSH levels falls (many time this gives false impression of hyperthyroidism). Therefore, by ↑TBG and ↑hCG, TSH values are affected, which dip down from normal. Hence, normal values of TSH in pregnancy are taken as:
- *First trimester*: 1–2.5 mU/L
- *Second trimester*: 2–3 mU/L
- *Third trimester*: 3–3 mU/L

Therefore TSH values above this level with normal T4 values will fall under SCH during pregnancy.

For nonpregnant adults, an elevated serum TSH is defined as a TSH concentration above the upper limit of the normal TSH reference range, which is typically 4–5 mU/L in most laboratories. These is considerable controversy over the appropriate upper limit of normal serum TSH. Some experts have suggested that the true upper limit is only 2.5 or 3 mU/L in healthy individuals without thyroid disease, while other argue that the serum TSH distribution shifts toward higher values with age, independent of the presence of antithyroid antibodies. In this case, the upper limit of normal could be as high as 6–8 mU/L in healthy octogenarians (80-89 years age).

Therefore, the TSH values with advancing age increases and it must be kept in mind while diagnosing and treating hypothyroidism.

For women trying to conceive who have ovulatory dysfunction or infertility, elevations in TSH can be defined using first trimester—specific TSH reference range (0.1–2.5 mU/L).

DIFFERENTIAL DIAGNOSIS

There are several causes of a high serum TSH concentration that do not properly fit in the definition of SCH. These include the following circumstances:
- During the period of recovery from nonthyroidal illness, where a transiently elevated serum TSH is seen after a period of TSH suppression.
- In viral and postpartum thyroiditis, there is initial thyrotoxic phase due to release of thyroxin from thyroid gland which lasts for 2–6 weeks. Following this the sick thyroid secrets less thyroxine and consequently TSH is raised—making hypothyroid phase for 2–6 months. In this phase, many times only TSH is raised and T3 and T4 is normal making the diagnosis of SCH.
- Assay variability
- Rheumatoid factors may cause similar interference in immunometric assays
- Untreated adrenal insufficiency
- Morbid obesity, where high TSH is mediated centrally by leptin and TSH falls with weight loss (e.g., after bariatric surgery).

IDENTIFYING THE CAUSE

Most patients with SCH have chronic autoimmune (Hashimoto's) thyroiditis. However, we do not routinely measure anti-TPO antibodies in patients with SCH unless the decision to treat or to monitor is not obvious, in which case the presence of antibodies may be useful in making management decisions.

CONSEQUENCES OF SUBCLINICAL HYPOTHYROIDISM

Progression to overt hypothyroidism—a substantial proportion of patients with SCH eventually develop overt hypothyroidism. In prospective studies with nearly 10–20 years of follow-up, the cumulative incidence of overt hypothyroidism ranges from 33 to 55%. The annual rate of progression to overt hypothyroidism ranges from 2 to 5%.

Spontaneous recovery has also been described in patients with SCH, although the frequency of this phenomenon is unclear. In a study of 422, 242 persons without known thyroid disease, serum TSH was elevated (5.5 to ≤10 mU/L) in 3%. During the 5 year follow-up period, TSH levels became normal without treatment in 62% of patients. Normalization of serum TSH concentrations is more likely to occur in patients with negative antithyroid antibodies, serum TSH levels <10 mU/L, and within the first 2 years after diagnosis.

CORONARY HEART DISEASE

Some but not all observational studies report an increased risk of coronary heart disease (CHD) in subjects with SCH. A meta-analysis of patients-level data from seven prospective cohort studies (25,977 participants, 2,020 with SCH) showed a significant trend of increased risk of CHD events (nonfatal myocardial infarction, CHD death, and hospitalization for acute coronary syndrome) at higher serum TSH concentrations. Compared with euthyroid individuals, patients with TSH ≥ 10 mU/L had a significant increase in CHD events (38.4 vs. 20.3 events per 1,000 person-years). In contrast, minimal TSH elevations (4.5–6.9 mU/L) were not associated with an increased risk. The risk estimates did not differ according to age, gender, or presence of preexisting cardiovascular disease (CVD). In a separate meta-analysis, risk estimates did not differ by TPO antibodies status.

HEART FAILURE

In a pooled analysis of patient-level data from six prospective cohort studies (25,390 participants, 2,068 with SCH), there was a significant trend for increased risk of heart failure events at higher TSH concentrations. Compared with euthyroid controls, patients with a TSH between 10 and 19.9 mU/L had a significant increase in heart failure [40 events in 224 participants (17.9%) vs. 1,762 events in 22,674 controls (7.8%)]. The increased risk of heart failure in those with a serum TSH between 7.0 and 9.9 mU/L was not statistically significant (54 events in 422 participants (12.8%); and minimal TSH elevations (4.5–6.9 mU/L) were not associated with an increased risk.

STROKE

Overall, there does not appear to be an association between SCH and risk of stroke. However, in predefined subgroup analysis, there was an increased risk of stroke events in patients 18–49 years of age and an increased risk of fatal stoke in patients 18–49 years and 50–64 years. There was no increased risk for those 65–79 years or ≥80 years. There was a nonsignificant pattern of increased risk of fatal stroke with higher TSH concentrations.

LIPIDS

Some, but not all, studies show an association between elevated TSH and total and low-density lipoprotein (LDL) and cholesterol concentrations. In one of the largest cross-sectional studies to date (25,862 participants, median age 56 years), patients with modest elevations of serum TSH (between 5.1 and 10 mU/L) had significantly higher mean total cholesterol concentrations than those who were euthyroid (223 vs. 216 mg/dL).

In addition, SCH has been associated with an increase in a number of other cardiovascular risk factors and CHD, including markers of inflammation, vascular reactivity, endothelial function, and carotid intima-media thickness. Some patients with SCH also have diastolic dysfunction and increased peripheral vascular resistance, as noted in patients with overt hypothyroidism.

REPRODUCTIVE ABNORMALITIES

In one study that evaluated the prevalence of SCH among 244 women with infertility (approximately half of whom had ovulatory dysfunction), SCH was diagnosed in 13.9%, compared with 3.9% of control women (healthy women with confirmed fertility). Whether women with preconception SCH [TSH levels above the usual normal range (e.g., >5 mU/L)] have decreased fertility remains uncertain.

In some studies (but not all) women with SCH were reported to be at increased risk for severe preeclampsia, preterm delivery, placental abruption, and pregnancy loss compared with euthyroid women.

Assessment of antibody status is important because women with SCH and positive anti-TPO antibodies tend to have the higher risk of adverse pregnancy outcomes, and adverse outcomes occur at a lower TSH than in women without TPO antibodies. In the American Thyroid Association (ATA) systematic review (ATA guidelines on thyroid disease during pregnancy), the risk of pregnancy-specific complications was apparent in TPO-positive women with TSH >2.5 mU/L but was not consistently apparent in TPO-negative women until TSH values exceeded 5–10 mU/L.

COGNITIVE IMPAIRMENT

It is uncertain if the children of women with SCH are at risk for neuropsychological impairment. Observational studies suggest an association between SCH in pregnancy and impaired cognitive development in children.

OBESITY AND DIABETES MELLITUS

Experimentally induced acute weight gain has significant effects on T4 to T3 conversion. A recent review of cohort studies of obese subjects suggests that serum TSH concentrations positively correlate with weight. Two longitudinal studies are particular importance in supporting a significant positive association between increase in TSH levels and change in body mass index (BMI). One of these studies that stringently corrected for age, smoking habits, and menopausal status indicated that for every unit increase in log TSH, there was 2.3 kg greater weight in females and 1.1 kg in men. Conversely, substantial weight loss appears to be associated with a decrease in TSH levels as shown in several studies in children and adolescents, and also in adults following bariatric procedures such as gastric banding or gastric bypass surgery. Currently there have been no randomized trials of the impact of L-thyroxine therapy in patients with obesity-related elevation of TSH serum levels. However, as observational studies are consistent in showing that TSH levels revert to normal upon weight reduction.

The prevalence of overt thyroid dysfunction in patients with type 1 diabetes mellitus (T1DM) is around 10% and manifestations such as SCH and raised serum thyroid autoantibody concentrations are found in up to 30% of females. This leads to the widespread recommendation that thyroid function should be monitored on a yearly basis in patients with T1DM. If autoimmune Addison's disease is present, the risk of subclinical or overt hypothyroidism is as high as 50% and this combination of disorders frequently co-exists with T1DM (known as the autoimmune polyglandular syndrome type 2). However, in the presence of untreated or inadequately replaced insufficiency, there is frequently an elevation in serum TSH, and judgment about the possibility of SCH should be delayed by at least 4 weeks from the institution of adequate steroid replacement in such patients.

Hypothyroidism is associated with a significant decrease in insulin sensitivity, most likely owing to a combination of effects including those on down regulation of plasma membrane glucose transporters and also direct effects on insulin secretion and clearance. Therefore, overt hypothyroidism is, and by extension SCH may, be associated with insulin resistance and components of the metabolic syndrome.

LIVER AND GALLBLADDER

In a cross-sectional study, nonalcoholic fatty liver disease (NAFLD) was correlated with serum TSH levels. 30 and 36% of individuals with subclinical or overt hypothyroidism, respectively, had typical ultrasonographic findings of NAFLD (vs. 20% of controls), while 20 and 26% of individuals with subclinical or overt hypothyroidism had abnormal liver enzymes.

In one study, patients with SCH were more likely to have common bile duct stones, thought to be secondary to sphincter of Oddi dysfunction.

NEUROPSYCHIATRIC SYMPTOMS

Several reports suggest that SCH is associated with neuropsychiatric diseases. However, other studies (including a large study of primary care patients in England that failed to demonstrate an association of SCH with depression, anxiety, or cognitive dysfunction) do not support this observation.

POTENTIAL CONSEQUENCES

In middle-aged adults, increasing serum TSH concentrations within the normal range or slightly above normal were associated with a modest increase in body weight. In older women (>65 years), SCH (mean TSH 6.7 mU/L) compared with euthyroidism (TSH 2.2 mU/L) was associated with a slightly higher baseline weight. There was no relationship between TSH and weight in older men.

In one study, 21 of 33 patients (64%) with SCH had a higher frequency of neuromuscular symptoms (weakness, fatigue, paresthesias, and cramps), as compared with 6 of 44 normal subjects (14%). SCH may also be associated with defects in verbal memory and executive functioning. These defects correct with T4 therapy and are thought to reflect abnormal hippocampal function rather than general cognitive slowing. In a population-based study, SCH was associated with an increased risk of Alzheimer disease in women but not in men.

EFFECT OF THYROID HORMONE REPLACEMENT

Based upon the natural history alone, most experts and all professional groups recommend that treatment should be started to prevent progression to overt hypothyroidism in patients with serum TSH values ≥10 mU/L.

The treatment of patients with TSH values between 4.5 and 10 mU/L remains controversial. The results of the meta-analyses and subsequent trials, in which most patients had TSH <10 mU/L, suggest that treatment of SCH with T4 does not result in clinically significant improvement in quality of life, depression, and cognitive function.

In patients with SCH and goiter, T4 treatment may decrease the size of the goiter.

CARDIOVASCULAR DISEASE

Although T4 replacement has been shown to improve a number of cardiovascular risk factors and surrogate cardiovascular endpoints in patients with SCH, including dyslipidemia, markers of inflammation, vascular smooth muscle proliferation, vascular reactivity, ventricular function, endothelial function, and carotid intima media thickness, data demonstrating its ability to decrease cardiovascular events are limited.

Those under age 65 years who were treated with T4 had reduced overall mortality compared with those who were not treated. For patients over age 65 years, there was no difference in overall mortality between treated and untreated patients.

In several randomized trials of patients with SCH treated with T4 versus placebo, serum total and LDL cholesterol and apolipoprotein B-100 concentrations decreased significantly, whereas serum high-density lipoprotein (HDL) cholesterol, triglyceride, and lipoprotein(a) concentrations did not change.

FERTILITY

There are few data showing improved fertility outcomes in women with SCH treated with thyroid hormone. In observational studies of women with infertility and SCH, 44–84% of women treated with T4 successfully conceived during treatment.
- In a study of 113 patients with chronic kidney disease and SCH, progression of renal failure was attenuated by treatment with T4.
- Patients with coexisting iron-deficiency anemia and SCH had a greater increase in hemoglobin when given both iron and thyroid hormone replacement when compared with those given iron alone.

MANAGEMENT

Thyroid hormone should not be prescribed for patients with hypothyroid symptoms but normal thyroid function.

Candidates for T4 Replacement

Although virtually all experts recommend treatment of patients with serum TSH concentrations >10 mU/L, the routine treatment of asymptomatic patients with TSH values between 4.5 and 10 mU/L remains controversial.
- *TSH ≥ 10 mU/L*: In view of data linking SCH with atherosclerosis and myocardial infarction and the increased risk of progression to overt hypothyroidism, we suggest treatment of patients with SCH and TSH levels ≥10 mU/L.

This recommendation is consistent with that of a clinical consensus group comprised of representatives from the ATA and the American Association of Clinical Endocrinologists (AACE), and with the European Thyroid Association guidelines.
- *TSH 7–9.9 mU/L*: In view of the report of increased cardiovascular mortality in younger individuals with TSH in this range, we treat most patients under age 65–70 years with TSH 7.0 or higher. However, due to the absence of treatment trials showing a benefit of treating older patients, the absence of a benefit of treatment in older patients in the analyses of large databases and the concern that older patients may have complications from unintended overtreatment, we consider treatment only in those older patients (i.e., those age > 65–70 years) who have convincing symptoms suggestive of hypothyroidism.
- *TSH above upper limit of normal to 6.9 mU/L*: We suggest T4 therapy in patients <65–70 years who have convincing symptoms suggestive of hypothyroidism and who have serum TSH values above the upper limit of normal to 6.9 mU/L. Patients with high titers of anti-TPO antibodies, who may rapidly progress to overt hypothyroidism, and patients with goiter may also benefit from early treatment.

We suggest not treating older patients (>65–70 years) with SCH and TSH above the upper limit of normal to 6.9 mU/L, since TSH values in this range are age appropriate, and we prefer to avoid treatment of patients over age 80 years.

Infertility or Attempting Pregnancy

We suggest initiating T4 replacement in women with SCH who are trying to conceive and who have ovulatory dysfunction or infertility.

Arguments for Treatment

Treatment will prevent progression to overt hypothyroidism, especially in those with serum TSH concentrations >10 mU/L and high serum anti-TPO antibody concentrations.

Arguments against Treatment

Arguments against T4 treatment include its cost (for both the hormone and for monitoring its efficacy), the lifelong commitment to daily medication in asymptomatic patients, the potential risk of overtreatment and inducing symptoms from excess thyroid hormone, and the possible induction or exacerbation of angina pectoris or cardiac arrhythmia in susceptible patients. We do recommend a higher TSH threshold for treating older patients.

Dosing and Monitoring

There are two approaches to initiate T4 therapy:
1. One option is to start with the lowest dose necessary to normalize the serum TSH concentration, typically 25–50 μg daily. This approach will avoid overtreatment and is most appropriate in older adults or in patients with underlying CVD.

2. An alternative approach for younger patients with Hashimoto's thyroiditis who do not have autonomy (e.g., a prior history of toxic adenoma or Graves' disease treated with radioiodine) and who have normal negative feedback is to initiate treatment at slightly below full replacement doses (1.6 µg/kg/day). This approach obviates the need for periodic dose increases, should there be progressive autoimmune destruction of their gland. Alternatively, younger patients could be started on low-dose therapy, as is recommended for older patients.

The goal of therapy is to reduce the patient's serum TSH concentration into the normal reference range. Since the mean serum TSH for the general population is around 1.4 mU/L, with 90% having serum TSH levels <3.0 mU/L, many experts recommend a therapeutic TSH target of 0.5–2.5 mU/L in young and middle-aged patients.

In patients aged ≥ 65–70 years who are treated, whether with initial serum TSH levels > 10 mU/L or between 7 and 9.9 mU/L, a target serum TSH of 3–6 mU/L, consistent with the normal age-related increase in serum TSH, is appropriate.

Serum TSH should be evaluated 6 weeks after initiation of therapy, and if the target TSH has not been reached, the dose of thyroxin should be increased by 12.5–25 µg/day. If the serum TSH is too low, the thyroxin should be decreased by the same amount. Once the correct dose has been achieved, serum TSH levels can be assessed annually.

In addition, if there was hypercholesterolemia or other dyslipidemia before L-thyroxine was commenced, then it is worthwhile to recheck the serum lipid profile to see whether there has been adequate improvement, or whether additional therapy for dyslipidemia is necessary. At this stage, it is also worthwhile to re-evaluate the symptoms of hypothyroidism in those SCH individuals who were started on therapy for symptoms suggestive of hypothyroidism. Although most studies suggest little or no symptomatic benefit from treatment of SCH. If symptoms have improved, then lifelong treatment may be considered. If there has been no improvement in symptoms, or even some side effects perceived from the medication, then L-thyroxine may be stopped after a 3–6-month therapeutic trial.

When to Take Thyroxin

For optimal absorption, L-thyroxine should be taken on an empty stomach. Studies show different results with regard to the optimal time for its administration. One study of US patients showed optimal serum TSH control when L-thyroxine was taken in the fasting state, 60 minutes before breakfast. However, a Dutch study showed that L-thyroxine taken at bedtime was superior to that taken 30 minutes before breakfast. Several foods specifically impair L-thyroxine absorption, including milk (due to the calcium content), coffee, soya products, and papaya. Indeed, many medications including iron salt, calcium salt, and antacids (including sucralfate, H2-receptor blockers, and proton pump inhibitors) also hamper absorption.

■ FOLLOW-UP OF UNTREATED PATIENTS

A proportion of patients with SCH will progress to overt hypothyroidism, 2–5% per year depending on the degree of serum TSH elevation. On the other hand, thyroid function may normalize in 6–35% of SCH patients depending on initial TSH levels, thyroid autoantibody status and length and frequency of follow-up. Hence, in the majority, SCH remains stable.

Once SCH has been diagnosed then a repeat thyroid function test should be rechecked within 8–12 weeks along with thyroid auto antibodies. If thyroid function has normalized, then no further testing is required in those who are asymptomatic, have negative thyroid auto antibodies or do not have goiter. In those who have persistent SCH, thyroid function should be tested 6 monthly at least for the first 2 year and then yearly thereafter. This is to follow the tendency to progression and to detect consequent overt hypothyroidism.

CONCLUSION

- SCH is defined biochemically as a normal serum free T4 concentration in the presence of an elevated serum TSH concentration. SCH may occur in the presence or absence of mild symptoms of hypothyroidism.
- For nonpregnant adults, an elevated serum TSH is defined as a TSH concentration above the upper limit of the normal TSH reference range, which is typically 4–5 mU/L in most laboratories.
- For pregnant women, elevations in TSH should be defined using population and trimester-specific TSH reference ranges. For women trying to conceive who have ovulatory dysfunction or infertility, elevations in TSH can be defined using first trimester-specific TSH reference ranges (0.1–2.5 mU/L).
- A substantial proportion of patients with SCH eventually develop overt hypothyroidism.
- The annual rate of conversion into overt hypothyroidism is 2–5% annually.
- SCH may be associated with an increased risk of CVD (e.g., coronary artery and heart failure), particularly when the serum TSH concentration is above 10 mU/L.
- For patients with SCH and TSH concentrations ≥10 mU/L, we suggest treatment with thyroid hormone [T4 (levothyroxine)].
- For patients with TSH of 7.0–9.9 mU/L who are <65–70 years, we also suggest treatment with thyroid hormone. However, for patients >65–70 years, we suggest treatment only if they have convincing symptoms of hypothyroidism.
- For patients with TSH above the upper limit of normal to 6.9 mU/L, we suggest treatment in patients <65–70 years who have symptoms of hypothyroidism. Treatment with T4 can also be considered in such patients with TSH above the upper limit of normal to 6.9 mU/L who have high titers of TPO antibodies, which predict progression to overt hypothyroidism or goiter.
- For older patients (>65–70 years) with SCH and TSH above the upper limit of normal to 6.9 mU/L, we suggest not treating in view of the uncertain benefits and the potential for both cardiovascular and skeletal morbidity associated with inadvertent overtreatment.
- For women with SCH (TSH values above first trimester-specific normal reference range with normal free T4) who are trying to conceive and who have ovulatory dysfunction or infertility, we suggest initiating T4 replacement.

- Synthetic T4 is the treatment of choice for correction of hypothyroidism. For older patients and those with underlying CVD, the initial dose of T4 is typically 25–50 µg/day. This approach will avoid overtreatment. For younger patients without a history of thyroid autonomy, an alternative approach is to initiate treatment at slightly below full replacement doses (1.6 µg/kg/day).
- For younger patients, the goal of therapy is to reduce the patient's serum TSH concentration into the lower half of the age-adjusted normal reference range.
- For patients aged >65–70 years who are treated, whether with initial serum TSH levels >10 mU/L or 7–9.9 mU/L, the goal of therapy is a serum TSH of 3–6 mU/L, consistent with the normal age-related increase in serum TSH.
- If there is no improvement in symptoms or any parameters and if some side effects perceived from medication then thyroxine may be stopped after 3–6 months therapeutic trial.

SUGGESTED READINGS

1. Bemben DA, Hamm RM, Morgan L, et al. Thyroid disease in the elderly. Part 2. Predictability of subclinical hypothyroidism. J Fam Pract. 1994;38:583-8.
2. Tunbridge WM, Evered DC, Hall R, et al. The spectrum of thyroid disease in a community: the Whickham survey. Clin Endocrinol (Oxf). 1977;7:481-93.
3. Biondi B, Cooper DS. The clinical significance of subclinical thyroid dysfunction. Endocr Rev. 2008;29:76-131.
4. Canaris GJ, Manowitz NR, Mayor G, et al. The Colorado thyroid disease prevalence study. Arch Intern Med. 2000;160:526-34.
5. Cooper DS, Biondi B. Subclinical thyroid disease. Lancet. 2012;379:1142-54.
6. Despres N, Grant AM. Antibody interference in thyroid assays: a potential for clinical misinformation. Clin Chem. 1998;44:440-54.
7. Moulin de Moraes CM, Mancini MC, de Melo ME, et al. Prevalence of subclinical hypothyroidism in a morbidly obese population and improvement after weight loss induced by Roux-en-Y gastric bypass. Obes Surg. 2005;15:1287-91.
8. Huber G, Staub JJ, Meier C, et al. Prospective study of the spontaneous course of subclinical hypothyroidism: prognostic value of thyrotropin, thyroid reserve, and thyroid antibodies. J Clin Endocrinol Metab. 2002;87:3221-6.
9. Kabadi UM. 'Subclinical hypothyroidism'. Natural course of the syndrome during a prolonged follow-up study. Arch Intern Med. 1993;153:957-61.
10. Meyerovitch J, Rotman-Pikielny P, Sherf M, et al. Serum thyrotropin measurements in the community: five-year follow-up in a large network of primary care physicians. Arch Intern Med. 2007;167:1533-8.
11. Díez JJ, Iglesias P, Burman KD. Spontaneous normalization of thyrotropin concentrations in patients with subclinical hypothyroidism. J Clin Endocrinol Metab. 2005;90:4124-7.
12. Imaizumi M, Akahoshi M, Ichimaru S, et al. Risk for ischemic heart disease and all-cause mortality in subclinical hypothyroidism. J Clin Endocrinol Metab. 2004; 89:3365-70.
13. Walsh JP, Bremner AP, Bulsara MK, et al. Subclinical thyroid dysfunction as a risk factor for cardiovascular disease. Arch Intern Med. 2005;165:2467-72.
14. Rodondi N, Newman AB, Vittinghoff E, et al. Subclinical hypothyroidism and the risk of heart failure, other cardiovascular events, and death. Arch Intern Med. 2005; 165:2460-6.
15. Hyland KA, Arnold AM, Lee JS, et al. Persistent subclinical hypothyroidism and cardiovascular risk in the elderly: the cardiovascular health study. J Clin Endocrinol Metab. 2013;98:533-40.
16. Rodondi N, den Elzen WP, Bauer DC, et al. Subclinical hypothyroidism and the risk of coronary heart disease and mortality. JAMA. 2010;304:1365-74.

17. Collet TH, Bauer DC, Cappola AR, et al. Thyroid antibody status, subclinical hypothyroidism, and the risk of coronary heart disease: an individual participant data analysis. J Clin Endocrinol Metab. 2014;99:3353-62.
18. Gencer B, Collet TH, Virgini V, et al. Subclinical thyroid dysfunction and the risk of heart failure events: an individual participant data analysis from 6 prospective cohorts. Circulation. 2012;126:1040-9.
19. Chaker L, Baumgartner C, Ikram MA, et al. Subclinical thyroid dysfunction and the risk of stroke: a systematic review and meta-analysis. Eur J Epidemiol. 2014;29:791-800.
20. Canaris GJ, Manowitz NR, Mayor G, et al. The Colorado thyroid disease prevalence study. Arch Intern Med. 2000;160:526-34.
21. Monzani F, Caraccio N, Kozàkowà M, et al. Effect of levothyroxine replacement on lipid profile and intima-media thickness in subclinical hypothyroidism: a double-blind, placebo- controlled study. J Clin Endocrinol Metab. 2004;89:2099-106.
22. Cikim AS, Oflaz H, Ozbey N, et al. Evaluation of endothelial function in subclinical hypothyroidism and subclinical hyperthyroidism. Thyroid. 2004;14:605-9.
23. Abalovich M, Mitelberg L, Allami C, et al. Subclinical hypothyroidism and thyroid autoimmunity in women with infertility. Gynecol Endocrinol. 2007;23:279-83.
24. Danforth E Jr, Horton ES, O'Connell M, et al. Dietary-induced alterations in thyroid hor-mone metabolism during overnutrition. J Clin Invest. 1979;64:1336-47.
25. De Moura Souza A, Sichieri R. Association between serum TSH concentration within the normal range and adiposity. Eur J Endocrinol. 2011;165:11-5.
26. Kitahara CM, Platz EA, Ladenson PW, et al. Body fatness and markers of thyroid function among US men and women. PLoS One. 2012;7:e34979.
27. Nyrnes A, Jorde R, Sundsfjord J. Serum TSH is positively associated with BMI. Int J Obes (Lond). 2006;30:100-5.
28. Fox CS, Pencina MJ, D'Agostino RB, et al. Relations of thyroid function to body weight: cross-sectional and longitudinal observations in a community-based sample. Arch Intern Med. 2008;168:587-92.
29. Wolters B, Lass N, Reinehr T. TSH and free triiodothyronine concentrations are associated with weight loss in a lifestyle intervention and weight regain afterwards in obese children. Eur J Endocrinol. 2013;168:323-9.
30. Chikunguwo S, Brethauer S, Nirujogi V, et al. Influence of obesity and surgical weight loss on thyroid hormone levels. Surg Obes Relat Dis. 2007;3:631-5.
31. Kadiyala R, Peter R, Okosieme OE. Thyroid dysfunction in patients with diabetes: clinical implications and screening strategies. Int J Clin Pract. 2010;64:1130-9.
32. Boelaert K, Newby PR, Simmonds MJ, et al. Prevalence and relative risk of other autoimmune diseases in subjects with autoimmune thyroid disease. Am J Med. 2010;123:183.e1-9.
33. Perros P, McCrimmon RJ, Shaw G, et al. Frequency of thyroid dysfunction in diabetic patients: value of annual screening. Diabet Med. 1995;12:622-7.
34. Kahaly GJ. Polyglandular autoimmune syndrome type 2. Presse Med. 2012;41:e663-70.
35. Napier C, Pearce SH. Autoimmune Addison's disease. Presse Med. 2012;41:e626-35.
36. Stryker TD, Molitch ME. Reversible hyperthyrotropinemia, hyperthyroxinemia, and hyperprolacti-nemia due to adrenal insufficiency. Am J Med. 1985;79:271-6.
37. Dimitriadis G, Mitrou P, Lambadiari V, et al. Insulin action in adipose tissue and muscle in hypothyroidism. J Clin Endocrinol Metab. 2006;91:4930-7.
38. Roos A, Bakker SJ, Links TP, et al. Thyroid function is associated with components of the metabolic syndrome in euthyroid subjects. J Clin Endocrinol Metab. 2007;92:491-6.
39. Chung GE, Kim D, Kim W, et al. Non-alcoholic fatty liver disease across the spectrum of hypothyroidism. J Hepatol. 2012;57:150-6.
40. Laukkarinen J, Kiudelis G, Lempinen M, et al. Increased prevalence of subclinical hypothyroidism in common bile duct stone patients. J Clin Endocrinol Metab. 2007;92:4260-4.

41. Laukkarinen J, Sand J, Nordback I. The underlying mechanisms: how hypothyroidism affects the formation of common bile duct stones-a review. HPB Surg. 2012; 2012:102825.
42. Baldini IM, Vita A, Mauri MC, et al. Psychopathological and cognitive features in subclinical hypothyroidism. Prog Neuropsychopharmacol Biol Psychiatry. 1997; 21:925-35.
43. Tappy L, Randin JP, Schwed P, et al. Prevalence of thyroid disorders in psychogeriatric inpatients. A possible relationship of hypothyroidism with neurotic depression but not with dementia. J Am Geriatr Soc. 1987;35:526-31.
44. Haggerty JJ Jr, Stern RA, Mason GA, et al. Subclinical hypothyroidism: a modifiable risk factor for depression? Am J Psychiatry. 1993;150:508-10.
45. Engum A, Bjøro T, Mykletun A, et al. An association between depression, anxiety and thyroid function—a clinical fact or an artefact? Acta Psychiatr Scand. 2002;106:27-34.
46. Jorde R, Waterloo K, Storhaug H, et al. Neuropsychological function and symptoms in subjects with subclinical hypothyroidism and the effect of thyroxine treatment. J Clin Endocrinol Metab. 2006;91:145-53.
47. Pasqualetti G, Pagano G, Rengo G, et al. Subclinical Hypothyroidism and Cognitive Impairment: Systematic Review and Meta-Analysis. J Clin Endocrinol Metab. 2015;100:4240-8.
48. Monzani F, Caraccio N, Del Guerra P, et al. Neuromuscular symptoms and dysfunction in subclinical hypothyroid patients: beneficial effect of L-T4 replacement therapy. Clin Endocrinol (Oxf). 1999;51:237-42.
49. Samuels MH, Schuff KG, Carlson NE, et al. Health status, mood, and cognition in experimentally induced subclinical hypothyroidism. J Clin Endocrinol Metab. 2007;92:2545-51.
50. Correia N, Mullally S, Cooke G, et al. Evidence for a specific defect in hippocampal memory in overt and subclinical hypothyroidism. J Clin Endocrinol Metab. 2009; 94:3789-97.
51. Tan ZS, Beiser A, Vasan RS, et al. Thyroid function and the risk of Alzheimer disease: the Framingham Study. Arch Intern Med. 2008;168:1514-20.
52. Meier C, Staub JJ, Roth CB, et al. TSH-controlled L-thyroxine therapy reduces cholesterol levels and clinical symptoms in subclinical hypothyroidism: A double blind, placebo-controlled trial (Basel Thyroid Study). J Clin Endocrinol Metab. 2001;86:4860-6.
53. Razvi S, Ingoe L, Keeka G, et al. The beneficial effect of L-thyroxine on cardiovascular risk factors, endothelial function, and quality of life in subclinical hypothyroidism: randomized, crossover trial. J Clin Endocrinol Metab. 2007;92:1715-23.
54. Iqbal A, Jorde R, Figenschau Y. Serum lipid levels in relation to serum thyroid-stimulating hormone and the effect of thyroxine treatment on serum lipid levels in subjects with subclinical hypothyroidism: the Tromsø Study. J Intern Med. 2006;260:53-61.
55. Shin DH, Lee MJ, Lee HS, et al. Thyroid hormone replacement therapy attenuates the decline of renal function in chronic kidney disease patients with subclinical hypothyroidism. Thyroid. 2013;23:654-61.
56. Cinemre H, Bilir C, Gokosmanoglu F, et al. Hematologic effects of levothyroxine in iron-deficient subclinical hypothyroid patients: a randomized, double-blind, controlled study. J Clin Endocrinol Metab. 2009;94:151-6.
57. Garber JR, Cobin RH, Gharib H, et al. Clinical practice guidelines for hypothyroidism in adults: cosponsored by the American Association of Clinical Endocrinologists and the American Thyroid Association. Thyroid. 2012;22:1200-35.
58. Pearce SH, Brabant G, Duntas LH, et al. 2013 ETA Guideline: Management of Subclinical Hypothyroidism. Eur Thyroid J. 2013;2:215-28.
59. Razvi S, Weaver JU, Butler TJ, et al. Levothyroxine treatment of subclinical hypothyroidism, fatal and nonfatal cardiovascular events, and mortality. Arch Intern Med. 2012;172:811-7.
60. Andersen MN, Olsen AM, Madsen JC, et al. Levothyroxine Substitution in Patients with Subclinical Hypothyroidism and the Risk of Myocardial Infarction and Mortality. PLoS One. 2015;10:e0129793.
61. Jaeschke R, Guyatt G, Gerstein H, et al. Does treatment with L-thyroxine influence health status in middle-aged and older adults with subclinical hypothyroidism? J Gen Intern Med. 1996;11:744-9.

62. Bach-Huynh TG, Nayak B, Loh J, et al. Timing of levothyroxine administration affects serum thyrotropin concentration. J Clin Endocrinol Metab. 2009;94:3905-12.
63. Bolk N, Visser TJ, Nijman J, et al. Effects of evening vs. morning levothyroxine intake: a randomized double-blind crossover trial. Arch Intern Med. 2010;170:1996-2003.
64. Benvenga S, Bartolone L, Pappalardo MA, et al. Altered intestinal absorption of L-thyroxine caused by coffee. Thyroid. 2008;18:293-301.
65. Surks MI, Ortiz E, Daniels GH, et al. Subclinical thyroid disease: scientific review and guidelines for diagnosis and management. JAMA. 2004;29:228-38.
66. Karmisholt J, Andersen S, Laurberg P. Variation in thyroid function in subclinical hypothyroidism: importance of clinical follow-up and therapy. Eur J Endocrinol. 2011;164:317-23.

CHAPTER 34

Physical Activity and Exercise Plan in a Patient with Type 2 Diabetes Mellitus

Sirshendu Pal

■ INTRODUCTION

Physical activity involves any movement that enhances use of energy, while exercise is planned structured activity. The blood glucose level in type 2 diabetes mellitus (T2DM) is improved and it also helps in weight reduction. Physical activity can also prevent falls and improves memory in older adults and helps one to sleep better.

Naresh (pseudonym), aged 65 years, having weight 80 kg and body mass index (BMI) 30 kg/m² attended our Diabetes Wellness Clinic (pseudonym). He was also suffering from T2DM with hypertension with mild peripheral neuropathy and mild parkinsonism.

■ PHYSICAL ACTIVITY PLAN

Pre-exercise assessment was done to evaluate for conditions that may predispose to injury.
- Neuropathy (autonomic and peripheral)
- Retinopathy
- Coronary artery disease— electrocardiogram (ECG) → exercise stress test
- Peripheral arterial disease

Medication history was taken as some medicines increase risk and sometimes doses are required to be adjusted. Evening prandial doses of insulin were reduced and on resistance exercise days, dose of insulin secretagogues were reduced.

Sedentary Time Reduction and Physical Activity

Postretirement he was experiencing a lot of leisure time which led to increased TV viewing and prolonged sitting. He was asked to interrupt sitting time by getting up briefly every 20–30 minutes. We asked him to play and spend time with his grandchildren and take up gardening, which was his hobby in morning and evenings.

If unstructured physical activity is increased (e.g., errands, household tasks, dog walking, or gardening) the daily energy expenditure is increased and this helps in weight management. With unstructured activity the daily sitting time is reduced. Raising nonexercise activity even briefly (3–15 min) is helpful in diminishing postprandial hyperglycemia and bettering blood glucose control[4].

Pedometer as Activity Monitor

He was asked to self-monitor physical activity with a pedometer or accelerometer. He was asked to record values, review at visits, set step count targets (initially set at 5,000 steps/day and then increased to 7,000 steps/day and finally to 10,000 steps/day). The recommendations were formalized with a written prescription. Use of pedometer leads to increased participation, even if there are self-selected step goals.

Supervised Training

As our patient was 65 years of age and also obese, we asked him to undergo supervised training. We encouraged his wife to accompany him which further motivated him. In T2DM, supervised training reduces A1c whether or not they include dietary cointervention, but unsupervised exercise reduces A1c only if there is concomitant dietary intervention. Similarly, patients undergoing supervised aerobic and resistance exercise achieved better improvements in waist circumference, BMI, blood pressure, A1c, high-density lipoprotein (HDL) cholesterol, fitness, and muscle strength.

Technology

We took the help of technology to improve outcome. We have had Whatsapp group for patients and we also followed up with phone and e-mail. It is well-known that internet delivered promotional interventions for physical activity is more efficient than normal care. Through internet-based programs, physical activity monitoring, goal setting, feedback and coach support by phone or email is possible.

Exercise schedule of Naresh consisted the following:
1. Aerobic exercises
2. Resistance exercises
3. Flexibility and balance exercises

He was advised to practice yoga during very hot and humid days to avoid dehydration or during the rainy season when the exercise schedule is often disrupted from June to August in India. Yoga may lead to improvement in blood glucose control, lipid levels and body composition in patients with T2DM. He was asked to drink lots of water prior to exercise to prevent dehydration.

Aerobic Exercise

Naresh was asked to start gradually while walking at a gentle pace for as little as 5–15 minutes at one time. He was asked to progress slowly over 12 weeks to up to 50 minutes per session (including 20 minutes of warm up and cool down) of brisk walking.

He was advised for at least 150 min/week of moderate intensity exercises with no >2 consecutive days without exercise. The aerobic exercises could also be jogging, cycling, or swimming.

Aerobic exercise improves insulin sensitivity, compliance and reactivity of blood vessels, mitochondrial density, oxidative enzymes, immune function, cardiac output, and lung function. For patients of T2DM, regular training reduces insulin resistance, glycated hemoglobin (HbA1c), blood pressure, and triglycerides.

Resistance Exercise

Our patient Naresh was advised to choose 6-8 exercises targeting the major muscle groups of arms, chest, back, legs, and abdomen. He was to increase the resistance gradually until he could perform 3 sets of 8-12 repetitions for each exercise, with 1-2 minutes of rest between sets. Resistance exercises were to be done on minimum 2 nonconsecutive days per week.

At the beginning, we ensured that he received initial instruction and supervision by a qualified physiotherapist to maximize benefits and minimize risk of injury.

If aerobic and resistance exercises were done together, resistance exercises would be done first to ensure less hypoglycemia. The health benefits of resistance exercises include better muscle strength, muscle mass, physical function, body composition, bone mineral density, mental health, insulin sensitivity, lipid profile, blood pressure, and cardiovascular status. Resistance exercise for T2DM patients include improvements in insulin resistance, blood glucose control, blood pressure, strength, lean body mass, and fat mass. Resistance training improves strength by 50%.

Flexibility, Balance, and Other Training

Our patient was advised static or dynamic stretch for 10-30 seconds with 2-4 repetitions of each exercise. He was to do flexibility exercises for 2-3 days/week.

Balance exercises of light to moderate intensity like standing on 1 leg or standing on toes or heels of any duration for 2-3 days/week. The duration and frequency were to be increased over time.

Doing flexibility exercises for each of the major muscle tendon groups on 2 or more days/week helps to maintain range of movement. Though flexibility training is desirable for all patients with diabetes, it should not replace other recommended activities (e.g., aerobic and resistance exercises) as flexibility exercises do not affect glucose control, body composition or insulin action. Adult patients with diabetes (50 years or older) should do training that maintains/improves balance 2-3 times/week particularly if they have peripheral neuropathy as in our patient.

Hypoglycemia

Exercise induced hypoglycemia may occur in T2DM patients on insulin or insulin secretagogues. A maximal intensity sprint done before or after a moderate intensity exercise besides insulin regimen and carbohydrate intake changes can protect against hypoglycemia.

Hyperglycemia

The risk is lessened if intense training is interspersed between moderate intensity aerobic exercises.

Behavioral Change Strategies

We also tried behavioral intervention to improve participation in physical activity and A1c improvements by such methods are sustained up to 24 months. The technique may include focus on past success, barrier identification/problem solving, use of follow-up prompts, provision of information, education, communication, and regular review of goals.

■ CONCLUSION

Sedentary time reduction, physical activity along with aerobics, resistance, flexibility and balance exercises besides the use of technology and behavioral change strategies shall go a long way in maintaining wellness in T2DM.

■ SUGGESTED READINGS

1. Chen L, Pei JH, Kuang J, et al. Effect of life style intervention in patients with type 2 Diabetes: a meta-analysis. Metabolism. 2015;64(2):338-47.
2. Lin X, Zhang X, Guo J, et al. Effects of exercise training on cardiorespiratory fitness and biomarkers of cardiometabolic health: a systematic review and meta-analysis of randomized control trials. J Am Heart Assoc. 2015;4(7):e002014.
3. Levin JA, Eberhardt NL, Jensen MD. Role of non-exercise activity thermogenesis in resistance and fat gain in humans. Science 1999;283(5399):212-4.
4. Thorpe AA, Kingwell BA, Sethi P, et al. Alternating bouts of sitting and standing attenuate post prandial glucose responses. Med Sci Sports Exerc. 2014;46(11):2053-61.
5. Qui S, Cai X, Chen X, et al. Step counter use in type 2 Diabetes: a meta-analysis of randomized control trial. BMC med. 2014;12:36.
6. Umpierre D, Ribeiro PA, Kramer CK, et al. Physical activity advice only or structured exercise training and association with HbA1C levels in type 2 diabetes: a systemic review and meta-analysis. JAMA. 2011;305(17):1790-9.
7. Balducci S, Zanuso S, Niccolucci A, et al. Italian Diabetes Exercise Study (IDES) Investigators (2010). Effect of an intensive exercise intervention strategy on modifiable cardio-vascular risk factors in subjects with type 2 diabetes mellitus: a randomized control trial: the Italian Diabetes and Exercise Study (IDES). Arch Intern Med. 2010;170(20):1794-803.
8. Connelly J, Kirk A, Mastoff J, et al. The use of technology to promote physical activity in type 2 Diabetes management: a systematic review. Diabet Med. 2013;30(12):1420-32.
9. Innes KE, Selfe TK. Yoga for adults with type 2 Diabetes: a systemic review of controlled trials. J Diabetes Res 2016;2016:6979370.
10. Garber CE, Blissmer B, Deschenes MR, et al.; American College of Sports Medicine. American College of Sports Medicine position stand. Quantity and quality of exercise for developing and maintaining cardiorespiratory, musculoskeletal and neuromotor fitness in apparent healthy adults: guidance for prescribing exercise. Med Sci Sports Exerc. 2011;43(7):1334-59.
11. Snowling NJ, Hopkins WG. Effects of different modes of exercise training on glucose control and risk factors for complication in type 2 diabetic patients: a meta-analysis. Diabetes Care. 2006;29(11):2518-27.
12. Yardley JE, Kenny GP, Perkins BA, et al. Effects of performing resistance exercise before versus after aerobic exercise on glycemia in type 1 diabetes. Diabetes care. 2012;35(4):669-75.

13. Gordon BA, Benson AC, Bird SR, et al. Resistance training improves metabolic health in type 2 Diabetes: a systemic review: Diabetes Res Clin Pract. 2009;83(2):157-75.
14. Colberg SR, Sigel RJ, Fernhall B, et al.; American College of Sports Medicine; American Diabetes Association. Exercise and type 2 Diabetes: The American College of Sports Medicine and the American Diabetes Association: joint position statement Diabetes Care. 2010;33(12):e147-67.
15. Morrison S, Colberg SR, Mariano M, et al. Balance training reduces fall risk in older individuals with type 2 Diabetes. Diabetes Care. 2010;33(4):748-50.
16. Fahey AJ, Paramalingam N, Davy RJ, et al. The effect of a short sprint on post exercise whole body glucose production and utilization rates in individuals with type 1 diabetes mellitus. J Clin Endocrinol Metab. 2012;97(11):4193-200.
17. Guelfi KJ, Jones TW, Fournier PA. The decline in blood glucose levels is less with intermittent high-intensity compared with moderate intensity exercise in individuals with type 1 Diabetes. Diabetes Care. 2005;28(6):1289-94.
18. Avery L, Flynn D, Van Wersch A, et al. Changing physical activity behavior in Type 2 Diabetes: a systematic review and meta-analysis of behavioral interventions. Diabetes Care. 2012;35(12):2681-9.
19. Muller N, Stengel D, Kloos C, et al. Improvement of HbA(1C) and stable weight loss 2 year after an out-patient treatment and teaching program for patients with type 2 diabetes without insulin therapy based on urine glucose self-monitoring. Int J Gen Med. 2012;5:241-7.
20. Ekong G, Kavookijan J. Motivational interviewing and outcomes in adults with type 2 Diabetes: a systematic review. Patient Educ Couns. 2016;99(6):944-52.

CHAPTER 35

Physiology of Yoga and Its Effect on Body

Arun Chaturvedi

■ HISTORY

The practice of yoga is believed to have started with the very dawn of civilization. Lord Shiva is seen as the first *"yogi"* or *"adiyogi"* and the first *guru* or *adiguru*.

History of yoga starts with *"yogasutra"* written by Patanjali, Vedas, ancient text record yogic technique in between 1800 and 300 BC.

Yoga entered the western mainstream through the work of Swami Vivekanand.

■ WHAT IS YOGA?

Yoga is a Sanskrit word for "yoke" or "union". It is spiritual and self-discipline method of body breath and mind.

■ COMPONENT OF BODY

According to yogic science body has five layers of *koshas* (chambers).
1. *Annamaya kosha*: Musculoskeletal body
2. *Pranamaya kosha*: Organic body
3. *Manomaya kosha*: Mental body
4. *Vijnanamaya kosha*: Body of intelligence
5. *Anandamaya kosha*: Body of bliss

■ PURPOSE OF YOGA

- To achieve highest potential.
- To experience enduring health and happiness.
- To improve the quality of life.
- To extend healthy, productive years far beyond the accepted norms.

ELEMENTS OF YOGA
- *Asanas*: Poses (posture)
- *Pranayama*: Breathing tactics
- Meditation
- *Kriyas*: Cleansing processes. They should be done in professional centers.

EIGHT LIMBS OF YOGA
1. *Yama*
2. *Niyam*
3. *Asana*
4. *Pranayama*
5. *Pratyahara*
6. *Dharana*
7. *Dhyana*
8. *Samadhi*

Yama
Five ethical guidelines regarding moral behavior toward others.
- *Ahimsa*: Nonviolence
- *Satya*: Truthfulness
- *Asteya*: Non-stealing
- *Brahmacharya*: No lust or sexual activity within marriage.
- *Aparigraha*: Do not collect things that are not necessary.

Niyam
Five ethical guidelines regarding moral behavior for self.
- *Sauch*: Cleanliness
- *Santosh*: Contentment
- *Tapas*: Sustained practice
- *Swadhyaya*: Self-study
- *Ishvara pranidhana*: Surrender to God

Asana
Practice of yoga postures.

Pranayama
Practice of breathing exercises.

Pratyahara
Withdrawal of the senses, meaning that the exterior world is not a distraction from the interior world within oneself.

Dharana

Concentration: The ability to focus on something uninterrupted by external or internal distraction.

Dhyana

Meditation.

Samadhi—Bliss

Building upon *Dhyana*, the transcendence of the self through meditation. The merging of self with the universe.

For doing yoga practice always use exercise mat, room should be well-ventilated and clean, there should be no talk while doing yoga and should be done on an empty stomach in peaceful surrounding slowly, gently, and smoothly.

Yoga helps the body by constant blood supply and proper nourishment to endocrine glands to produce their adequate secretions.

Cultural poses are fully capable of fulfilling of the following conditions:
- Effective removal of waste products.
- Healthy functions of nerve connections.

EFFECT OF YOGA ON DIFFERENT SYSTEMS OF BODY

On Cardiovascular System
- Heart rate and systemic blood pressure decreases.
- Cardiovascular efficiency increases due to increase in baroreflex sensitivity.

On Respiration
- Respiratory rate decreases.
- Tidal volume increases.
- Vital capacity increases.
- Breath-holding time increases.
- Respiratory efficiency increases and respiration becomes smoother.

Effect on Metabolic Rate
- Metabolism is a good indicator of the rate at which we live. Yoga exercise slow down metabolism by decreasing the oxygen consumption. The fall in the metabolic rate is much greater and steeper than during sleep, further, there is no fall in the internal body (core) temperature.
- Higher maximum oxygen consumption can be achieved due to increase in cardio respiratory efficiency.

Effect on Neurohumoral Activity

Regular yogic practice results in reduction in intrinsic neurohumoral activity, such as:
- Increase in urinary excretion of catecholamines.
- Serum catecholamines, testosterone, and luteinizing hormone levels decrease.
- Increase in the urinary excretion of cortisol.
- Thyroxin increases.
- Prolactin increases.
- Oxytocin increases.
- Decrease in fasting blood glucose level.

Effects on Musculoskeletal System

- Electromyography (EMG) activity decreases.
- Musculoskeletal flexibility and joint range of movement increases.
- Strength and resiliency increases.
- Endurance increases.
- Energy level increases.

Effect on Digestive System

- Increases blood flow to gastrointestinal tract (GIT).
- Stimulate peristalsis.
- Relax digestive system and leads to more effective elimination.

YOGA VERSES CONVENTIONAL EXERCISE

Yoga	Conventional Exercise
1. Performed with the right/positive attitude proceeded by purification of behavior.	1. Performed without any such attitude (*Note*: Any conventional exercise performed with spiritual aim may be considered yogic.)
2. Parasympathetic nervous system dominates.	2. Sympathetic nervous system dominates
3. Subcortical region of brain dominates.	3. Cortical region of brain dominates.
4. Provides normalization of muscles tone, low risk of injuring muscles and ligaments.	4. Associated with increased muscle tension with higher risk of injury.
5. Low caloric consumption.	5. Moderate to high caloric consumption.
6. Effort is minimized and relaxed.	6. Effort is maximized.
7. Energizing (breathing is natural or controlled).	7. Fatiguing.
8. Balanced activity of opposing muscles group.	8. Imbalanced activity of opposing muscles group.
9. Noncompetitive and process-oriented.	9. Competitive and goal-oriented.
10. Awareness is internal, e.g., focus is on breath and infinite.	10. Awareness is external, e.g., focus is on reaching the finish line.
11. Limitless possibilities for growth in self-awareness.	11. Boredom factor.

CONCLUSION

Yoga is a holistic scientific and perfect approach for healthy living. This is an ancient art which must be practiced for healthy life.

CHAPTER 36

Enjoy Your Exercise

KK Pareek

Exercise is a Medicine "physicians should prescribe it, patients should take it!"

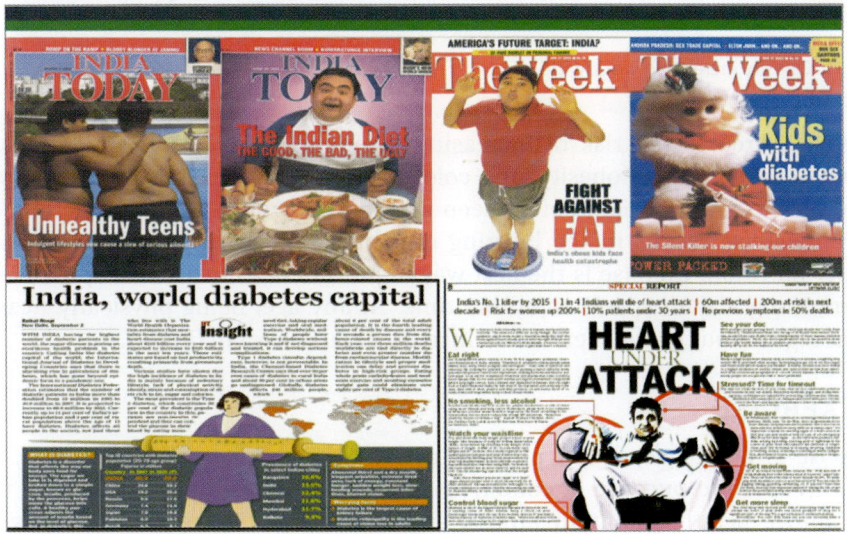

INTRODUCTION

Physical activity can be defined as any bodily movement produced by skeletal muscles which require energy expenditure. The term "physical activity" is not equal to "exercise". Exercise is a part of physical activity which is structured, repetitive, and purposeful. Exercise does not mean to go to gym or some club for daily activity but it only means to do some physical activity no matter how and where. Strengthening exercises provide appropriate resistance to the muscles to increase endurance and strength. A well-balanced exercise program can improve general health, build endurance, and slow many of the effects of aging. The benefits of exercise not only improve physical health, but also enhance emotional well-being. Regular physical

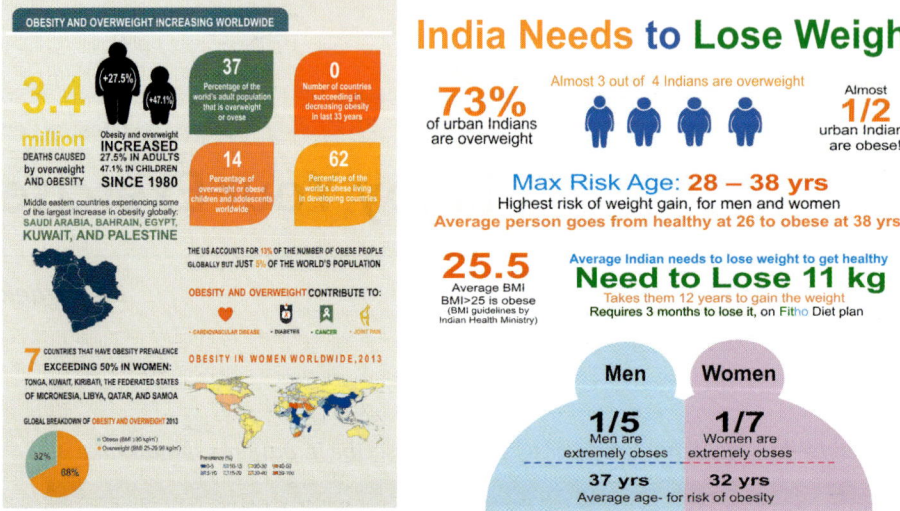

FIG. 1: Obesity increasing worldwide.

activity decreases the risk of increasing coronary heart disease, hypertension, diabetes, osteoporosis, obesity, and colon cancers. Daily exercise improves your skin, increased relaxation, better sleep and mood, strong immune function, and more. Exercise results in the burning of calories and when supplemented with proper nutrition, exercise is the best way to prevent obesity. Exercise provides an entertaining way to spend enjoyable time. At any age, being physically fit is an advantage to your overall health and increases your life span **(Fig. 1)**.

EXERCISE

Exercise is a subcategory of physical activity that is planned, structured, and repetitive for the purpose of conditioning any part of the body. Exercise is used to improve health, maintain fitness, and is important as a means of physical rehabilitation. Exercise can also be defined as any bodily movement—performed in order to develop or maintain physical fitness and overall health.

Types of Exercise

Exercise and physical activity are of four basic categories:
1. Endurance
2. Strength
3. Balance
4. Flexibility

Each type of exercise is different, but if you do all of them you will be benefited more **(Fig. 2)**.

- **Physical**
  - Anaerobic
  - Aerobic
  - Flexibility or starching
  - Balancing
- **Mental**
  - Yoga and meditations
  - Increases congenital ability

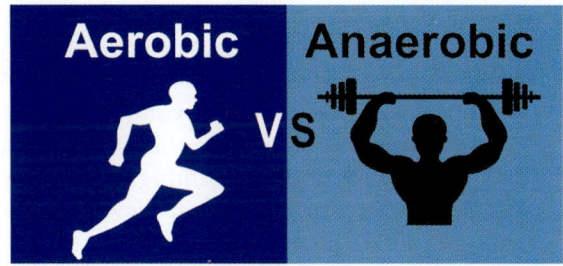

FIG. 2: Types of exercise.

Endurance (Aerobic)

Endurance, or aerobic, activities increase your breathing, heart rate, and overall fitness. Building your endurance makes easier to do many of your everyday activities. Walking, jogging, mowing, raking, digging, and dancing are examples of aerobic exercises.

Strength

Strength exercises build your muscles stronger and even little increase in strength can make a lot off difference in your work ability. We can find this type of exercise in lifting weights, using a resistance band with your own body weight.

Balance

Balance exercises help you in preventing falls, which is a public problem in older populations. Lower-body strength exercises will also improve balance. This type can be noticeable in standing on one foot, heel-to-toe walk, and tai chi.

Flexibility

Flexibility exercises stretch your muscles and can help your body stay limber. Being flexible gives you more freedom of movement for other exercises as well as for your everyday activities. Some examples for that in shoulder and upper arm stretch, calf stretch, and yoga.

Physical exercises can be grouped into two types depending on the overall effect on the human body:

1. *Aerobic exercise* is any physical activity that uses large muscle groups and causes the body to use more oxygen than it would while resting. The goal of aerobic exercise is to increase cardiovascular endurance. Examples of aerobic exercise include cycling, swimming, brisk walking, skipping rope, rowing, hiking, playing tennis, continuous training, and long slow distance training.
2. *Anaerobic exercise*, which includes strength and resistance training, can firm, strengthen, and tone muscles, as well as improve bone strength, balance, and coordination. Examples of strength moves are push-ups, lunges, and bicep curls using dumbbells. Anaerobic exercise also includes weight training, functional training, eccentric training, interval training, sprinting, and high-intensity interval training increase short-term muscle strength.

According to the intensities of the exercise, can also divide to three categories. Heart rate is typically used as a measure of intensity of exercise:

1. *Light exercise*: There is no obvious change in breathing patterns, sleeping, writing, desk work, typing, very slow walking, are examples for the first category.
2. *Moderate exercise*: It increases heart rate, breathe faster, and feel warm enough to start to sweat after performing the activity for about 10 minutes. Breathing becomes deeper and frequent. Bicycling, very light effort, calisthenics, home exercise, and light or moderate effort are examples of moderate exercise.
3. *Vigorous exercise*: It will make you breathe hard, increase your heart rate significantly and make you hot enough to sweat profusely after 3–5 minutes. Breathing is deep and rapid. Examples of this type are running, jogging, jogging in place, calisthenics (e.g., pushups, sit-ups, pull-ups, and jumping jacks), heavy vigorous effort, and rope jumping **(Table 1 and Box 1)**.

F-I-T for aerobic activity:
- F—three to five times each week
- I—keep heart rate between 60 and 80% maximum heart rate (MHR)
- T—exercise continuously for minimum of 20 minutes.

F-I-T for anaerobic activity:
- F—three to four times each week
- I—keep speed near 100% for 10 seconds to 2 minutes
- T—repeat your intervals 15–30 times with rest between

TABLE 1: Parts to a workout.

Phases	Constituent
Warm-up	At least 5–10 minutes of low to moderate intensity aerobic exercise or resistance exercise with lighter weights
Conditioning	0–60 minutes of aerobic, resistance, neuromuscular and/or sport activities
Cool-down	At least 5–10 minutes of low to moderate intensity aerobic exercises or resistance exercise with lighter weights
Stretching	At least 10 minutes of stretching exercise performed after the warm-up or cool-down phase

BOX 1: The FITT principle of prescribing resistance exercise.

- *Frequency (how often)*—the number of days per week
- *Intensity (how hard)*—"load" is the standard way to refer to the intensity of resistance exercises prescribed. "Load" refers to the amount of weight or resistance assigned to an exercise set
- *Time (how long)*—no specific amount of time is recommended for resistance exercise
- *Type (type)*—it is the mode of exercise performed
- The exercise regimen should include multijoint or compound exercises. Examples of multijoint exercises include the chest press, shoulder press, pull-down, dips, low-back extension, abdominal crunch/curl-up, and leg press while single-joint exercises include bicep curls, triceps extension, quadriceps extensions, leg curls, and calf raises. These usually take the form of free weights or weight machines

Need of Exercise

Everybody knows that the need of exercise in our daily lives, but we may not know why or what exercise can do for us. The daily practice of some physical work does not mean to take stress on body, but it is actually the stress relieving activity. Exercise not only makes you physically fitter but it also improves your mental health and general sense of well-being. Getting fit is not just about running on a treadmill for hours in your local gym, it can be a dance class or a new hobby like fencing or mountain biking. It could be a group or team activity like football or a karate class. Whatever form of exercise you choose, you'll practically certainly meet new people and may make new friendships. These recommendations can be achieved through 30–60 minutes of moderate-intensity exercise (five times a week) or 20–60 minutes of vigorous-intensity exercise (three times a week) or a combination of both types. One continuous session combined with multiple shorter sessions (of at least 10 minutes) is also acceptable.

Importance of Exercise

Exercising the body is one way of keeping it healthy. If we do not exercise then our muscles become weaker and we are less able to do things properly **(Fig. 3)**. Also the bones can become weaker and thus break easily. Frequent and regular physical exercise boosts the immune system and helps prevent "diseases of affluence" such as cardiovascular, type 2 diabetes mellitus (T2DM), and obesity. It may also help prevent stress and depression, increase quality of sleep, and act as a nonpharmaceutical sleep aid to treat diseases such as insomnia, help promote or maintain positive self-esteem, improve mental health, and maintain steady digestion. Exercise augments sex appeal or body image. Childhood obesity is a growing global concern, and physical exercise may help decrease some of the effects of childhood and adult obesity. Some care providers call exercise the *"miracle" or "wonder" drug*—alluding to the wide variety of benefits that it can provide for many individuals.

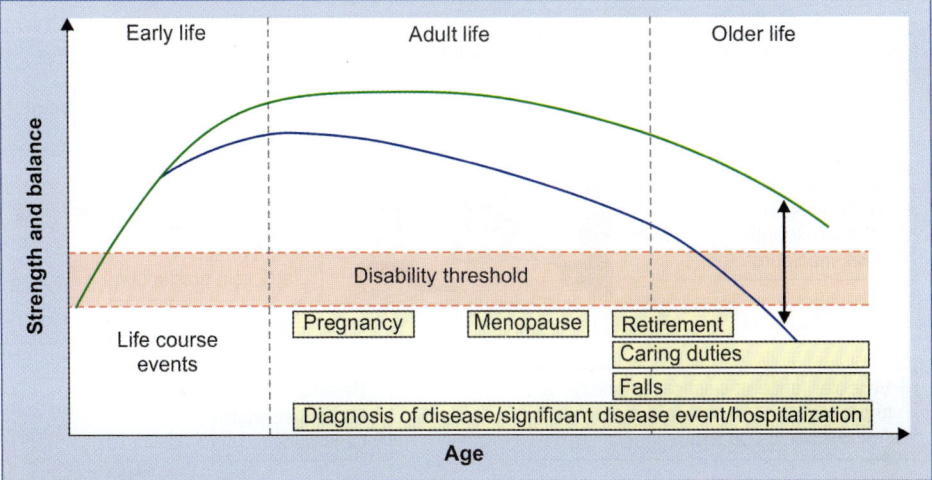

FIG. 3: Age versus strength and balance.

R-I-C-E (Rest, Ice, Compression, Elevation)

- Rest: Do not use/put weight on injured area
- Ice: 20–30 minutes. Every 2–3 hours for first 24–48 hours. Four stages of cold—cold, aching, burning, and numbness
- Compression: Use "ace" bandage; start below, and wrap upward
- Elevation: While I icing or compression—raise higher than heart to decrease swelling and pain

Benefits of Exercise

Regular exercise makes the heart stronger and the lungs fitter, enabling the cardiovascular system to deliver more oxygen to the body with every heartbeat and the pulmonary system to increase the maximum amount of oxygen that the lungs can take in. Exercise lowers blood pressure, slightly decreases the levels of total and low-density lipoprotein (LDL) cholesterol (the bad cholesterol), and increases the level of high-density lipoprotein (HDL) cholesterol (the good cholesterol). These helpful effects decrease the risk of heart attack, stroke, and coronary artery disease. In addition, colon cancer and some forms of diabetes are less likely to occur in people who exercise regularly. Every physical task requires muscle strength and some degree of range of motion in joints. Regular exercise can improve both of these qualities. Exercise stretches muscles and joints, which in turn can increase flexibility and help prevent injuries. Weight-bearing exercise, such as brisk walking and weight training, strengthens bones and helps prevent osteoporosis **(Fig. 4)**. Other health benefits include the following:

Reduce Stress and Anxiety

Regular exercise can help to decrease physical and mental stress. Exercise also increases concentrations of norepinephrine, a chemical that can moderate the brain's response to stress. Study suggests that 30 minutes exercise for 5 or more

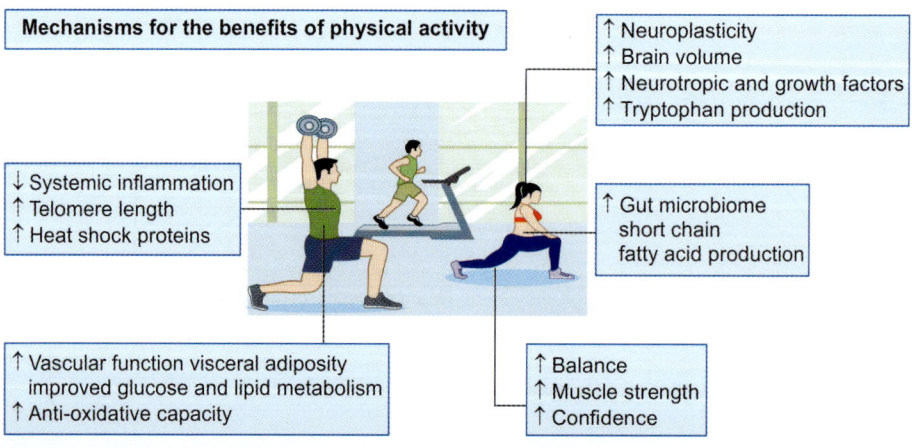

FIG. 4: Benefits of physical activity.

days in a week, make helps in lowering the depression and mental stress and also helps in having a good night sleep. Regarding anxiety, the warm and chemicals that are released during and after any physical exercise can help people with anxiety disorders calm down.

Boost Happy Chemicals

Exercise releases endorphins, which create feelings of happiness and euphoria. In some cases, exercise can be just as effective as antidepressant pills in treating depression. Higher energy levels resulting from exercise help a person in remaining fresh and happy. Working out for just 30 minutes a few times a week can instantly boost overall mood.

Improve Self-confidence and Self-image

Physical fitness can boost self-esteem and improve positive self-image regardless of weight, size, gender, or age, can elevate a person's perception of his or her attractiveness, that is, self-worth.

Increase Brainpower

Various studies on mice and men have shown that cardiovascular exercise can create new brain cells (aka neurogenesis) and improve overall brain performance. Studies suggest that a vigorous workout increases levels of a brain-derived protein (known as BDNF) in the body, believed to help with decision making, higher thinking, and learning.

Sharpen Memory

Regular physical activity increases memory and ability to learn new things. Getting sweaty increases production of cells in hippocampus responsible for memory and learning. For this reason, research has linked children's brain development with level of physical fitness, but exercise-based brainpower isn't just for kids, regular exercise can boost memory among adults, too.

Improves Muscles and Bones Strength

Exercise involves a series of sustained muscle contractions, of either long or short duration, depending on the nature of the physical activity. Muscle-strengthening activities can help you increase or maintain your muscle mass and strength. Strong muscles and ligaments reduce your risk of joint and lower back pain by keeping joints in proper alignment. Research shows that doing aerobics bone-strengthening physical activity of at least a moderately-intense level can slow the loss of bone density that comes with age, along with hip fracture is a serious health condition in older adult. But research shows that people who do 120–300 minutes of at least moderate-intensity aerobic activity each week have a lower risk of hip fracture.

Reduce the Risk of Heart Diseases

Daily physical activity reduces risk of stroke and heart disease. According to the American Heart Association (AHA), exercising 30 minutes a day, 5 days a week will improve your heart health and help reduce your risk of heart disease. You can even break it up into quick and manageable 10-minute sessions, three times a day.

Preventing Obesity

Obesity and overweight are associated with increased risk for hypertension, osteoarthritis, abnormal cholesterol and triglyceride levels, T2DM, coronary heart disease, stroke, gallbladder disease, sleep apnea, respiratory problems, and some cancers. Obesity is a significant health problem all over the world for all ages. The more you exercise, the easier it is to keep your weight under control. Excess calories are stored as fat in different parts of body. Exercise can help prevent excess weight gain and help in weight loss. When you engage in physical activity, you burn calories. The more intense the activity, the more calories you burn. Regular exercise (and proper nutrition) can help reduce body fat. Weight loss will achieve most effectively when we follow a cardiovascular exercise of moderate-intensity activity accumulated over 5–7 days/week. Eating a healthy diet is ways in which to combat obesity.

Exercise and Diabetes

Diabetes and exercise go hand in hand, at least when it comes to managing your diabetes. Exercise can help you improve your blood sugar control, boost your overall fitness, and reduce your risk of heart disease and stroke. To exercise safely, it's crucial to track your blood sugar before, during and after physical activity. Physical activity can lower your blood glucose up to 24 hours or more after your work out by making your body more sensitive to insulin.

Exercise and Cancer

Exercise is one of the most important activities to prevent against many types of cancer. Up to one-third of cancer-related deaths are due to obesity and a sedentary lifestyle, including two of the most common cancers in the United States, breast and colon cancer.

It is estimated that 30–60 minutes of moderate to vigorous physical activity per day is needed to protect against colon cancer, endometrial cancer, and lung cancer. Most studies suggest that 30–60 min/day of moderate-to-high-intensity physical activity is associated with a reduction in breast cancer risk also, there is one recent study suggested that regular vigorous activity could slow the progression of prostate cancer in men age 65 or older.

Exercise puts the spark back into your sex life:
- Do you feel too tired or too out of shape to enjoy physical intimacy? Regular physical activity can improve energy levels and increase your confidence about your physical appearance, which may boost your sex life.
- But there's even more to it than that. Regular physical activity may enhance arousal for women. And men who exercise regularly are less likely to have problems with erectile dysfunction than are men who don't exercise.

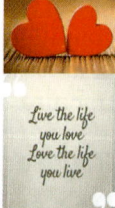

■ PRACTICAL RECOMMENDATIONS TO ENHANCE EXERCISE ADHERENCE

Clarify Individual Needs to Establish the Motive for Exercise

- Identify individualized attainable goals and objectives for exercise
- Identify safe, convenient, and well-maintained facilities for exercise
- Identify social support for exercise
- Identify environmental supports and reminders for exercise
- Identify motivational exercise outcomes for self-monitoring of exercise progress and achievements, such as step counters
- Emphasize and monitor the acute or immediate effects of exercise
- Emphasize variety and enjoyment in the exercise program
- Establish a regular schedule of exercise
- Provide qualified, personable, and enthusiastic exercise professionals
- Minimize muscle soreness and injury by participation in exercise of moderate intensity, particularly in the early phase of exercise adoption

Risk of Physical Activity

- Physical activity is safe and beneficial for almost all people, including those with disabilities.
- A safeguard against doing too much too soon is to start at low durations and intensities, build up over time as the body adjusts.
- Intensity and duration can be controlled, has defined cautions (such as known or suspected coronary artery disease) where increased hemodynamic load may cause myocardial ischemia.
- In pregnancy, impact activities causing trauma, prolonged supine lying, high altitude, or underwater activities are not advised.
- There is a greater risk of musculoskeletal injury with greater volumes of physical activity and injuries are more common with impact activities.

■ CONCLUSION

Exercise not only makes you physically fit but also improves your all body health and general sense of well-being. Physical activity or exercise can reduce the risk of developing several diseases like T2DM, cancer and cardiovascular disease. Daily exercise can reduce stress and anxiety, boost happy chemicals, improve self-confidence, increase the brain power, sharpen the memory, and increase our muscles and bones strength. Physical activity and exercise can have immediate and long-term health benefits. Most importantly, regular activity can improve your quality of life. A minimum of 30 minutes a day can allow you to enjoy these benefits.

■ SUGGESTED READINGS

1. World Health Organization (Regional office for Europe) WHO. (2016). Physical activity strategy for the WHO European Region. 2016–2025. [online] Available from https://www.euro.who.int/__data/assets/pdf_file/0010/282961/65wd09e_PhysicalActivityStrategy_150474.pdf [Last accessed October, 2022].

2. Jones DA, Ainsworth BE, Croft JB. Moderate leisure-time activity: who is meeting the public health recommendations? A national cross-sectional study. Arch Famy Med. 1998,7:285-9.
3. Vuori I. Exercise and physical health: Musculoskeletal health and functional capabilities. Res Q Exerc Sport. 1995;66:276-85.
4. Andersen LB, Haraldsdottir J. Tracking of cardiovascular disease risk factors including maximal oxygen uptake and physical activity from late teenage to adulthood: an 8 year follow-up study. J Int Med. 1993;234:309-15.
5. Kann L, Kinchen SA, Williams BI, et al. Youth risk behavior surveillance: United States, 1999. MMWR CDC Surveill Summ. 1999;49(5):1-32.
6. Trost SG, Pate RR, Sallis JF, et al. Age and gender differences in objectively measured physical activity in youth. Med Sci Sports Exerc. 2002;34:350-5.
7. National Institutes of Health, National Heart, Lung, and Blood Institute. Your Guide to Physical Activity and Your Heart (PDF). US: U.S. Department of Health and Human Services; 2006.
8. Wilmore J, Knuttgen H. Aerobic exercise and endurance improving fitness for health benefits. Phys Sports Med. 2003;31(5):45.
9. De Vos N, Singh N, Ross D, et al. Optimal load for increasing muscle power during explosive resistance training in older adults. J Gerontol. 2005;60A(5):638-47.
10. Levine BD. VO2max: what do we know, and what do we still need to know? J Physiol. 2008;1,586(1):25-34.
11. Hiilloskorpi HK, Pasanen ME, Fogelholm MG, et al. Use of heart rate to predict energy expenditure from low to high activity levels. Int J Sports Med. 2003;24(5):332-6.
12. Elmahgoub SS, Calders P, Lambers S, et al. The effect of combined exercise training in adolescents who are overweight or obese with intellectual disability: The role of training frequency. J Strength Cond Res. 2011;25(8):2274-82.
13. Gulhane TF. Benefits of exercises. Int J Phys Educ, Sports Health. 2015;1(4):105-6.
14. Skills You Need. (2022). The Importance of Exercise. [online] Available from https://www.skillsyouneed.com/ps/exercise.html [Last accessed October, 2022].
15. Stampfer MJ, Hu FB, Manson JE, et al. Primary prevention of coronary heart disease in women through diet and lifestyle. N Engl J Med. 2000;343(1):16-22.
16. Hu FB, Manson JE, Stampfer MJ, et al. Diet, lifestyle, and the risk of type 2 diabetes mellitus in women. N Engl J Med. 2001;345(11):790-7.
17. WHO. (2021). Obesity and overweight. [online] Available from https://www.who.int/news-room/fact-sheets/detail/obesity-and-overweight [Last accessed October, 2022].
18. Pimlott N. The miracle drug. Can Fam Physician. 2010;56:407-9.
19. Buckley JP, Hedge A, Yates T, et al. The sedentary office: a growing case for change towards better health and productivity. Expert statement commissioned by Public Health England and the Active Working Community Interest Company. Br J Sports Med. 2015;49(21):1357-62.
20. Meyers J. Exercise and cardiovascular health. Circulation. 2003;107:2e-5.
21. Dunn AL, Trivedi MH, Kampert JB, et al. Chambliss exercise treatment for depression: Efficacy and dose response. Am J Prevent Med. 2005;28(1):1-8.
22. Griffin EW, Mullally S, Foley C, et al. Aerobic exercise improves hippocampal function and increases BDNF in the serum of young adult males. Physiol Behav. 2011;104(5):934-41.
23. Broman-Fulks JJ, Berman ME, Rabian BA, et al. Effects of aerobic exercise on anxiety sensitivity. Behav Res Ther. 2004;42(2):125-36.
24. Craft LL, Perna FM. The benefits of exercise for the clinically depressed. Prim Care Companion J Clin Psychiatry. 2004;6(3):104-11.
25. Elavsky S. Longitudinal examination of the exercise and self-esteem model in middle-aged women. J Sport Exerc Psychol. 2010;32(6):862-80.
26. Esfahani N. The impact of sport on physical, anxiety, sleep disorder, social function and depression components of mental health in Azzahra University students. Harakat. 2002;(12):75-86.
27. Elmagd M, Abubakr M, Manal S, et al. The Impact of Physical Activity Participation on the Self-Esteem of the Students. A Cross Sectional Study from RAKMHSU–RAK–UAE. Int J Phys Edu Sports Health. 2015;2(1):87-91.

28. Pretty J, Peacock J, Sellens M, et al. the mental and physical health outcomes of green exercise. Department of Biological Sciences, University of Essex, Colchester, UK. Int J Environm Health Res. 2005;15(5):319-37.
29. Mustroph ML, Chen S, Desai SC, et al. Aerobic exercise is the critical variable in an enriched environment that increases hippocampal neurogenesis and water maze learning in male C57BL/6J mice. Neuroscience Program, the Beckman Institute for Advanced Science and Technology, University of Illinois at Urbana-Champaign, Urbana, IL, USA. Neuroscience. 2012;6(219):62-71.
30. Griffin EW, Mullally S, Foley C, et al. Aerobic exercise improves hippocampal function and increases BDNF in the serum of young adult males. Department of Physiology, School of Medicine, University of Dublin, Trinity College, Dublin, Ireland. Physiol Behav. 2011;24,104(5):934-41.
31. Erickson KI, Voss MW, Prakash RS, et al. Exercise training increases size of hippocampus and improves memory. Department of Psychology, University of Pittsgurgh, Pittsburgh, PA, USA. Proceed National Acad Sci. 2011;108(7):3017-22.
32. Winter B, Breitenstein C, Mooren FC, et al. High impact running improves learning. Department of Neurology, University of Muenster, Muenster, Germany. Neurobiol Learning Memory. 2007;87(4):597-609.
33. LiberTexts Medicine. (2020). Impacts of exercise on muscles. [online] Available from https://med.libretexts.org/Bookshelves/Anatomy_and_Physiology/Book%3A_Anatomy_and_Physiology_(Boundless)/9%3A_Muscular_System/9.5%3A_Exercise_and_Skeletal_Muscle_Tissue/9.5A%3A_Impacts_of_Exercise_on_Muscles [Last accessed October, 2022].
34. Paul B, Dahners LE. The effect of enforced exercise on the healing of ligament injuries. Am J Sports Med. 1990;18(4):376-8.
35. Fletcher GF, Balady G, Blair SN, Blumenthal J, Caspersen C, Chaitman B, et al. Statement on exercise: Benefits and recommendations for physical activity programs for all Americans a statement for health professionals by the committee on exercise and cardiac rehabilitation of the council on clinical cardiology, American heart association. Circulation. 1996;94(4):857-62.
36. Singh A. Essentials of Physical Education. New Delhi: Kalyani Publishers; 2007.
37. Burleson Jr MA, O'Bryant HS, Stone MH, Collins MA, Triplett-McBride T. Effect of weight training exercise and treadmill exercise on post-exercise oxygen consumption. Med Sci Sports Exercise. 1998;30(4):518-22.
38. Fred Hutch. (2022). Events and Seminars. [online] Available from https://www.fredhutch.org/en/events/healthy-living/Trim- Risk.html [Last accessed October, 2022].
39. Lee I, Oguma Y. Physical activity. In: Schottenfeld D, Fraumeni JF (Eds). Cancer Epidemiology and Prevention, 3rd edition. New York: Oxford University Press; 2006.
40. McTiernan A. Cancer prevention and management through exercise and weight control. Boca Raton: Taylor & Francis Group, LLC; 2006.
41. Giovannucci EL, Liu Y, Leitzmann MF, et al. A prospective study of physical activity and incident and fatal prostate cancer. Arc Intern Med. 2005;165(9):1005-10.

CHAPTER 37

Approach to a Patient of Dyspepsia

Avik Chakraborty

■ INTRODUCTION

Dyspepsia is often referred to as discomfort or pain in upper part of abdomen related to the problem of upper gastrointestinal tract. The prevalence of dyspepsia in community varies depending upon the definition used in the study population. Around 14–66% of the population from different community seek medical advice for dyspepsia. People with dyspepsia have significant poorer quality of life. Dyspepsia without any investigation is termed as uninvestigated dyspepsia, which is broadly classified into functional and organic dyspepsia. Functional dyspepsia is the most common cause of dyspepsia and may be found in up to 75–80% of the patients with dyspepsia. ROME IV criteria are used most to classify functional dyspepsia **(Box 1)**. Clinician's job is to identify organic cause of dyspepsia **(Box 2)** by focused history and examination and guide these group of patients toward relevant investigation for appropriate diagnosis.

■ PATHOPHYSIOLOGY

Polymorphisms of the G-protein β-polypeptide 3 *(GNB3)* gene have been associated with the risk of functional dyspepsia, which was found by *Holtmann G et al*. Frequency of dyspepsia in first-degree relatives of affected patients is increased compared with the frequency in their spouses. Variable proportion of patients with functional dyspepsia is infected with *Helicobacter pylori (H. pylori)* and statistically significant beneficial effect of eradication therapy for *H. pylori* on symptoms in patients with functional dyspepsia was found by *Moayyedi P et al*. Impaired accommodation of the proximal stomach, which was attributed to dysfunction at the level of gastric nitrergic neurons by *Tack J et al*. Psychosocial factors such as anxiety, depression, somatoform disorder, and recent or remote physical or sexual assault all contribute to visceral hypersensitivity and are linked to functional dyspepsia. Alteration in gut microbiome may also cause dyspepsia, as studies have observed development of dyspepsia after an episode of gastroenteritis.

BOX 1: ROME IV criteria for functional dyspepsia.

B1. *Functional dyspepsia*: Must fulfill criteria for PDS and/or EPS and diagnostic criteria fulfilled for the last 3 months with symptom onset at least 6 months prior to diagnosis
  1. *One or more* of the following:
     - Bothersome postprandial fullness
     - Bothersome early satiation
     - Bothersome epigastric pain
     - Bothersome epigastric burning

     and

  2. No evidence of structural disease (including at upper endoscopy) that is likely to explain the symptoms

  Subtypes of functional dyspepsia

B1a. *Postprandial distress syndrome*

  Diagnostic criteria must include one or both of the following at least 3 days a week for the last 3 months with symptom onset at least 6 months prior to diagnosis:
  1. Bothersome postprandial fullness (i.e., severe enough to impact on usual activities)
  2. Bothersome early satiation (i.e., severe enough to prevent finishing a regular size meal)

  No evidence of organic, systemic, or metabolic disease that is likely to explain the symptoms on routine investigations (including at upper endoscopy)

  Supportive criteria
  - Postprandial epigastric pain or burning, epigastric bloating, excessive belching, and nausea can also be present
  - Vomiting warrants consideration of another disorder
  - Heartburn is not a dyspeptic symptom but may often coexist
  - Symptoms that are relieved by evacuation of feces or gas should generally not be considered as part of dyspepsia
  - Other individual digestive symptoms or groups of symptoms (e.g., from GERD and IBS) may coexist with PDS

B1b. *Epigastric pain syndrome*

  Diagnostic criteria fulfilled for the last 3 months with symptom onset at least 6 months prior to diagnosis. Must include one or both of the following symptoms at least 1 day a week:
  1. Bothersome epigastric pain (i.e., severe enough to impact on usual activities)
  2. Bothersome epigastric burning (i.e., severe enough to impact on usual activities)

  No evidence of organic, systemic, or metabolic disease that is likely to explain the symptoms on routine investigations (including at upper endoscopy)

  Supportive criteria
  - Pain may be induced by ingestion of a meal, relieved by ingestion of a meal, or may occur while fasting
  - Postprandial epigastric bloating, belching, and nausea can also be present
  - Persistent vomiting likely suggests another disorder
  - Heartburn is not a dyspeptic symptom but may often coexist
  - The pain does not fulfill biliary pain criteria
  - Symptoms that are relieved by evacuation of feces or gas generally should not be considered as part of dyspepsia
  - Other digestive symptoms (such as from GERD and IBS) may coexist with EPS

(EPS: epigastric pain syndrome; GERD: gastroesophageal reflux disease; IBS: irritable bowel syndrome; PDS: postprandial distress syndrome)

Approach to a Patient of Dyspepsia

> **BOX 2: Differential diagnosis of dyspepsia.**
>
> Diagnosis
> Functional dyspepsia
> *Dyspepsia caused by structural or biochemical disease*:
> - Peptic ulcer disease
> - *Helicobacter pylori* gastritis
> - Gastroesophageal reflux disease (GERD)
> - Biliary pain
> - Chronic abdominal wall pain
> - Gastric or esophageal cancer
> - Gastroparesis
> - Pancreatitis
> - Carbohydrate malabsorption
> - Medications [including potassium supplements, digitalis, iron, theophylline, oral antibiotics (especially ampicillin and erythromycin), nonsteroidal anti-inflammatory drugs (NSAIDs), glucocorticoids, niacin, gemfibrozil, narcotics, colchicine, quinidine, estrogens, and levodopa]
> - Infiltrative diseases of the stomach (e.g., Crohn's disease and sarcoidosis)
> - Metabolic disturbances (hypercalcemia and hyperkalemia)
> - Hepatocellular carcinoma
> - Ischemic bowel disease, celiac artery compression syndrome, superior mesenteric artery syndrome
> - Systemic disorders (diabetes mellitus, thyroid and parathyroid disorders, and connective tissue disease)
> - Intestinal parasites (*Giardia* and *Strongyloidiasis*)
> - Abdominal cancer, especially pancreatic cancer

Initial Evaluation

Detailed history followed by focused physical examination and investigation is essential to distinguish between functional and organic causes of dyspepsia and most of the causes of organic dyspepsia. History should include duration, location, character and intensity of pain, radiation, and relationship to food. History must include presence of alarm features which include presence of weight loss, which is unintentional, difficulty in swallowing, painful swallowing, iron deficiency anemia without any identifiable cause, continuous vomiting, presence of lymphadenopathy or palpable mass, family history of upper gastrointestinal malignancy. Drug history of possible offending drugs should be included in history. Physical examination of organic disease includes presence of anemia, jaundice, lymphadenopathy including Virchow node, signs of malnutrition, and edema. Epigastric tenderness is the most common finding but does not distinguish functional from organic cause. Carnett's sign which is increased local tenderness on abdominal muscle tensing may help in differentiating the origin of pain from abdominal wall and intra-abdominal cause. Other abdominal signs of organic disease include presence of organomegaly or palpable mass, ascites, succussion splash, and a bruit (celiac artery compression syndrome). Most young patients without alarm features need not undergo any

investigation. Complete blood count, erythrocyte sedimentation rate (ESR), C-reactive protein (CRP), electrolytes including calcium, stool microscopic, and routine examination are done in others with suspected underlying organic cause or persistent dyspepsia. Upper gastrointestinal (UGI) endoscopy is advised for patients with alarm features and usually above the age of 65 years. However, the cut-off for endoscopy varies as per various guidelines. As per the European Consensus statement, endoscopy is advocated in adults of >45 years presenting with persistent dyspepsia. Endoscopic evaluation of patients <60 years is reserved for patients with any one of the following:
- Clinically significant weight loss (>5% usual body weight over 6–12 months)
- Overt gastrointestinal bleeding.
- >1 other alarm feature
- Rapidly progressive alarm features

Alarm features or red flag signs include:
- Unintentional weight loss
- Dysphagia
- Odynophagia
- Unexplained iron-deficiency anemia
- Persistent vomiting
- Palpable mass or lymphadenopathy
- Family history of upper gastrointestinal cancer

Noninvasive test for *H. pylori* like urea breath test, and stool antigen test is advocated by most of the guidelines as a part of "test and treat" approach. Though the Indian guideline does not advocate routine testing of *H. pylori* due to lack of local data.

TREATMENT

Treatment of organic causes of dyspepsia is to treat the underlying etiology. Functional dyspepsia patients without alarm features and of age <60 years a trial of antisecretory drugs may be given either H2 receptor antagonists (H2RA) or proton pump inhibitors (PPIS). Both are found to be effective than placebo in trials. PPI may have slight advantage over H2RA though the respective studies were quite different. Low FODMAP diet improve symptoms of PDS in functional dyspepsia patients and improved somatization and depression. Noninvasive *H. pylori* testing with urea breath test or stool antigen test may be advocated who fails to respond to antisecretory medications, *H. pylori* eradication therapy has small but statistically significant benefit in epigastric pain syndrome (EPS) subtype of functional dyspepsia. Patient remaining symptomatic may be offered prokinetic drugs followed by tricyclic antidepressants and psychotherapy **(Flowcharts 1 and 2)**. Acotiamide 100 mg TDS may be efficacious in postprandial distress syndrome.

Patient remaining symptomatic may be offered prokinetic drugs followed by tricyclic antidepressants. Acotiamide 100 mg TDS may be efficacious in postprandial distress syndrome.

338 Approach to a Patient of Dyspepsia

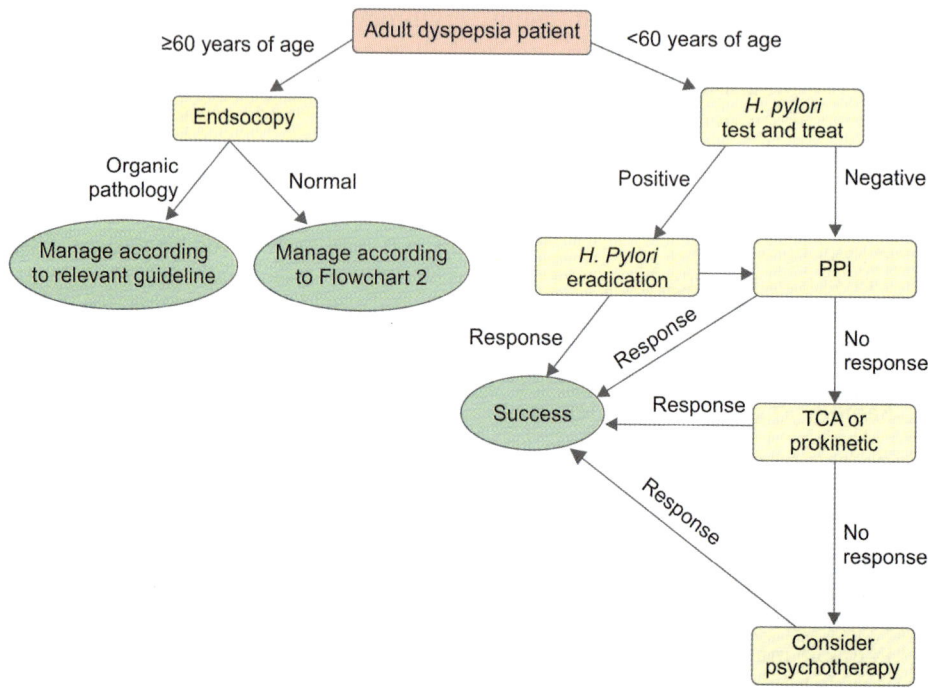

FLOWCHART 1: Algorithm for the management of undiagnosed dyspepsia.
(PPI: proton pump inhibitors; TCA: tricyclic antidepressant)

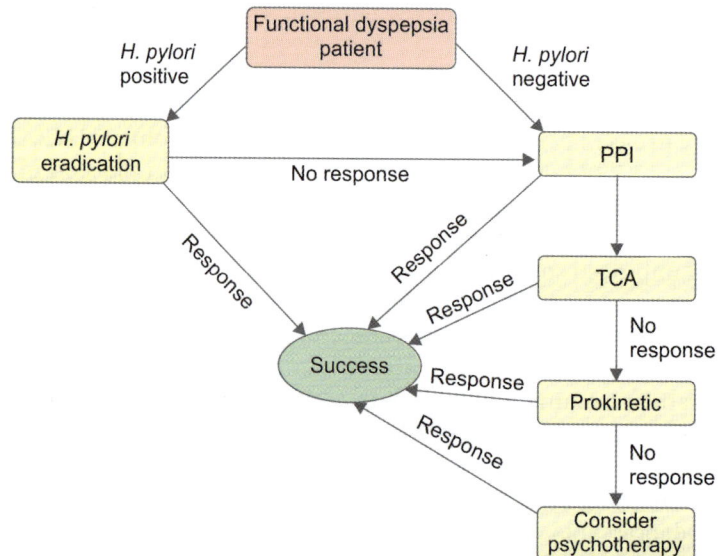

FLOWCHART 2: Approach algorithm to a patient of dyspepsia is depicted above as per Moayyedi et al.
(PPI: proton pump inhibitors; TCA: tricyclic antidepressant)

CONCLUSION

Dyspepsia is common clinical presentation in day to day practice. Good clinical history and examination with focused investigation can diagnose most of the cases of dyspepsia and can differentiate organic from functional cases. Though there are gray areas in testing and treatment of *H. pylori* in Indian context. Epigastric pain syndrome subset of functional dyspepsia do respond to *H. pylori* eradication therapy. *H. pylori* testing also becomes important in those who are contemplating long term PPI therapy. Acotiamide may play a role in postprandial distress syndrome. Psychotherapy and tricyclic antidepressant may be useful in other cases of functional dyspepsia.

SUGGESTED READINGS

1. Ford AC, Marwaha A, Sood R, et al. Global prevalence of, and risk factors for, uninvestigated dyspepsia: a meta-analysis. Gut. 2015;64(7):1049-57.
2. Hantoro IF, Syam AF, Mudjaddid E, et al. Factors associated with health-related quality of life in patients with functional dyspepsia. Health and Quality of Life Outcomes. 2018;16(1):1-6.
3. Talley NJ, Silverstein MD, Agreus L, et al. AGA technical review: evaluation of dyspepsia. Gastroenterology. 1998;114(3):582-95.
4. Fisher RS, Parkman HP. Management of nonulcer dyspepsia. N Engl J Med. 1998;339(19):1376-81.
5. Kim HG, Lee KJ, Lim SG, et al. G-protein beta-3 subunit C825T polymorphism in patients with overlap syndrome of functional dyspepsia and irritable bowel syndrome. J neurogastroenterol motil. 2012;18(2):205.
6. Locke III GR, Zinsmeister AR, Talley NJ, et al. Familial association in adults with functional gastrointestinal disorders. Mayo Clin Proceed. 2000;75(9):907-12.
7. Tack J, Piessevaux H, Coulie B, et al. Role of impaired gastric accommodation to a meal in functional dyspepsia. Gastroenterology. 1998;115(6):1346-52.
8. Ford AC, Thabane M, Collins SM, et al. Prevalence of uninvestigated dyspepsia 8 years after a large waterborne outbreak of bacterial dysentery: a cohort study. Gastroenterology. 2010;138(5):1727-36.
9. Anand P, Aziz Q, Willert R,et al. Peripheral, and central mechanisms of visceral sensitization in man. Neurogastroenterol Motil. 2007;19:29-46.
10. Malfertheiner P, Megraud F, O'Morain C, et al. Current concepts in the management of Helicobacter pylori infection: the Maastricht III Consensus Report. Gut. 2007;56(6):772-81.
11. Singh SP, Ahuja V, Ghoshal UC, et al. Management of Helicobacter pylori infection: The Bhubaneswar Consensus Report of the Indian Society of Gastroenterology. Indian J Gastroenterol. 2021;40(4):420-44.
12. Staudacher HM, Nevin AN, Duff C, et al. Epigastric symptom response to low FODMAP dietary advice compared with standard dietetic advice in individuals with functional dyspepsia. Neurogastroenterol Motil. 2021;33(11):e14148.
13. Moayyedi PM, Lacy BE, Andrews CN, et al. ACG and CAG clinical guideline: management of dyspepsia. Offic j Am Coll Gastroenterol ACG. 2017;112(7):988-1013.
14. Matsueda K, Hongo M, Tack J, et al. A placebo-controlled trial of acotiamide for meal-related symptoms of functional dyspepsia. Gut. 2012;61(6):821-8.

CHAPTER 38

Recent Advances in Management of Acute Pancreatitis

Gurinder Mohan, Arvinder Pal, Jagga Sankalp Harish

CASE SCENARIO

A 32-year-old male presented to emergency with sudden onset pain abdomen, severe in intensity radiating to back, associated with nausea, vomiting, and constipation followed by abdominal distention for 3 days. On examination—BP: 90/70 mm Hg, pulse rate (PR): 122 bpm, respiratory rate (RR): 22 breaths/min. Palpation per abdomen showed tenderness and guarding in the epigastric and right hypochondrium region.

What should be the management protocol for this patient?

INTRODUCTION

Acute pancreatitis (AP) is a disease of inflammation of the pancreas and is rising exponentially in the world. The human and financial burden of acute pancreatitis continues to grow, and it is now one of the most common reasons for hospitalization with a gastrointestinal condition. Numerous studies show an increasing but varying incidence across the globe often between 20 to 40 per 1,00,000 people. According to population-based cohort studies, AP is the most prevalent pancreatic disease worldwide. The overall mortality rate from AP has significantly decreased from >10% a few years ago to less than 2% in recent years.

Physiologically acute pancreatitis is best defined as an acute inflammatory process of the pancreas with varying involvement of other local tissues or distant organ systems. A patient is currently considered to have AP if they fulfill two of the following three criteria:

1. Symptoms of pancreatitis, such as sudden onset left upper quadrant and/or epigastric pain, which frequently radiates to the back
2. Blood amylase or lipase level that is three times higher than the laboratory's reference range, and
3. Radiologic imaging, often CT or MRI, that is consistent with pancreatitis.

TABLE 1: 2012 Atlanta Classification Revision of Acute Pancreatitis.
Mild acute pancreatitis
• No organ failure
• No local or systemic complications
Moderately severe acute pancreatitis
• Transient organ failure (<48 hours) and/or
• Local or systemic complications* without persistent organ failure
Severe acute pancreatitis
• Persistent organ failure (>48 hours)—single organ or multiorgan

*Local complications are peripancreatic fluid collections, pancreatic necrosis, and peripancreatic necrosis (sterile or infected), pseudocyst, and walled-off necrosis (sterile or infected).

TABLE 2: Causes of AP: (Mnemonic: I GET SMASHED).
• Gallstone
• Ethanol
• Trauma
• Scorpion venom
• Measles
• Autoimmune
• Mumps/Malignancy
• Hypertriglyceridemia or hypercalcemia
• Endoscopic retrograde cholangiopancreatography
• Drugs (didanosine, pentamidine, and azathioprine)

CLINICAL PRESENTATION

- Pancreatitis typically presents with rapid onset pain across upper abdomen and in most cases, reaches its peak intensity in 10–20 minutes.
- In half of the individuals, the pain radiates to back in a band-like pattern. The discomfort is mildly alleviated in forwarding bending position.
- About 90% of the people with pancreatitis experience nausea and vomiting.

PHYSICAL EXAMINATION

- Upper abdominal discomfort and guarding are more noticeable in pancreatitis, and a palpable epigastric mass may appear during the disease from a pseudocyst or a large inflammatory mass. Due to extravasation of hemorrhagic exudate to these locations, additional abdominal signs may include ecchymosis in one or both flanks (Gray Turner sign) or in the periumbilical region (Cullen sign).
- Typical fundus abnormalities associated with visual problems, including blindness, can result from microembolization in the retina, referred to as Purtscher retinopathy.

TABLE 3: Etiology of pancreatitis with their specific features.

Etiology	Clinical features
Alcoholic pancreatitis	Hepatomegaly, spider angiomas, and thickening of palmar sheaths
Hyperlipidemic pancreatitis	Eruptive xanthomas and lipemia retinalis
Mumps	Parotid pain and swelling
Hypercalcaemic pancreatitis	Band keratopathy

TABLE 4: Differential Diagnosis of AP.
- Biliary pain
- Acute cholecystitis
- Perforated hollow viscus
- Mesenteric ischemia
- Intestinal obstruction
- Ectopic pregnancy

LABORATORY INVESTIGATIONS

- *Serum amylase*: It rises within 6–12 hours of onset. In AP, the serum amylase concentration is usually more than three times the upper limit of normal, with a sensitivity of 85%. Pathologic events in other organs (such as the salivary glands and fallopian tubes) that typically generate amylase are among the nonpancreatic illnesses that cause hyperamylasemia.
- *Serum lipase*: It tends to have greater specificity to pancreatitis than serum amylase since serum lipase is increased on the first day of acute pancreatitis and stays elevated for a longer period than serum amylase.

IMAGING MODALITIES

Chest radiography: Patients with AP are 30% more likely to have abnormalities evident on the chest roentgenogram, such as an elevated hemidiaphragm, pleural effusion(s), basal atelectasis, and pulmonary infiltrates.

Abdominal ultrasonography: During the first 24 hours of admission, abdominal ultrasonography is utilized to look for ascites, choledocholithiasis-related bile duct dilatation, and gallstones.

Computed tomography (CT): The three main indications are:
1. To exclude other serious intra-abdominal conditions (e.g., mesenteric infarction or a perforated peptic ulcer)
2. Stage the severity of AP
3. Determine whether complications of pancreatitis are present (e.g., involvement of the gastrointestinal (GI) tract or nearby blood vessels and organs, including liver, spleen, and kidney).

MRI: Similar information is provided by MRI and CT on the severity of pancreatitis. However, MRI outperforms CT in evaluating fluid collections by more clearly displaying necrotic debris.

Endoscopic retrograde cholangiopancreatography (ERCP) and endoscopic ultrasound (EUS): Early on in AP, EUS is helpful in identifying common bile duct stones and enabling ERCP to be performed concurrently, hence avoiding ERCP if the bile duct is free of stones. By detecting changes in the pancreas echocardiography texture, EUS can also predict the severity of AP.[8]

Scoring System for Acute Pancreatitis

- For many years, APACHE II has been the most verified system. Most studies defined severe AP as a score of 8 or above.
- The classification system referred to as BISAP (Bedside Index for Severity in AP), assigns each parameter 1 point a possible total of 5 points.
- Organ failure AP is 7–12 times more likely to occur in those with BISAP scores of 4 or 5.

TABLE 5: BISAP score.

B	BUN > 25 mg/dL
I	Impaired mental status
S	SIRS
A	Age >60 years
P	Pleural effusion

TABLE 6: CT grading Balthazar–Ranson's grading system.

Grade	Features	Score
A	Normal appearing pancreas	0
B	Focal or diffuse enlargement of pancreas	1
C	Pancreatic organ abnormalities related to mild peripancreatic inflammatory changes (stranding)	2
D	Fluid collection in a single location, usually within anterior pararenal space	3
E	Two or more fluid collections near the pancreas and/or presence of gas in or adjacent to the pancreas	4
Necrosis	Score	
None	0	
<33%	2	
33–50%	4	
>50%	6	

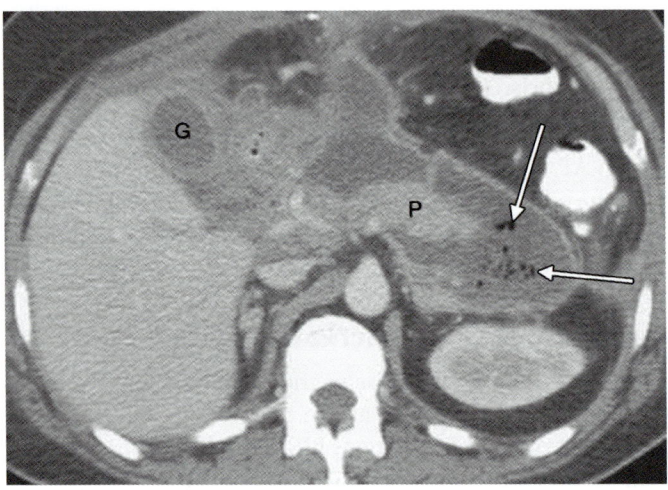

FIG. 1: CT showing acute necrotizing pancreatitis. The pancreas (P) is surrounded by peripancreatic inflammation that contains bubbles of air (arrows) due to sterile necrosis.

- Systemic inflammatory response syndrome (SIRS) is defined by 2 or more of the following four criteria: (i) pulse > 90 bpm, (ii) rectal temperature <36°C or >38°C, (iii) WBC count <4,000/mm^3 or >12,000/mm^3, and (iv) a respiratory rate > 20 breaths/min or an arterial PCO$_2$ < 32 mm Hg.
- APACHE II has stood the test of time and no score is convincingly superior to it, but it has the drawback of being cumbersome.

CT severity index (0–10)
CT grade (0–4) + Necrosis (0–6) = Total score

▮ TREATMENT

Initial management during the first week:
   The treatment of AP in first week is mainly supportive care.
- *Intravenous fluid and electrolyte resuscitation*: IV fluid at a rate of 5–10 mL/kg/h or 250–500 mL/h of probably lactated ringer solution preferably during the first few hours after admission is suggested.

   Lactated Ringer solution is supposed to reduce intracellular acidosis in the pancreas and thus the tryptic activity. A small RCT showed a benefit with lactated Ringer solution over normal saline with regard to a decrease in SIRS score as well as CRP levels.
- *Respiratory and cardiovascular care*: Supplemental oxygen is given to maintain oxygen saturation of well over 90%. If nasal or face mask oxygen fails to correct hypoxemia or if there is fatigue and borderline respiratory reserve, noninvasive PPV or endotracheal intubation and assisted mechanical ventilation can be required early.
- *Metabolic complications*: Hyperglycemia may be present for the first few days after having acute pancreatitis, but it normally goes away as the inflammation goes down. Because blood sugar levels might change, insulin needs to be used carefully.

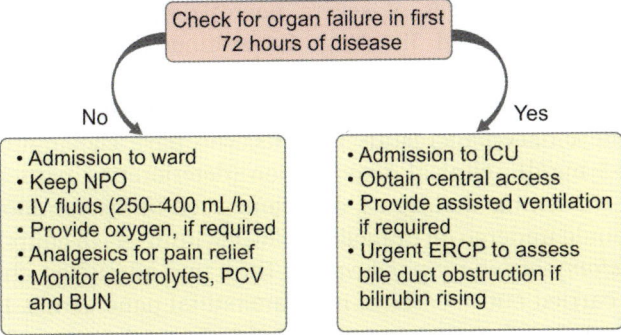

FIG. 2: Stepwise approach in management of AP in first 72 hours.

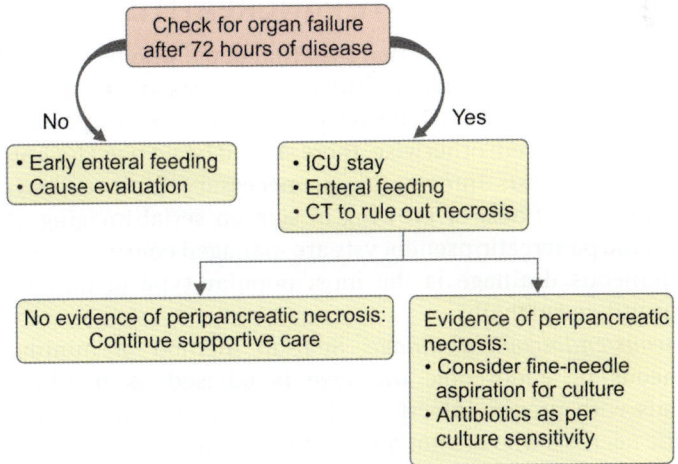

FIG. 3: Stepwise approach in management of AP after 72 hours.

As albumin-rich intravascular fluid extravasates into the peritoneum and retroperitoneum, as well as the negative phase reactant impact on lowering albumin synthesis during the acute disease phase, hypocalcemia is mostly caused by low serum albumin. The calcium that is typically linked to albumin is reduced as a result of albumin loss. The nonionized nature of this loss makes hypocalcemia mainly asymptomatic and without the need for special treatment.

Under the presence of hypomagnesemia, the release of parathyroid hormone is inhibited; magnesium replenishment should return blood calcium levels to normal in these circumstances.

- *Nutrition*: According to American Gastroenterological Association (AGA) recommendations, all patients with AP—mild, moderately severe, and severe—should start eating as soon as they are able to tolerate it (often within 24 hours). Early oral feeding has been demonstrated to reduce morbidity and mortality by protecting the gut mucosal barrier and preventing the transfer of micro-organisms from the intestinal lumen into circulation.

- *Antibiotics*: Even in cases of severe necrotizing pancreatitis, prophylactic antibiotics are not advised. The drugs that attained the greatest inhibitory concentrations in pancreatic tissue were imipenem/meropenem, fluoroquinolones (ciprofloxacin, ofloxacin, and pefloxacin), and metronidazole.
- *ERCP*: Acute biliary pancreatitis patients who have cholangitis, total serum bilirubin >5 mg/dL, clinical deterioration (deteriorating pain and white cell count and worsening vital signs), or a stone seen in the common bile duct on imaging should undergo an immediate ERCP within 24–48 hours.
- *Cholecystectomy in biliary pancreatitis*: The same admission cholecystectomy should be carried out in cases of mild interstitial pancreatitis. It is advised to have an interval cholecystectomy at around 6 weeks when the inflammation has subsided and all fluid collections have resolved in cases of moderately severe to severe necrotizing pancreatitis.

COMPLICATIONS OF ACUTE PANCREATITIS

- *Acute peripancreatic fluid collection (APFC)*: People who have APFC If there is a clinical or radiological suspicion of infected necrosis, image-guided FNAC with culture should be performed. If the results of the culture are positive, antibiotics should be administered; otherwise, there should be no need for antibiotics.
- *Pancreatic pseudocyst*: Intervention is necessary for pseudocysts that are symptomatic, infectious, or growing in size on serial imaging. Patients with asymptomatic pancreatic pseudocysts are managed conservatively.
    Percutaneous drainage is the most popular type of minimally invasive technique utilized globally.
- *Percutaneous/endoscopic drainage*: Step-up method of minimally invasive percutaneous or endoscopic drainage is advised as first-line therapy in individuals with proven infections of acute necrotic collection or walled-off pancreatic necrosis who are not responding to antibiotics.

TABLE 7: Complications of AP.

Local complications	Systemic complications
- Necrosis - Walled off necrosis - Pancreatic fluid collection - Pancreatic pseudocyst - Disruption of main pancreatic duct - Pancreatic ascites - Involvement of contiguous organs by necrotizing pancreatitis - Thrombosis of blood vessels (splenic vein, portal vein) - Pancreatic enteric fistula - Bowel infarction - Obstructive jaundice	- Respiratory failure - Renal failure - Shock - Hyperglycemia - Hypocalcemia - Disseminated intravascular coagulation (DIC) - Fat necrosis (subcutaneous nodules) - Retinopathy - Psychosis

Surgical Intervention

Surgery should be postponed (ideally for at least 4 weeks) to allow for the delineation of necrotic pancreatic tissue. It is recommended for patients who are not responding to minimally invasive treatment, those who have abdominal compartment syndrome, intestinal ischemia, bowel fistulas, or acute continuous bleeding when minimally invasive treatment fails.

▮ CONCLUSION

Acute pancreatitis is an emergency condition requiring immediate attention. Gallstones and alcohol are the leading causes of AP. In the management of acute pancreatitis, there is the main role of fluid resuscitation and enteral nutrition is always preferred over TPN and there is no role for prophylaxis of antibiotics. To handle AP complications, a multidisciplinary strategy with specialized persons, abilities, and equipment is necessary.

▮ SUGGESTED READINGS

1. Roberts SE, Morrison-Rees S, John A, et al. The incidence and aetiology of acute pancreatitis across Europe. Pancreatology 2017;17:155-65.
2. Banks PA, Bollen TL, Dervenis C, et al. Classification of acute pancreatitis—2012. Revision of classification and definitions by international consensus. Gut 2013;62:102–11.
3. Vege SS, Gardner TB, Chari ST, et al. Low mortality and high morbidity in severe acute pancreatitis without organ failure: a case for revising the Atlanta classification to include "moderately severe acute pancreatitis." Am J Gastroenterol 2009;104:710–5.
4. Wang Q, Wang H, Yang X, et al. A sensitive one-step method for quantitative detection of alpha-amylase in serum and urine using a personal glucose meter. Analyst 2015;140:1161–5.
5. Stimac D, Lenac T, Marusic Z. A scoring system for early differentiation of the etiology of acute pancreatitis. Scand J Gastroenterology 1998;33:209–11.
6. Balthazar EJ, Freeny PC, van Sonnenberg E. Imaging and intervention in acute pancreatitis. Radiology 1994;193:297–306.
7. Tsuji Y, Takahashi N, Fletcher JG, et al. Subtraction color map of contrast-enhanced and unenhanced CT for the prediction of pancreatic necrosis in early stage of acute pancreatitis. AJR Am J Roentgenol2014;202:W349–56.
8. McLatchie GR, Imrie CW. Acute pancreatitis associated with tumor metastases in the pancreas. Digestion 1981;21:13–7.
9. Tenner, S., Baillie, J., DeWitt, J. et al.American College of Gastroenterology guideline: management of acute pancreatitis. Am J Coll Gastroenterology.2013;108(9):1400-15.
10. Leppaniemi A, Tolonen M, Tarasconi A et al. 2019 WSES guidelines for management of severe acute pancreatitis . World J Emerg Surg. 2019 ;14:27.

CHAPTER 39

Chronic Pancreatitis: Newer Concepts in Management

Rajesh Gopalakrishna

■ INTRODUCTION

Chronic pancreatitis (CP) is defined as a continuing inflammatory disease of the pancreas characterized by irreversible morphological changes typically causing pain and/or permanent CP can produce a variety of symptoms and complications that require therapy. Abdominal pain is the most common symptom, the most common reason for intervention and hospitalization, and has the maximum impact on quality of life in these patients. As CP progresses, patients may develop exocrine pancreatic insufficiency (steatorrhea and maldigestion) as well as diabetes (pancreatic diabetes or type 3C diabetes mellitus) due to destruction of pancreatic islet cells. The time to disease progression in CP is variable, and is dependent on the age at presentation, presence of environmental risk factors, genetic mutations, integrity of the main pancreatic duct, and individual variability. The progression to exocrine and endocrine insufficiency appears to vary by etiology, and particularly due to differences in the natural history of alcoholic and idiopathic (nonalcoholic) CP.

The key issues in management of CP include treatment of abdominal pain, treatment of pancreatic exocrine insufficiency, and treatment of pancreatic diabetes. Complications of CP such as pancreatic pseudocyst, gastric or biliary obstruction, gastric varices, and splanchnic venous thromboses need special considerations.

■ GENERAL MEASURES

Cessation of Alcohol and Tobacco

Abstinence from alcohol can variably delay the progression of CP. Smoking cessation can delay onset of clarification and lower the risk of pancreatic cancer. Some patients will experience some degree of pain relief with abstinence alone.

Dietary Measures

Patients with CP are advised to consume low-fat meals. Usually, the patients will restrict fat in diet as it helps in reducing recurrences of pain or acute exacerbations. However, it is essential to ensure good nutrition. Very low-fat diets are to be avoided due to increased risk for fat-soluble vitamin deficiencies (A, E, D, and K). Vitamin supplementation is often required especially for vitamin D. Dietary counseling can be effective alternative to use of expensive dietary replacements. Medium chain triglycerides (MCTs) may be helpful in some patients. The concerns of those with diabetes need extraconsideration.

MANAGEMENT OF PAIN

Pain is the most common symptom of CP (seen in >90% patients). However, some patients with CP may present with exocrine insufficiency or diabetes only rather than pain. Pancreatic pain is most commonly epigastric in location, boring in character with radiation to the back; it is alleviated by leaning forward and is worse within 5-10 minutes of eating. Pancreatic pain may initially be episodic and tends to become more continuous over time. During the initial phases, elevations in amylase and lipase are common with painful flares, but as the disease progresses, pancreatic enzymes are often not elevated during painful flares. There is a natural variability of pain over time in CP.

The mechanisms of pain in patients with CP are complex and multiple mechanisms may coexist in same patient. Some mechanisms of pain include pancreatic ductal obstruction, pancreatic inflammation and ischemia, pancreatic neuropathy, altered nociception with sensitization, and altered central pain processing.

Pain is the most common reason for intervention or hospitalization. Chronic or continuous pain in particular has the most negative impact on quality of life. Predicting patient response to a particular therapy for pain is not currently possible. One confusing feature of this disease is that the amount of damage to the pancreas [pancreatic morphology on computed tomography (CT) scan] does not correlate with the severity or even presence of pain. Assessment of pain frequency and accurate identification of pain patterns is crucial. However, it is usually difficult to identify the dominant pain mechanism in individual patients. Interventions which provide remission from pain likely to be more beneficial than which only decrease pain severity.

Evaluation to Rule Out Other Etiologies

Prior to initiating therapy in a patient with CP who presents with abdominal pain, it is necessary to confirm that the symptoms are in fact due to CP and not an alternative etiology. This is particularly challenging in the early stages of CP when abdominal pain may be significant, but characteristic and diagnostic imaging features may be absent.

Initial evaluation should include a detailed history to assess for the presence of abdominal pain associated with CP at baseline, the character of pain (constant or intermittent, usual triggers for pain), severity, and impact on their quality of life. Patients with established CP may develop worsening abdominal pain for many other reasons (peptic ulcer disease; superimposed pancreatic carcinoma; or local complications like pancreatic pseudocyst, duodenal, or biliary obstruction).

Cross-sectional abdominal imaging CT or magnetic resonance imaging (MRI) is useful in identifying alternative etiologies of pain especially local complications or malignancy. Assessment of the pancreatic duct morphology may be useful when considering possible endoscopic or surgical therapy for pain.

Medical Management for Pain

Analgesics

First-line analgesics are paracetamol and nonsteroidal anti-inflammatory drugs (NSAIDs). This is followed by low potency opioids like tramadol (a dual-action analgesic, with mu-opioid agonistic and monoaminergic properties) and has similar efficacy as stronger opioids in painful CP. Efforts should be made to minimize use of opioids, especially chronic narcotic use.

Adjunctive Agents

Adjunctive agents including tricyclic antidepressants, serotonin and norepinephrine reuptake inhibitors (SSRIs), and combined SSRIs (duloxetine) or gabapentinoids (pregabalin or gabapentin) are useful agents as they target neuropathic pain. Use of these agents may allow opioid dose to be minimized.

Antioxidants

Antioxidant therapy can be utilized for initial management of abdominal pain due to CP, although the benefit of pain reduction is likely small. Etiology of CP and the nutritional status prior to antioxidant therapy are some factors which determine response to antioxidants. A combination of vitamin E (200 IU), vitamin C (500 mg), beta-carotene (5,000 IU), selenium (500 μg), and methionine (1,000 mg) is ideal.

Pancreatic Enzymes

Pancreatic enzyme supplementation may reduce pain in selected patients. Delivering high doses of pancreatic proteases to the duodenum would reduce cholecystokinin (CCK) levels, which would reduce the stimulation of the pancreas by CCK. The nonenteric enzyme preparations with high protease contents are preferred; however, lack of response after 6 weeks suggests that this approach may not be beneficial.

Alternative approaches for managing pain in CP include acupuncture, acupressure, cognitive behavioral therapy, mindfulness, meditation, and yoga.

Interventions for Pain in CP

In patients with pain due to CP who fail to respond to medical management alone, the subsequent management includes endoscopic or surgical interventions with a limited role of neurolytic procedures.

Patients with refractory pain due to CP and a dilated pancreatic duct require drainage of the obstructed pancreatic duct. This may be performed endoscopically or surgically. Endoscopic drainage procedures in patients with a symptomatic, obstructed pancreatic duct as first-line therapy with surgery reserved for patients who fail endoscopic treatment or are unable or unwilling to undergo endoscopic treatment is attractive option. Surgical therapy is more effective and more durable than endoscopic approaches.

The primary goal of endoscopic therapy is to improve the flow through the pancreatic duct by eliminating obstructing ductal strictures or ductal stones. Careful patient selection based on pancreatic ductal anatomy is the key determinant to better outcomes. Those patients most amenable for endoscopic therapies are those with ductal obstruction especially a dilated main pancreatic duct with an obstructing stricture or stone in the head of the pancreas.

Endoscopic therapy for pain usually involves endoscopic retrograde cholangiopancreatography (ERCP) with pancreatic sphincterotomy, dilatation of strictures, pancreatic stone removal, and pancreatic duct stents. Large pancreatic calculi may need to be crushed by extracorporeal shock wave lithotripsy (ESWL) or by intraductal lithotripsy (laser or electrohydraulic lithotripsy) before removal. Multiple endoscopic procedures are usually necessary to achieve ductal clearance and resolution of strictures.

Surgical therapy can be directed at improving pancreatic ductal flow. Patients with a dilated main pancreatic duct (≥6-7 mm) and pain are candidates for a drainage procedure most commonly the modified Puestow procedure which is a lateral pancreaticojejunostomy (LPJ). It may be combined with coring of the pancreatic head (Frey's procedure). These are the commonly performed procedures.

Surgical management in patients with a nondilated main pancreatic duct (<6-7 mm) involves resection of the involved pancreas. In CP, patients with inflammatory mass in pancreatic head, pancreatoduodenectomy, or modified Whipple's procedure may be needed. Patients with diffuse parenchymal involvement may require a total pancreatectomy, ideally with islet autotransplantation.

Celiac plexus blockade is an option for pain relief in patients with refractory pain due to CP. Injection of an anesthetic (bupivacaine) with a steroid (triamcinolone) into the celiac plexus is performed under CT or endoscopic ultrasound (EUS) guidance. Pain relief is transient, lasting for 1-6 months.

Experimental therapies for CP include agents such as ketamine, antipsychotics, clonidine; cannabinoids; nerve growth factor inhibitors; lacosamide; and pirfenidone.

MANAGEMENT OF PANCREATIC EXOCRINE INSUFFICIENCY

Patients with mild exocrine pancreatic insufficiency may be asymptomatic or have mild abdominal discomfort and bloating with normal-appearing bowel movements. Advanced exocrine pancreatic insufficiency results in maldigestion of fat and protein and weight loss. Overt steatorrhea does not occur until approximately 90% of glandular function has been lost. Patients with steatorrhea report loose, greasy, foul-smelling stools that are difficult to flush. Other symptoms include bloating, cramping, and increased flatulence. Deficiencies of vitamins (especially fat-soluble vitamins A, D, E, and K) are common. In particular, vitamin D deficiency and subsequent osteopenia and osteoporosis are exceedingly common.

Pancreatic Enzyme Replacement Therapy

Fat maldigestion is usually controlled by oral pancreatic enzymes (pancreatin/pancrelipase) with high lipase content typically 30,000 lipase units with each meal. However, patients often do relatively well with smaller doses. Both enteric and nonenteric-coated preparations are available. Minimicrosphere preparations may be superior.

The effectiveness of enzyme supplementation is generally gauged clinically by an improvement in stool consistency, loss of visible fat in the stool and gain in weight, or absence of weight loss.

Failure of enzyme therapy is usually due to inadequate dosage of enzymes or due to noncompliance (often due to high cost of therapy). Patients with refractory symptoms should be advised to eat more frequent, smaller meals. Changing the enzyme preparation or increasing the dose or addition of an agent to suppress acid (PPIs or H_2 blockers) may be helpful. Evaluation and treatment of alternative causes of maldigestion such as small intestinal bacterial overgrowth (SIBO) are helpful.

■ MANAGEMENT OF PANCREATIC DIABETES (FLOWCHART 1)

Patients with CP may have type 2 diabetes mellitus (T2DM) but are more often prone to secondary diabetes due to destruction of pancreatic islets. This type of diabetes, termed type 3C diabetes mellitus or pancreatic diabetes is characterized

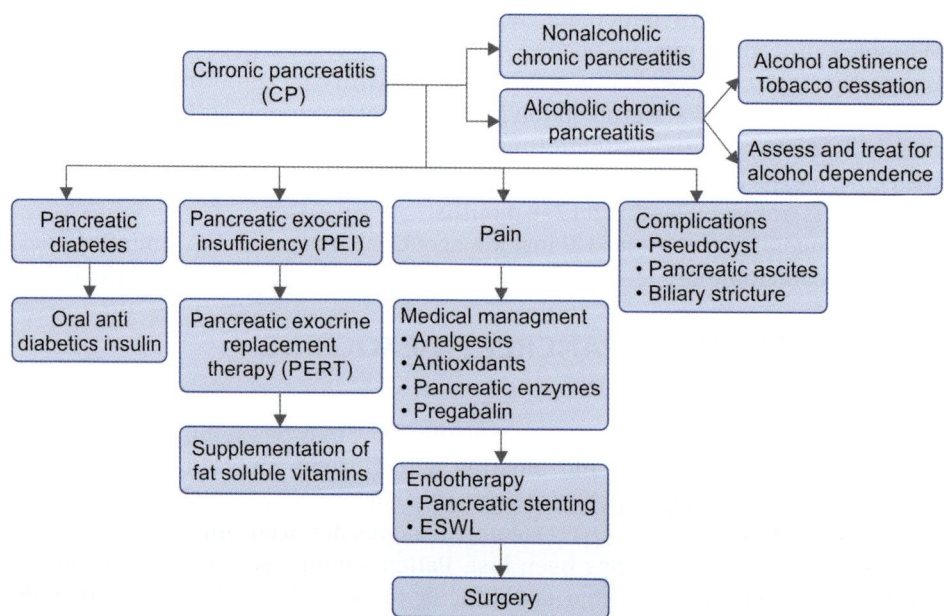

FLOWCHART 1: Algorithm for management of chronic pancreatitis.

by loss of insulin as well as loss of other counter-regulatory islet hormones (glucagon, pancreatic polypeptide) and carries a higher risk of treatment-induced hypoglycemia as compared to T2DM and caution needs to exercise in attempting very tight control of blood sugars. Although microvascular complications are more common, macrovascular complications have also been reported in pancreatic diabetes.

Metformin is the preferred first therapy, as in addition to its antidiabetic effects, it may lower the risk of pancreatic cancer in CP patients. However, insulin is often needed eventually in most CP patients. Patients with CP tend to have lower insulin requirements than patients with type 1 diabetes mellitus (T1DM). Glucagon-like peptide (GLP)-1 analogs and dipeptidyl peptidase-4 (DPP4) inhibitors need to be used with caution in CP patients and are generally avoided due to some reports of increased risk of acute pancreatitis.

SCREENING FOR PANCREATIC CANCER

Development of obstructive jaundice in a patient of CP is highly suggestive of malignancy. Rapid weight loss and sudden worsening of pain in absence of other complications are indicative of malignancy. New onset of diabetes mellitus (NODM) or recent worsening of glycemic control in a CP patient could be pointers to development of pancreatic cancer. Elevated levels of serum CA 19-9, especially in the absence of jaundice are also a useful marker.

CONCLUSION

In conclusion, current treatment options for CP are generally limited to symptomatic management of disease manifestations. Interventions to favorably alter the natural course of CP and reduce development of functional derangements and morphologic destruction of the pancreas are awaited.

SUGGESTED READINGS

1. Vege SS, Chari ST. Chronic pancreatitis. N Engl J Med. 2022;386:869-78.
2. Beyer G, Habtezion A, Werner J, et al. Chronic pancreatitis. Lancet. 2020;396(10249):499-512.
3. Singh VK, Yadav D, Garg PK. Diagnosis and management of chronic pancreatitis: A Review. JAMA. 2019;322(24):2422-243.
4. Kleeff J, Whitcomb DC, Shimosegawa T, et al. Chronic pancreatitis. Nat Rev Dis Primers. 2017;3:17060.
5. Rajesh G, Veena AB, Menon S, et al. Clinical profile of early-onset and late-onset idiopathic chronic pancreatitis in South India. Indian J Gastroenterol. 2014;33(3):231-6.
6. Rajesh G, Girish BN, Panicker S, et al. Time trends in the etiology of chronic pancreatitis in South India. Tropical Gastroenterol. 2014;35(3):164-7.
7. Balakrishnan V, Rajesh G. Chronic pancreatitis: a Southern Indian perspective. In: Garg P (Ed) Chronic Pancreatitis. New Delhi: Elsevier; 2010.
8. Balakrishnan V, Rajesh G. Chronic pancreatitis. In: Balakrishnan V, Rajesh G (Eds). Practical Gastroenterology, 2nd edition. New Delhi: Jaypee Brothers Medical Publishers Pvt Ltd.; 2015.
9. Forsmark CE. Management of chronic pancreatitis. Gastroenterology. 2013;144(6):1282-91.

CHAPTER

40

Clinicopathological Approach in a Case of Chronic Diarrhea

Ashish Kumar Saha

■ INTRODUCTION

Healthy adult daily excretes 100–200 g stool containing 100–200 mL fluid; number of defecation is 2–3 times/day. So, diarrhea can be defined as daily stool weight of >200 g and water content of >200 mL. Diarrhea may be acute when lasts for <2 weeks and chronic when lasts >4 weeks.

■ CLASSIFICATION

Watery Diarrhea

- *Secretary diarrhea (fecal osmolar gap < 50 mOsm/kg)*: Bacterial enterotoxins of *Vibrio cholerae*, bile aid malabsorption, medications, hyperthyroidism, microscopic colitis, neuroendocrine tumor (VIPoma, carcinoid tumor, gastrinoma, mastocytosis), laxatives such as senna, postsurgery such as cholecystectomy, vagotomy, intestinal resection
- *Osmotic diarrhea (fecal osmolar gap >125 mOsmol/kg*: Sugar-based alcohol such as sorbitol and mannitol, malabsorption of lactose and fructose, celiac disease, osmotic laxatives such as magnesium phosphate, and sulphate salts
- *Functional diarrhea*: This differentiates secretary type by its small volumes, hyperosmolarity, and improvement of symptoms by fasting.

Fatty Diarrhea

- Loss of absorptive capacity due to damage of intestinal mucosa leading to lactose intolerance, celiac disease, tropical sprue, Whipple's disease, mesenteric ischemia, small bowel syndrome, lymphoma, and congestive cardiac failure
- Maldigestion due to pancreatic insufficiency, decreased secretion of bile acids, and hepatobiliary disorders

Inflammatory Diarrhea

Inflammatory bowel disease, diverticulitis, radiation colitis, bacterial infections from tuberculosis, yersinia enterocolitis, amebic colitis, cytomegalovirus, or herpes simplex virus infection. Lymphoma, villus adenoma, and colonic carcinoma.

■ CLINICAL APPROACH

From Present History

- *Age*:
  - *Younger age*: Lactose deficiency, irritable bowel syndrome (IBS), inflammatory bowel disease (IBD), celiac disease
  - *Elderly*: Colonic cancer, IBD, human immunodeficiency virus (HIV)
- *Frequency of stool*:
  - *More*: Colonic pathology
  - *Less*: Ileal pathology
- *Stool volume*:
  - More from small intestine
  - Less from colonic involvement
- *Consistency*:
  - *Watery, soupy, or greasy stool*: Small intestine
  - *Small in quantity mixed with blood or mucus*: Large intestine
  - *Presence of oily particles*: Maldigestion
- Associated with fever in IBD, HIV, lymphoma, and Whipple's disease
- *Relation with meals*:
  - *After prolonged fasting diarrhea stops*: Secretory or osmotic diarrhea
  - *Even after prolonged fasting diarrhea continues*: Inflammatory or secretary diarrhea
- *Diurnal variation*: Nocturnal diarrhea with symptoms in diabetic diarrhea or IBS with diarrhea (IBS-D)
- *Excessive flatus*:
  - Malabsorption of carbohydrate
  - Bacterial overgrowth
  - Poorly absorbed carbohydrate
- *Gradual loss of weight*:
  - Intestinal bacterial overgrowth
  - IBD
  - Hyperthyroidism
  - Malignancy
- *Continuous or nocturnal diarrhea for <3 months with significant weight loss*:
  - IBD
  - Diabetic diarrhea
  - Microscopic colitis
- *Malodorous, bulky, and pale stool with or without abdominal pain*: Chronic pancreatitis
- *Bloody diarrhea following antibiotic therapy*: Clostridium difficile infection

- *Postprandial cramping pain in abdomen*:
  - Chron's disease
  - Radiation enterocolitis
  - Tubercular enteritis
  - Carbohydrate malabsorption
- *Dietary history*:
  - *Excessive intake of coffee and milk*: Lactose deficiency
  - Food additives such as sorbitol
  - Fructose and FOODMAPS, i.e., fermentable oligo, di, monosaccharide, and polyols
- Intake of drugs such as nonsteroidal anti-inflammatory drugs (NSAIDs), theophylline, antibiotics, antiarrhythmic drugs, antineoplastic agent, biologics such as anti-interleukin 2 (IL-2) therapy
- Alcohol abuse
- *History of systemic disease*:
  - Diabetes mellitus
  - Hyperthyroidism
  - Adrenal disease
  - Amyloidosis
  - Hypoparathyroidism
  - Systemic sclerosis

From Past History

- Neoplastic disease
- Tuberculosis
- Pancreatic disease

From Family History

- Neoplastic disease
- IBD
- Celiac disease
- Lactase deficiency

From Personal History

Exposure to infected animal or contaminated water: Tuberculosis, giardiasis, and amoebiasis

From Travel History

Travel to overseas: Giardiasis, postinfectious IBS

From Sexual History

History of contact: HIV infection

From Operative History
- *Short resection of terminal ileum, jejunoileal bypass for treating obesity*: Bacterial overgrowth
- *Extensive resection of right colon and ileum*: Short bowel syndrome
- *Sphincter damage due to perineal trauma*: Fecal incontinence

PHYSICAL EXAMINATION
- *Anemia*:
    - *Iron deficiency*: Pallor, koilonychias, cheilosis
    - *Vitamin B12 deficiency*: Macroglossia, glossitis, peripheral neuropathy
    - *Protein energy malnutrition*: Pedal edema, white nails
- *Jaundice*: Lymphoma, alcohol, IBD
- *Clubbing*: Whipple's disease, tuberculosis
- *Few specific features*:
    - *Urticaria pigmentosa*: Mastocytosis
    - *Flushed face, right-sided heart failure, tender enlarged liver*: Carcinoid syndrome
    - *Macroglossia, pinch purpura, waxy papule*: Amyloidosis
    - *Dermatitis herpetiformis*: Celiac disease
    - *Increased pigmentation in the creases, inner lip, pressure points*: Addison's disease
    - *Pyoderma gangrenosum*: Ulcerative colitis
    - *Thyroid nodules with cervical lymphadenopathy*: Malignant thyroid nodules
    - *Fine tremor, tachycardia, warm moist hand, stare look, sweating*: Thyrotoxicosis
    - *Hepatosplenomegaly, lymphadenopathy*: HIV infection, lymphoma
    - *Arthritis, sacroiliitis*: IBD, Whipple's disease, enteric infection
    - *Chronic liver disease, primary sclerosing cholangitis*: IBD
- *Abdominal examination*:
    - Localized or generalized tenderness in IBD or pseudomembranous enterocolitis
    - Abdominal masses in tuberculosis, lymphoma, Chron's disease, and diverticulitis

PATHOLOGICAL APPROACH
- *Chronic small bowel diarrhea with*:
    - *Thrombocytosis*: Chron's disease, celiac disease associated with reversible hyposplenism
    - *Lymphopenia*: Associated with HIV infection or intestinal lymphangiectasia
    - *Eosinophilia*: Strongyloidiasis, eosinophilic gastroenteritis

Red Blood Cells
- *Microcytic hypochromic anemia*:
    - Celiac disease
    - Whipple's disease

- Colonic cancer
- Ischemic colitis
- *Macrocytic anemia*:
  - Extensive ileal resection
  - Ileal disease
  - Intestinal bacterial overgrowth
- *Normocytic anemia*:
  - Ulcerative colitis
  - Chron's disease
  - Intestinal lymphoma

White Blood Cells

- *Leukocytosis*: Inflammatory diarrhea
- *Hypersegmented neutrophil containing more than five lobes*: Vitamin B12 deficiency

Biochemistry

- Serum iron profile is low in iron deficiency anemia.
- Low serum vitamin B12, folic acid are low in macrocytic anemia.
- Serum calcium, vitamin B12, and albumin levels are low in intestinal mucosal diseases
- *Low thyroid-stimulating hormone (TSH), high T_4*: Hyperthyroidism
- *Raised blood sugar and glycosylated hemoglobin*: Diabetes mellitus
- Abnormal liver function test (LFT), raised international normalized ratio (INR), and PT: IBD or celiac disease
- *Raised adrenocorticotropic hormone (ACTH) and low cortisol*: Addison's disease
- *Raised serum vasoactive intestinal peptide (VIP)*: VIPoma
- *Lipase level reduced to 10% of its normal value*: Chronic pancreatitis
- *Serum gastrin level is >1,000 pg/mL in the absence of achlorhydria*: Gastrinoma. In case of equivocal result, after injection of secretin if serum gastrin level > 200 pg/mL—diagnostic of gastrinoma
- *Gastric pH <2 with gastric fluid volume of >140 mL in 1 hour*: Gastrinoma

Serological Tests

- *C-reactive protein (CRP)*: Suggests infective or noninfective inflammatory disorders
- *Antinuclear antibody (ANA)*: Raised in collagen vascular disease
- *Perinuclear antineutrophil cytoplasmic antibody (p-ANCA)*: Positive in ulcerative colitis
- *Antisaccharomyces cerevisiae antibody (ASCA)*: Positive in Chron's disease
- Antitransglutaminase (ttG) antibody IgA, antiendomysial antibody raised in celiac disease, but at the same time serum IgA level should also be measured.

Serum Protein Electrophoresis

Serum protein electrophoresis is done in HIV infection, intestinal lymphoma, immunoproliferative disease in intestine, and giardiasis (IgA deficiency).

Stool Tests

- *Volume*:
  - Large in small intestine
  - Small in large intestine
- *Frank or occult blood in stool*:
  - IBD
  - Ischemic colitis
  - Amebic dysentery
  - Colonic carcinoma
- *Microscopy*:
  - *White blood cell (WBC) in stool*:
    - IBD
    - Ischemic colitis
    - Parasitic invasion of intestinal wall
  - *Absence of WBC in the stool*:
    - Osmotic diarrhea
    - Giardiasis
    - Drugs
  - *Ova/parasite*:
    - Giardiasis
    - Amebic dysentery
    - Helminth infestation
- *Fecal calprotectin level*: According to the National Institute for Health and Care Excellence (NICE) guideline:
  - *More than 50 mg/g*: Inflammatory diarrhea
  - *Less than 50 mg/g*: IBS
- *Fecal lactoferrin*: Raised in lactose deficiency
- *Fecal elastase-1*:
  - Normal is 200–500 mg/g
  - *100–200 mg/g*: Mild pancreatic insufficiency
  - *<100 mg/g*: Severe pancreatic insufficiency
- *Stool osmolality and osmotic gap* [290 − 2 × (serum sodium + potassium)]:
  - *If it is <290 mOsmol/kg, it suggests*:
    - Urinary contamination
    - Dilution with water
    - Excess water intake
  - In secretary diarrhea osmotic gap is <50 mOsmol/kg due to the presence of a large amount of unabsorbed electrolytes in the lumen.
  - In case of secretary diarrhea osmotic gap is >125 mOsmol/kg due to the presence of a large amount of nonelectrolytes in the lumen.

- *pH of stool*:
  - If <6: Suggests carbohydrate malabsorption due to excessive fermentation in intestine
  - If 6–7.5: Suggests loss of fatty acids and amino acids in the stool
- *Stool fat screening*: >100 globules of 6 µg diameter fat globule/HPF – steatorrhea.
- *Estimation of stool fat*: Intake of 80–100 g of fat for 2 days, which is followed by collection of stool for the next 48–72 hours:
  - <8–9% excretion: Suggests steatorrhea
- *Clostridium difficile toxins A and B in the stool*: Pseudomembranous enterocolitis
- *Reverse transcriptase polymerase chain reaction (RT-PCR) of stool*: Microsporidia, tuberculosis
- *ELISA test*: Giardia and cryptosporidium
- *CD4 count in stool if >200/mL with positive culture*:
  - *Bacteria*: Tuberculosis, bacterial overgrowth
  - *Virus*: Herpes simplex virus (HSV), cytomegalovirus (CMV)
  - *Protozoa*: Microsporidium, cryptosporidium, *Entamoeba histolytica*
  - *Fungus*: Cryptococcus, histoplasma, candida
- *CD4 count < 200/mL and culture negative*:
  - HIV
  - Lymphoma
  - Kaposi's sarcoma
  - Protease inhibitors

Special Tests

- *D-xylose absorption test*: After the intake of 25 g of D-xylose, blood samples are collected at first and third hours and urine sample at fifth hour. Normal value is ≥5 g. Low excretion occurs in:
  - Celiac disease
  - Small intestine bacterial overgrowth
- *Hydrogen breath test*: Test dose is 2 g/kg. Normal value <10 ppm. In lactase deficiency, it will be 20 ppm.
- *Carbon dioxide breath test*: Following substrates are used:
  - C14 triolein absorption test assesses fat absorption and lipolysis.
  - C14 mixed chain triglyceride assesses intraluminal pancreatic lipase activity.
  - C13 cholesterol octanoate assesses pancreatic exocrine activity in severe pancreatic insufficiency.
- *Schilling test*:
  - It is positive in ileal disease with or without intrinsic factor.
  - This is abnormal in case of deficient intrinsic factor.
  - In the presence of intrinsic factor, in intestinal bacterial overgrowth, this test will be normal after administration of a course of antibiotic.
- *75-selenium homocholic acid taurine (SeHCAT) test*: This synthetic bile acid conjugate detects bile acid diarrhea at the seventh day:
  - *Retention of 10–15%*: Mild
  - *Retention of 5–10%*: Moderate
  - *Retention of <5%*: Severe

- *Serum bile aid precursor 7-α-hydroxy-4-cholesten-3-one, intermediary product in synthesis of bile acid if >47.1 ng/mL*: Bile acid diarrhea
- *Metyrapone test*: Abnormal in case of Addison's disease

Radiological Investigations
- *Straight X-ray of abdomen*: Calcification in pancreatic region—chronic and alcoholic pancreatitis
- *Small intestinal follow through*:
  - *Coarsening and normal mucosal pattern obliteration, flocculation, fragmentation, dilatation of small intestine*: Celiac disease
  - *Segmental narrowing, string, and fistula formation*: Chron's disease
- *Barium enema*:
  - *Lead pipe appearance*: Ulcerative colitis
  - *Skip lesion, rectal sparing*: Crohn's disease
- *Endosonography*: It can diagnose chronic pancreatitis if 5 out of 10 above criteria are positive:
  - *Parenchymal features*: Atrophy, stranding cyst, lobularity, hyperechoic foci
  - *Ductal features*: Dilatation, narrowing, irregularity, cyst, dilatation of side branches, hyperechoic walls

Gastrointestinal Endoscopy
- *Upper gastrointestinal endoscopy*:
  - *Flattening of duodenal mucosa*: Small intestinal bacterial overgrowth
  - *If duodenal aspirates contain $>10^6$ CFU/mL bacteria*: Bacterial overgrowth
- Double balloon enteroscopy diagnoses tuberculosis, Chron's disease, carcinoid syndrome, and celiac disease
- *Colonoscopy*:
  - *Exudates, ulceration, mucosal erythema with friability, pseudopolyp formation*: Ulcerative colitis
  - *Colonic or ileal ulcers, skip lesions with normal intervening mucosa, and rectal sparing*: Chron's disease
  - *Ulcerations stricture at ileocecal junction, thickening*: Tuberculosis
  - *Yellowish white raised 2–10 mm plaques over edematous sigmoid and rectal mucosa*: Clostridium colitis

Biopsy of Small and Large Intestines
- *Lamina propria is infiltrated with periodic acid–Schiff (PAS)-positive macrophages containing Tropheryma whipplei*: Whipple's disease, acid fast bacilli—tuberculosis
- *Flat mucosa in lamina propria diminished plasma cells, presence of trophozoite form of giardia*: Giardiasis
- *Presence of noncaseating granuloma with inflammation of submucosa and lamina propria*: Chron's disease
- *Presence of endarteritis, bizarre appearing fibroblast, and fibrosis*: Radiation enteritis

- *Presence of shortened villi, hyperplastic crypts with coccidial forms on absorptive cell surface*: Cryptosporidiosis
- *Evidence of thickening of subepithelial collagen layer of >10 μm in the lamina propria*: Collagenous colitis

CONCLUSION

Diarrhea is always a serious concern, because any loose motion of more than 4 weeks duration, proper investigation and treatment should be undertaken so that the patient can be cured. In some cases severe disease can be diagnosed by taking proper history, clinical examination, routine and specific investigations which help the clinician to think of the future management.

SUGGESTED READINGS

1. Loscalzo J, Fauci AS, Kasper DL, et al. Harrison's Principle of Internal Medicine, 21st edition. New York: McGraw Hill; 2022.
2. Kumar SS, Deenadayalan MD, Pari L, et al. Differential Diagnosis in Clinical Medicine, 1st edition. Delhi: Jaypee Brothers Medical Publishers; 2012.
3. Stern SDC, Cifu AS, Altkorn D. Symptoms to Diagnosis: An Evidence-Based Guide, 4th edition. New York: McGraw Hill; 2019.
4. Siegenthaler W. Differential Diagnosis in Internal Medicine: From Symptom to Diagnosis. Noida: Thieme; 2011.

CHAPTER 41

Ascites: Diagnostic and Management Issues

Rajesh Upadhyay, Amrit Yog Datley, VS Gaurav Narayan

■ INTRODUCTION

Ascites is defined as the abnormal accumulation of fluid in the peritoneal cavity. The word ascites is of Greek origin (*askos*), and means bag or sac. Patients with ascites usually present with abdominal swelling. Ascites has a number of causes listed in **Table 1**.

Common causes in India are cirrhosis, abdominal tuberculosis, malignancy, and others such as heart failure and nephrotic syndrome. The Indian data on etiology of ascites by Patel et al. is summarized in **Table 2**.

TABLE 1: Causes of ascites.	
Normal peritoneum	**Diseased peritoneum**
Portal hypertension: • Cirrhosis • Constrictive pericarditis • Tricuspid regurgitations • Budd–Chiari syndrome	*Infections*: • Tubercular peritonitis
Hypoalbuminemia: • Nephrotic syndrome • Protein-losing enteropathy • Severe malnutrition with anasarca	*Malignant conditions*: • Peritoneal carcinomatosis • Pseudomyxoma peritonei • Primary mesothelioma
Miscellaneous: • Chylous ascites • Pancreatic ascites • Bile ascites • Ovarian diseases	*Other rare conditions*: • Vasculitis • Granulomatous peritonitis • Eosinophilic peritonitis

TABLE 2: Etiology of ascites in India.	
Etiology	Number (total 150)
Liver cirrhosis	88 (58.9%)
Tuberculosis	21 (14.1%)
Malignancy	11 (7.2%)
Cardiac	12 (8.1%)
Renal	10 (6.4%)
Inconclusive	8 (5.3%)

■ PATHOGENESIS

In cirrhosis, portal hypertension results in sodium and water retention, leading to ascites. There is systemic and splanchnic vasodilation and intrahepatic vasoconstriction. This occurs due to increased systemic nitric oxide (NO) and decreased intrahepatic NO. There is also increase in levels of vascular endothelial growth factor and tumor necrosis factor. All these changes lead to the release of antidiuretic hormone and activation of sympathetic nervous system and the renin–angiotensin–aldosterone system (RAAS), resulting in sodium and water retention and ascites.

In the absence of cirrhosis, ascites results from peritoneal disease-like infection, e.g., tuberculosis, peritoneal carcinomatosis, and pancreatic ascites. Peritoneal carcinomatosis results from either primary peritoneal malignancy such as mesothelioma and sarcoma or due to metastasis from abdominal malignancy such as gastric cancer and colonic malignancy or from breast and lung cancers. These metastatic deposits secrete protein-rich fluid, leading to ascites. Tubercular peritonitis causes ascites via similar mechanism.

■ CLINICAL PRESENTATION

Patients with ascites may complain of abdominal bloating and fullness, and may note gradually increasing abdominal girth as appreciated by progressive tightening of clothes and increasing belt size. Abdominal discomfort may be present but pain is not the predominant feature and if present, suggests infection of ascitic fluid. Patients with ascites may complain of dyspnea and new-onset inguinal and umbilical hernias.

■ DIAGNOSTIC WORKUP

History and Physical Examination

Diagnosis of ascites and its cause requires meticulous history-taking and physical examination. Cirrhosis remains the most common cause of ascites, hence questions regarding symptoms and risk factors for cirrhosis should be specifically asked. If a patient consumes alcohol, then the pattern of alcohol consumption should be assessed. Questions regarding symptoms of heart failure should also be asked. Fever, night sweats, anorexia, and weight loss can be present both in tuberculosis and in malignancy. History of acute or recent pancreatitis may be suggestive of pancreatic origin of ascites.

In physical examination, signs of other systemic diseases should be assessed. Raised jugular venous pressure (JVP), Kussmaul's sign (elevation of JVP during inspiration), and murmur of tricuspid regurgitation suggest cardiac origin of ascites whereas enlarged lymph node, particularly Virchow's node (supraclavicular lymph node), is suggestive of metastatic abdominal malignancy. Stigmata of liver disease such as spider angioma, palmar erythema, enlarged parotid gland, caput medusa, gynecomastia, and testicular atrophy suggest chronic liver disease and hepatic origin of ascites.

Inspection of the abdomen shows symmetrical distension with fullness of flanks. An enlarged spleen may be palpable in portal hypertension. On abdominal percussion, patients have dull percussion note, and may demonstrate shifting dullness. However, an absence of dullness does not exclude ascites because a minimum 1,500 mL of fluid is required for detection on physical examination. On auscultation, the presence of umbilical venous hum is suggestive of the presence of portal hypertension. Hepatic bruit may be present in hepatocellular carcinoma.

Laboratory Investigations

In new-onset ascites, the following laboratory tests should be done—complete blood count, liver function test, renal function test, urine routine and microscopy, serum electrolytes, and ultrasound of the abdomen. Other tests which may be of diagnostic value include chest X-ray, if there is a suspicion of tubercular peritonitis, and in selected cases high-resolution computed tomography (HRCT) chest. An electrocardiogram (ECG) and echocardiogram may be required if cardiac origin of ascites is suspected. If there is significant urinary protein loss, 24 hours urinary protein should be done to look for nephrotic syndrome.

Abdominal Paracentesis

Paracentesis is a procedure in which a needle or catheter is inserted into the peritoneal cavity to obtain ascitic fluid for diagnostic or therapeutic purposes. Ascitic fluid examination is crucial and helps to determine the etiology of ascites.

Indications

Diagnostic tap is used for the following:
- *To evaluate new-onset ascites*: Fluid evaluation helps to determine etiology, differentiate transudate versus exudate, detect the presence of cancerous cells, or address other considerations.
- Suspected spontaneous bacterial peritonitis (SBP) or secondary bacterial peritonitis

Therapeutic tap is used for the following:
- Respiratory compromise secondary to ascites
- Abdominal pain or pressure secondary to ascites (including abdominal compartment syndrome)
- Refractory ascites

Contraindications

An acute abdomen that requires surgery is an absolute contraindication. Severe thrombocytopenia (platelet count <30 × 103/μL) and coagulopathy [international normalized ratio (INR) >2.5] are relative contraindications. Many patients with chronic liver disease have baseline coagulopathy and thrombocytopenia, but the risk of clinically significant bleeding is very low (<0.2%). Hence, routine use of fresh frozen plasma (FFP) or platelet transfusion is not recommended. The risk of bleeding is increased in patients with higher serum creatinine. Paracentesis should be avoided in patients with disseminated intravascular coagulation (DIC) and should be done with caution in pregnancy, bowel obstruction, organomegaly, intra-abdominal adhesions, or distended urinary bladder. Paracentesis catheter should not pass through cutaneous infection, visibly engorged cutaneous vessels, surgical scars, or abdominal wall hematoma.

Site of Paracentesis

Recommended needle insertion sites include a point 2 cm below the umbilicus in the midline or in the right or left lower quadrant, 2–4 cm medial and cephalad to the anterior superior iliac spine. The advantage of midline tapping is that linea alba is devoid of any blood vessels. If lower quadrants are preferred for tapping, needle insertion should be lateral to rectus sheath to avoid puncture of inferior epigastric artery. Left lower quadrant is preferred because abdominal wall is thin and depth of ascitic fluid is deeper.

Complications of Paracentesis

Common complications of paracentesis are persistent leak from puncture site, abdominal wall hematoma, wound infection, perforation of hollow viscus, laceration of major blood vessel, and postparacentesis circulatory dysfunction (PPCD). PPCD is characterized by further reduction in arterial blood volume, activation of RAAS resulting in rapid reaccumulation of ascites, hyponatremia, high risk of hepatorenal syndrome (HRS), and high mortality. The risk of PPCD is high after large volume paracentesis (LVP—removal of >5 L of ascitic fluid). It can be best prevented by administration of 20% intravenous albumin after LVP. Dose of intravenous albumin is 8 g/L fluid removed. Avoid diuretics and beta blocker on the day of tapping and diuretics should also be avoided on the next day of tapping. Tapping more than 5–6 L should be avoided. Midodrine was found to be equally effective in preventing PPCD in one study.

■ ANALYSIS OF ASCITIC FLUID

Once the ascitic fluid is aspirated, gross appearance of the fluid should be examined. Turbid fluid may result from infection or due to the presence of malignant cells. Milky fluid suggests high level of triglyceride (usually >1,000 mg/dL), which is a hallmark of chylous ascites. Chylous ascites results from lymphatic disruption, which may be due to trauma, tumor, tuberculosis, cirrhosis, and some congenital anomaly. Bloody aspirate may be present in trauma, tumor rupture, or malignancy. Aspirated fluid should immediately be sent for laboratory investigations. A tube without additives should be used for measurement of albumin and protein in fluid. Ethylenediaminetetraacetic acid (EDTA)-treated tube should be used for cell count and differential count. Aerobic and anaerobic culture bottles should be inoculated at the bedside. Simultaneous measurement of serum albumin should be done to facilitate calculation of serum ascitic albumin gradient (SAAG).

Serum Ascitic Albumin Gradient Versus Exudative/Transudative Concept

There is conceptual shift from transudative and exudative ascitic fluid to SAAG. Traditionally, ascitic fluid is classified as exudative if ascitic fluid total protein is ≥2.5 mg/dL and transudative if ascitic fluid protein is <2.5 mg/dL. Occasionally, 3 mg/dL is used for discrimination. However, in numerous studies it has been found that SAAG has higher discriminatory value for determination of portal hypertension, and ascitic fluid total protein concentration has adjunctive role to identify the cause of ascites.

Serum ascitic albumin gradient is calculated by subtracting ascitic fluid albumin level from serum albumin level. It is helpful in distinguishing the etiology of ascitic fluid, and whether it is related to portal hypertension or not. SAAG value ≥1.1 g/dL suggests that the ascitic fluid is due to portal hypertension. The causes of ascites based upon SAAG and fluid protein level are shown in **Table 3**.

Additional testing of ascitic fluid may be done in certain clinical situations. Fluid glucose and lactate dehydrogenase (LDH) levels are usually done in suspected hollow viscus perforation. Fluid glucose is often <50 mg/dL, and fluid LDH is higher than the serum LDH level. Fluid amylase is increased in pancreatic ascites and usually >1,000 mg/dL. Tubercular peritonitis has elevated fluid lymphocyte count. Fluid adenosine deaminase (ADA) is frequently used to diagnose tubercular peritonitis; it has sensitivity of >95% when a cutoff 35–40 U/L is used. 50–100 mL of fluid is typically used to assess malignant cells in ascitic fluid. In low SAAG ascites, it

TABLE 3: Diagnoses of ascites according to SAAG and fluid protein level.

SAAG level	Ascitic fluid protein level	Etiology
SAAG ≥1.1 g/dL	Ascitic fluid protein <2.5 g/dL	• Cirrhosis • Late Budd–Chiari syndrome • Massive liver metastases
	Ascitic fluid protein ≥2.5 g/dL	• Heart failure/constrictive pericarditis • Early Budd–Chiari syndrome • IVC obstruction • Sinusoidal obstruction syndrome
SAAG <1.1 g/dL		• Biliary leak • Nephrotic syndrome • Pancreatitis • Peritoneal carcinomatosis • Tuberculosis

(IVC: inferior vena cava; SAAG: serum ascitic albumin gradient)

is also prudent to test for tumor markers such as Ca-125, carcinoembryonic antigen (CEA), and Ca-19.9. Ultrasonography of the abdomen is a useful initial screening tool to ascertain the cause of ascites, but often fails to differentiate between different causes. However, it may be useful in diagnosing advanced cirrhosis of the liver. In the presence of ascites, FibroScan values are often spuriously high, hence LVP should be done before performing this test. Contrast-enhanced CT (CECT) scan should also be done if ascitic fluid analysis report is inconclusive. CECT abdomen may identify characteristic radiological features of tuberculosis and malignancy as a cause of ascites. When the cause of ascites cannot be ascertained by using the above-mentioned laboratory tests, laparotomy or laparoscopy with peritoneal biopsies for histology and culture is the gold standard for diagnosis.

TREATMENT

Treatment of ascites mainly depends upon the underlying etiology. Cirrhotic ascites is mainly treated with daily salt restriction to 2 g/day and diuretics. Combination of furosemide, a loop diuretic, and spironolactone, which is an aldosterone antagonist, is preferred in the ratio of 40:100. Maximum daily dose is 160 mg and 400 mg, respectively. However, most Indians are not able to tolerate high dosage of diuretics and therefore, one should be cautious while increasing the dosage with regular monitoring of renal function and serum electrolytes.

Abdominal tuberculosis is managed with antitubercular drugs. The presence of malignant ascites is a poor prognostic marker and usually signifies metastatic disease. Patients with malignant ascites usually require repeated paracentesis, and an expert consultation with an oncologist should be considered.

Refractory ascites is defined as the persistence of ascites despite sodium restriction and maximum (maximum tolerated) dose of diuretics. Hypovolemia; vascular complications such as portal, hepatic vein thrombosis, and arteriovenous (AV) fistula; intake of drugs such as amiodarone and methotrexate; congestive cardiac failure; and infections such as tuberculosis and spontaneous bacterial peritonitis should be ruled out before labeling a patient as having refractory ascites. In refractory ascites, another pharmacological agent that can be used is midodrine, an α-1-adrenergic agonist, which has vasoconstrictory properties that counteract splanchnic vasodilation. When pharmacological treatment is ineffective, LVP can be done with simultaneous infusion of intravenous albumin (6–8 g/L of ascites).

Transjugular intrahepatic portosystemic shunt (TIPS) is a radiologically placed portosystemic shunt. TIPS may be considered in patients of refractory ascites but it has its own complications, especially hepatic encephalopathy in advanced cirrhosis. Hence, careful selection of patients is very important. Refractory ascites is the most important indication for TIPS. Important contraindications for the TIPS procedure are advanced liver failure [Child–Turcotte–Pugh (CTP) score >13, model for end-stage liver disease (MELD) score >20], cardiac failure, technical and anatomical complications, pulmonary hypertension, hepatic malignancy, and unrelieved biliary obstruction. Definitive treatment for ascites due to cirrhosis is liver transplant and should be considered in all patients.

Alfa Pump System

Alfa pump system is a new technology that was introduced for patients with refractory ascites in recent years. This device is subcutaneously implanted and battery-powered, and moves ascites from the peritoneal cavity to the urinary bladder to facilitate removal of fluid by urination. It is mainly used in patients who are unsuitable for TIPS, those who have previously failed TIPS, or patients with portal thrombosis-associated cardiac dysfunction. After alfa pump placement, there is significant reduction in the frequency of LVP (median number per month, 3.4 vs. 0.2, $p < 0.01$). However, it is a potential source of infection, and cost and availability are the major limitations.

COMPLICATIONS

Spontaneous Bacterial Peritonitis

Spontaneous bacterial peritonitis occurs in 10–30% of patients with cirrhotic ascites. Patients with SBP may present with abdominal pain, fever, increase in abdominal girth, abdominal tenderness, and hepatic encephalopathy. SBP is defined by the presence of ≥250/µL polymorphonuclear neutrophil (PMN) in the ascitic fluid. The presence of multiple pathogens in ascitic fluid culture suggests perforation of hollow viscus. Most common pathogens are gram-negative rods. The treatment is started with third-generation cephalosporins and can be modified according to culture report.

Hepatic Hydrothorax

Hepatic hydrothorax occurs when ascitic fluid migrates to pleural space through fenestration present in diaphragm. The patient presents with shortness of breath, hypoxia, and spontaneous bacterial infection of pleural fluid. Diagnostic thoracentesis should be done to rule out cardiopulmonary causes. Diagnostic criteria for spontaneous bacterial infection is same as for SBP. The treatment is same as for ascites and includes salt restriction, diuretics, thoracentesis, and TIPS. Patients with hepatic hydrothorax have reduced survival, and such patients should be considered for liver transplantation.

Abdominal Wall Hernia

Abdominal wall hernia is common in patients with ascites and more common in patients with refractory ascites. Umbilical hernia is more common than inguinal hernia. Elective surgical repair may be considered on an individual basis.

CONCLUSION

The development of ascites is an important landmark in the natural history of any disease particularly in cases of cirrhosis and malignancy. In cirrhosis, development of ascites is the time when a patient should be assessed for suitability for liver transplant which is the definitive treatment for ascites and its complications. Similarly, development of ascites in cases of malignancy suggest inoperability with limited survival. In most cases the cause of ascites is straightforward, in difficult cases diagnostic ascitic tap provides the clue and it should be done in every patient whenever there is doubt regarding etiology or there is suspicion of overlap as in cirrhosis with tubercular ascites. Treatment of ascites is mainly directed toward the underlying etiology.

SUGGESTED READINGS

1. European Association for the Study of the Liver. EASL clinical practice guidelines for the management of patients with decompensated cirrhosis. J Hepatol. 2018;69:406-60.
2. Runyon BA, AASLD Practice Guidelines Committee. Management of adult patients with ascites due to cirrhosis: an update. Hepatology. 2009;49:2087-107.
3. Marx JA. Peritoneal procedures. In: Roberts JR, Hedges J (Eds). Clinical Procedures in Emergency Medicine, 4th edition. Philadelphia: Saunders; 2004. pp. 851-6.
4. Pache I, Bilodeau M. Severe hemorrhage following abdominal paracentesis for ascites in patients with liver disease. Aliment Pharmacol Ther. 2005;21:525-9.
5. Runyon BA, Montano AA, Akriviadis EA, et al. The serum-ascites albumin gradient is superior to the exudate-transudate concept in the differential diagnosis of ascites. Ann Intern Med. 1992;117:215-20.
6. Runyon BA. Cardiac ascites: a characterization. J Clin Gastroenterol. 1988;10:410-2.
7. Ginès P, Cárdenas A, Solà E, et al. Liver disease and the kidney. In: Schrier RW (Ed). Schrier's Diseases of the Kidney. Philadelphia: Lippincott Williams & Wilkins; 2012. pp. 2179-205.
8. Sanyal AJ, Freedman AM, Luketic VA, et al. The natural history of portal hypertension after transjugular intrahepatic portosystemic shunts. Gastroenterology. 1997;112:889-98.
9. Riggio O, Angeloni S, Salvatori FM, et al. Incidence, natural history, and risk factors of hepatic encephalopathy after transjugular intrahepatic portosystemic shunt with polytetrafluoroethylene-covered stent grafts. Am J Gastroenterol. 2008;103:2738-46.
10. Bellot P, Welker MW, Soriano G, et al. Automated low flow pump system for the treatment of refractory ascites: a multicenter safety and efficacy study. J Hepatol. 2013;58:922-7.
11. Piano S, Borcca A, Mareso S, et al. Infections complicating cirrhosis. Liver Int. 2018;38(Suppl 1): 126-33.
12. Xiol X, Tremosa G, Castellote J, et al. Liver transplantation in patients with hepatic hydrothorax. Transpl Int. 2005;18:672-5.
13. Patel AB, Patel AJ, Patel MB. A study of 150 cases of ascites: etiology and diagnostic evaluation. IJSER. 2020;5:2347-3878.

CHAPTER 42

Peripheral Blood Smear: Clues to Diagnosis

Nandini Chatterjee, Nabanita De

■ INTRODUCTION

The peripheral blood smear (PBS) examination is an invaluable tool, which is relevant despite the availability of automated counter reports, in making a diagnosis. Clinical suspicion and automated blood counts are to be supplemented and cross-checked by information provided by a good smear report. At times it may point to a definite diagnosis, at others it gives clues for further investigations to reveal a diagnosis.

■ WHEN TO ORDER A PERIPHERAL BLOOD SMEAR?

- Unexplained cytopenias or leukocytosis, lymphocytosis, or monocytosis reported by automated counter
- Clinical suspicion of chronic hemolytic anemias or myeloproliferative disease, e.g., chronic myeloid leukemia with findings such as organomegaly jaundice, pallor
- Suspected organ failure such as liver failure with signs such as ascites and caput medusae jaundice; clues of renal failure such as edema, pallor, and hypertension
- Features of hyperviscosity syndrome such as headache, blurring of vision, and congested conjunctiva
- Clues of bacterial sepsis or parasitic infections such as fever, rigor, dysuria, cough, and altered sensorium
- Clues to disseminated intravascular coagulation (DIC) such as oozing from vascular ports and ecchymosis
- Hematological malignancies with possible bone marrow involvement—lymphadenopathy, organomegaly bony tenderness
- *Suspected cases of nutritional anemia*: In vegans, malabsorption syndrome, alcoholics, history of bariatric surgery

Peripheral Blood Smear: Clues to Diagnosis

■ HOW TO MAKE A GOOD BLOOD SMEAR?

Blood is drawn from peripheral veins and mixed with anticoagulant, namely ethylene diamine tetra-acetic acid (EDTA). It is important to prepare the smear in time so that samples may be analyzed within 2 hours of blood collection. Delay in this process leads to degeneration of the cells and formation of platelet aggregates. This results in pseudothrombocytopenia.

Slide preparation is an art to be mastered by meticulous training. Slides, pipette, and blood spreader are required to make PBS. There are two methods, "push" (wedge) or coverslip method, though the former is favored. The smear is made with the spreader inclined at an angle of about 30–45° to the blood. An ideal smear should cover two-thirds of the base slide with an oval feathered end. The smear should be air dried. Absolute methanol or ethyl alcohol are used to fix the slide; the process of fixation should not take more than 4 hours. Thereafter it is stained by suitable stains, such as Leishman stain, May–Grunwald Giemsa, or Wright–Giemsa stain.

■ HOW TO EXAMINE A SLIDE?

The head of the smear should be avoided as the cell density is greater than the tail where cells are in a monolayer. The feathered end may be examined for platelet clumps and large cells like monocytes and blasts. Examination of erythrocytes at the border of the feathered edge reveals red blood cell (RBC) without central pallor, while in thick areas of the slide the morphology of the erythrocytes is distorted by contact between cells. A good area for examination is selected in low power and then the slide is examined under the oil immersion lens, about 1 mm away from the tail of the smear.

■ WHAT ARE THE COMPONENTS OF A PERIPHERAL BLOOD SMEAR TO BE STUDIED?

The distribution, size, shape, color, cellular inclusions of the RBC, and other major cell lines should be carefully assessed.

The cellular components include:
- RBC
- White blood cell (WBC)
- Platelets
- Special cells

Red Blood Cell Morphology and Aberrations (Fig. 1)

The normal red cell is a biconcave disc about 7–8 μm in diameter. There is a central pallor (approximately a third of the red cell diameter) without intracytoplasmic inclusions.

The size of a normal red cell is roughly about the size of the nucleus of a small lymphocyte. A wide variation in cell size in a peripheral blood film (PBF) is called anisocytosis. Abnormalities of cell size can be microcytic (smaller) or macrocytic (larger RBC). Microcytosis is found in iron deficiency anemia, thalassemia, sideroblastic anemia, and lead poisoning. Macrocytes usually reflect abnormal

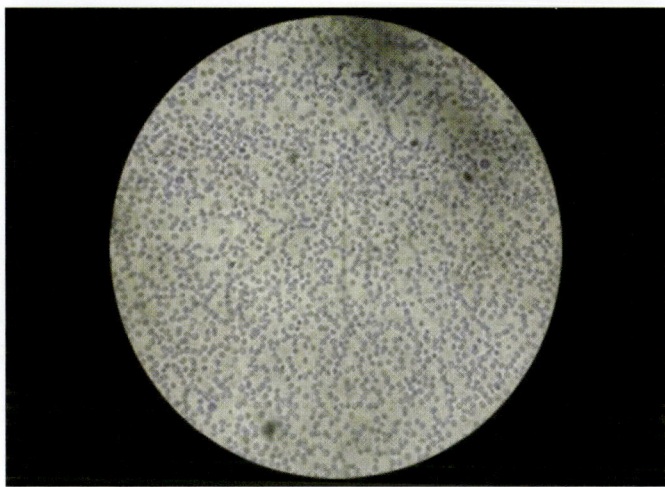

FIG. 1: Microcytic hypochromic anemia.

erythropoiesis in which there is a defect in nuclear maturation and cell division of erythroid precursors. Oval macrocytosis is associated with megaloblastic anemias (folate or cobalamin deficiency) and myelodysplasia while round macrocytes are seen in liver disease and alcoholism.

The color of the red cells is a reflection of its hemoglobin content. Increased hemoglobinization is termed hyperchromia found in microspherocytes, and decreased hemoglobination, that is hypochromia, is found in iron deficiency.

Shape Abnormalities and Special Cells

Spherocytes can be due to an inherited membrane abnormality of erythrocytes (hereditary spherocytosis) or can also result from the action of phagocytes on erythrocytes sensitized with antibodies wherein the phagocytes remove portions of the red cell membrane as in immune hemolytic anemia. Also, both spherocytes and schizocytes result from the action of abnormal physical forces in the circulation (particularly shear stress) that cause fragmentation of normal erythrocytes.

Stomatocytes are overhydrated cells found in chronic liver disease and alcoholism.

The target cell is found in chronic hemolytic anemia and obstructive liver disease where a significant increase in the total membrane content of cholesterol leads to the increase in cell surface area.

The spur cells (acanthocytes) have irregular projections from the membrane and are found in chronic liver disease while the echinocytes with regularly spaced projections are found in uremia.

Sickle cells are produced by deposits of deoxygenated hemoglobin S in which valine is substituted for glutamic acid at the sixth amino acid position of the beta chain of hemoglobin.

Bite cells arise when a phagocyte removes a portion of the red cell along with a Heinz body.

Rouleaux formation, i.e., stacking of the red cells, suggests paraproteinemia/plasma cell dyscrasia.

RBC Inclusions and their Implications

Red cell inclusions are the result of defective maturation of the erythrocytes, oxidant injury to the cells, or infections.

Loss of pitting action of spleen leads to Howell–Jolly bodies that are deoxyribonucleic acid (DNA) remnants in RBCs in splenectomized patients and in anatomical or functional asplenia.

Basophilic stipplings are denatured ribonucleic acid (RNA) fragments dispersed within the cytoplasm and are associated with hemoglobinopathies (thalassemias), lead or arsenic poisoning, and sideroblastic anemia.

Siderotic granules or Pappenheimer bodies look purple on Romanowsky stain, found in disorders of iron utilization like sideroblastic anemias.

Heinz bodies are denatured hemoglobin seen in oxidant injury and glucose-6-phosphate dehydrogenase (G6PD) deficiency.

Reticulocytes appear as polychromatic cells due to bluish reticular fragments (ribosomal proteins and RNA) in supravital staining. They are immature red cells that undergo full maturation after 1 or 2 days in circulation. Nucleated red cells are not part of normal blood picture but their presence suggests a premature release from bone marrow. Leukoerythroblastosis is the presence of leukocyte precursors in association with RBC precursors found in marrow fibrosis, severe sepsis, and marrow infiltrations (due to leukemia, lymphoma, myeloma, or secondary metastasis).

White Blood Cell Morphology and Aberrations (Fig. 2)

Leukocytosis is said to be present if WBC > 5 leukocytes/hpf and leukopenia < 2 cells/hpf (normal 2–5).

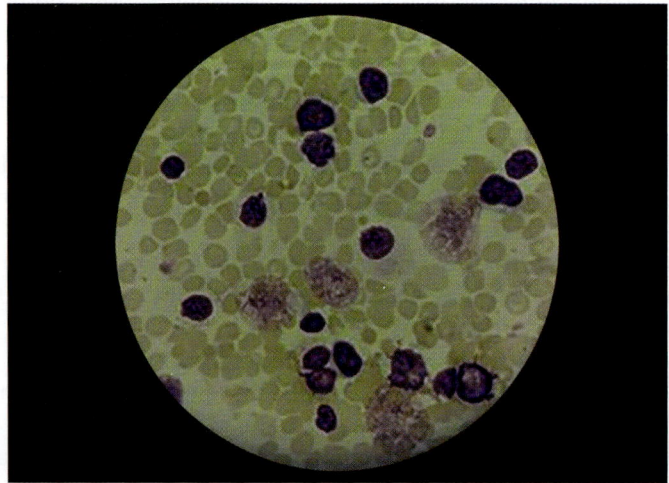

FIG. 2: Acute myeloid leukemia (AML).

Falsely elevated leukocyte count may be generated by the automated or manual counts due to circulating nucleated red cells. A PBF examination may be of help to correct the error. Corrected WBC may be calculated by [estimated WBC/(100 + number of nucleated RBCs among 100 WBCs)] × 100%. Hence, blood film remains a means of cross-checking high counts generated manually or from automated particle counters.

Mature neutrophils have segmented nucleus with 2-5 lobes joined by a thin filament. Less mature forms include bands forms, metamyelocyte, myelocyte, promyelocyte, and myeloblast.

Normally, mature segmented neutrophils are seen with band neutrophil population being less than 8% and metamyelocytes less than 0.5%.

However, an increase in the proportion of myeloid precursors is termed left shift. Severe neutrophilia with left shift is termed leukemoid reaction.

Neutrophil hypersegmentation is a diagnostic feature of megaloblastic anemia. It is defined by the presence of at least one neutrophil with six or more nuclear segments or at least 5% of circulating neutrophils with five nuclear segments. The Pelger–Huët anomaly, on the other hand, is an inherited disorder characterized by impaired nuclear segmentation of mature neutrophilic granulocytes, with bilobed nuclei.

Neutrophilia is commonly a response to bacterial infections, especially pyogenic infections. Other associations of neutrophilia include any form of acute inflammation (such as myocardial infarction), burns, corticosteroid use (inhibits neutrophil margination), malignancy, and chronic myelogenous leukemia.

Eosinophils are larger than neutrophils with bilobed nucleus and orange-red granules in the cytoplasm. Significant eosinophilia may be seen in allergies and parasitic infections. However, marked eosinophilia (>1,500/mL) suggests hypereosinophilic syndrome (especially with associated tissue damage) or a neoplastic entity, especially when there is an associated cellular dysplasia as in chronic eosinophilic leukemia.

Basophils are smaller than neutrophils and have large basophilic granules. Basophilia is seen in hypersensitivity states, lymphomas, and chronic myeloid leukemia.

Monocytes are the largest WBCs with blue-grey ground glass cytoplasm. Monocytosis is seen in tuberculosis, Crohn's disease, chronic myeloid leukemia, and acute myeloid leukemia.

Lymphocyte

The small lymphocytes are round with high nuclear cytoplasmic ratio (N:C ratio) and scanty, pale, dark blue cytoplasm, which is the most common type found in the normal film. Large lymphocytes have lower N:C ratio. When large lymphocytes have cytoplasmic granules, they are termed large granular lymphocytes and they represent cytotoxic T lymphocytes or natural killer (NK) cells. Reactive lymphocytes are usually larger and at times have deep blue staining of the periphery of the cytoplasm with bean-shaped nuclei.

Relative lymphocytosis is normally seen in children aged <5 years, acute viral infections, connective tissue diseases, thyrotoxicosis, and adrenocortical insufficiency.

Causes of absolute lymphocytosis include infectious mononucleosis syndromes, hepatitis, pertussis, tuberculosis, brucellosis, and lymphatic leukemias. Neoplastic lymphoid blasts are large with a high N:C ratio.

WBC Inclusions and Implications

Toxic granulation refers to small, dark blue-staining granules in bacterial sepsis.

Döhle bodies are light blue cytoplasmic inclusions; 1–2 μm in diameter, they are remnants of rough endoplasmic reticulum seen in myeloid left shifts.

Platelets and their Abnormalities

Platelets are approximately 2–4 μm in diameter with coarse cytoplasmic granules. A platelet/hpf is equivalent to approximately 15,000–20,000 platelets in circulation.

Platelets with diameters >3 μm are considered "large," which normally occur in <5% of the platelets. They may also be found in idiopathic thrombocytopenic purpura, myeloproliferative and myelodysplastic disorders, and Bernard–Soulier syndrome.

Thrombocytopenia mechanisms are reduced production (aplastic anemia), increased peripheral destruction (disseminated intravascular coagulopathies, thrombotic microangiopathies), or increased splenic sequestration (hypersplenism). Thrombocytopenia may be spurious (pseudothrombocytopenia) in EDTA-induced platelet aggregation or presence of clots in the blood specimen.

■ ARTIFACTS THAT WE SHOULD BE AWARE OF

Many artifacts may be found in a peripheral film and we should be aware of them.

Cytoplasmic vacuoles of red cells are an artifact, and granulocytes of blood anticoagulated with EDTA may acquire cytoplasmic vacuoles.

Echinocytes (crenated red cells) may be caused by hypertonicity or alkalinity of the staining solution while stomatocytes may be a result of a too-acidic staining solution. Naturally occurring target cells are distributed uniformly throughout the slide but if found localized, are an artifact.

Leukocytes may rupture during the smear preparation, producing an amorphous nuclear material-forming "basket" cell. The lymphocytes of chronic lymphocytic leukemia are particularly prone to rupture.

■ PARASITE DETECTION IN PERIPHERAL BLOOD SMEAR (FIGS. 3 AND 4)

A very important use of a PBS is the diagnosis of intracellular parasites in Giemsa-stained thick and thin blood films, although other stains such as a Wright stain, a Wright-Giemsa stain, or a rapid stain such as a Field stain are options. The use of inexpensive, easily available resources (staining materials and high-quality microscopes) is an advantage but the diagnosis also requires well-trained and

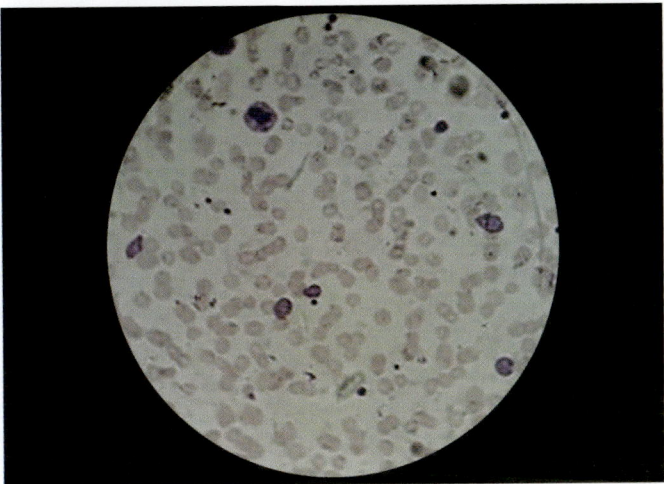

FIG. 3: Malarial schizonts.

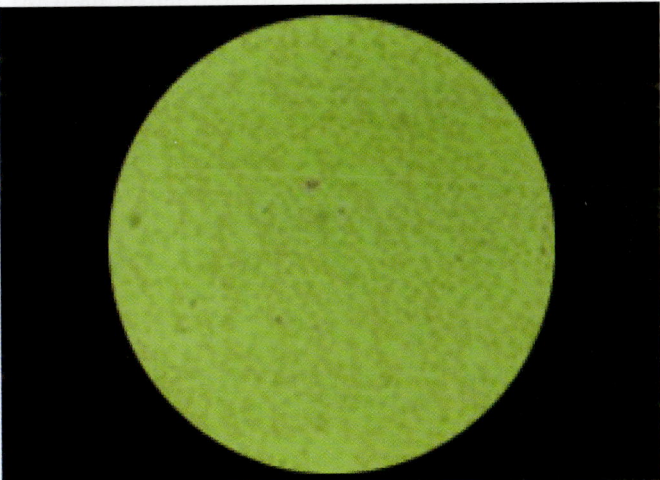

FIG. 4: Malarial gametocyte.

experienced technologists. Timely examination of the slide by 2–3 hours of sample collection is imperative for the diagnosis of malaria. Also, if blood is collected in tubes containing EDTA, parasite morphology may be distorted if preparation of the slides is delayed. Thick blood films are ideal for the detection of parasites consistent with either *Plasmodium* or *Babesia*, but identification of a particular species of *Plasmodium* needs thin film evaluation along with determination of the level of parasitemia.

Fallacy: The Simian parasite *Plasmodium knowlesi* has morphologic features similar to those of *Plasmodium malariae*, but the severity may be manifold. Because of difficulty in differentiation, molecular testing may be required.

Babesia and *Plasmodium* species may at times look similar on smears and both can be transmitted by transfusion. The quantitative buffy coat method detects fluorescently stained parasites within RBCs and requires specialized equipment. Still preparation of a thin blood smear is required if a quantitative buffy coat sample is positive for parasites, for specific identification and level of parasitemia.

The standard method for diagnosis of lymphatic filariasis is microscopy of thick and thin blood or buffy coat films stained with Giemsa or other appropriate stains Well-trained personnel are needed for the preparation and examination of these slides. The quantitative buffy coat system may increase sensitivity but thin smears would be required to determine identification of any microfilaria present. Concentration methods can increase the sensitivity of light microscopy. *Wuchereria bancrofti* and *Brugia malayi* may have nocturnal periodicity (depending on the geographic origin of the infection), and blood may be best examined from 10 PM to 2 AM.

CONCLUSION

Peripheral blood smear examination has many advantages. It helps in the diagnosis of some diseases such as malaria, chronic myeloid leukemia (CML), and sickle cell anemia. At times, it gives direction for further workup in nutritional anemias, malignancies, and myeloproliferative diseases. Investigations like cytochemistry, flow cytometry, cytogenetics, or molecular techniques may be indicated according the clues given by a smear. Some fallacies/errors in automated counters may be corrected. Most importantly, it is a low cost, simple procedure with easy availability. Hence, the importance of PBS examination cannot be undermined even in the presence of modern investigations, especially in a resource-limited country like ours.

SUGGESTED READINGS

1. Bain BJ. Diagnosis from the blood Smear. N Engl J Med. 2005;353:498-507.
2. Peterson LC, Sandhaus LM, Spier CM, Ward PCJ. Physician review of the peripheral blood smear: when and why. Lab Hematol. 2001;7:175-9.
3. Ryan DH. Examination of the blood. In: Beutler E, Lichtman MA, Coller BS, et al. (Eds). Williams Hematology, 6th edition. New York: McGraw-Hill; 2001. pp. 12-14.
4. Constantino BT, Cogionis B. Nucleated RBCs: significance in the peripheral blood film. Lab Med. 2000;31(4):223-9.
5. Bainton DF. Morphology of neutrophils, eosinophils, and basophils. Williams Hematology, 7th edition. New York: McGraw-Hill; 2006.
6. Bain BJ. Blood cell morphology in health and disease. Dacie and Lewis Practical Hematology, 11th edition. London: Churchill Livingstone; 2012. pp. 69-100.
7. Bessis M, Lessin LS, Beutler E. Morphology of the erythron. In: Williams WJ, Beutler E, Ersler AJ, et al. (Eds). Hematology, 3rd edition. New York: McGraw-Hill; 1983. pp. 257-79.
8. Zeigler Z, Murphy S, Gardner FH. Microscopic platelet size and morphology in various hematologic disorders. Blood. 1978;51:479-86.

Approach to Lymphadenopathy

Alladi Mohan, Srishti Ahluwalia, Saumya Ahluwalia, G Bindhu Madhavi

■ INTRODUCTION

The lymphatic system is composed of lymphatic vessels and lymphoid organs, such as the lymph nodes, tonsils, thymus, and spleen. These play a role in acquired and innate immunities. Lymph nodes are small, kidney-shaped structures around 1–2 cm located along the course of lymphatic vessels, mainly at the convergence of major blood vessels. The hilum is the point where blood vessels enter and leave the lymph node. Normal size depends upon the location as well as the axis, which is being measured. The long axis should be 1 cm or less. They are considered abnormal if there is change in size or shape, loss of the hilar fat, or an asymmetrical thickening of the cortex. Lymph node enlargement generally results from cellular proliferation of lymph node components associated with the normal immune response to antigens. This is also caused by infiltration of the lymph node by malignant cells or substance deposition.

■ PERIPHERAL LYMPHADENOPATHY

In normal healthy individuals, peripheral lymph nodes are seldom palpable. Peripheral lymphadenopathy is said to be present if the lymph nodes are abnormal in size, consistency, or number. Significantly enlarged lymph nodes are generally greater than 1 cm in diameter. However, subcentimeter lymph nodes that are palpable in supraclavicular, popliteal, and epitrochlear regions are also considered abnormal. In India, barefoot walking is a common practice; therefore, clinical significance of inguinal lymphadenopathy in barefoot walkers is to be interpreted with caution.

Diagnostic Approach

A careful history and physical examination, associated symptoms, and distribution of the lymphadenopathy will aid in the clinical diagnosis. Some of the frequently encountered causes of lymphadenopathy in adults are listed in **Table 1**.

Approach to Lymphadenopathy

TABLE 1: Some of the common causes of lymphadenopathy.	
Etiology	**Common causes**
Infections	
Bacterial	*Staphylococcus*, *Streptococcus*, cat-scratch fever, chancroid, melioidosis, tuberculosis, nontuberculous mycobacterial infections, primary and secondary syphilis
Viral	Infectious mononucleosis (EBV), CMV, hepatitis, postvaccinial lymphadenitis, adenovirus, herpes zoster, HIV/AIDS, HTLV-1
Others	Lymphogranuloma venereum, toxoplasmosis, histoplasmosis, coccidioidomycosis, scrub typhus, filariasis, *Cryptococcus* infections
Malignancy	
Hematological	Hodgkin's disease, NHL, acute and chronic leukemia, Waldenström macroglobulinemia, multiple myeloma (rarely), systemic mastocytosis, Kaposi's sarcoma
Metastatic "solid" tumors	Breast, lung, renal cell, prostate, other malignancies
Hypersensitivity syndromes	Serum sickness, drug-sensitivity
Connective tissue diseases	Rheumatoid arthritis, SLE, dermatomyositis, MCTD, Sjögren's syndrome, Castleman disease, lymphomatoid granulomatosis, granulomatosis with polyangiitis (Wegener's granulomatosis)
Other granulomatous disorders	Sarcoidosis, silicosis, berylliosis
Drugs, medications	Allopurinol, atenolol, carbamazepine, phenytoin, quinidine
Others	Kawasaki disease, Kikuchi–Fujimoto disease, Kimura disease, SHML, LCH, HLH, AOSD

(AOSD: adult-onset Still's disease; CMV: cytomegalovirus; EBV: Epstein–Barr virus; HIV–AIDS: human immunodeficiency virus/acquired immunodeficiency syndrome; HLH: hemophagocytic lymphohistiocytosis; HTLV-1: human T-lymphotropic virus type 1; LCH: Langerhans cell histiocytosis; MCTD: mixed connective tissue disease; NHL: non-Hodgkin's lymphoma; SLE: systemic lupus erythematosus)

History and Physical Examination

A detailed history is the most important step in evaluation of the patient with lymphadenopathy. This includes age of the patient, duration of lymphadenopathy, travel history, exposure to toxins or infections or exposure to animals, sexual history, recent immunization history, current medication, and history of fever and other associated symptoms such as fatigue, weight loss, night sweats, joint pain or swelling, and rash. In children, lymphadenopathy is most likely physiological or infectious in etiology. Lymphadenopathy lasting <2 weeks or >12 months without change in size has a low likelihood of being neoplastic.

Physical examination in a patient with peripheral lymphadenopathy would include careful examination of the Waldeyer's ring [nasal-associated lymphoid tissue (NALT)] consisting of palatine tonsils, nasopharyngeal tonsil (adenoid) and lingual tonsils, the tubal tonsils, and lateral pharyngeal bands. The Waldeyer's ring belongs to the mucosa-associated lymphoid tissue (MALT) and is located at the gateway of the respiratory and alimentary tract.

Assessment of the lymph nodes on physical examination would also include the distribution of lymphadenopathy, consistency of lymph nodes, warmth, overlying redness, tenderness, mobility, consistency, and fluctuation. It is imperative to carefully examine the draining area of the lymph nodes to look for clues for the causation of lymphadenopathy, such as, evidence of infection, among others.

Clinically, lymphadenopathy is classified as *localized* (when lymphadenopathy is present in only one region) and *generalized* when it involves two or more noncontiguous sites. Lymphadenopathy can also be categorized as acute or chronic.

Acute Lymphadenopathy

In patients presenting with acute lymphadenopathy, the lymph nodes enlarge rapidly and are usually painful and tender. Bacterial, viral, and rarely fungal infections are common causes of acute lymphadenitis. Other noninfectious cases also present with acute lymphadenitis such as systemic lupus erythematosus and Kikuchi–Fujimoto disease (KFD), among others. KFD is a self-limiting, acute, lymphadenitis more frequently seen in young women. It involves cervical lymph nodes most frequently, and clinically mimics bacterial lymphadenitis. Kawasaki disease, a medium vessel vasculitis of childhood, should be considered in case of acute lymphadenopathy not resolving with antibiotics; it is known to present with acute-onset or chronic lymphadenopathy.

Chronic Lymphadenopathy

Patients with tuberculosis (TB) lymphadenopathy usually present with slowly enlarging lymph nodes. Isolated cervical lymphadenopathy is the most common clinical presentation. Axillary and inguinal lymph nodes may also be involved. Associated intrathoracic (hilar, mediastinal) and intra-abdominal (mesenteric, porta hepatis, retroperitoneal) lymphadenopathies may also be present sometimes. In patients with peripheral lymph node TB, fever, and constitutional symptoms are rare. Cough may be a prominent symptom in patients with mediastinal lymphadenopathy; clinical presentation as fever of unknown origin (FUO) is increasingly being seen in adults. Matting is a characteristic feature of periadenitis in TB lymphadenopathy. Later on in the course of the disease, cold abscess, collar-stud abscess, and sinus formation are seen. In human immunodeficiency virus (HIV)-seropositive patients, multifocal lymphadenopathy and suppurative and nonreactive histopathological types are more common.

Lymphadenopathy is a common feature in patients with HIV/acquired immunodeficiency syndrome (AIDS). Lymphadenopathy can result from primary HIV-induced pathology and from diseases, such as TB lymphadenitis, nontuberculous mycobacterial lymphadenitis, nodal Kaposi's sarcoma, and nodal lymphoma, among others. Patients with leukemia and lymphoma can present with either acute or chronic lymphadenopathy.

Lymphadenopathy presenting as a painless, hard, irregular mass or a firm lesion that is immobile or fixed may be the feature of malignancy. Rubbery consistency of the lymph nodes may be seen in Hodgkin's disease. No specific lymph nodal size is indicative of malignancy and the tissue diagnosis should be ascertained by cytopathological/histopathological methods.

Chronic lymphadenopathy is also seen in case of infections, such as, cytomegalovirus (CMV), chlamydia, and treponema. It is also seen in certain autoimmune diseases like, sarcoidosis, Kawasaki disease, angiofollicular lymph node hyperplasia (Castleman disease).

Other Causes

Drugs and medications are known to cause lymphadenopathy. Some of the common drugs causing lymphadenopathy are listed in **Table 1**.

Some of the uncommon causes of lymphadenopathy are described below. Kimura disease is a rare disorder of unknown etiology that involves the lymph nodes of the head and neck region and is common in middle-aged Asian men. Associated laboratory abnormalities include elevated serum immunoglobulin E levels and peripheral blood eosinophilia. Sinus histiocytosis with massive lymphadenopathy (SHML, Rosai–Dorfman disease), Langerhans cell histiocytosis, hemophagocytic lymphohistiocytosis (HLH), adult-onset Still's disease (AOSD) also present with significant peripheral lymphadenopathy.

Laboratory Diagnosis, Imaging Studies, Endoscopic Methods

Laboratory evaluation consists of complete blood picture including peripheral smear, serum biochemistry, lactate dehydrogenase, specific investigations for infectious diseases. Various imaging modalities include ultrasonography, computed tomography (CT), ^{18}fluorodeoxyglucose positron emission tomography-computed tomography (^{18}FDG PET-CT). Pursuit of the cause of lymphadenopathy can sometimes be rewarding as it can facilitate recognition of underlying etiology in uncommon sites (e.g., myocardial TB). Image-guided FNAC, biopsy mediastinoscopy, video-assisted thoracoscopy, endobronchial ultrasound-guided transbronchial needle aspiration (EBUS-TBNA), laparoscopy can facilitate sampling and diagnostic testing.

In case of incidentally detected lymphadenopathy follow-up imaging in short intervals is done to establish a lesion to be unchanged and provide reassurance of its benign nature. Imaging studies are useful in determining the location of lymphadenopathy, pattern, and size of lymph nodes. They are also used to guide a biopsy, if needed.

Fine Needle Aspiration, Cytopathological Examination, Excision Biopsy

Fine needle aspiration, a cytopathological examination from the most accessible peripheral lymph node, is done for investigation of infectious causes. Early biopsy of palpable lymph nodes will lead to early diagnosis; excision biopsy is the *gold standard* and is preferred if malignancy is suspected.

Treatment

Most of the causes of lymphadenopathy are of infectious and malignant etiologies in adults. Management is based upon etiology, and institution of specific treatment is life-saving.

Inadequately worked-up lymphadenopathy may lead to deterioration of the underlying condition, which can result in significant morbidity and mortality. Thus, there is a need for a systematic clinical approach and early confirmation of diagnosis and treatment of lymphadenopathy. Patients with "reactive lymphadenopathy" should be followed-up for the emergence of other causes of lymphadenopathy subsequently.

CONCLUSION

Lymphadenopathy is caused by various infectious, noninfectious and malignant causes. A detailed history and a thorough clinical examination and appropriate laboratory investigations will guide in arriving at the aetiological diagnosis. Imaging modalities facilitate disease extent mapping and facilitated image-guided procedures for procuring lymph node tissue for diagnostic testing. In chronic lymphadenopathy procuring tissue from the representative lymph node followed by histopathological molecular and microbiological examination remains the gold standard for diagnosis. However, despite all the possible tests a few cases of lymphadenopathy can still remain undiagnosed and constitutes a diagnostic challenge. Careful clinical follow-up is helpful in this situation.

SUGGESTED READINGS

1. Gaddey HL, Riegel AM. Unexplained lymphadenopathy: evaluation and differential diagnosis. Am Fam Physician. 2016;94:896-903.
2. Bontumasi N, Jacobson JA, Caoili E, et al. Inguinal lymph nodes: size, number, and other characteristics in asymptomatic patients by CT. Surg Radiol Anat. 2014;36:1051-5.
3. King D, Ramachandra J, Yeomanson D. Lymphadenopathy in children: refer or reassure? Arch Dis Child Educ Pract Ed. 2014;99:101-10.
4. Bazemore AW, Smucker DR. Lymphadenopathy and malignancy. Am Fam Physician. 2002;66: 2103-10.
5. Chau I, Kelleher MT, Cunningham D, et al. Rapid access multidisciplinary lymph node diagnostic clinic: analysis of 550 patients. Br J Cancer. 2003;88:354-61.
6. Mohan A, Reddy MK, Phaneendra BV, et al. Etiology of peripheral lymphadenopathy in adults: analysis of 1,724 cases seen at a tertiary care teaching hospital in southern India. Natl Med J India. 2007;20:78-80.
7. Zeppa P, Cozzolino I. Lymphadenitis and lymphadenopathy. Monogr Clin Cytol. 2018;23:19-33.
8. Perry AM, Choi SM. Kikuchi–Fujimoto disease: a review. Arch Pathol Lab Med. 2018;142:1341-6.
9. Rife E, Gedalia A. Kawasaki disease: an update. Curr Rheumatol Rep. 2020;22:75.
10. Jindal SK, Aggarwal AN, Gupta D, et al. Tuberculous lymphadenopathy: a multicenter operational study of 6-month thrice weekly directly observed treatment. Int J Tuberc Lung Dis. 2013;17:234-9.
11. Habermann TM, Steensma DP. Lymphadenopathy. Mayo Clin Proc. 2000;75:723-32.
12. Mohan A, Sharma MC, Pande I, et al. Sinus histiocytosis with massive lymphadenopathy. A case report. J Assoc Physicians India. 1996;44:418-9.
13. Allen CE, Merad M, McClain KL. Langerhans-cell histiocytosis. N Engl J Med. 2018;379:856-68.
14. Ramos-Casals M, Brito-Zerón P, López-Guillermo A, et al. Adult hemophagocytic syndrome. Lancet. 2014;383:1503-16.
15. Giacomelli R, Ruscitti P, Shoenfeld Y. A comprehensive review on adult onset Still's disease. J Autoimmun. 2018;93:24-36.
16. Solav SV. FDG PET/CT in evaluation of pyrexia of unknown origin. Clin Nucl Med. 2011;36:e81-6.
17. Mohan A, Thachil A, Sundar G, et al. Ventricular tachycardia and tuberculous lymphadenopathy: sign of myocardial tuberculosis? J Am Coll Cardiol. 2015;65:218-20.
18. Mohan A, Prabath Kumar D, Harikrishna J. Isolated mediastinal lymphadenopathy in a young adolescent. In: Kar M (Ed). Clinical Medicine Update—2010. Agra: Indian Academy of Clinical Medicine; 2010. pp.193-204.

CHAPTER 44

Approach to Pancytopenia

BL Bhardwaj

INTRODUCTION

Cytopenia is a reduction in the number of each type of peripheral blood cell. A reduction in all the three types of cellular components in peripheral blood is termed pancytopenia and this involves anemia, neutropenia, and thrombocytopenia.

Initially, mild impairment in marrow function is inapparent and pancytopenia may become apparent only during times of stress or increased demand (e.g., bleeding or infection). More severe degrees of cytopenias affect the peripheral blood count even in the steady state.

Severe pancytopenia is defined as follows:
- Absolute neutrophil count <500/mm^3
- Platelet count <20,000/mm^3
- Corrected reticulocyte count <1%

What is Normal Marrow Activity?

The normal adult marrow produces about 1.7×10^{11} RBC, 1.0×10^{11} neutrophils, and 2×10^{11} platelets each day and thus it has a tremendous capacity to substantially increase the output of these cells when necessary with the help of growth factors and other cytokines. All peripheral blood cells arise from common progenitor cells known as pluripotent stem cells which have enormous capacity of self-renewal that ensures their continuous supply throughout the lifetime of the individual. Whenever necessary, a pluripotent stem cell can begin to differentiate (thus gradually losing its capacity of self-renewal) leading to individual clone of differentiated cells. The circumstances that lead to pancytopenia due to bone marrow failure include both defects in the stem cells (i.e., seed) or defects in the stromal cells or micro-environment (i.e., soil). However, quite obviously majority of the defects are in the stem cells.

WHAT IS THE ETIOPATHOGENESIS OF PANCYTOPENIA?

Aplastic anemia is one of the most serious causes of pancytopenia. Marrow failure leading to pancytopenia may result from immune-mediated or nonimmune-mediated damage or suppression of either pluripotent stem cells or committed progenitor cells. Fortunately, serious damage to pluripotent cells is less common because these cells are relatively resistant to the effects of most cytotoxic agents (notable exceptions are radiation and the drug busulfan which mainly affect pluripotent stem cells). Interestingly, most cytotoxic drugs used in the treatment of malignancies exert their major effects on committed progenitor cells. Ablation of these cells result in marrow hypoplasia but recovery is still possible by regeneration from the pluripotent stem-cell compartment.

Pancytopenia from bone marrow failure is also an important feature of acute leukemias, the later stages of chronic leukemias, myeloproliferative disorders, and myelodysplasias. The mechanisms of marrow failure in these diseases are unclear but probably involve active suppression of normal hematopoiesis as well as bone marrow infiltration by these abnormal cells.

The different causes of pancytopenia due to bone marrow failure are enumerated in **Box 1**.

OVERVIEW OF COMMON CAUSES OF PANCYTOPENIA

Megaloblastic anemia: Megaloblastic hematopoiesis is a hypercellular bone marrow failure due to deficiency of vitamin B12 (cobalamin) and folate. These nutrients have important role in synthesis of DNA.

Megaloblastic anemia is a predominant cause of pancytopenia in India because of high prevalence of nutritional anemia in Indian subcontinent. Vitamin B12 deficiency may also cause subacute combined degeneration of cord and psychiatric

---

BOX 1: Causes of pancytopenia.

Bone marrow failure
Hypoplastic/aplastic anemia: Inherited, idiopathic, viral, drugs

Bone marrow infiltration
- Acute leukemia
- Carcinoma
- Lymphoma
- Myeloma
- Hemophagocytic syndrome
- Myelodysplastic syndromes

Ineffective hematopoiesis
- Megaloblastic anemia
- Acquired immunodeficiency syndrome (AIDS)

Peripheral pooling/destruction
- Hypersplenism: Portal hypertension, malaria, Felty's syndrome, myelofibrosis
- Systemic lupus erythematosus

illness (megaloblastic madness). The degree of bone marrow suppression is inversely related to presence and severity of neurological dysfunction.

Hypersplenism: Hypersplenism is characterized by splenomegaly, cytopenia(s), normal or hyperplastic bone marrow, and a response to splenectomy. In hypersplenism, there is peripheral pooling and destruction of cells in enlarged spleen resulting in pancytopenia. Causes of hypersplenism include congestive splenomegaly (cirrhosis, congestive heart failure), malaria, hyper-reactive malarial splenomegaly, leishmaniasis, thalassemia, and Hodgkin's disease. Hypersplenism can rarely be idiopathic.

Infections: Hematological abnormalities have been frequently observed in patients with HIV infection. Pancytopenia is usually seen in advanced stage of HIV infection. Etiology of pancytopenia in advanced HIV stage is multifactorial in nature and includes high viral load, use of antiretroviral therapy, and presence of acute or chronic opportunistic infection. Viral hepatitis has been known to cause transient pancytopenia during the course of illness and has also been associated with aplastic anemia. Hepatitis associated with pancytopenia and aplastic anemia is usually fatal. Whereas hepatitis B and hepatitis C are common causes—Epstein-Barr virus, cytomegalovirus, and rarely hepatitis A and dengue virus can also cause pancytopenia. Mild blood count depression is common in course of many viral and bacterial infections but resolves with the resolution of infection. Sepsis and enteric fever continue to be important public health problems in India and have been associated with pancytopenia which has been attributed to bone marrow suppression, disseminated intravascular coagulation, and infection associated hemophagocytic syndrome. Tuberculosis is a common disease in India. Disseminated miliary tuberculosis is known to cause pancytopenia. Although pancytopenia is a rare presentation of tuberculosis, it should always be considered in patients presenting with pancytopenia, unexplained pyrexia and weight loss. Both tuberculous bacilli and antituberculous therapy have been implicated in pathogenesis of pancytopenia. *Wuchereria bancrofti* is an endemic filarial nematode spread by a mosquito vector. The clinical manifestations vary from asymptomatic microfilaremia to lymphedema. Cases of microfilaria in bone marrow aspirate presenting as pancytopenia in peripheral blood have been reported. Though, etiopathological correlation of pancytopenia with microfilaria infection is not clear.

Aplastic anemia: Aplastic anemia is defined as pancytopenia with hypocellular marrow in absence of abnormal infiltrate or increased fibrosis. It is a normocytic normochromic anemia that results from a loss of blood cell precursors, causing hypoplasia of bone marrow leading to pancytopenia. Severe aplastic anemia is defined as a bone marrow cellularity <25% with at least two of the three criteria, i.e., neutrophils <500/µL, platelets <20,000/µL, and reticulocyte count <20,000/µL. It is a potentially life-threatening failure of bone marrow. Most cases of aplastic anemia are acquired and T-cell mediated autoimmune disease. Triggering factors may include drugs, viruses, and toxins but most cases are idiopathic. In some cases radiation, drugs, toxic chemicals, and viruses induce depletion of hematopoietic stem cells by direct toxicity.

Paroxysmal nocturnal hemoglobinuria (PNH): PNH is an acquired chronic hemolytic anemia characterized by persistent intravascular hemolysis with recurrent exacerbations due to activation of complement C. In addition to hemolysis, there is often pancytopenia and a risk of venous thrombosis. Hemolysis in PNH is due to an intrinsic abnormality of the red cell, which makes it sensitive to activated complement C. Diagnostic gold standard of PNH is flow cytometry which can be carried out on granulocytes as well as on RBC. A bimodal distribution of cells with a discrete population that is CD59 and CD55 negative is diagnostic of PNH.

Acute leukemias: Acute myeloid leukemia occurs in all age group but predominantly in older adults. Acute lymphoblastic leukemia is the most common acute leukemia in childhood. Clinical history and symptoms usually indicate bone marrow failure. These include fatigue, dyspnea, dizziness, bleeding, easy bruising, and recurrent infections. Cytogenetic abnormalities are prognostically important and affect patient management. In all cases of severe pancytopenia (symptomatic anemia, WBC <500/µL, and platelets <20,000/µL) investigations are mandatory within first 24-49 h. Supportive therapy with RBC, platelets, and broad spectrum antibiotics may be initiated before underlying cause has been ascertained.

Myelodysplastic syndrome: Myelodysplastic syndromes (MDS) are the common hematological diseases characterized by cytopenias associated with abnormal appearing cellular marrow producing ineffective red blood cells The incidence of MDS increases with advancing age, median age at disease onset is 70 years with only about 10% of the patients below 50 years MDS are diseases of hematopoietic stem cells. They are characterized by disturbance of differentiation and maturation, and by changes in the bone marrow stroma. MDS are accompanied not only by reducing blood cell counts but also with an increased risk (20-25%) of developing acute myeloid leukemia.

Systemic lupus erythematosus (SLE): Hematologic abnormalities such as anemia, leukopenia, and thrombocytopenia secondary to peripheral destruction are commonly seen in SLE. Most frequent hematologic manifestation of SLE is normocytic and normochromic anemia. Leukopenia is also common and almost always consists of lymphopenia and not granulocytopenia. Thrombocytopenia may be a recurring problem in SLE. Cytopenias from autoimmune myelofibrosis are also uncommonly seen in SLE.

Drug-induced pancytopenia: Drugs are the common causes of pancytopenia. Drug-induced pancytopenia can be dose dependent or immune mediated (idiosyncratic). Chloramphenicol can cause pancytopenia by both the mechanisms. Azathioprine, an immunosuppressant drug. Neomercazole used for treatment of various diseases, usually causes leukopenia and rarely *pancytopenia.*

Congenital causes: Fanconi's anemia is an autosomal recessive disorder and manifests as congenital developmental anomaly, progressive pancytopenia, and an increased risk of malignancy. Patients typically have short stature, café-au-lait spots, and anomalies involving thumb, radius, and genitourinary tract. Dyskeratosis congenita is characterized by mucous membrane leukoplakia, dystrophic nails, reticular hyperpigmentation, and development of aplastic anemia during childhood.

APPROACH TO A CASE OF PANCYTOPENIA

Evaluation of pancytopenia requires a careful history and physical examination. The causes of pancytopenia are diverse. Attention must be paid to history of the patient and the family. Nutritional history, drug history and history of alcohol intake should always be assessed. History suggestive of previous pancytopenia, aplastic anemia, inherited bone marrow failure syndrome, repeated early fetal loss, cancer, liver disease, metabolic disorders, or connective tissue disorder is important. Cytotoxic chemotherapy and radiotherapy are the important causes of transient pancytopenia. History of weight loss and anorexia may suggest underlying infection or malignancy. Recurrent oral ulcers and chronic diarrhea may point toward HIV infection. Recurrent oral ulcers, malar rash and joint pain may suggest SLE. Bone pain and loss of height indicate multiple myeloma. A thorough physical examination is of paramount importance in evaluation of pancytopenia. It should include assessment of jaundice, clubbing of fingers, lymphadenopathy, and splenomegaly (underlying infection, infectious mononucleosis, lymphoproliferative disorder, and malignancy), loss of height (suggestive of multiple myeloma), malar rash, retinal hemorrhage, oral petechiae, gingival hyperplasia, stomatitis or cheilitis, oropharyngeal candidiasis, right upper quadrant (RUQ) abdominal tenderness, signs of chronic liver disease. *Laboratory evaluation:* A routine complete blood count (CBC) is required as a part of initial evaluation of pancytopenia. CBC should include red cell indices, peripheral blood film, reticulocytes count, and absolute reticulocyte count. A very high MCV (>110 fl) indicates megaloblastic anemia. In addition liver function test, viral markers for hepatitis, coagulation profile, fibrinogen, D-dimer, serum B12, folate levels, HIV serology, antinuclear antibodies (ANA) should be done. Serum ferritin levels should also be assessed. Low levels of serum ferritin along with low serum B12 and/or folate levels may indicate mixed anemia/pancytopenia. Peripheral blood smear provides important information in pancytopenia and it should always be done prior to transfusion of blood. Blood smear may reveal polychromasia-red cells that are slightly larger than normal and grayish blue in color. These cells are reticulocytes that have been prematurely released from the bone marrow.

These cells may appear in circulation due to architectural damage of the bone marrow caused by fibrosis or malignant cell infiltration. Bone marrow examination is almost always indicated in cases of pancytopenia unless the cause is otherwise apparent (e.g., chronic liver disease with portal hypertension, deficiency of vitamin B12 or folate). In megaloblastic anemia, bone marrow shows megaloblastic erythroid hyperplasia, sieved nuclear chromatin, asynchronous nuclear maturation, bluish cytoplasm with cytoplasmic blebs. Giant metamyelocytes and band forms are predominant in granulocyte series. Bone marrow in aplastic anemia is hypocellular with suppression of erythropoiesis, myelopoiesis, and megakaryopoiesis with relative lymphoplasmacytosis. In acute leukemias, bone marrow is hypercellular with reduced erythroid and megakaryocytic series and majority of cells are myeloblast or lymphoblast. Bone marrow aspiration in AML shows myeloblasts with Auer rods.

Absolute Reticulocyte Count

An accurate reticulocyte count is the key to initial evaluation of pancytopenia. Normally, reticulocytes are the red cells that have been recently released from the bone marrow. Normal reticulocyte count ranges from 1 to 2% and reflects the daily replacement of 0.8–1% of the circulating RBC population. Reticulocyte count provides reliable measure of RBC production. Reticulocyte count and absolute reticulocyte count (ARC) should be done on day one along with CBC in order to avoid therapy related changes in reticulocyte count particularly with nutritional anemia. Absolute reticulocyte count is a calculated index derived from the product of reticulocyte count percentage and RBC count (Normal: Male: 4.32–5.72 million/mm, Female: 3.90–5.03 million/mm). ARC is a marker of red cell production by bone marrow. It plays important role in establishing the cause of pancytopenia and helps in distinguishing between hypoproliferative and hyperproliferative anemias. Normal range of absolute reticulocyte count is 50,000–100,000/mm. All cases of pancytopenia with very low ARC (<25,000/ mm) should be examined by bone marrow aspiration for aplastic anemia. All cases of pancytopenia with high ARC (>100,000/mm) should also be evaluated by bone marrow aspiration unless there is a history suggestive of sepsis or malaria. Pancytopenia with ARC 25,000–50,000/mm should initially be evaluated with serum B12, folate and ferritin assays and if any one of these is found to be low, bone marrow aspiration is not needed.

Specific Evaluation

- *Lymphoproliferative disorders:* Immunophenotyping, cytogenetics, lymph node biopsy
- *Multiple myeloma:* Serum electrophoresis, bone marrow aspiration
- *Paroxysmal nocturnal hemoglobinuria:* Flow cytometry (CD55, CD59)
- *Cytomegalovirus (CMV) infection:* Serology for CMV (IgG, Ig/M)
- *Epstein-Barr virus:* Serum monospot, viral capsid antigen, EB nuclear antibody
- *Leishmaniasis:* Blood and bone marrow culture, LD bodies
- *Carcinoma prostate:* Serum PSA
- *Fanconi's anemia:* Diepoxybutane test for chromosomal breakage in peripheral blood lymphocyte

CONCLUSION

The basic management of patients with pancytopenia involves identification and reversal of the underlying cause and adequate supportive care until normal counts are restored. It must be emphasized that bleeding and infection due to cytopenias is a medical emergency. Anemia is corrected by transfusion of packed red cells to maintain hemoglobin (Hb) level above 8–9 g/dL. The scope of granulocyte transfusions for the management of neutropenia is very limited as well as controversial because of inconsistent rise in leucocyte count, prohibitive cost, unreliability in the homing of infused granulocytes at the sites of infection, possibility of allosensitization, and GVHD. Reverse barrier isolation is one of the most cost-effective measures in the management of pancytopenia. Scrupulous hand washing by medical and healthcare personnel routinely before examining any patient of pancytopenia is a simple modality for infection prophylaxis. The availability of recombinant growth factors like granulocyte colony macrophage colony stimulating factor (GM-CSF), and recombinant erythropoietin (rhu EPO) have enabled more specific management with improved outcome of the pancytopenic patients. Immunosuppressive therapy with anti-lymphocyte globulin (ALG) and/or cyclosporine has proved to be effective in achieving remission in aplastic anemia.

SUGGESTED READINGS

1. Kar M, Ghosh A. Pancytopenia. J Ind Acad Clin Med. 2002;3:29-34.
2. Gayatri BN, Rao KS. Pancytopenia: A clinico-haematological study. J Lab Physician. 2011;3:15-20.
3. Kumar R, Kalra SP, Kumar H, et al. Pancytopenia--a six year study. J Assoc Physician India. 2001;49:1078-81.
4. Jain A, Naniwadekar M. An etiological reappraisal of pancytopenia-largest series reported to date from a tertiary care teaching hospital. BMC Hematol. 2013;13(1):10.
5. Khunger JM, Arulselvi S, Sharma U, et al. Pancytopenia- A Clinico Haematological study of 200 cases. Indian J Pathol Microbiol. 2002;45:375-9.
6. Priya PP, Subhashree AR. Role of absolute reticulocyte count in evaluation of Pancytopenia: A Hospital based study. J Clin Diagn Res. 2014;8: FC01-03.
7. Eduardo J, Rodriguez S, Mayer AM, et al. Profile of HIV infected Hispanics with Pancytopenia. Int J Environ Res Public Health. 2016;13:38.
8. Martinez Faci C, Ros Arnal I, Martines de Zabarte Fernandes JM, et al. Azathioprine induced pancytopenia: case series. Arch Argent Pediatr. 2016;114:e252-5.
9. Jain M, Shukla A, Kumar A, et al. *Wuchereria bancrofti*: Unusual presentation as Pancytopenia. J Clin Diagn Res. 2016;10:ED05-6.
10. Ungprasert P, Chowdhary VR, Davis M, et al. Autoimmune myelofibrosis with pancytopenia as a presenting manifestation of SLE responsive to mycophenolate mofetil. Lupus. 2016;25:427-30.
11. Azad MA, Le Y, Zhang Q, et al. Detection of pancytopenia associated with clinical manifestation and their final diagnosis. Open J Blood Dis. 2015;5:17-30.

CHAPTER 45

Updated Antiretroviral Therapy Guidelines: 2022 and Beyond

BB Rewari

INTRODUCTION

Antiretroviral therapy (ART) has been a panacea for people living with HIV (PLHIV), saving lives, and improving the quality of life of those infected. ART has helped millions of people across globe in returning to their work and reduced hospitalizations and consequent massive economic and social benefits. Over the years, newer drugs have been discovered which are less toxic, have lesser pill burden, and are available at lower costs. Most countries have scaled up free ART programs and wider coverage has led to HIV being regarded as a chronic manageable disease just like other chronic conditions such as diabetes and hypertension.

WHAT IS ANTIRETROVIRAL THERAPY AND HOW TO TAKE IT?

Antiretroviral therapy consists of use of combination of three drugs from different groups to inhibit the replication of HIV and reduce viremia to undetectable levels. The suppression of viral replication leads to restoration of immune response and slowing of the disease progression reflected by increase in CD4 cell count, reduced frequency of opportunistic infections (OIs), improvement in the quality of life, and increased longevity. The ART besides treating those with HIV infection is also used for prevention of transmission of HIV from an infected pregnant woman to her child (PMTCT) and also for prevention of infection among healthcare workers accidentally exposed to HIV while caring for their patients [postexposure prophylaxis (PEP)]. The antiretroviral (ARV) drugs are also approved for pre-exposure prophylaxis (PrEP) among high-risk groups for prevention of HIV.

The ARV drugs act by blocking the replication of HIV at different stages of HIV life cycle but cannot eradicate the latently infected CD4 cells that are established during the earliest stages of acute HIV infection and persist long half-life in the lymphoid tissue in gut, spleen, lymph nodes, and brain. The moment ART is withdrawn in a person who has shown viral suppression, the latent virus in reservoir starts replicating again and becomes detectable again. Hence, the basic purpose of providing ART is to keep virus replication suppressed so that the CD4 cell destruction is stopped and a person gets immune restoration. So, it is important to take ART lifelong with good adherence so that the virus remains suppressed. This also helps in preventing the transmission of virus.

■ WHAT ANTIRETROVIRAL DRUGS ARE AVAILABALE AND HOW DO THESE ACT?

Ever since the first ARV drug, Zidovudine (AZT), was approved in 1985, there has been a rapid expansion of the drug portfolio and now more than 26 ARV drugs and combinations are available; most of these are available in India. These drugs act on various stages of replication of HIV in the body and interrupt the process of viral replication. **Figure 1** depicts various enzymes involved in viral replication and the points where ARVs target the virus and **Table 1** shows various groups of ARV drugs

■ WHEN TO START ANTIRETROVIRAL THERAPY AND FOR WHOM?

There has been a debate for quite some time on optimal time to start ART based on the CD4 count or the World Health Organization (WHO) clinical stage of the person infected with HIV. The guidelines have been evolving based on the results from

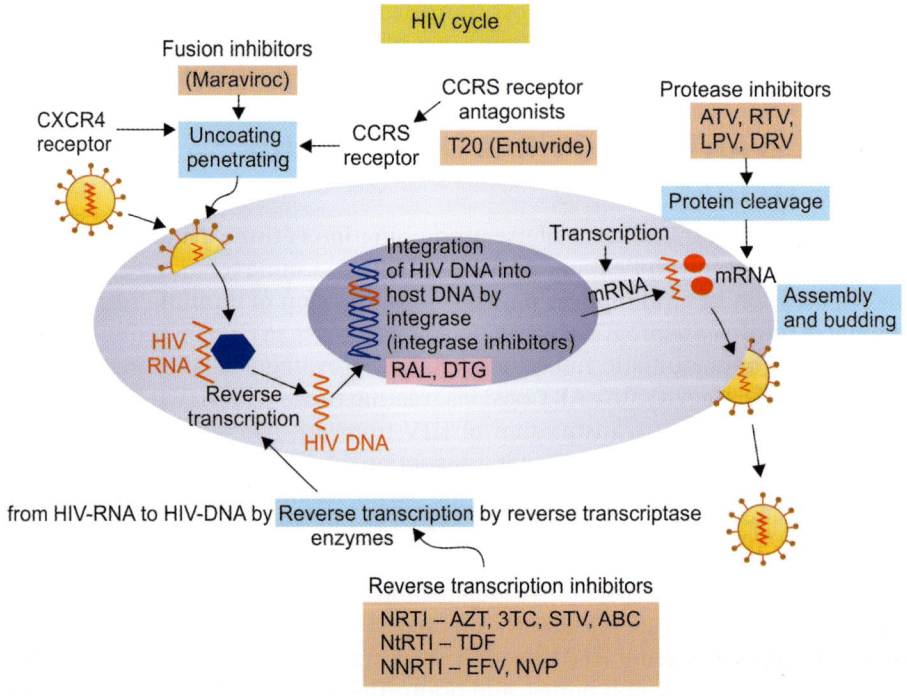

FIG. 1: Sites of action of antiretroviral (ARV) drugs.

various randomized controlled trials (RCTs) and long observational studies. Over the years, the trend has been toward earlier initiation of ART in view of its benefits in terms of prevention of various OIs such as tuberculosis (TB) and overall risk reduction when started earlier and since the 2016 guideline has been to provide ART to all irrespective of clinical stage, viral load, or CD4 count **(Table 2)**.

TABLE 1: Classes of antiretroviral drugs.

Nucleoside reverse transcriptase inhibitors (NRTIs)	Non-nucleoside reverse transcriptase inhibitors (NNRTIs)	Protease inhibitors (PIs)
Zidovudine (AZT)*	Nevirapine (NVP)*	Saquinavir (SQV)
Stavudine (d4T)	Efavirenz (EFV)*	Ritonavir (RTV)*
Lamivudine (3TC)*	Delavirdine (DLV)	Nelfinavir (NFV)
Abacavir (ABC)*	Rilpivirine (RPV)	Amprenavir (APV)
Didanosine (ddI)	Etravirine (ETV)	Indinavir (INV)
Zalcitabine (ddC)	Doravirine (DOR)	Lopinavir (LPV)*
Emtricitabine (FTC)	Integrase inhibitors	Fosamprenavir (FPV)
Nucleotide reverse transcriptase inhibitors (NtRTI)	Dolutegravir (DTG)*	Atazanavir (ATV)*
	Raltegravir (RGV)*	Tipranavir (TPV)
	Elvitegravir (EVG)	Darunavir (DRV)*
Tenofovir disoproxil fumarate (TDF)*	Bictegravir (BIC)	
Tenofovir alafenamide (TAF)	Cabotegravir (CAB)	
Fusion inhibitors (FI)	CCR5 entry inhibitor	Postattachment maturation inhibitor
Enfuvirtide (T-20)	Maraviroc (MVC)	Ibalizumab (IBA)

*Available in the national program.

TABLE 2: Changing the cutoff for ART initiation.

1995–2005	2005–2010	2010–2013	2015
Several ACTG and CPCRA studies (early post-HAART era): ART initiation CD4 <200 cells/mm^3—impact on AIDS mortality and major OIs incidence	Observational studies (ART initiation at CD4 >350 cells/mm^3) impact on mortality, disease progression, and non-AIDS events		TEMPRANO and START studies: (ART initiation at CD4 >500 cells/mm^3) impact on severe HIV morbidity and disease progression, without increase in severe adverse events. 44% less deaths, IPT 35%. Start 53% decline
CIPRA and SMART studies (ART initiation at CD4 <350 cells/mm^3): Impact on HIV mortality, disease progression, and comorbidities (TB)-CIPRA-70% decline in death and 50% in TB. Similar in SMART		HPTN 052: 96% reduction of HIV transmission among HIV serodiscordant couples and risk of TB in adults (impact on HIV incidence)	

(AIDS: acquired immunodeficiency syndrome; ART: antiretroviral therapy; HAART: highly active antiretroviral therapy; HIV: human immunodeficiency virus; TB: tuberculosis)

National AIDS Control Organisation (NACO) ART guidelines have also been changing accordingly. The current NACO guidelines on when to start ART are given in the following text.

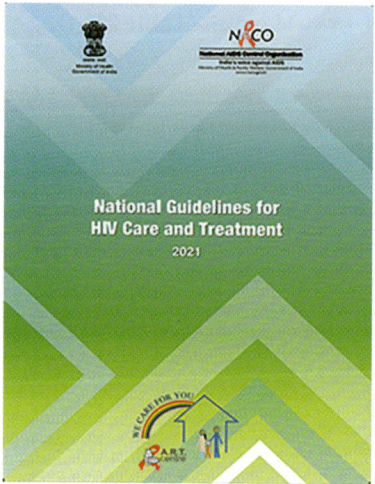

WHAT DRUGS TO START WITH? WHICH IS THE BEST REGIMEN?

The decision around what to start is governed by the efficacy of drugs, toxicity profile, pill burden, drug–drug interaction, and other medications for comorbidities/coinfections. The WHO recommendations over the years have been to move toward simpler more efficacious and less toxic regimen with minimal pill burden to increase adherence potential. In 2018, the WHO recommended the use of Dolutegravir (DTG) in the first-line ART in place of efavirenz (EFV) in view of the fact that viral suppression with DTG containing regimen is faster than with EFV (average 4 weeks for DTG vs. 12 weeks for EFV), DTG has fewer side effects, fewer drug–drug interactions, and above all has a higher threshold for resistance.

In line with WHO guidelines, NACO has also revised its ART guidelines to include DTG based regimen as preferred regimen for first line ART in ART naïve patients and also to transition existing patients on other sub optimal regimen to DTG based regimen. It is now recommended that all PLHIV with HIV-1 infection be initiated on a regimen consisting of

Moving toward simpler treatment with less toxic drugs:

Tenofovir (TDF 300 mg) + Lamivudine (3TC 300 mg) + Dolutegravir (DTG 50 mg) as fixed-dose combination (FDC) in a single pill once a day

For those with TB, the dose of DTG needs to be increased to 50 mg twice a day for the period of Rifampicin containing ATT. DTG is effective against HIV-2 also, so this also simplifies the ART regimen for those with HIV-2 and they need not use LPV/r (ritonavir boosted lopinavir) in first-line ART.

TABLE 3: NACO-recommended first-line ART regimen.

PLHIV group	ARV regimen
Preferred first-line ART for ART initiation for those more than 10 years of age and weight more than 30 kg (including pregnant women)	Tenofovir 300 mg plus Lamivudine 300 mg plus Dolutegravir 50 mg (in a FDC) once a day
Preferred first-line ART for ART initiation for those more than 10 years of age and weight less than 30 kg	Abacavir plus Lamivudine in FDC as per weight band plus Dolutegravir 50 mg once a day
Women of childbearing potential not on effective contraception	Preferred regimen is the same as all other adults (TLD). Should be counseled on immense benefits of TLD, namely a very small risk of neural tube defects. If they do not want to use TLD, should be offered Tenofovir 300 mg plus Lamivudine 300 mg plus Efavirenz 400 mg (in a FDC) once a day

(ART: antiretroviral therapy; FDC: fixed-dose combination; NACO: National Aids Control Organization; PLHIV: people living with HIV; TLD: Tenofovir 300 mg plus Lamivudine 300 mg plus Dolutegravir 50 mg)

The *current guidelines* on the ART regimen in first-line ART by NACO are depicted in **Table 3**.

Before starting ART, it is of utmost importance to ensure that the patient is well prepared for the therapy. The preparedness includes that the patient has adequate understanding of the disease, is aware of the treatment regimen, importance of high levels of adherence to therapy, and is willing to take the treatment on a long-term basis. All patients found HIV positive should be subjected to a detailed workup before ART is considered.

HOW TO FOLLOW PATIENTS INITIATED ON ANTIRETROVIRAL THERAPY?

The patients started on ART must be seen every month during the initial few months and looked for adherence, drug toxicity, and any clinical manifestations such as OIs and immune reconstitution inflammatory syndrome (IRIS). The various monitoring indicators are as follows:
- *Clinical monitoring*
    - Monthly clinical evaluation
        - Weight, overall well-being, any fresh symptoms, routine four-symptom screening for TB on every visit
    - Monthly treatment adherence evaluation, pill count, self-reported
    - For adverse reactions of ART/OI drugs
    - For drug interactions, look for concomitant drugs
    - For IRIS
- *Immunological monitoring*
    - CD4 count (every 6 months but for virologically suppressed patients, frequency can be reduced or stopped)
- *Virological monitoring* (at 6, 12, and every 12 months)

WHEN TO CHANGE THE REGIMEN?

The adherence to ART is one of the most crucial determinants of success of ART on a long-term basis. The adherence of 95% or more is crucial for patients to achieve desirable suppression of viral replication. However, even with good adherence levels, resistance occurs to ARV drugs over a period due to viral mutation and this requires change of ARV drugs. The virological failure appears first followed by immunological failure which finally leads to clinical failure. Any decline in CD4 count of a detectable viral load of more than 1,000 copies after at least 6 months of ART is considered as treatment failure. It is desirable to switch the entire regimen from first- to second-line ART as soon as virological failure is detected. **Table 4** depicts the criteria for suspecting and confirming treatment failure.

The second-line regimen for patients failing on DTG-based first-line ART is AZT + Lamivudine (3TC) + ATV/r for those on TDF in first-line regimen [and TDF + 3TC + ATV/r for those on AZT or stavudine (d4T)-based regimen in the first line]. For those failing on FEV-based first line ART, the regimen of choice includes DTG.

Use of ARV Drugs for Postexposure Prophylaxis following Needle Stick Injury

Postexposure prophylaxis refers to the comprehensive management instituted to minimize the risk of infection following potential exposure to blood-borne

TABLE 4: WHO criteria for defining treatment failure.

Failure	Definition	Comments
Clinical failure	• Adults and adolescents • New or recurrent clinical event indicating severe immunodeficiency (WHO clinical stage 4 condition) after 6 months of effective treatment	• The condition must be differentiated from immune reconstitution inflammatory syndrome occurring after initiating ART • For adults, certain WHO clinical stage 3 conditions (pulmonary TB and severe bacterial infections) may also indicate treatment failure
Immunological failure	Adults and adolescents CD4 count at or below 250 cells/mm^3 following clinical failure† or persistent CD4 levels below 100 cells/mm^3	• Without concomitant or recent infection to cause a transient decline in the CD4 cell count • Current WHO clinical and immunological criteria have low sensitivity and positive predictive value for identifying individuals with virological failure
Virological failure	Viral load above 1,000 copies/mL based on two consecutive viral load measurements in 3 months, with adherence support following the first viral load test	An individual must be taking ART for at least 6 months before it can be determined that a regimen has failed

†Previous guidelines defined immunological failure based on a fall from baseline, which is no longer applicable in the context of CD4-independent treatment initiation. The option of CD4 cell count at or below 250 cells/mm^3 following clinical failure is based on an analysis of data from Uganda and Zimbabwe.

(ART: antiretroviral therapy; WHO: World Health Organization)

pathogens (HIV, HBV, HCV). This includes first-aid, counseling, risk assessment, relevant laboratory investigations based on informed consent of the source and exposed person and depending on the risk assessment, the provision of short-term (4 weeks) antiretroviral drugs, with follow-up and support including maintaining confidentially.

A designated person/trained doctor must rapidly assess the risk of HIV and HBV transmission following an accidental exposure to blood (AEB). The first dose of PEP should be administered ideally within 2 hours (but certainly within the first 72 hours) of exposure. The currently recommended drug for PEP is Tenofovir plus 3TC plus DTG 50 mg once daily for 28 days.

ANTIRETROVIRAL THERAPY: LOOKING BEYOND 2022

A number of newer options are becoming available which include:
- Starting with a two-drug regimen
- Switching patients stable on a three-drug regimen to a two-drug regimen
- Using long-acting injectable options: One- or three-monthly injections
- Using broadly neutralizing antibodies
- Potential toward sterilizing "HIV cure"

The results from GEMINI 1 and 2 studies have shown that a two-drug combination of DTG + 3TC is noninferior to DTG + TDF + 3TC in treatment-naïve patients. These studies also provided evidence on supporting long-term durability of a two-drug regimen and there were no differences in outcomes by age, sex, race, or baseline VL or CD4 count.

In terms of switching from triple to dual therapy, TANGO study showed that at week 96, switching to DTG + 3TC was noninferior to continuing a tenofovir alafenamide (TAF)-based three-drug regimen in maintaining viral suppression.

The ATLAS 2M study using long-acting injectable cabotegravir showed that results at week 48 and 96 revealed that the efficacy of long-acting cabotegravir plus rilpivirine given every 8 weeks continued to be noninferior to administration every 4 weeks.

The FLAIR study enrolled people who were newly diagnosed with HIV infection. They were administered induction therapy with DTG/abacavir/3TC and then randomized to the long-acting cabotegravir/rilpivirine versus continuing that induction regimen. The results were found to be comparable in both the arms.

Islatravir is another potent and long-acting nucleoside reverse transcriptase inhibitor (NNRTI), with a half-life of 177–209 hours in healthy adults offering hope of less-frequent dosing.

In pipeline are drugs such as MK-8591, a nucleoside reverse transcriptase translocation inhibitor (NRTTI) in phase II study. Preclinical data show potent activity against wild-type and multidrug resistance HIV-1. A long half-life may allow weekly or longer dosing intervals. Another investigational agent is a capsid inhibitor GS-6207, which is also extremely potent in vitro and can be given every 12 weeks as a subcutaneous injection.

CONCLUSION

Antiretroviral therapy has been a boon for PLHIV and has changed the way clinicians looked at HIV in pre-HAART era. It has prolonged lives of millions of people, given them many more productive years, reduced their hospitalizations and OIs thus preventing them from sliding into poverty. Every single paisa spent on ART scale-up has been rewarded by better quality of life of PHLIV, prolongation of their lives, and reduction in new infections. However, issues of adherence, toxicity, emerging resistance, and cost of newer drugs are emerging areas of concern. The HIV care is rapidly evolving and becoming complex as people live longer. The future options include new groups of drugs and better strategies but at higher costs. The therapy is no doubt panacea for those already infected, but HIV prevention messages and probably newer tools such as HIV self-testing hope for more and more people knowing their status to reach first 95 of 95–95–95 targets for 2020 and also while PrEP offers an opportunity for people at high risk to protect themselves from acquiring HIV.

SUGGESTED READINGS

1. Panel on Antiretroviral Guidelines for Adults and Adolescents. Guidelines for the use of antiretroviral agents in HIV-1-infected adults and adolescents. Department of Health and Human Services, USA. 2021. [online] Available from https://clinicalinfo.hiv.gov/sites/default/files/guidelines/archive/AdultandAdolescentGL_2021_08_16.pdf [Last accessed October, 2022].
2. National Technical Guidelines on ART, NACO. Ministry of Health and Family Welfare, December 2021. (2022). [online] Available from http://naco.gov.in/sites/default/files/National_Guidelines_for HIV Care and_Treatment_2021.pdf [Last accessed October, 2022].
3. World Health Organization. (2019). Policy brief: update of recommendations on first- and second-line antiretroviral regimens. [online] Available from https://apps.who.int/iris/handle/10665/325892. [Last accessed October, 2022].
4. World Health Organization. (2018). Updated recommendations on first-line and second-line antiretroviral regimens and post-exposure prophylaxis and recommendations on early infant diagnosis of HIV interim guidance (July 2018). [online] Available from https://www.who.int/hiv/pub/guidelines/ARV2018update/en/ [Last accessed October, 2022].
5. World Health Organization. (2021). WHO consolidated guidelines on HIV prevention, testing, treatment, service delivery and monitoring: recommendations for a public health approach, July 2021. [online] Available from https://www.who.int/publications/i/item/9789240031593 [Last accessed October, 2022].
6. What's new in treatment monitoring: viral load and CD4 testing. July 2017. [online] Available from http://www.who.int/publications/i/item/WHO-HIV-2017.22 [Last accessed October, 2022].
7. World Health Organization. (2017). WHO guidelines for managing advanced HIV disease and rapid initiation of antiretroviral therapy, July 2017. [online] Available from http://www.who.int/hiv/pub/guidelines/advanced-HIV-disease/en/ [Last accessed October, 2022].
8. Key considerations for differentiated antiretroviral therapy delivery for specific populations: children, adolescents, pregnant and breastfeeding women and key populations. July 2017. [online] Available from https://apps.who.int/iris/handle/10665/258506 [Last accessed October, 2022].

Pre- and Post-exposure HIV Prophylaxis

Naval Chandra

PRE-EXPOSURE HIV PROPHYLAXIS

Oral pre-exposure prophylaxis (PrEP) is highly effective in preventing HIV in adherent, high-risk individuals, and is well-tolerated.

Pre-exposure prophylaxis programs have addressed key groups such as sex workers, intravenous drug users and men who have sex with men (MSM); however, the critical group that requires intervention within Southern Africa is young women, and PrEP programs addressing them have only recently been developed. These programs include provision of care outside of the school environment, due to perceived resistance from school management and parents. PrEP reduces the risk of getting HIV from sex by about 99%. PrEP reduces the risk of getting HIV from injection drug use by at least 74%.

Based on evidences from randomized trials, open-label extension studies and demonstration projects, World Health Organization (WHO) recommended daily oral PrEP containing tenofovir as an additional prevention choice for people at substantial risk of HIV infection. In 2019, WHO published a technical brief updating the WHO recommendation on oral PrEP to include the option of event-driven (ED) dosing for cisgender men who have sex with men. This consists of the use of a double dose of oral PrEP 2–24 hours before sex, followed by a third dose 24 hours after the first two doses and a fourth dose 48 hours after the first two doses. This has been described as 2+1+1. No cases of renal failure have yet been seen after a normal screening test, using tenofovir-containing PrEP, but most guidelines recommend continuing monitoring **(Tables 1 and 2)**.

Whenever possible, people in their social and sexual networks should be offered HIV testing, treatment and prevention services. PrEP should be considered, in combination with other prevention services, for HIV uninfected partners of recently diagnosed people.

TABLE 1: Recommended oral PrEP regimen.

Drug name	Dose	Frequency
F/TDF	200 mg/300 mg	Once a day
F/TAF	200 mg/25 mg	Once a day

TABLE 2: Summary of clinician guidance for daily oral PrEP use.

	Sexually-active adults and adolescents[1]	Persons who inject drug[2]
Identifying substantial risk of acquiring HIV infection	Anal or vaginal sex in past 6 months *and* any of the following: • HIV-positive sexual partner (especially if partner has an unknown or detectable viral load) • Bacterial STI in past 6 months[3] • History of inconsistent or no condom use with sexual panned (s)	HIV-positive injecting partner *or* Sharing injection equipment
Clinically eligible	All of the following conditions are met: • Documented negative HIV Ag/Ab test result within 1 week before initially prescribing PrEP • No signs/symptoms of acute HIV infection • Estimated creatinine clearance ≥30 mL/min[4] • No contraindicated medications	
Dosage	• Daily, continuing, oral doses of F/TDF (TRUVADA®), ≤90-day supply or • For men and transgender women at risk for sexual acquisition of HIV; daily, continuing, oral doses of F/TAF (DESCOVY®), ≤90-day supply	
Follow-up care	Follow-up visits at least every 3 months to provide the following: • HIV Ag/Ab test and HIV-1 RNA assay, medication adherence and behavioral risk reduction support • Bacterial STI screening for MSM and transgender women who have sex with men[3]- oral, rectal, urine, blood • Access to clean needles syringes and drug treatment services for PWID Follow-up visits every 6 months to provide the following: • Assess renal function for patients aged ≥50 years or who have an eCrCl <90 mL/min at PrEP initiation • Bacterial STI screening for all sexually-active patients[3] - (vaginal, oral, rectal, urine- as indicated), blood Follow-up visits every 12 months to provide the following: • Assess renal function for all patients • *Chlamydia* screening for heterosexually active women and men - vaginal, urine • For patients on F/TAF, assess weight, triglyceride and cholesterol levels	

[1] Adolescents weighing at least 35 kg (77 lb).

[2] Because most PWID are also sexually active, they should be assessed for sexual risk and provided the option of CAB for PrEP when indicated.

[3] Sexually transmitted infection (STI): Gonorrhea, *Chlamydia*, and syphilis for MSM and transgender women who have sex with men including those who inject drugs; Gonorrhea and syphilis for heterosexual women and men including persons who inject drugs.

[4] Estimated creatine clearance (eCrCl) by Cockcroft–Gault formula ≥60 mL/min for F/TDF use, ≥30 mL/min for F/TAF use.

Operational research is especially needed in diverse settings on how to generate demand for prevention services and support effective PrEP use among adolescents and young people. It is recognized that many PrEP users will not choose to take PrEP continuously for several years. Therefore, support to start, stop and restart PrEP related to periods of sexual risk is an important part of PrEP counseling. This includes innovative platforms such as using social media and mobile applications to engage with potential and existing PrEP users. Efforts are needed to simplify provision of the intervention, to make delivery as efficient as possible.

Globally, the largest numbers of PrEP users have been among cisgender men who have sex with men and cisgender women at risk of acquiring HIV. More research is needed on the specific needs of transgender women, transgender men, and non-binary people, including additional support for adherence in this population and integration of gender-affirming care with HIV services, including PrEP. Research involving transgender men and non-binary people is particularly lacking, including how to improve awareness and uptake of and adherence to PrEP.

POST-EXPOSURE PROPHYLAXIS

The term "post-exposure prophylaxis or PEP" refers to the prophylactic use of antiretrovirals to prevent establishment of HIV infection after an occupational exposure to HIV. The average risk of HIV infection after percutaneous exposure to HIV-infected blood is 0.3%. The nonoccupational (nPEP) can be offered for cases such as unprotected sexual exposure, sexual assault survivors, injecting drug users (IDUs) sharing equipment, etc. While considering PEP, evaluation of exposure, exposure source, and exposed person is to be done. PEP must be started as soon as possible to be effective—and always within 72 hours of a possible exposure. Initiating therapy after a longer interval (e.g., 1 week) might still be considered for exposures that represent an extremely high risk of transmission. PEP should be administered for 4 weeks, if tolerated.

The following types of exposure may warrant HIV PEP:
- *Body fluids*: Blood, blood-stained saliva, breast milk, genital secretions; cerebrospinal, amniotic, peritoneal, synovial, pericardial or pleural fluids. Although these fluids carry a high risk of HIV infection, this list is not exhaustive. All cases should be assessed clinically, and the healthcare workers should decide whether the actual exposure constitutes a significant risk.
- *Types of exposure*: (1) Mucous membrane from sexual exposure; splashes to the eye, nose, or oral cavity; and (2) parenteral exposures.

Exposure that does not require HIV PEP includes:
- When the exposed individual is already HIV positive
- When the source is established to be HIV negative; and
- Exposure to bodily fluids that do not pose a significant risk: tears, nonblood-stained saliva, urine, and sweat.

A regimen for PEP for HIV with two antiretroviral drugs (ARV) drugs is effective, but three drugs are preferred.
- Post-exposure prophylaxis ARV regimens for adults and adolescents:
  - TDF + 3TC (or FTC) as the preferred backbone regimen (strong recommendation, low-quality evidence)

- LPV/r or ATV/r as the preferred third drug (conditional recommendation, very low-quality evidence)
  - Where available, RAL, DRV/r, or EFV can be considered as alternative options
- Post-exposure prophylaxis ARV regimens for children ≤10 years:
  - AZT + 3TC as the preferred backbone regimen
  - ABC + 3TC or TDF + 3TC (or FTC) can be considered as alternative regimens (strong recommendation, low-quality evidence)
  - LPV/r as the preferred third drug (conditional recommendation, very low-quality evidence)
  - An age-appropriate alternative regimen can be identified among ATV/r, RAL, DRV, EFV and NVP

Antiretroviral therapy (ART) should be initiated urgently among all pregnant and breastfeeding women living with HIV, even if they are identified late in pregnancy or postpartum, because the most effective way to prevent HIV vertical transmission is to reduce maternal viral load.

People with established chronic hepatitis B infection should be monitored for hepatic flare after discontinuing PEP. Among people with unknown hepatitis B status and where hepatitis B testing is readily available, people started on TDF-, 3TC- or FTC-based PEP should be tested for hepatitis B to detect active hepatitis B infection and the need for ongoing hepatitis B therapy after discontinuing PEP.

Universal precautions should be followed that include:
- Wash hands immediately if contaminated with body fluids.
- Wear gloves when contamination with body substances is anticipated.
- Protective eyewear and mask should be worn when splashing with body substance is anticipated.
- All healthcare workers should take precautions to prevent injuries during procedures and when cleaning or during disposal of needles and other sharp instruments.
- Needle should not be recapped.
- Needles should not be purposely bent or broken by hand, nor removed from the disposable syringe or manipulated by hand.
- After use, disposable syringes and needles, scalpel blades and other sharp items should be placed in a puncture-resistant container.
- Healthcare workers who have exudative lesions or dermatitis should refrain from direct patient care and from handling equipment.
- Clean and disinfect blood/body substances' spills with appropriate agents.
- Adhere to the disinfection and sterilization standards.
- Regard all waste soiled blood/body substance as contaminated and dispose-off according to the relevant standards.
- Vaccinate all clinical and laboratory workers against hepatitis B, other measures such as double gloving, changing surgical techniques to avoid "exposure prone" procedures use of needle, less systems and other safe devices should be encouraged.

CHAPTER 47

What is New in Current Guidelines of Management of Hypertension?

Hem Shanker Sharma, Reeja Antony

■ INTRODUCTION

Hypertension is a common condition in which the long-term force of the blood against your artery walls is high enough that it may eventually cause health problems such as heart disease.

Blood pressure (BP) is determined both by the amount of blood your heart pumps and the amount of resistance to blood flow in your arteries. The more blood your heart pumps and the narrower your arteries, the higher is your blood pressure. A blood pressure reading is given in millimeters of mercury (mm Hg). It has two numbers.

1. *Systolic pressure*: The first, or upper, number measures the pressure in the arteries when the heart beats.
2. *Diastolic pressure*: The second, or lower, number measures the pressure in your arteries between beats.

Hypertension is becoming a global health problem. The criteria for diagnosis are when systolic blood pressure >140 mm Hg and diastolic blood pressure >90 mm Hg as per all the latest guidelines. The important aspect in hypertension is to identify person with high blood pressure to prevent complications. Drug therapy should be initiated for patient with confirmed hypertension.

■ DIAGNOSTIC THRESHOLD FOR HYPERTENSION

As per US guideline BP level is 130/80, European Society of Hypertension (ESH) Guideline BP is 140/90, International Society of Hypertension (ISH) Guideline BP is 140/90, Asian guideline BP is 140/90, Indian Guidelines on Hypertension (IGH) guideline BP is 140/90.

MANAGEMENT OF HYPERTENSION

Nonpharmacological Management

Lifestyle Modification

- *Salt intake*: Increased salt intake corelates with increased blood pressure. Salt restriction is advised.
- *Healthy diet*: Eating whole grains, fruits, vegetables, polyunsaturated fats and reducing sugars, and saturated and trans-fat [Dietary Approaches to Stop Hypertension (DASH) diet].
- *Healthy drinks*: Green and black tea
- *Alcohol consumption*: About 10 g of alcohol/standard. Avoid binge drinking.
- *Weight reduction*: Avoiding obesity, abdominal obesity in particular should be controlled.
- Smoking cessation
- *Regular physical activity*: Regular moderate intensity aerobic exercise such as walking, jogging, cycling, yoga, swimming for 30 minutes on 5–7 days/week may be beneficial
- *Reduce stress and induce mindfulness*: Transcendental meditation/mindfulness practices lower blood pressure.

GUIDELINE RECOMMENDATIONS

American College of Cardiology/American Heart Association 2017 Guideline Recommendations

- Systolic blood pressure (SBP) <120 and diastolic blood pressure (DBP) <80 is considered normal BP
- SBP between 120 and 129 and DBP <80 is elevated BP.
- SBP between 130 and 139 or DBP 80–89 is stage 1 hypertension.
- SBP between 140 and 159 or DBP 90–99 is stage 2 hypertension.
- SBP ≥160 or DBP ≥100 is stage 2 hypertension.
- Monotherapy of angiotensin-converting enzyme inhibitors (ACEI), angiotensin II receptor blocker (ARB), thiazide diuretic or combination of thiazide diuretic with ACEI is considered useful in-patient having transient ischemic attack (TIA) or stroke.
- In patients having symptomatic heart failure (HF), loop diuretics such as furosemide, bumetanide, or torsemide are desired. Loop diuretic have higher preference over Thiazide diuretics in patients having glomerular filtration rate (GFR) <30 mL/min [patients having moderate-to-severe chronic kidney disease (CKD)].
- On the basis of a long half-life and cardiovascular disease (CVD) risk reduction trial and chlorthalidone has been given preference.
- Amiloride and triamterene (potassium sparing diuretic) are used as monotherapy and they are considered as antihypertensive agents with minimum effectiveness.

- In patients having hypokalemia, thiazide diuretic as monotherapy or combination with potassium sparing diuretic can be suggested. Try to avoid them in patients with impaired GFR [<45 mL/min].
- Aldosterone antagonist such as eplerenone and spironolactone have preference for use in resistant hypertension and primary aldosteronism.

European Society of Cardiology/European Society of Hypertension 2018 Guidelines Recommendations

Based on office BP hypertension ≥140/90 mm Hg.

Initial Drug Treatment

Dual therapy single pill combination for most patients. Usually, ACEI + calcium channel blocker (CCB) or ACEI + diuretics β-blockers when indicated. Other drugs for specific indication.

Triple Therapy

Further drug treatment using triple therapy can be used ACEI + CCB + diuretics. Ideally used as a single pill combination.
- *Spironolactone* can be added, in case of uncontrolled bp with triple combination therapy.

Among all the antihypertension (anti-HTN) drugs, diuretic (thiazide and thiazide-like drugs such as chlorthalidone and indapamide] have demonstrated an effective reduction in BP and CV events in randomized clinical trials, and hence these are indicated as a basis for an effective anti HTN regimen.

In case of reduced GFR (GFR <45 mL/min), thiazide is considered as less effective anti-HTN agents and they become inefficient when the GFR <30 mL/min. In such condition, loop diuretic such as furosemide or torsemide like loop diuretic should be used instead of thiazide diuretic to achieve an anti-HTN effect.

Treatment Targets

For 18–65 years age target is <140/90–130/80 mm Hg or lower if tolerated 65+ years age target is <140/90 mm Hg down to 130/80 mm Hg, if possible and if tolerated.

For monitoring purposes aim for BP control within 3 months, monitor for side effects. Check adherence if BP not controlled.

Statins for all high-risk patients for moderate/low-risk patients. Antiplatelets for secondary prevention.

INDIAN HYPERTENSION GUIDELINES 2019

- *Step 1*:
    - Age 55 years, nonblack: Start with ACEI or ARB
    - Age 55 years nonblack: Start with CCB
    - If CCB not suitable then Thiazide-like diuretic or indapamide
    - *Nondiabetic blacks*: CCB
    - *Diabetic*: ARB/ACEI
    - *Evidence of heart failure*: Thiazide-like diuretic or indapamide

- *Step 2*:
  Before moving into step 2, check whether the patient is compliant with step 1:
  - If started on ARB/ACEI add CCB or thiazide-like diuretic
  - If started on CCB add ARB/ACEI or thiazide-like diuretic

  In black use ARB instead of ACEI
- *Step 3*:
  - Compliance with step 2 to be checked
  - ARB/ACEI + CCB + thiazide-like diuretic
- *Step 4*:
  - Consider as resistant hypertension
  - Consider low dose spironolactone, if side effects then use eplerenone add α or β-blockers taking potassium levels into account. In special situation add centrally acting drugs or direct vasodilators.
  - Consider adding β-blocker at any step when there is a specific indication such as heart failure, angina, and postpregnancy.

  A—ACEI or ARB
  C—DHP-CCB
  D—thiazide-like diuretic

CONCLUSION

The various hypertension guidelines are almost similar. They differ in their BP levels for the diagnosis of hypertension, target BP, and some guidelines suggests that drugs should be customized as per patient's clinical profile.

SUGGESTED READINGS

1. Lawes CM, Vander Hoorn S, Rodgers A, et al. Global burden of blood-pressure-related disease, 2001. Lancet. 2008;371(9623):1513-8.
2. Lozano R, Naghavi M, Foreman K, et al. Global and regional mortality from 235 causes of death for 20 age groups in 1990 and 2010: a systematic analysis for the Global Burden of Disease Study 2010. Lancet. 2012;380(9859):2095-128.
3. Falaschetti E, Chaudhury M, Mindell J, et al. Continued improvement in hypertension management in England: results from the Health Survey for England 2006. Hypertension. 2009;53(3):480-6.
4. National Institute for Health and Care Excellence (NICE). (2011). Hypertension: Clinical Management of Primary Hypertension in Adults. Clinical Guideline 127 (CG 127). [online] Available from http://guidance.nice.org.uk/cg127 [Last accessed October, 2022].
5. Kannel WB, McGee D, Gordon T. A general cardiovascular risk profile: the Framingham Study. Am J Cardiol. 1976;38(1):46-51.
6. JBS3 Board. Joint British Societies' consensus recommendations for the prevention of cardiovascular disease (JBS3). Heart. 2014;100(Suppl 2):ii1-67.

CHAPTER 48

Calcium Channel Blockers and Angiotensin Receptor Blockers: A Friendly Duo

Kamlesh Tewary

■ INTRODUCTION

Scientific investigations comparing the long-term implications of calcium channel blockers (CCBs) and angiotensin II type 1 receptor blockers (ARBs) on hypertensive patients found that both antihypertensive drugs have similar favorable impacts on lowering the risk of cardiovascular (CV) morbidity and mortality, as predicted by a similar decrease in pulse wave velocity (PWV). Different mechanisms, however, were thought to be contributing to the benefits of CCBs and ARBs. Amlodipine, an L-type CCB, had a greater effect on lowering blood pressure (BP) and its variability than ARBs such as valsartan and candesartan, and its pleiotropic effects on lowering oxidative stress and urinary albumin excretion (UAE) may contribute significantly to improving the CV benefits of valsartan and candesartan.

A new generation of CCBs and ARBs was recently developed and is now being used to treat hypertensive patients. Cilnidipine is an N-type CCB which can restrict sympathetic nerve function and lower intraglomerular tension by dilatation of the efferent arterioles. However, telmisartan is an ARB that can attach to the peroxisome proliferator-activated receptor-alpha (PPAR-α). Recent research found that reductions in UAE as a result of lower intraglomerular pressure were significantly associated with a lower risk of micro- and macrovascular events. Furthermore, the PROactive study found that PPAR-stimulation significantly reduced the secondary endpoints of all-cause mortality, nonfatal myocardial infarction and stroke. Thus, hypertensive patients may benefit from the use of the new CCB Cilnidipine and the new ARB telmisartan. The purpose of this study was to see how Cilnidipine or telmisartan affected markers for vascular complications in hypertensive patients.

■ CILNIDIPINE

Background

Cilnidipine is a newly developed CCB that inhibits both L-type and N-type calcium channels. Because N-type calcium is distributed along nerves and in the

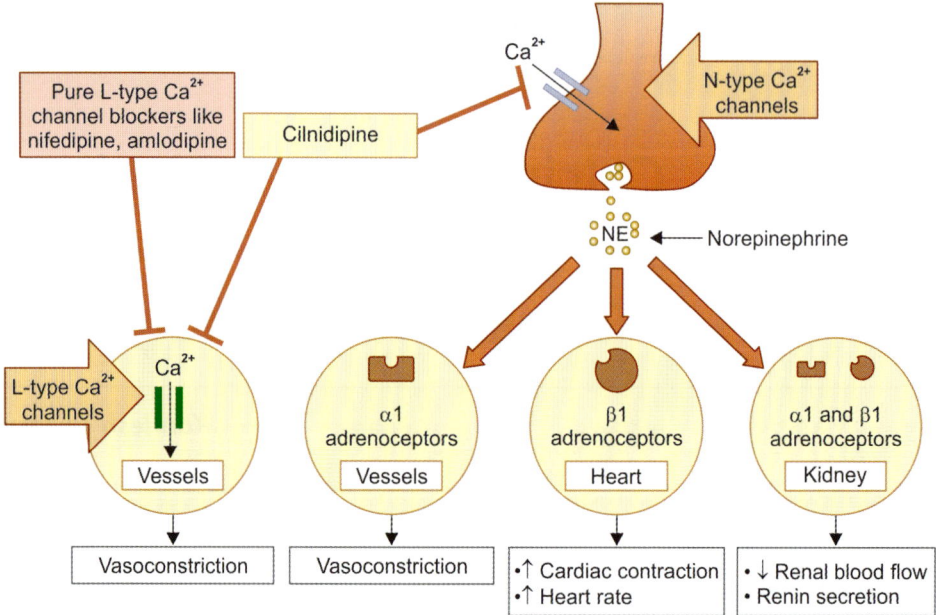

FIG. 1: Pharmacology of Cilnidipine.

brain, it is expected that Cilnidipine will have a specific effect on nerve activity, such as inhibition of the sympathetic nervous system. Cilnidipine has a unique dihydropyridine derivative CCB that inhibits sympathetic N-type calcium channels and has renoprotective, neuroprotective, and cardioprotective effects. Cilnidipine is a fourth-generation drug because it directly inhibits sympathetic neurotransmitter release via its N-type calcium channel-blocking property.

Cilnidipine at submicro molecular concentrations significantly inhibited N-type Ca^2 channel currents in isolated sympathetic neurons **(Fig. 1)**. They also compared the inhibitory effect of various dihydropyridines on cardiac L-type Ca^2 channels in isolated ventricular myocytes to that of N-type Ca^2 channels in Wistar rats' superior cervical ganglion neurons. It was discovered that the selectivity for L-type and N-type Ca^2 channels varied significantly among the compounds tested, with Cilnidipine blocking both L-type and N-type Ca^2 channels. Takahara A et al. demonstrated that Cilnidipine inhibits N-type channels in IMR32 human neuroblastoma cells. Cilnidipine inhibits N-type Ca^2 channels more potently as compared to other Ca^2 channel blockers. Another study by Nap A et al. discovered that in vitro, Cilnidipine diminishes norepinephrine secretion from sympathetic nerve endings.

Cilnidipine's cardioprotective action was investigated in a rabbit model of myocardial infarction, in which Cilnidipine reduced myocardial interstitial norepinephrine levels during ischemia and reperfusion, resulting in a reduction in myocardial infarct size and the incidence of ventricular premature beats. Furthermore, in vivo data show that Cilnidipine possesses antianginal influence in a vasopressin-induced angina experimentally induced model and strengthens ventricular repolarization abnormality in a canine model of long QT syndrome.

The patholytic patterns of Cilnidipine reported in vivo and in vitro are confirmed in clinical practice. Cilnidipine's antihypertensive effect has been established in clinical studies performed in hypertensive patients in addition to patients with severe hypertension by Iimura O et al. and Nagahama S et al. In a study of 2,920 hypertensive patients, diagnosis with Cilnidipine and ARBs led to significant decreases in heart rate, in those with a significantly elevated heart rate of 75 beats per min with few adverse consequences due to central nervous functions.

Renoprotection and Proteinuria

Cilnidipine, an L-type and N-type CCB, has been shown to be more effective than amlodipine, an L-type CCB, in preventing proteinuria progression in hypertensive patients. By facilitating efferent arteriole vasodilation, N-type calcium channel blockade, which impedes renal sympathetic nerve function, might minimize glomerular hypertension. In sympathetic nerves that innervate renal tubules, N-type Ca channels are abundant. Data suggest that N-type calcium channels contribute to multiple steps of renal fibrosis, and that blocking them may be a useful therapeutic approach for renal fibrosis prevention. In the general population, microalbuminuria is a well-known risk factor for CV morbidity and mortality. Low-grade albuminuria (30 mg/g) is thought to be a marker for subclinical vascular damage, which predisposes to future CV disease and death. Lowering albumin excretion in the urine lowers the risk of CV disease.

Calcium channel blockers are said to control glomerular pressure by altering afferent and efferent arteriole tone. Zhou et al. found that Cilnidipine reduced glomerular capillary pressure, afferent and efferent arteriole resistance, and proteinuria in nitric oxide synthase inhibited spontaneously hypertensive rat (SHR), indicating that Cilnidipine reduced glomerular hypertension and prevented proteinuria. In dog kidneys and hydronephrotic SHR, similar arteriole responses were observed. Notably, Konno, and Kimura observed that nifedipine, another L-type CCB, enlarged only afferent arteries but not efferent arteries, whereas Cilnidipine enlarged both afferent and efferent arteries, insinuating that Cilnidipine's N-type calcium channel inhibition may induce efferent vasodilation.

As a result, the influence of Cilnidipine on glomerular hemodynamics is expected to explain a portion of the renoprotective influence of Cilnidipine in SHR/ND in the current study. However, Hayashi et al. discovered that Cilnidipine and amlodipine had significant implications on efferent/afferent ratio arteriole dilation in hydronephrotic kidney. It appears likely that Cilnidipine induces renoprotection by regulating glomerular hemodynamics. However, whether this effect is responsible for the difference between Cilnidipine and amlodipine in the current study is unknown. As a result, Cilnidipine suppressed proteinuria development in SHR/ND patients more than amlodipine, presumably by impeding N-type calcium channels in the podocyte.

■ RENIN-ANGIOTENSIN-ALDOSTERONE SYSTEM

The renin-angiotensin-aldosterone system (RAAS) is a key mediator in the pathophysiology of hypertension, and its overexpression contributes to end-organ damage such as coronary artery disease and myocardial infarction, congestive

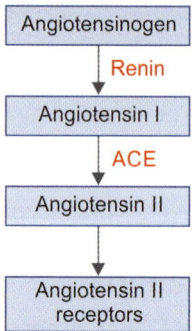

FLOWCHART 1: Renin-angiotensin-aldosterone system.

heart failure, and renal disease. Because of the close relationship between the RAAS and hypertension, there are compelling reasons to block angiotensin II (Ang II), formation or activity with angiotensin-converting enzyme (ACE) inhibitors and angiotensin II receptor blockers (ARBs) **(Flowchart 1)**. It regulates BP, fluid volume, and sodium-potassium balance, and is one of the most important hormonal mechanisms in controlling hemodynamic stability. As a result, any change in the molecules that make up RAAS contributes to the development of AH.

Renin is synthesized as an inactive form in the kidneys and released into circulation in response to low-intratubular sodium levels, hypotension in the afferent arterioles of the renal glomerulus, and sympathetic activation. Prorenin is activated in the bloodstream by proteolytic and nonproteolytic mechanisms to produce the active form. Here, active renin catalyzes the cleavage of the glycoprotein angiotensinogen, resulting in the formation of angiotensin I.

The ACE cleaves angiotensin I to produce Ang II, the main effector in the RAAS. Whereas neutral endopeptidases (EP) cleave angiotensin I to produce angiotensin-(1–7), another active peptide in this system that usually works against the implications of Ang II. The majority of Ang II's known proliferative and profibrotic effects are via the angiotensin type 1 receptor (AT1-R), but it can also bind to the Ang II type 2 receptor (AT2-R), causing the opposite effects as the AT1-R. Angiotensin-(1–7) can also be produced by cleaving Ang II by ACE2, reducing the concentration in favor of Ang II, which promotes vasodilation in cardiac and vascular tissues.

■ TELMISARTAN

Telmisartan is a long-acting ARB with a superior pharmacodynamic profile when compared to other ARBs, and it is the only ARB with an indication for the prevention of CV disease progression that is available in combination with CCB. In CV high-risk patients and those with evidence of renal disease, clinical studies indicate that ARB/CCB combinations may be preferable to ARB/hydrochlorothiazide (HCTZ) combinations. Telmisartan is an insurmountable antagonist at the AT1-R, which means the blockade is semi-irreversible and characterized by the antagonist's slow release from its receptor **(Fig. 2)**. This antagonism reduces the maximal response to Ang II; when the receptor is preincubated with telmisartan, the Ang II dose-response curve shifts nonparallel rightward.

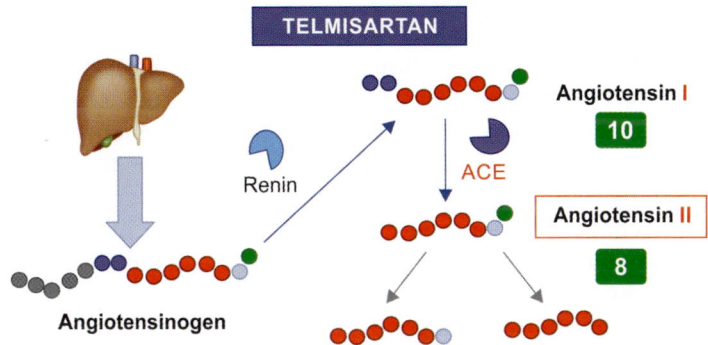

FIG. 2: Mechanism of action of ARB.

The insurmountable antagonism is caused by telmisartan's slow dissociation from the AT1-R. Telmisartan has the highest affinity for the AT1-R of any ARB currently available. Telmisartan had a dissociation half-life of 213 minutes when tested in an in vitro preparation of human AT1-R, whereas the other ARBs ranged from 166 minutes with olmesartan to 67 minutes with losartan. Another in vitro study using a different methodology discovered that telmisartan has a faster dissociation half-life than olmesartan. Telmisartan's AT1 binding properties are likely to be important for its long-lasting antihypertensive effects.

In a number of studies, the efficacy of telmisartan in controlling BP was compared to that of other ARBs. It demonstrated comparable (or noninferior) efficacy in controlling BP values, while a peculiar and significant finding was the consistently documented better control of BP during the 6 hours preceding the next dose and a better 24-hour BP control. It is well known that high BP in the early morning is linked to an increased risk of CV disease. To reduce this risk, it is critical that antihypertensive medication control BP.

In a recent meta-analysis of six randomized, controlled trials (including 3,762 patients), Zheng et al. found no significant difference in lowering systolic blood pressure (SBP) and diastolic blood pressure (DBP) between telmisartan 80 mg daily and valsartan 160 mg daily, but when combined with HCTZ, telmisartan showed a significant benefit on lowering SBP and DBP compared to valsartan. More studies are needed to compare the efficacy of telmisartan versus valsartan in this setting, based on evidence that early morning BP surge and 24-hour mean BP are linked to target organ damage and CV events.

Lacourciere et al. discovered that telmisartan ($n = 447$) significantly reduced mean DBP and SBP in the last 6 hours compared to valsartan ($n = 430$; $p = 0.0044$ and 0.0066, respectively for DBP and SBP). Similarly, after a missed dose, telmisartan ($n = 437$) significantly reduced 24-hour mean DBP and SBP compared to valsartan ($n = 431$; $p = 0.0004$ and 0.0024, respectively). Furthermore, telmisartan had greater 24-hourly mean reductions in DBP and SBP than valsartan. Other trials confirmed these findings, as summarized by Galzerano et al.

CONCLUSION

This study discovered that controlling hypertension reduces CV outcomes by doubling CV risk with BP increases of 20/10 mm Hg, and that lower is better because the relationship between BP and CV risk is continuous. The majority of patients require more than two medications to achieve their BP goals. It was also discovered that the combination of Cilnidipine and telmisartan is superior to other combinations (renal protection and cardiac protection). It has been discovered that patient response to fixed dose combinations is predictable. Combinations representing several antihypertensive classes, not just thiazide combinations, achieved incremental efficacy with good tolerability.

SUGGESTED READINGS

1. Page IH. The mosaic theory of arterial hypertension—its interpretation. Perspect Biol Med. 1967;10:325e333.
2. Frolich BD. The first Irvine H. Page lecture. The mosaic of hypertension: past, present and future. J Hypertens Suppl. 1988;6(4):S2-11.
3. Frolich ED. Mechanisms contributing to high blood pressure. Ann Intern Med. 1983;98:709e714.
4. Chatzikyrkoyu C, Menne J, Haller H. [Hypertension 2007-2008]. Med Klin (Munich). 2009;104(8):614-21.
5. Chobanian AV, Bakris GL, Black HR, et al. The seventh report of the Joint National Committee on prevention, detection, evaluation, and treatment of high blood pressure: The JNC 7 Report. JAMA. 2003;289(19):2560-72.
6. Julius S, Schork N, Schork A. Sympathetic hyperactivity in early stages of hypertension: The Ann Arbor data set. J Cardiovasc Pharmacol. 1988;12 Suppl 3·S121-9.
7. Frishman WH. Calcium channel blockers: Differences between subclasses. Am J Cardiovasc Drugs. 2007;7 (Suppl 1):17-23.
8. Aoum K, Berdeaux A. Dihydropyridines from the first to fourth generation: Better effects and safety. Therapie. 2003;58(4):333-9.
9. Mohammed MS. Spctrophotometric method for the estimation of cilnidipine in bulk and pharmaceutical dosage forms. Orient. J Chem. 2013;29(1):131-4.
10. Singh BN. The mechanism of action of calcium antagonists relative to their clinical applications. Br J Clin Pharmacol. 1986;21(Suppl 2):109S-21S.
11. Vekariya PP, Joshi HS. Development and validation of RP-HPLC method for azilsartan medoxomil potassium quantitation in human plasma by solid phase extraction procedure. ISRN Spectroscopy. 2013;2013(572170).
12. Singh S, Singh B, Bahuguna R, et al. Stress degradation studies on ezetimibe and development of a validated stability-indicating HPLC assay. J Pharm Biomed Anal. 2006;41(3):1037-40.
13. Bakshi M, Singh S. Development of validated stability indicating assay methods—critical review. J Pharm Biomed Anal. 2002;(6):1011-40.
14. Niranjan CD, Patil SM, Sabaji JK, et al. Development of UV spectrophotometric method for estimation and validation of telmisartan as a pure API. J Pharm Res. 2012;5(6):3331-3.
15. Pradhan KK, Mishra US, Sahoo A, et al. Method development and validation of telmisartan in bulk and pharmaceutical dosage forms by UV spectrophotometric method. Int J Pharm Sci. 2011;2(4):526-30.
16. Takahara A, Fujita S, Moki K, et al. Neuronal calcium channel blocking action of antihypertensive drug, cilnidipine in IMR32 human neuroblastoma cells. Hypertens Res. 2003;26:743-47.
17. Nap A, Mathy MJ, Balt JC, et al. The evaluation of N type channel blocking properties of cilnidipine and other voltage dependent calcium antagonists. Fundam Clin Pharmacol. 2004;18(3):309-19.
18. Iimura O, Ishi M, Inagaki Y, et al. Study of FRC-8653 (cilnidipine) in patients with severe hypertension. Jpn Pharmacol Ther. 1993;21:S155-70.

19. Nagahama S, Norimatsu T, Maki T, et al. The effect of combination therapy with L/N type calcium channel blocker cilnidipine, and an angiotensin II receptor blocker on blood pressure and heart rate in Japanese hypertensive patients: An observational study conducted in Japan. Hypertens Res. 2007;30(9):815-22.
20. Mahathi G, Reddy YR, Prasad PU. Development and validation of telmisartan and atorvastatin calcium in combined dosage form by RP-HPLC. Int J Pharm Technol. 2011;3(3):3370-89.
21. Zhou X, Ono H, Ono Y, et al. N- and L-type calcium channel antagonist improves glomerular dynamics, reverses severe nephrosclerosis, and inhibits apoptosis and proliferation in an l-NAME/SHR model. J Hypertens. 2002;20:993-1000.
22. Konno Y, Kimura K. Vasodilatory effect of cilnidipine, an L-type and N-type calcium channel blocker, on rat kidney glomerular arterioles. Int Heart J. 2008;49:723-32.
23. Hayashi K, Wakino S, Sugano N, et al. Ca^{2+} channel subtypes and pharmacology in the kidney. Circ Res. 2007;100:342-53.
24. Brunner HR. The new oral angiotensin II antagonist olmesartan medoxomil: a concise overview. J Hum Hypertens. 2002;16(Suppl 2):S13-6.
25. Zheng Z, Lin S, Shi H. A systematic review and meta-analysis of telmisartan vs valsartan in the management of essential hypertension. J Clin Hypertens. 2010;12:414-21.
26. Lacourciere Y, Lenis J, Orchard R, et al. A comparison of the efficacy and duration of action of the angiotensin II receptor blocker telmisartan to amlodipine. Blood Press Monit. 1998;3:295-302.
27. Galzerano D, Capogrosso C, Michele SD, et al. New standards in hypertension and cardiovascular risk management: focus on telmisartan. Vasc Health Risk Manag. 2010;6:113-33.

CHAPTER 49

Management of Hypertension in Chronic Kidney Disease

Mritunjay Kumar Singh

■ INTRODUCTION

Studies from India and abroad have provided concordant data on high prevalence of chronic kidney disease (CKD) worldwide. Up to 1 in 10 people world wide has CKD. It is a silent killer like other metabolic diseases and engages major human and economical resources. Association of hypertension and CKD is unique. There is a cause and effect relationship between them. Hypertension is considered as most important modifiable risk factor for CKD. Managing hypertension effectively not only retards the progression of CKD, but also reduces the cardiovascular risk significantly.

■ PATHOPHYSIOLOGY OF HYPERTENSION IN CKD

Pathophysiology of hypertension in CKD is multifactorial. It contains components of neural and hormonal pathways. The important mechanisms include:
- *Impaired sodium excretion*: Guyton and his team have shown that hypertension can be generated in partially nephrectomized dog (renal mass reduced to 30%) with salt loading. The elevated blood pressure (BP) in this setting is induced by increased cardiac output (volume expansion) initially, and later on sustained by increased peripheral resistance which is due to autoregulatory peripheral vascular bed vasoconstriction in response to increase peripheral perfusion due to extracellular volume expansion. So sodium retention can induce hypertension in two ways: at first by volume-dependent mechanism (extracellular fluid expansion) and later on mainly through volume-independent mechanism like increased peripheral vascular resistance.
- *Increased renin-angiotensin-aldosterone (RAAS) activity*: Hypersecretion of renin in a sclerosed kidney leads to increased angiotensin II and RAAS activity leading to increased systemic vascular resistance, sodium retention, and high BP.

- *Increased activity of systemic nervous system (SNS)*: The kidney is a richly innervated sensory organ. Several studies from animal and human subjects establish the kidney–brain axis theory. Sensory inputs from kidney transmitted to central nervous system in turn leads to increased activity of SNS leading to vasoconstriction, rennin secretion, sodium retention, and hypertension.
- *Endothelin dysfunction*: CKD is a chronic low-grade inflammatory state and so endothelial dysfunctions are commonly observed in CKD. Endothelial dysfunction leads to impaired nitrous oxide production and increased endothelin level leading to increased peripheral vasoconstriction and hypertension.
- *Vascular stiffness*: The distensibility of resistance arteries is affected by certain functional and morphological changes. It includes intimal hyperplasia, medial calcification, smooth muscle cell hyperplasia, and endothelial dysfunction. These changes are largely contributed by disturbed calcium-phosphorus balance, secondary hyperparathyroidism, and other neurohumoral components discussed above. Vascular stiffness leads to increased systolic BP and wide pulse pressure, which is a strong predictor of cardiovascular mortality in CKD.
- The erythropoietin-induced hypertension and obstructive sleep apnea (OSA) are important causes of hypertension in CKD, especially in dialysis population. The erythropoietin or erythropoietin-stimulating agents used for treatment of anemia in CKD can induce hypertension or require change in antihypertensive regimen in approximately 30% of the cases. Besides rapid and over correction of anemia, hypertension in this subset is thought to be caused by vasoconstrictor effect of erythropoietin which is independent of hemoglobin. OSA is common in advanced CKD population. Chronic intermittent nocturnal hypoxemia provoke sympathetic nervous system activity, RAAS activity, and increases nocturnal BP.
- Medications like over the counter nonsteroidal anti-inflammatory drugs, herbal supplements, steroids, and decongestants can provoke hypertension in the CKD population.
- The worsening of hypertension has been reported in CKD patients with the use of potent antituberculosis drug rifampicin. Rifampicin is a potent enzyme inducer and decreases the level of commonly used antihypertensive drugs: amlodipine, metoprolol, and prazosin. So, it is advisable to monitor hypertension in CKD patients, once they have been put on rifampicin.
- Hypertension is the most common complication of CKD as well as major factor responsible for progression of CKD. Renal autoregulatory mechanism protects renal vasculatures from elevated BP. Maintenance of afferent arteriole tone in response to elevated systemic pressure and increased sodium chloride delivery to macula densa are part of this autoregulatory mechanism. However, it is impaired in patients with diabetes and nondiabetics CKD, thus leads to progressive renal damage with even moderate elevation of BP.

MEASUREMENT OF BP IN CKD

The proper BP measurement is the first step toward the effective blood pressure management in CKD. BP measurement can vary depending on the setting (e.g., casual office, standardized office, or home) and type of device used (e.g., aneroid or Oscillometric). Standardized office BP (SOBP) is 5–10 mm Hg lower than casual office BP. Most of the recent trials on optimum BP goals have used SOBP as a method of measurement. For SOBP measurement certain preparations are required (e.g., 5 minutes of quite rest/no nicotine, caffeine, and exercise 30 minutes prior to measurement/well validated and periodically calibrated device/correct cuff size/middle of the cuff should be placed at the level of right atrium/average of more than two readings obtained on two occasions) as laid down by 2017 ACC/AHA high BP guidelines.

The out of office BP measurement (ambulatory BP and home BP monitoring) is required to diagnose white-coat hypertension (defined as elevated office BP with controlled out of office BP, prevalence in CKD ranges from 2 to 41%) and masked hypertension (defined as controlled office BP and elevated out of office BP, prevalence in CKD ranges from 6 to 51%). Additionally, 24 hour ambulatory BP gives clue about the nocturnal BP. Physiological nocturnal dipping is absent in 14–75% of the CKD population. Thus in CKD out of office BP accurately define the clinical problem and predicts more accurately about the cardiovascular and renal outcomes than office BP.

KDOQI (Kidney Disease Outcome Quality Initiative) US commentary on the 2017 ACC/AHA hypertension guideline commented that home BP monitoring (HBPM) can accurately predict target organ damage and better placed than ambulatory BP monitoring and office BP monitoring. HBPM can also help to overcome the therapeutic inertia.

In our limited resource setting we should prefer standardized office BP, because it requires nothing but our little patience (premeasurement preparation as mentioned above).

■ TARGET BLOOD PRESSURE IN CKD

The management of hypertension in CKD is a dynamic process, as estimated glomerular filtration rate, comorbidities, and risk changes with time. Due to presence of vascular stiffness and wide pulse pressure in CKD, achieving a BP target rapidly may lead to postural hypotension. So a cautious and gradual approach is required to reach a desired BP target.

From 1994 to 2010, there were four landmark trials compared the standard versus intensive BP control in patients with CKD. These were:
- MDRD (Modification of Diet in Renal Disease), year 1994
- AASK (Africans American Study of Kidney Disease and Hypertension), year 2002
- REIN-2 (Ramipril Efficacy in Nephropathy-2), year 2005
- ACCORD (Action to Control Cardiovascular Risk in Diabetes), year 2010.

    Results of all these trials favored standard BP control rather than intensive control in most of the CKD patients, exceptions are patients with proteinuria >1 g/day, which were benefited from intensive control of BP. On the basis of these trials KDIGO (Kidney Disease Initiative Global Outcome) 2012 suggested a lower BP for significant proteinuria.
- Albuminuria (<30 mg/24 h): ≤140/90 (1B)
- Albuminuria (>30 mg/24 h): ≤130/80 (2D)

Till year 2015 it was thought that controlling blood pressure to <140/90 is likely to be beneficial in CKD population. But with the advent of SPRINT (systolic blood pressure intervention trial) study in 2015, intensive control of systolic blood pressure (<120 mm Hg) has gained momentum. SPRINT has included data from 9,361 adults age 50 or older with systolic blood pressure of 130 mm Hg or higher and at least one additional cardiovascular disease risk factor. 28% of participants had CKD without significant proteinuria. The highlights of SPRINT study are:
- Intensive reduction in SBP reduces cardiovascular events.
- Intensive reduction in SBP has mortality benefit in CKD population.
- The sub group analysis of older patients with CKD in SPRINT has also favorable outcome.
- With adoption of SBP <120 mm Hg in all CKD population, separate blood pressure target for proteinuria is not required.

However, it should be noted that more than 50% of participants in intensive arm of SPRINT had not achieved SBP target after 1 year. So targeting and achieving a lower SBP is a big challenge. Additionally the benefit of lower BP is less certain in diabetic CKD and advanced CKD population. The 2017 American College of Cardiology (ACC) has adopted the result of SPRINT and suggested more intensive BP control in CKD population. In light of SPRINT and other newer studies KDIGO controversies conference 2017 has also suggested for revision in BP diagnosis threshold and BP treatment target.

In our setting, we should target lower BP:
- If SOBP/HBPM is the method used for measurement of BP.
- If patient is tolerating the target BP well without postural hypotension or other adverse effect.
- If patient is having non diabetic CKD.

■ SECONDARY HYPERTENSION IN CKD

Secondary causes of HTN are potentially treatable and should be searched in following conditions:
- If the onset of elevated BP occurred before puberty and preceded the development of CKD.
- Severe or malignant hypertension that is out of proportion to the degree of CKD is present.
- Acute worsening of BP control occurs in a previously hypertensive patient with good BP control, or resistant hypertension is present.
- Persistent hypokalemia off diuretic treatment (primary aldosteronism)
- Development of tremor and palpitation (pheochromocytoma)
- Flash pulmonary edema (renal artery stenosis)

■ NONPHARMACOLOGICAL THERAPY

Early institution of nonpharmacological therapy in form of dietary modification and lifestyle modification is the fist step to the treatment of hypertension in CKD.
- Dietary salt restriction (sodium intake <1.5 g/day) – reduce BP and proteinuria; potentiate the action of ACEI/ARB.

- DASH (Dietary approach to stop hypertension) diet: Diet rich in fruits and vegetables, low in saturated and unsaturated fat can lead to modest reduction in BP. But it is not appropriate to use DASH Diet in advanced CKD because of the potential for hyperkalemia.
- Modest physical activity of 150 min duration/week is useful for CKD population. It can be modified depending on the cardiorespiratory fitness status and physical limitation of the individual.
- Other lifestyle interventions include weight loss in obese people, limiting alcohol intake and avoidance of over the counter medications such as nonsteroidal anti-inflammatory drugs.

CHOOSING ANTIHYPERTENSIVE DRUGS IN CKD

Most of the CKD patients require multiple antihypertensives for adequate control of hypertension. Certain classes of antihypertensives are preferred because of their renoprotective, cardioprotective and diuretics actions apart from antihypertensive effects. Before choosing antihypertensives agents in CKD we should look for comorbidities, risk benefit ratio of individual drug, volume status, and age of the patient.

Angiotensin-converting Enzyme Inhibitors/Angiotensin Receptor Blockers (ACEI/ARBs)

- ACEI/ARB are the agent of choice to treat hypertension in diabetic CKD with severely increased proteinuria (>300 mg/day). But the superiority of ACEI/ARB over other agents (calcium channel blockers, diuretics) is questionable in nonproteinuric CKD. However as majority of CKD patients require multiple agents to achieve adequate control of hypertension, it is reasonable to include ACEI/ARB as add on therapy in nonproteinuric CKD patients.
- The common side effect of ACEI/ARB is hyperkalemia particularly in advanced CKD hence limiting their use despite their proven benefit. Novel potassium binding agents (patiromer and sodium zirconium cyclosilicate) in combination with ACEI/ARB could change the way of pharmacotherapy in hypertension in CKD. But further research is required before their routine clinical use.
- Another potential problem with the use of ACEI/ARB is acute kidney injury. Recent guidelines suggest that up to 30% increase in serum creatinine in first few weeks and later on stabilization is an acceptable physiological change which confers long term renoprotection.
- Combination therapy (ACEI+ARB) has failed to show any cardioprotection and renoprotection in major studies. Additionally this combination is associated with increase risk of hyperkalemia, acute kidney injury, and hypotension.

Calcium Channel Blockers (CCB)—Dihydropyridine (DHP)-CCB (Amlodipine)

These are frequently prescribed antihypertensives in CKD because:
- They are the potent antihypertensive agents.
- Can work synergistically with ACEI/ARB.

- Work well in volume expanded states and
- Minimal side effect (pedal edema)

Diuretics
- Sodium retention and volume overload are the main concerns of the majority of CKD patients. Diuretics act by natriuresis (promote sodium excretion through kidney), thus reduce extracellular volume and has been shown to improve left ventricular mass index (LVMI) and arterial stiffness in CKD patients. Diuretics also enhance the blood pressure lowering effect of ACEI/ARB. Thiazide diuretics (hydrochlorothiazides, chlorthalidone) are less effective at lower glomerular filtration rate so switching to loop diuretics (furosemide, torsemide) with frequent dosing is done in advanced CKD. Sometimes loop diuretics can be combined with thiazide diuretics to treat refractory edema in advanced CKD.
- Diuretics should be avoided in end stage renal disease with no residual function and poly cystic kidney disease as they can lead to accelerated cyst growth and decreased renal function. The major adverse effects of diuretics are volume depletion and electrolyte imbalance.
- Mineralocorticoid receptor antagonists (MRA) are effective drugs for resistant hypertension but may cause hyperkalemia in patients with low estimated glomerular filtration rate, so better to avoid at estimated glomerular filtration rate below 45 mL/min/m^2.

Beta Blockers
- Although beta blockers has lost credential in treatment of primary hypertension in general population, but still they are found to be useful adjunctive therapy in CKD population because they decrease sympathetic over activity and are cardioprotective. A recent trial named HDPAL (hypertension in hemodialysis patients treated with atenolol or lisinopril) has concluded that atenolol arm has less cardiovascular events and better blood pressure control than lisinopril arm in hemodialysis patients.
- Other antihypertensive agents for patients with CKD include direct vasodilator (minoxidil and hydralazine), centrally acting alpha adrenergic agonist (clonidine), alpha blockers (prazosin), and direct rennin inhibitors (aliskiren).

Resistant and Refractory Hypertension in CKD
The prevalence is up to 40% as shown in CRIC Study. It has got poor prognosis—increases the risk of death by 30% and the risk of heart failure by 59%. The selection of complementary medications and ensuring drug adherence often resolve treatment resistance. Thiazide and thiazide like diuretics in combination with ACE/ARB or MRA can be very effective in treatment of CKD populations with apparent drug resistant hypertension.

Adherence

Adherence to therapy is poor due to frequent dosing of pills, pill burden, drug interaction, and adverse effects. Strategies to improve adherence include:
- Patients should be communicated regarding treatment and its importance
- Use of combination pill and whenever possible long acting, once a day medication to be used.

Nocturnal Therapy

Nondipping is detected more frequently in later stages of CKD and associated with significant CV death. Multiple clinical trials have shown an improvement in nocturnal dipping of BP by dosing at least 1 antihypertensive medication at bedtime.

MANAGEMENT OF HTN IN PATIENTS ON DIALYSIS

The relationship between BP and CVD in this group is more complex. There is U-shaped relationship between 24 hours ambulatory SBP and all cause mortality as noted by Mayer et al. So BP treatment should be individualized in this group keeping in mind of comorbid conditions. Besides pharmacotherapy these are the novel measure to treat HTN in dialysis patients:
- Dry weight reduction (DRIP trial)
- Dietary sodium restriction
- Dialysate sodium restriction
- Adequate time on dialysis
- Consideration of frequent dialysis

MANAGING HYPERTENSION FOLLOWING KIDNEY TRANSPLANTATION

Hypertension is common in post-transplant period. It has been reported that HTN is prevalent in >90% of calcineurin inhibitors treated kidney transplant recipient. The higher BP is associated with poor graft survival, increased CVD risk, and most common cause of death post-transplant. KDIGO and the ACC/AHA guidelines currently recommend a BP target <130/80 mm Hg. Some useful tips to manage HTN following kidney transplants are:
- Weight control
- Steroid and CNI dose optimization
- During 1st year after transplant, CCB (DHP) is the preferred antihypertensive agent over ACEI/ARBs.
- In patient with mild graft dysfunction with proteinuria ARBs are the preferred drug.
- In case of post transplant hyperuricemia losartan is the preferred drug.

FUTURE PROSPECTIVE

In recent years the underlying mechanism and unmet therapeutic needs to halt the progression of CKD and CVD have been better understood. Due to this few promising therapeutic measures have emerged. They are:

- Sodium-glucose cotransporter-2 (SGLT-2) inhibitors: Interest in molecules of this group has intensified following the result of EMPA-REG OUTCOME (Empagliflozin Cardiovascular Outcome Event Trial in Type 2 Diabetes Mellitus Patients) and CREDENCE (Canagliflozin and Renal Outcomes in Type 2 Diabetes and Nephropathy) trials, which demonstrated significant slowing of CKD progression and a reduction in the composite outcome of death from CVD. Combining ACEI/ARB with SGLT-2 inhibitors may further reduce intraglomerular pressure by their synergistic effects.
- The DUET (Dual Endothelin Receptor and Angiotensin Receptor Blocker) trials with sparsentan and irbesartan have shown promising results in control of hypertension and proteinuria in IgA nephropathy and Focal Segmental Glomerulosclerosis (FSGS).
- *Renal denervation therapy (RDN)*: After initial hiccups this radio frequency energy-based therapy for ablation of the networks of nerves around renal arteries has shown promising results in newer trials. However, this strategy is still in experimental stage.

CONCLUSION

The Prevalence of HTN in CKD is very high, but HTN control rate is far from optimal. When CKD and HTN coexist, CV morbidity and mortality is substantially increased. Personalized and individualized hypertension therapy using HBPM holds great promise. ACEIs or ARBs, appropriate diuretic therapy, and dietary salt restriction make up the foundation for the treatment of HTN in CKD.

SUGGESTED READINGS

1. Jhonson RJ, Feehally J, Floege J (Eds). Comprehensive Clinical Nephrology, 5th edition. Elsevier Saunders; 2014.
2. Pugh D, Gallacher PJ, Dhaun N. Management of Hypertension in Chronic Kidney Disease. Drugs. 2019;79(4):365-79.
3. Elaine Ku, Lee BJ, Wei J, Matthew R. Weir Hypertension in CKD: Core Curriculum. Am J Kidney Dis. 2019;74(1):120-31.
4. Coleman TG, Guyton AC. Hypertension Caused by Salt Loading in the Dog III. Onset transients of Cardiac output and other circulatory variables. Circ Res. 1969;25(2):153-60.
5. Krapf R, Hulter HN. Arterial hypertension induced by erythropoietin and erythropoiesis-stimulating agents (ESA). Clin J Am Soc Nephrol. 2009;4:470-80.
6. Agrawal A, Agarwal SK, Kaleekal T, et al. Rifampicin and anti-hypertensive drugs in chronic kidney disease: Pharmacokinetic interactions and their clinical impact. Indian J Nephrol. 2016;26:322-8.
7. Whelton PK, Carey RM, Aronow WS, et al. 2017 ACC/AHA/AAPA/ABC/ACPM/ AGS/APhA/ASH/ASPC/NMA/PCNA Guideline for the Prevention, Detection, Evaluation, and Management of High Blood Pressure in Adults: Executive Summary: A Report of the American College of Cardiology/American Heart Association Task Force on Clinical Practice Guidelines. Hypertension. 2018;71(6):1269-324.
8. AK Cheung, Chang TI, Cushman WC, et al. Blood pressure in kidney disease: A KDIGO conference report. Kidney Int. 2019;95:1027-36.
9. Kramer HJ, Townsend RR, Griffin K, et al. KDOQI US Commentary on the 2017 ACC/AHA Hypertension Guideline. Am J Kidney Dis. 2019;73(4):437-58.

10. Klahr S, Levey AS, Beck GJ, et al. The effects of dietary protein restriction and blood pressure control on the progression of chronic renal disease. Modification of Diet in Renal Disease Study Group. N Engl J Med. 1994;330:877-84.
11. Wright JT Jr, Bakris G, Greene T, et al. Effect of blood pressure lowering and antihypertensive drug class on progression of hypertensive kidney disease: results from the AASK trial. JAMA. 2002;288:2421-31.
12. Ruggenenti P, Perna A, Loriga G, et al. Blood-pressure control for renoprotection in patients with non-diabetic chronic renal disease (REIN-2): multicentre, randomised controlled trial. Lancet. 2005;365:939-46.
13. Cushman WC, Evans GW, Byington RP, et al. Effects of intensive blood-pressure control in type 2 diabetes mellitus. N Engl J Med. 2010;362:1575-85.
14. Wright JT Jr, Williamson JD, Whelton PK, et al. A randomized trial of intensive versus standard blood-pressure control. N Engl J Med. 2015;373:2103-16.
15. Sinha AD, Agarwal R. Clinical Pharmacology of Antihypertensive Therapy for the Treatment of Hypertension in CKD. CJASN. 2019;14(5):757-64.
16. Muntner P, Anderson A, Charleston J, et al. Hypertension awareness, treatment, and control in adults with CKD: results from the Chronic Renal Insufficiency Cohort (CRIC) Study. Am J Kidney Dis. 2010;55(3):441-51.
17. Judd E, Calhoun DA. Management of hypertension in CKD: beyond the guidelines. Adv Chronic Kidney Dis. 2015;22(2):116-22.
18. Hermida RC, Ayala DE, Mojon A, Fernandez JR. Bedtime dosing of antihypertensive medications reduces cardiovascular risk in CKD. J Am Soc Nephrol. 2011;22:2313-21.
19. Mayer CC, Matschkal J, Sarafidis PA, et al. Association of ambulatory blood pressure with all-cause and cardiovascular mortality in hemodialysis patients: effects of heart failure and atrial fibrillation. J Am Soc Nephrol. 2018;29:2409-17.
20. Agarwal R, Alborzi P, Satyan S, et al. Dry-weight reduction in hypertensive hemodialysis patients (DRIP): a randomized, controlled trial. Hypertension. 2009;53:500-7.
21. Wanner C, Lachin JM, Inzucchi SE, et al. on behalf of the EMPA-REG OUTCOME Investigators. Empagliflozin and Clinical Outcomes in Patients With Type 2 Diabetes, Established Cardiovascular Disease and Chronic Kidney Disease. Circulation. 2018;137(2):119-29.
22. Perkovic V, Jardine MJ, Neal B, et al. Canaglifloin and Renal Outcomes in Type2 Diabetes and Nephropathy. N Engl J Med. 2019;380:2295-306.
23. Herrington WG, Preiss D, Haynes R. The potential for improving cardio-renal outcomes by sodium-glucose co-transporter-2 inhibition in people with chronic kidney disease: a rationale for the EMPA-KIDNEY study. Clin Kidney J. 2018;11(6):749-61.
24. Komers R, Gipson DS, Nelson P, et al. Efficacy and safety of sparsentan compared with irbesartan in patients with primary focal segmental glomerulosclerosis: randomized, controlled trial design (DUET). Kidney Int Rep. 2017;2:654-64.
25. Townsend RR, Mahfoud F, Kandzari DE, et al. Catheter-based renal denervation in patients with uncontrolled hypertension in the absence of antihypertensive medications (SPYRAL HTN-OFF MED): a randomised, sham-controlled, proof-of-concept trial. Lancet. 2017;390:2160-21.

CHAPTER 50

Antimicrobial Stewardship Program

Amit Aggarwal

■ INTRODUCTION

Antimicrobials are the only medications that become less useful over a period of time, even if they are used correctly. Antibiotics that were in use 50 years ago are no longer as effective. While drug resistance is an inevitable evolutionary process, two factors have accelerated the development of multidrug resistant (MDR) infections—first, lesser new classes of antimicrobial agents developed in recent times and secondly, irrational or inappropriate use and abuse of antimicrobials by the medical professionals, the agricultural industry, and the society in general. In order to effectively deal with this issue, Antimicrobial Stewardship Program (ASP) has emerged as one of the mechanisms to regulate antimicrobial usage in healthcare systems. The aim of antimicrobial stewardship is to restrict inappropriate antibiotic therapy in order to reduce the development of drug resistance, avoid associated adverse effects, and optimize clinical outcomes.

■ PRINCIPLES OF OPTIMAL ANTIBIOTIC THERAPY

There are several key tenets of ASPs, which begin with optimal antibiotic utilization. Selection of appropriate empirical antibiotic begins with an accurate differential diagnosis that includes a likely bacterial etiology. Even in a patient with an obvious bacterial infection, antimicrobial therapy should only be initiated when it is expected to favorably alter the patient's clinical course. There should be a lower threshold for instituting empirical therapy in critically ill patients. One should not unnecessarily treat "colonizers" in endotracheal tube aspirates, nonpurulent wounds, or bacteriuria associated with chronic indwelling urinary catheters, in asymptomatic individuals. The predicament with needlessly "covering" colonizers in bodily fluids is that these organisms are often of the MDR variety and prolonged therapy associated with trying to eradicate such microbes is frequently complicated by further increase in antimicrobial resistance.

Another consideration in the selection of appropriate antibiotic is to take into account the spectrum of activity against the presumptive pathogens, which is usually related to the resident flora at the particular anatomical site. Antibiotic regimen with inadequate spectrum of activity results in therapeutic failure or selection of drug-resistant organisms. Multiple host factors and comorbidities affect the breadth of empirical therapy by altering the probabilities of the likely infective agents.

Pharmacokinetic-pharmacodynamic (PK/PD) principles are important in dosing and assessing antibiotic penetration at the site of infection. Tissue-serum PK principles, i.e., serum/tissue concentration gradient, lipid solubility, pKa, local pH, and estimated local tissue concentrations should be considered by the "infectious disease" consultant before making an antibiotic selection.

The shortest defined duration of antimicrobial therapy that eliminates the infection should be used in order to minimize both the potential adverse effects and antibiotic resistance potential. Early de-escalation of therapy is of paramount importance, based on microbiology results and clinical or biomarker responses. In cases of therapy failure, the clinician should consider source control and/or alternative diagnoses before blaming drug resistance and broadening the therapy. Also, new infection should be distinguished from the failure of initial therapy. The distinction between bacteriostatic and bactericidal antimicrobial agents is an in-vitro construct and clinical trial data does not support any difference in intrinsic clinical efficacy between the two. Antimicrobial combination therapy may be beneficial in only a few clinical situations, and its routine use is not supported by clinical evidence in most cases. It also results in increased drug-related toxicity, disruption of the host microbiome, and selection of antimicrobial resistance. Another method to control resistance is by restricting "high-resistance potential" antibiotics, e.g., imipenem (not meropenem or ertapenem), ceftazidime (not other third or fourth generation cephalosporins), and gentamicin/tobramycin (not amikacin). Some antibiotics may be restricted for other reasons; e.g., excessive vancomycin use (IV not PO) predisposes to VRE emergence, and it also causes cell wall thickening in *Staphylococcus aureus* (*S. aureus*), resulting in permeability-related resistance (to vancomycin and other antibiotics, e.g., daptomycin).

WHAT DOES ANTIMICROBIAL STEWARDSHIP MEAN?

Stewardship is described as careful and responsible management of something, entrusted with one's care. Antibiotic stewardship has been defined in a consensus statement from the Infectious Diseases Society of America (IDSA), the Society for Healthcare Epidemiology of America (SHEA), and the Pediatric Infectious Diseases Society (PIDS) as "coordinated interventions designed to improve and measure the appropriate use of (antibiotic) agents by promoting the selection of the optimal (antibiotic) drug regimen including dosing, duration of therapy, and route of administration".

Antimicrobial stewardship (AMS) is one of the three pillars of an integrated approach to strengthening the healthcare system. The other two include infection prevention and control (IPC) and patient safety.

The AMPs have the following goals:
- To work with healthcare practitioners to prescribe 5 "D"s of antimicrobial therapy, which is the right *D*rug, correct *D*ose, right *D*rug-route, suitable *D*uration, timely *D*e-escalation to pathogen-directed therapy.
- To prevent antimicrobial overuse, misuse, and abuse in inpatient, outpatient, and community settings, including the agriculture industry.
- To reduce antibiotic-related adverse effects, e.g., *Clostridioides difficile (C. difficile)* infection, organ-specific injury.
- To minimize drug resistance.
- To reduce healthcare-associated cost.

Core members of the ASP team should ideally include:
- An infection disease consultant/physician.
- A clinical pharmacist.
- A clinical microbiologist.
- An infection prevention nurse.

Support Staff
- Clinicians.
- Department heads.
- Pharmacy and Therapeutics Committee.
- Infection preventionists and hospital epidemiologists.
- Quality control, patient safety, and regulatory staff.

KEY REQUIREMENTS OF ANTIMICROBIAL STEWARDSHIP PROGRAM

- Creation of a multidisciplinary inter-professional AMS team that is physician directed or supervised. Minimum, one or more members of the team should have training in AMS. The number of team members may vary on the basis of the size and complexity of the facility.
- A formulary limited to non-duplicative antibiotics with demonstrated clinical needs.
- Institutional guidelines for the management of common infection syndromes.
- Processes to measure and monitor antimicrobial use at the institutional level for internal benchmarking.
- Periodic distribution of a facility-specific antibiogram indicating the rates of relevant antibiotic susceptibilities to key pathogens.
- Additional interventions to improve the antimicrobial usage, including those designed to detect and eliminate:
  - Multidrug regimens with unnecessarily redundant antimicrobial spectra
  - Antibiotic therapy for the management of non-bacterial syndromes or cultures that represent contamination or routine colonization.
  - Empiric regimens that are either inadequately or excessively broad spectrum for infection syndromes.

- Regimens that do not adequately treat infections caused by culture-confirmed pathogens.

CORE ELEMENTS OF ANTIMICROBIAL STEWARDSHIP PROGRAM

Hospital Leadership Commitment

The availability of requisite dedicated human, financial, and information technology resources should be ensured with the ASP team in any healthcare facility. ASP leadership should dedicate adequate time to report stewardship activities, resources, and outcomes to senior executives and hospital board. There must be regular meetings within leaders of the stewardship program to assess the resources needed to accomplish the hospital's goals for improving antibiotic use. A senior executive/leader should serve as a point of contact or "champion" for the stewardship program.

Accountability

Appoint infectious disease specialist/physician, clinical pharmacist, and clinical microbiologist as co-leaders for responsibility of program management and outcome. ASP co-leaders should have a clear delineation of responsibilities and expectations. Regular "stewardship rounds" of the co-leaders or the nonphysician lead and the supporting physician can strengthen program leadership. Expanding these rounds to include discussions with prescribers (also called "handshake stewardship") has been shown to improve antibiotic use and is an effective way to enhance the visibility and support of the stewardship program.

Pharmacy/Drug Expertise

A clinical pharmacist must lead the implementation part to improve and rationalize the pharmacological aspect of antibiotic management. Pharmacy-based interventions are initiated by pharmacists and embedded into pharmacy sections of electronic health records and include:
- Documentation of indications for antibiotics.
- Automatic changes from intravenous to oral antibiotic therapy, whenever possible.
- Dose adjustment in case of organ dysfunction.
- Dose optimization as in the administration of beta-lactams and carbapenems as slow extended infusions, especially in the critically ill.
- Duplicative therapy alerts can prevent simultaneous use of multiple agents with overlapping microbiological spectra.
- Time-sensitive automatic stop orders of antibiotics can be issued in certain specific situations, as in surgical prophylaxis.
- Detection and prevention of antibiotic-related drug–drug interactions.

Action/Implementation of Program

Implementation of ASP includes key interventions such as—preauthorization (formulary restriction) or prospective audit and feedback (PAF) (post-prescription approach) in order to improve antimicrobial use.
- Preauthorization, PAF, and facility-specific treatment recommendations are the most high priority interventions in any ASP.
- Antibiotic timeout is a useful supplemental intervention, but it should not be a substitute for PAF.
- Nursing-based actions, such as prompt and proper collection of culture samples prior to starting first dose of antimicrobials, timely collection of specimen reports for early de-escalation and improving the evaluation of penicillin allergies, are of immense importance in the hospital stewardship efforts. Nurses can contribute significantly in prompting antibiotic timeouts and in deciding intravenous to oral drug shifts. Also, decisions regarding early removal of central vascular and urinary catheters can be greatly influenced by them.
- Microbiology-based interventions in the form of selective reporting of antimicrobial susceptibility results help in documenting antibiotics that are consistent with hospital treatment guidelines recommended by the stewardship program. Also, microbiology laboratory can guide the provider about which pathogens might represent colonization or contamination.

Preauthorization requires prescribers to obtain prior approval for the use of certain antibiotics based on clinical indications. This allows for expert input on antibiotic selection and dosing, which can be lifesaving in severe sepsis. It prevents unnecessary or inappropriate initiation of antibiotics, as it optimizes empiric choices and influences downstream use. There is review of clinical data and prior cultures at the time of initiation of therapy. This approach has few disadvantages too, as there is a loss of prescriber autonomy resulting in delay of therapy. Also, there is potential for manipulation of system by presenting a request in a biased manner to gain approval. It may possibly result in shifting to other agents and thereby select different antibiotic-resistance patterns, as it impacts use of restricted agents only.

Prospective audit and feedback is an external review of antibiotic therapy by the expert in antibiotic use, accompanied by suggestions to optimize use, at some point after the drug has been prescribed. It is different from an "antibiotic timeout" because the ASP team rather than the primary treating team conducts the audit. It can help in reviewing more complex antibiotic treatment regimens for better clinical outcome. In contrast, it preserves prescriber autonomy and addresses de-escalation as well as duration of therapy. There is greater flexibility in timing of recommendations but the compliance is voluntary, as the success depends on delivery method of feedback to the prescribers. One of the potential drawbacks could be that the prescriber may be reluctant to change therapy if the patient is doing well.

Facility-specific treatment guidelines enhance the effectiveness of both PAF and preauthorization by establishing lucid recommendations for optimal antibiotic use at the healthcare facility and by comparing the prescriptions with these guidelines. They reflect hospital treatment preferences based on local susceptibilities, formulary options, and patient cohorts. The recommendations must also address diagnostic approaches, such as when to send diagnostic samples and what tests to perform, including indications for rapid diagnostics and nonmicrobiologic tests (e.g., imaging and procalcitonin).

Antibiotic timeout is a provider-led reassessment of the need to continue and choice of antibiotics when the clinical picture is more clear and more diagnostic information, like results of cultures and rapid diagnostics, is available.

Tracking

It involves monitoring of antibiotic selection/prescription, impact of key interventions, and other important outcomes like *C. difficile* infection and drug resistance patterns.

Antibiotic Use Measures

- Excess days of therapy (DOTs) (i.e., unnecessary DOTs avoided based on accepted targets and benchmarks).
- Days of therapy or defined daily doses (DDDs).
- Standardized Antimicrobial Administration Ratio (SAAR), which compares observed antibiotic use to predicted use, where predicted use is based on risk-adjusted data models.
- Proportion of patients compliant with facility-based guideline or treatment algorithm.
- Proportion of patients with revision of antibiotics based on microbiology data.
- Proportion of patients converted to oral therapy.

Clinical Outcome Measures

- Duration of hospitalization.
- 30-day mortality.
- Proportion of patients with clinical failure (e.g., need to escalate therapy to broader spectrum; percentage of patients developing MDR super-infections like—VRE, MRSA; recurrence of infection).
- Proportion of patients diagnosed with hospital-acquired *C. difficile* infection or other adverse event(s) related to antibiotic therapy.
- Unplanned hospital re-admission within 30 days.
- Delay in antibiotic therapy due to preauthorization interventions.

Reporting

Regular reporting of accumulated information on antibiotic use and resistance patterns to the prescribers, pharmacists, nurses, and hospital leadership is one of the most crucial intervention for further improving antimicrobial prescription practices.

Education

Imparting continuous education about adverse reactions from antibiotics, antibiotic resistance and optimal prescribing practices to the prescribers, pharmacists, and nurses forms the backbone of any stewardship program. This can be even more effective when the case-based education is provided in person. There are many options for providing education on antibiotic use such as power-point presentations in formal or informal settings, messaging through posters, flyers, and newsletters, or electronic communication to staff groups.

CONCLUSION

Antimicrobial agents revolutionized the practice of medicine, resulting in dramatic reduction in deaths from a variety of infectious diseases. As a result, deaths from infections declined from approximately 280 per 100,000 population in 1936 (pre-sulfa) to approximately 60 per 100,000 population by 1950 (post-penicillin), with virtually no further decline ever since. Antibiotic efficacy is lost with every use of these drugs due to developing resistance, rendering them ineffective for any subsequent exploit. Thus, antibiotics are a shared societal trust. ASPs need to adapt as per the requirements of limited resource settings, as in low- and middle-income countries for addressing the issue of antimicrobial resistance successfully, since these nations have more unregulated antibiotic consumption. There should be specific national health policies, addressing antimicrobial resistance as one of the key issues and prioritizing development of guidelines regarding antibiotic usage, limiting over-the-counter use of antibiotics, and restricting their utilization as growth promoters in livestock. In 1945 during his Nobel Prize lecture, Alexander Fleming admonished that those who so abused penicillin would be "morally responsible" for the deaths of patients due to resistant bacteria who could no longer be treated with it. This clarion call for antibiotic stewardship, >70 years ago, went unheeded. We will never win the war against microbes, which outnumber us by a factor of 10^{22}, outweigh us by 100 million times, can replicate 500,000 times faster than we can, and have been doing this for 10,000 times longer than our species has existed. These facts place an extraordinary responsibility upon the infectious disease experts as stewards and also the society in general, to protect antibiotics from further abuse and misuse.

SUGGESTED READINGS

1. Lutters M, Harbarth S, Janssens JP, et al. Effect of a comprehensive multidisciplinary, educational program on the use of antibiotics in a geriatric university hospital. J Am Geriatr Soc. 2004;52: 112-6.
2. Cunha CB, Varughese CA, Mylonakis E. Antimicrobial stewardship programs (ASPs): the devil is in the details. Virulence. 2013;4:147-9.
3. Cunha BA. Effective antibiotic-resistance control strategies. Lancet. 2001;357:1307-8.
4. Fishman N. Policy statement on antimicrobial stewardship by the Society for Healthcare Epidemiology of America (SHEA), the Infectious Diseases Society of America (IDSA), and the Pediatric Diseases Society (PIDS). Infect Control Hosp Epidemiol. 2012;33:322-7.
5. Dellit TH, Owens RC, McGowan JE Jr, et al. Infectious Diseases Society of America and the Society for Healthcare Epidemiology of America guidelines for developing an institutional program to enhance antimicrobial stewardship. Clin Infect Dis. 2007;44:159-77.
6. Davey P, Brown E, Charani E, et al. Interventions to improve antibiotic prescribing practices for hospital inpatients. Cochrane Database Syst Rev. 2013;4:CD003543.

CHAPTER 51

Systemic Fungal Infections

Vipin Mediratta

■ INTRODUCTION

Medical mycology is the study of fungi that have an impact on human health. Its importance has increased in recent times because of increased use of immunosuppressive drugs and increase in incidence of opportunistic fungal infections. Initially medical mycology dealt with medical dermatological conditions mainly, but now it also deals with systemic diseases with considerable morbidity and mortality.

Fungi can be classified either morphologically or according to site of infection. In latter classification, mycoses can be classified as superficial or deep mycoses. Deep mycoses include subcutaneous and systemic mycoses; systemic fungal infections will be the main topic of our discussion here.

Systemic mycoses are of two types—*primary systemic* or *opportunistic systemic*.
1. Primary systemic infections are due to dimorphic endemic fungi that live normally in soil or rotting vegetation. They usually infect healthy individuals, and often cause mild infection. It includes: Blastomycoses, paracoccidiomycoses, coccidiomycoses, histoplasmoses.
2. Opportunistic systemic fungal infections are due to fungi that are part of normal commensal flora of body. They infect only those who are sick or have immunodeficiency disorder. It includes aspergillosis, penicilliosis, zygomycosis, candidosis, cryptococcosis, *Pneumocystis jirovecii*.

In non-neutropenic, 70–90% infections due to *Candida*, 10–20% due to *Aspergillus* and around 5% due to others (cryptococcosis).

Important *risk factors* for systemic fungal infections: Antimicrobial agents (number and duration), chemotherapy, hematological, or solid organ malignancy, neutropenia, corticosteroids or immunosuppressive therapy, hospitalization or ICU stay, TPN, malnutrition, surgery, etc.

Diagnosis of invasive fungal infection can be done via: (1) Microscopy, (2) Culture, (3) Serology, (4) Histopathology, and (5) Imaging.
a. Direct microscopy: Calcofluor white stain mixed with 10-20% KOH-stains fungal cell wall or wet mounts or gram stains of sputum, BAL fluid, tissue.
b. Culture: Commonly SDA (sabouraud dextrose agar) used. Confirmation of microscopic findings by culture is always desirable, for definitive identification of organism.
c. Serology:
   i. Galactomannan-polysaccharide antigen that exists primarily in cell wall of Aspergillus species. Sensitivity and specificity in serum is 60-80% and 80-95%, while in serum it is 85-90% and 90-95% respectively. Therefore, it is relatively Aspergillus specific, non-diagnostic assay.
   ii. 1,3 β-D-glucan assay—important cell wall component of *Candida, Aspergillus,* etc. It has high degree of sensitivity and specificity in diagnosis of invasive candidiasis (78-97% and 88-100%) and invasive aspergillosis (50-87% and 81-89%).
   iii. Nucleic acid detection: PCR has also been used successfully for early detection of *Aspergillus* DNA in peripheral blood and BAL fluid.
d. Histopathology/Cytology: Tissue and fluid specimens should be submitted in adequate quantities for simultaneous histopathologic/cytologic and culture examination. However, no histopathologic finding can definitively diagnose the pathogen, therefore, confirmation by culture or non-culture methods needed.
e. Imaging: CT scan in recommended, whenever there is clinical suspicion for invasive pulmonary infection, regardless of chest regardless of chest radiograph results. Imaging can also help to direct diagnostic procedures BAL/CT guided biopsy to appropriate areas.

■ TREATMENT OF INVASIVE FUNGAL INFECTIONS

Anti-fungal drugs can be classified according to chemical structures or according to site of action/mechanism of action, and they are: (1) antibiotics, (2) azoles, (3) echinocandins, (4) antimetabolites, (5) allylamines, and (6) others.
1. Antibiotics: It includes polyenes—*Amphotericin, Nystatin,* and *Natamycin* and these agents act via binding ergosterol in fungal cell wall and causing leakage of materials and fungal death. And heterocyclic benzofuran—*Griseofulvin,* disrupt mitotic spindle and inhibit fungal mitosis.
    Of these most important is amphotericin-B. Fungicidal agent, IV administration @0.6-1 mg/kg/day. It has broadest spectrum of action against most clinically important fungi and *Leishmania*. It is 90% bound to plasma proteins, therefore, longer half-life of 15 days. Important adverse effects are—nephrotoxicity and hypokalemia. To lower these side effects liposomal amphoterin B is used. It is 20-50 times costlier than amphotericin B and can be used in higher doses.
2. Azoles: These are most used antifungal agents, oral/topical. These are broad spectrum synthetic antifungals, fungicidal/fungistatic depending on drug

concentration. It is classified as imidazoles and triazoles. Both groups are structurally related, with similar spectrum with same mechanism of action of interfering with ergosterol synthesis.

Imidazoles have two nitrogens in structure and include: *Ketoconazole, Butaconazole,* etc. Triazoles have three nitrogens in structure and include: *Fluconazole, Itraconazole, Voriconazole, Posaconazole,* etc.

Ketoconazole is used less these days due to more side effects like hepatotoxicity, anti-androgenic or other endocrine effects, drug interactions due to CYP3A4 inhibition, etc.

Fluconazole has broad antifungal activity with good CSF penetration, but not effective against aspergillosis and mucormycosis. It is used in oral/vaginal candidiasis, tinea infection, meningitis (preferred agent), etc.

Itraconazole has broadest activity spectrum including aspergillosis, but poor CSF penetration. It is DOC for paracoccidiomycosis, chromoblastomycoses, histoplasmosis, blastomycosis. It can also be used for coccidiosis, aspergillosis, etc.

Voriconazole is DOC for invasive aspergillosis, most useful for esophageal candidiasis, first line for moulds like fusarium, etc., and useful in resistant *Candida* infections.

Posaconazole is also broad-spectrum agent and used in prophylaxis against aspergillosis and candidiasis in severely immunocompromised individuals, resistant candidiasis, mucormycosis, etc.
3. Echinocandins: New parenteral antifungal agents, act by inhibiting beta (1,3) glucan in fungal cell wall. It includes: *Caspofungin, Micafungin, Anidulafungin.* Fungicidal against *Candida*, fungistatic against *Aspergillus* species. They have no cross-resistance with azoles. They have no renal or hepatic toxicity and do not cross blood brain barrier.

Caspofungin used as 70 mg IV loading dose followed by 50 mg OD. It is used in treatment of refractory invasive aspergillosis, candidiasis (esophageal, peritoneal), empirical therapy in neutropenic patients, etc.
4. Antimetabolite—*5-flucytosine* acts by interfering with protein synthesis.
5. Allylamines—*Terbinafine, Butenafine,* etc., act by inhibiting ergosterol + lanosterol synthesis.

SOME SPECIFIC TREATMENTS FOR SYSTEMIC MYCOSES

1. Invasive candidiasis: Fluconazole is DOC for empirical therapy in patients with candidemia without sepsis/shock/recent exposure to azoles. Amphotericin B or caspofungin used in patients with previous azole exposure or neutropenia. Caspofungin is DOC in severe sepsis and septic shock.
2. Invasive aspergillosis: DOC/primary therapy is voriconazole. For combination therapy, caspofungin + voriconazole or liposomal amphotericin B used in critically ill patients.
3. Cryptococcosis: For CNS/disseminated cryptococcosis in HIV patients, amphotericin B (0.7–1 mg/kg/day) + flucytosine 1,100 mg/kg/day orally used for 2 weeks, followed by fluconazole/itraconazole 400 mg for 8 weeks, followed

by secondary prophylaxis with 200 mg of fluconazole, until start of HAART, symptom free or CD4 >200.

For asymptomatic/mild disease: Fluconazole/Itraconazole 400 mg for 6–12 months, followed by secondary prophylaxis.
4. Mucormycosis: Surgical resection and debridement, followed by high doses of liposomal amphotericin B (5–10 mg/kg/day) for 6 months. In intolerable/refractory cases, posaconazole used.

Antifungal Prophylaxis

It is indicated for patients with neutropenia, high-risk patients in ICU or using *Candida* score. *Candida* score is a bedside index, used to decide early antifungal treatment when *Candida* infection is suspected in critically ill patients. It includes—TPN, surgery, *Candida* colonization, and severe sepsis.

If needed, fluconazole 400 mg/day is drug of choice. Itraconazole, voriconazole, posaconazole, caspofungin, etc., can also be used.

SUGGESTED READINGS

1. Jameson JL, Fauci A, Kasper D, et al. Harrison's Principles of Internal Medicine. 20th edition. McGraw Hill; 2018.
2. Bennett JE, Dolin R. Blaser MJ. Mandell, Douglas and Bennett's Infectious Diseases. 9th edition. Elsevier; 2019.
3. Anaissie EJ, McGinnis MR, Pfaller MA. Clinical Mycology. Elsevier Health Sciences. 2008.

CHAPTER 52

Approach to Tropical Fever

Anusha Singhania, Vikas Loomba

INTRODUCTION

Tropical fevers are prevalent in tropical and subtropical regions. In a patient presenting with an acute febrile illness in a tropical region, the causes may include acute undifferentiated fevers or chronic medical problems unrelated to tropical exposure such as inflammatory or malignant conditions. At the same time, common infections such as influenza or tuberculosis may also occur in tropics and have atypical presentation thereby confusing the clinician.

Tropical fever or acute undifferentiated fever is a very important cause of fever in India, especially between June and September. Unlike pyrexia of unknown origin (PUO) which has a clear-cut definition, tropical fever lacks a consensus definition. The accepted definition of acute undifferentiated fever states fever of less than 2 weeks duration without any localizing signs or symptoms.

Tropical fever poses a diagnostic and therapeutic challenge to the healthcare workers, especially in limited resource settings like in most of India. These diagnostic challenges lead to irrational use of antimalarials and antibiotics. Another point to reckon is the fact that acute undifferentiated fevers with associated features such as rash, arthralgias, myalgias, hemorrhage, or jaundice may have overlapping etiologies, posing bigger challenges in the management of these patients.

The common causes of tropical fevers are malaria, viruses, rickettsial infections, leptospirosis, and enteric fever. Since malaria is one of the most common causes of tropical fever, patients who test negative for malaria are categorized as nonmalarial tropical fevers. However, depending on the laboratory support, we may fail to reach the diagnosis in nearly 25–50% patients.[4]

APPROACH TO A PATIENT WITH TROPICAL FEVER

Whenever a patient in tropical regions presents with fever of less than 2 weeks' duration, always look for any comorbidities that may increase the risk of infections such as diabetes mellitus, HIV, malignancy, pregnancy, or postsplenectomy. We should also elicit occupational history, drug and immunization history, any history of exposure to animals or birds, and sexual history—these can have direct or indirect bearing on the patient's present condition. At the same time, also look for travel history—recent or past. In India, which is a vast country, having updated knowledge of recent outbreaks can help us in reaching a diagnosis. Some of the infections are seasonal, particularly common during or after monsoon season. We have to remember that the classical clinical picture of various conditions may be masked by the use of antipyretics and may be misleading. Therefore, absence of the classical clinical picture should not be the criteria to rule out any particular infection. After evaluating the history, clinical examination should be focused on skin rash, lymphadenopathy, jaundice, anemia, conjunctivitis, hepatomegaly, and splenomegaly.

After having evaluated the signs and symptoms, a syndromic diagnosis should be made and this will serve as a broad outline in the management of tropical fever. Tropical fever can have five major syndromes:

1. *Acute undifferentiated fever*: Fever without any localizing signs. Common infections are malaria, rickettsial infections, leptospirosis, enteric fever, and viral fevers.
2. *Fever with skin rash or thrombocytopenia* (platelet count <1,00,000/mm^3): Common infections are viral infections, especially dengue fever, rickettsial infections, meningococcal infections, malaria, and leptospirosis.
3. *Fever with respiratory distress* (ARDS): It is defined as PaO_2/FiO_2 ratio <200 or oxygen saturation <90% at room air. Common infections include malaria, rickettsial infections, viral infections such as COVID-19, swine flu, and influenza.
4. *Acute febrile encephalopathy*: Common infections are rickettsial infections such as scrub typhus, malaria, especially falciparum, enteric fever, leptospirosis, and viruses such as Japanese encephalitis.
5. *Fever with multiorgan failure*: Malaria, scrub typhus, leptospirosis, dengue fever, hantavirus infection, etc.

Many infections can have overlapping presentation making the job of the clinician even more challenging. To overcome this, we should follow an algorithm based on scientific rationale, logic, and prevalent clinical practices. This algorithmic approach is based on:
- Prevalence of infectious disease in the area
- Severity of febrile illness
- Availability of diagnostic tests
- Response to drug therapy

Various steps include the following:
1. *Assess severity of the illness and look for any evidence of sepsis*: Clinical evaluation of the patient should be done to look any evidence of sepsis—fever, tachycardia, tachypnea, and hypotension. Two to four blood cultures should be sent before initiating any antimicrobials, and each culture should contain at least 20 mL of blood. C-reactive protein and calcitonin should also be sent at the beginning

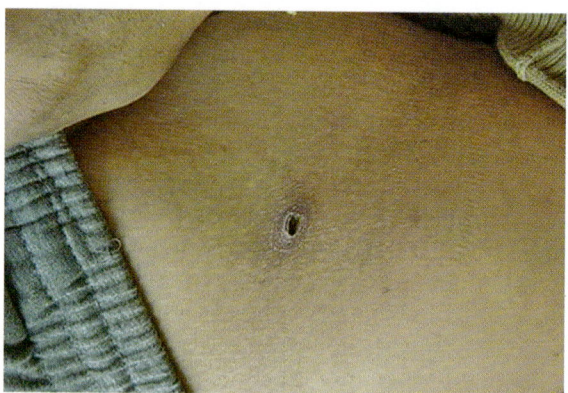
FIG. 1: Eschar in scrub typhus.

2. *Try to localize the fever*: Detailed history and clinical examination should be done to look for the cause of fever. Unfortunately, history and clinical examination may be helpful in a limited number of patients as most of the conditions have overlapping features. Hepatomegaly, splenomegaly, and lymphadenopathy may be present in malaria, dengue fever, leptospirosis, scrub typhus, or enteric fever. Eschar is a localized necrotic skin lesion at the site of the infected chigger bite usually found in scrub typhus. In a study conducted at CMC, we found that the prevalence of eschar in scrub typhus was 14.5% patients. The eschar may develop before the onset of systemic symptoms and can be seen at multiple sites. Thrombocytopenia and mild transaminitis (up to 200 IU/L) are nonspecific markers in tropical fever. A moderate rise in liver enzymes is found in leptospirosis and rise of more than 25 times the normal is found in viral hepatitis **(Fig. 1)**.
3. *Use of rapid diagnostic tests*: All patients of tropical fever should be subjected to rapid diagnostic tests (RDTs) for malaria and dengue fever. RDTs are immunochromatographic lateral flow devices offering qualitative diagnosis, based on detection of parasite antigens in patient blood. Histidine-rich protein 2 (HRP2) is expressed by *Plasmodium falciparum* and pLDH (*Plasmodium* lactate dehydrogenase) is expressed by all human malaria species. RDTs are relatively easy to use and provide a result within 30 minutes. HRP2-based RDT has very high sensitivity and specificity for falciparum malaria. On the other hand, pLDH-based RDT for vivax malaria has high specificity but the sensitivity is around 75–80%, necessitating the need for peripheral smear examination after negative RDT. Similarly, NS1 antigen for dengue fever appears positive on the first day and may stay positive till the ninth day. When NS1 antigen is combined with IgM enzyme-linked immunosorbent assay (ELISA), the sensitivity reaches 93% and specificity around 83%.
4. *Use simple antipyretics only* if the fever is of <3 days' duration and initial RDTs are negative.

5. *Further management if fever persists for more than 3 days and initial RDTs are negative*: If fever persists beyond 3 days and the RDTs are negative, common causes include leptospirosis, scrub typhus, and enteric fever. Specific investigations such as blood culture, serological tests, or polymerase chain reaction assays need to be planned now.

   After sending these tests, empirical treatment with doxycycline or azithromycin is advocated in patients with nonmalarial acute undifferentiated fevers. Both of them have comparable efficacy against salmonella, rickettsial infections, and leptospirosis. Phimda et al. found that 3-day azithromycin and 7-day doxycycline had similar efficacy in tropical fever, but patients receiving doxycycline had more adverse events. In a meta-analysis of 17 randomized controlled trials (RCTs), Fang et al. found that in the treatment of scrub typhus, doxycycline and azithromycin were comparable in efficacy but doxycycline yielded more adverse events. Fluoroquinolones should not be used in the management of scrub typhus due to the presence of gyrase A mutation in the organism. For treatment of enteric fever, a meta-analysis by Trivedi and Shah revealed that azithromycin and cephalosporins had comparable efficacy but azithromycin was superior with respect to relapse rates. Seeing these studies, azithromycin is a reasonable empirical choice for these three infections. The dosage schedule as advised for enteric fever—1,000 mg on day 1 and 500 mg/day for the next 5 days—may be useful in scrub typhus and leptospirosis.
6. *Acute undifferentiated fever with negative cultures that persists despite empirical antibiotic therapy*: Susilawati and McBride found that 95% of the fevers resolved within 3 weeks and only 5% progressed to PUO. However, there is no consensus on treatment of fevers that persist beyond 2 weeks and do not respond to the empirical antibiotic therapy. At times, the diagnosis is also not clear. If the patient continues to have fever without any other criteria meeting the definitions of severity such as systemic inflammatory response syndrome (SIRS) and quick Sequential Sepsis-related Organ Failure Assessment (qSOFA), most physicians stop antibiotics and reinvestigate with blood chemistry, cultures (of urine, blood, or body fluids), imaging, bone marrow, etc., and try to find out the cause of fever.
7. If fever persists beyond 3 weeks, then investigations are planned as per the workup of PUO **(Flowchart 1)**

CONCLUSION

- Tropical fever should be kept as a possibility in patients presenting with fever in tropical and sub-tropical regions, especially during or immediately after rainy season.
- During first 3 days, only give paracetamol, awaiting the rapid diagnostic test reports.
- If RDTs are negative, then give empirical course on ceftriaxone and doxycycline.
- If fever persists even after 3 weeks, then investigate as for PUO.

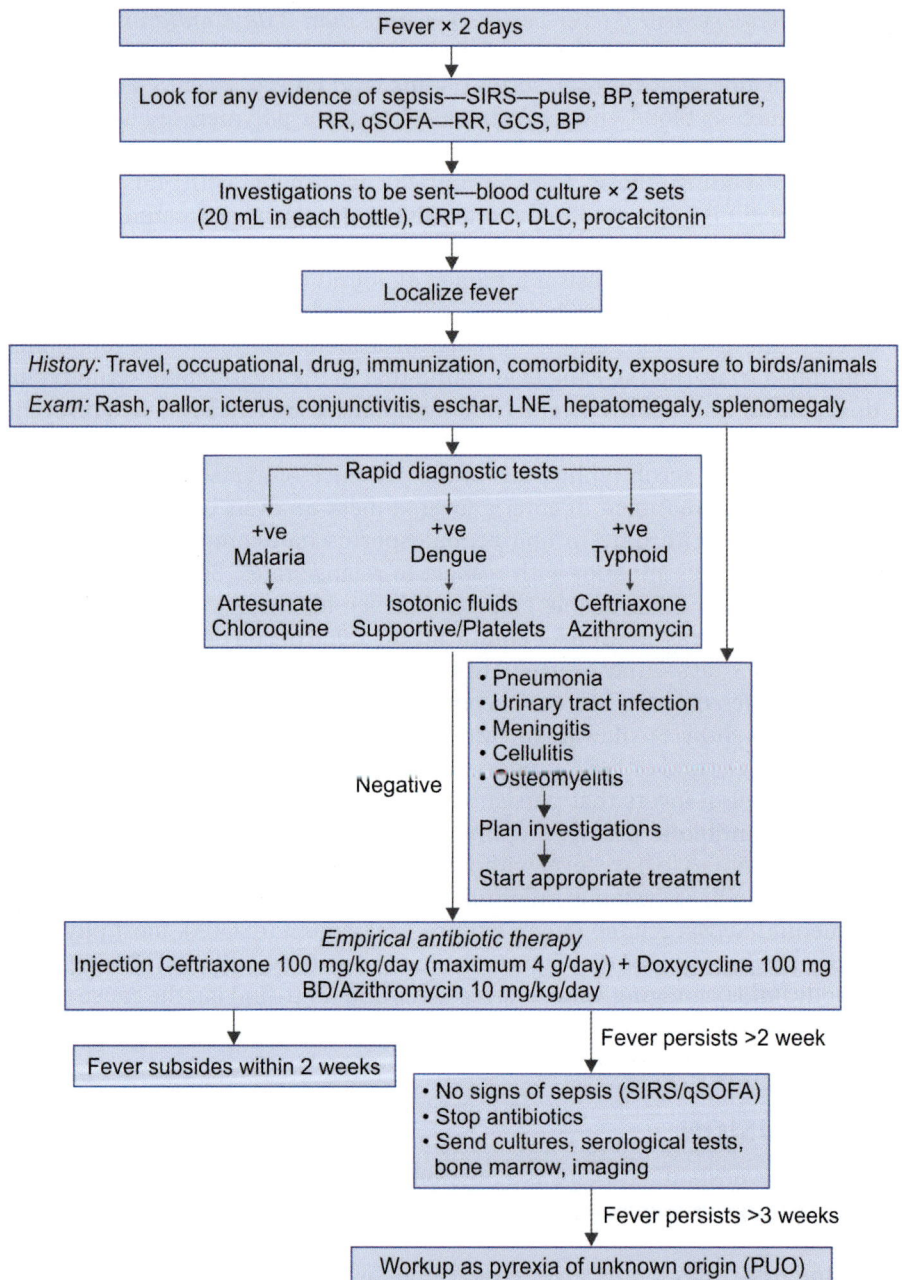

FLOWCHART 1: Algorithm for approach to tropical fever.

(CRP: C-reactive protein; DLC: differential leukocyte count; GCS: Glasgow Coma Score; qSOFA: quick Sequential Sepsis-related Organ Failure Assessment; SIRS: systemic inflammatory response syndrome; TLC: total leukocyte count)

SUGGESTED READINGS

1. Susilawati TN, McBride WJ. Acute undifferentiated fever in Asia: a review of the literature. The Southeast Asian Journal of tropical medicine and public health. 2014;45(3):719-26.
2. Joshi R, Colford JM, Jr, Reingold AL, et al. Nonmalarial acute undifferentiated fever in a rural hospital in central India: diagnostic uncertainty and overtreatment with antimalarial agents. Am J Trop Med Hyg. 2008;78(3):393-9.
3. Crump JA. Time for a comprehensive approach to the syndrome of fever in the tropics. Trans R Soc Trop Med Hyg. 2014;108(2)61-2.
4. Muller TC, Siv S, Khim N, et al. Acute undifferentiated febrile illness in rural Cambodia: a 3 year prospective observational study. PLoS One. 2014;9(4):e95868.
5. Dellinger RP, Levy MM, Rhodes A, et al. Surviving sepsis campaign international guidelines for management of severe sepsis and septic shock: 2012. Crit Care Med. 2013;41(2):580-637.
6. Loomba V, Mani A, John M, et al. Scrub typhus in Punjab: an acute febrile illness with multisystem involvement. Trop Doct. 2014;44(3):152-5.
7. Chang ML, Yang CW, Chen JC, et al. Disproportional exaggerated aspartate transaminase is a useful prognostic parameter in late leptospirosis. World J Gastroenterol. 2005;11(35):5553-6.
8. Moody A. Rapid diagnostic tests for malaria parasites. Clin. Microbiol Rev. 2002;15:66-78.
9. Lacksell SD, Jarman RG, Bailey MS, et al. Evaluation of six commercial point-of-care tests for diagnosis of acute dengue infections: the need for combining NS1 antigen and IgM/IgG antibody detection to achieve acceptable levels of accuracy. Clin Vaccine Immunol. 2011;18(12):2095-2101.
10. Phimda K, Hoontrakul S, Suttinont C, et al. Doxycycline versus azithromycin for treatment of leptospirosis and scrub typhus. Antimicrob Agents Chemother. 2007;51(9):3259-63.
11. Fang Y, Huang Z, Tu C, et al. Meta-analysis of drug treatment for scrub typhus in Asia. Intern Med J. 2012;51(17):2313-20.
12. Jang HC, Choi SM, Jang MO, et al. Inappropriateness of quinolone in scrub typhus treatment due to gyr A mutation in Orientia Tsutsugamushi Boryong strain. J Korean Med Sci. 2013;28(5):667-71.
13. Trivedi NA, Shah PC. A meta-analysis comparing the safety and efficacy of azithromycin over the alternate drugs used for the treatment of uncomplicated enteric fever. J Postgrad Med. 2012;58(2):112-8.
14. Susilawati TN, McBride WJ. Undiagnosed undifferentiated fever in Far North Queensland, Australia: a retrospective study. Int J Infect Dis. 2014;27:59-64.

CHAPTER

53

Sepsis Management: Current Update

Shankha S Sen

■ INTRODUCTION

"SEPSIS" is not a specific illness but a "syndrome".

It is one of the leading causes of mortality accounting for 19.7% of all global deaths.

Constant amendments and refinements have been going on to "define sepsis" more comprehensively. In 1991, 2001, and 2014, initiatives were taken to define sepsis.

SEPSIS 3 (2014 Definition)

"SEPSIS" is defined as life-threatening organ dysfunction caused by a dysregulated host response to infection.

"Septic shock" is a subset of sepsis in which profound circulatory, cellular, and metabolic abnormalities are associated with a greater risk.

Quick Sequential Organ Failure Assessment (qSOFA)	
• RR > 22 bpm • sBP < 100 mm Hg • Altered GCS	• 0 = Mortality < 1% • 1 = Mortality 2–3% • ≥2 = Mortality ≥ 10%
Screening for outcome rather than diagnosis	

(GCS: Glasgow Coma Scale; RR: respiratory rate)

Poor sensitivity of quick sequential organ failure assessment (qSOFA) leads to higher reporting of *false negative* cases and *delay* in diagnosis and treatment.
- But, it is apprehended that SEPSIS-3 might miss early and less severe form of "Sepsis" which ultimately might lead to a catastrophe. SEPSIS-3, however, failed to achieve overall consensus due to-early detection of sepsis, before the development of organ failure was not given enough importance in SEPSIS-3 as

it gives alarm only when life-threatening organ dysfunction is present which exposes so-called milder cases to vulnerability.

Noninclusion of lactate in SOFA score, a sensitive marker of severity, is another criticism.

- The use of systemic inflammatory response syndrome (SIRS) criteria has been suggested as a better screening tool as compared to qSOFA. However, the combination of SIRS and qSOFA could be advantageous for early detection of SEPSIS as SIRS will offer higher sensitivity and qSOFA will provide more specificity. Harnessing qSOFA and SIRS together for early detection in non-ICU setup could be a worth trying experience in future.

Problems with SIRS: The terminology used does not promote an understanding the underlying problem or disease process (lack of face validity)
- SIRS lacks sensitivity for defining sepsis
- SIRS not specific (Kaukonnen et al., NEJM 2015)
- SIRS does not reflect the severity of the disease process (lack of construct validity)
- SIRS may detract from the search for an infection prognosis varies depending on how the sepsis definitions are applied (lack of edictive validity)
- SIRS criteria do not account for the dynamic time-course of sepsis.

Surviving Sepsis Guidelines 2021 *recommends against* using qSOFA compared with SIRS, NEWS (National Early Warning Score), or MEWS (Modified Early Warning Score) as a single screening tool for sepsis or septic shock **(Fig. 1)**. (Strong recommendation, moderate-quality evidence.)

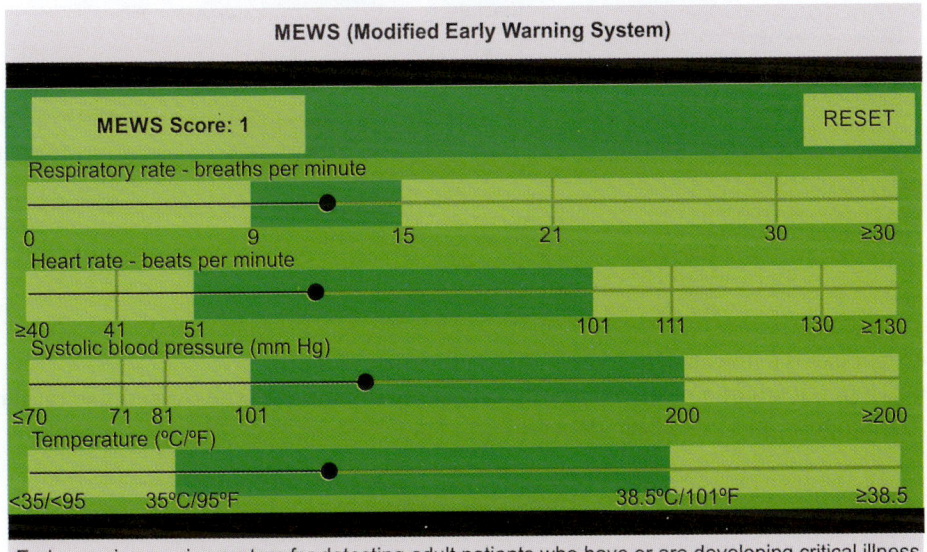

FIG. 1: Modified Early Warning Score (MEWS)—a screening tool.

Serum lactate level has been recommended as an adjunctive test to modify the pretest probability in patients with suspected sepsis.

SEPSIS MANAGEMENT (FLOWCHART 1)

Start resuscitation early with—source control, intravenous fluids, and antibiotics. Frequent assessment of the patients' volume status is crucial throughout the resuscitation period.

The Surviving Sepsis Guidelines suggest guiding resuscitation to normalize lactate in patients with elevated lactate levels as a marker of tissue hypoperfusion.

As it increases significantly in tissue hypoperfusion and hypoxia, lactate can be a surrogate marker of severe infection as an independent predictor of mortality in sepsis.

- Intermediate lactate levels (2–4 mmol/L) are at a significant risk compared to those with normal lactate values. Early clearance of lactate is associated with better outcome.

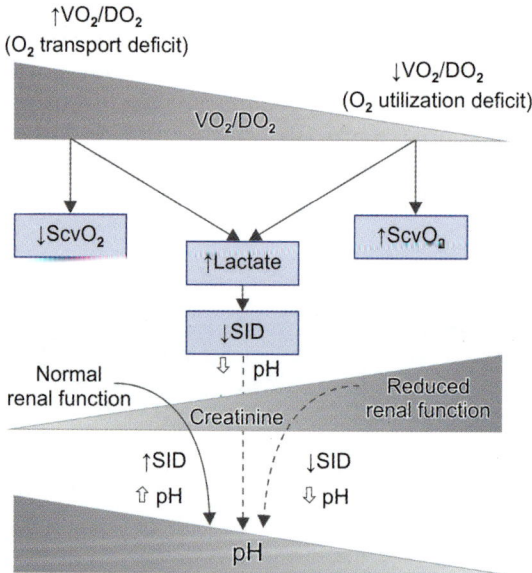

- Lactate is a powerful marker of illness severity.
- Hyperlactatemia more frequently caused by impaired tissue oxygen use rather than by impaired oxygen delivery.

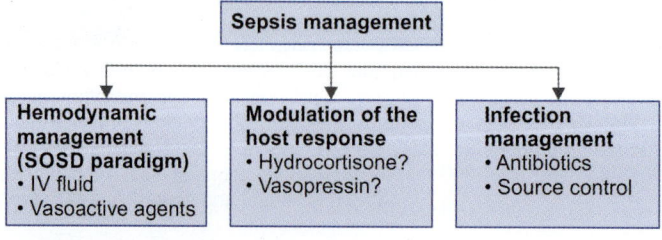

FLOWCHART 1: Sepsis management.

- Acidemia only observed in the presence of renal dysfunction.
- Clinical significance—patients with impaired oxygen delivery benefit from goal-directed therapy. However, the majority of patients with good O_2 delivery but impaired cellular O_2 use may have worse outcome after aggressive fluid replacement.

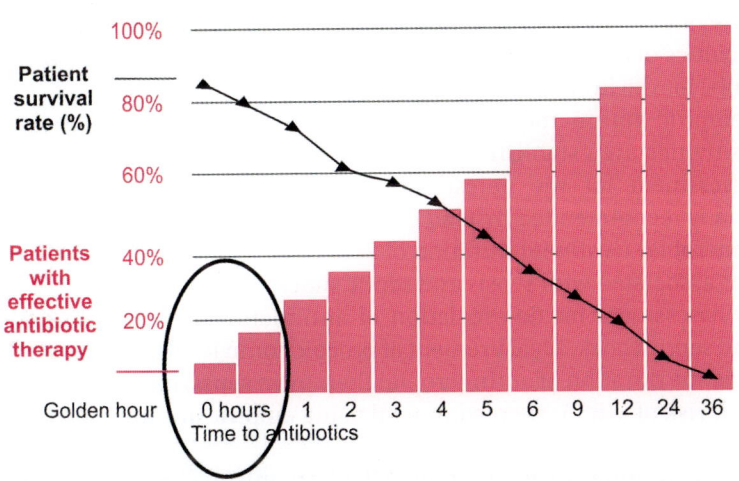

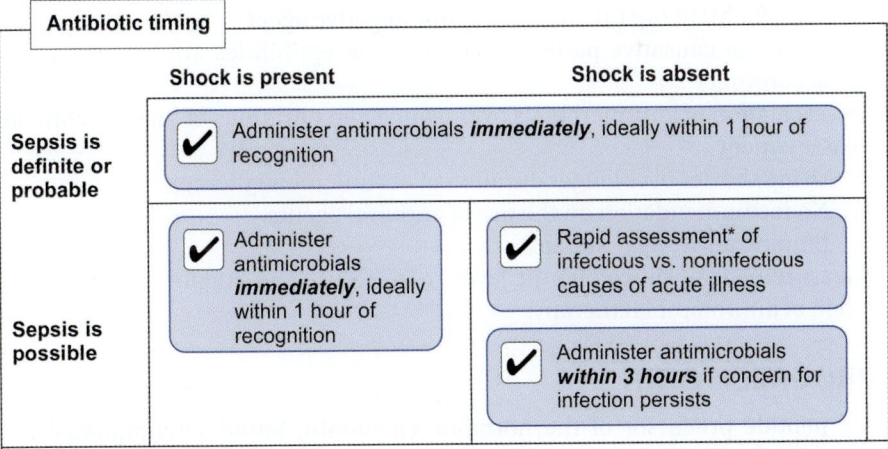

*Rapid assessment includes history and clinical examination, tests for both infectious and noninfectious causes of acute illness and immediate treatment for acute conditions that can mimic sepsis. Whenever possible, this should be completed within 3 hours of presentation so that a decision can be made as to the likelihood of an infectious cause of the patient's presentation and timely antimicrobial therapy provided if the likelihood is thought to be high

The SSG recommends that appropriate routine microbiologic cultures (including blood) be obtained before starting antimicrobial therapy in patients with suspected sepsis and septic shock if doing so results in no substantial delay in the start of antimicrobials.

Appropriate routine microbiologic cultures always include at least two sets of blood cultures (aerobic and anaerobic).

Early administration of antibiotics ideally within 1 hour of recognition of "Sepsis" is imperative. SSG suggests empiric combination therapy (using at least two antibiotics of different antimicrobial classes) aimed at the most likely bacterial pathogen(s) for the initial management of septic shock.

The empiric antimicrobial therapy be narrowed once pathogen identification and sensitivities are established and/or adequate clinical improvement is noted. Daily assessment for the de-escalation of anti-microbials guided by clinical evaluation is recommended instead of using a fixed duration of antibiotic therapy. An antimicrobial treatment duration of 7-10 days is adequate for the most serious infections associated with sepsis and septic shock.

Daily assessment for de-escalation of antimicrobial therapy in patients with sepsis and septic shock. Measurement of procalcitonin levels can be used to support shortening the duration of antimicrobial therapy in sepsis patients.

- At high risk of MRSA, we recommend using empiric antimicrobials with MRSA coverage.
- High risk for multi-drug resistant (MDR) organisms—two antimicrobials with gram-negative coverage empirically
- Low risk for MDR organisms—one gram-negative agent
    - Once the causative pathogen and the susceptibilities are known—change accordingly
- De-escalation of antimicrobials over using fixed durations of therapy with daily reassessment
    - Using shorter over longer duration of antimicrobial therapy.
    - No recommendation on the use of antiviral agents.
    - Empiric antifungal therapy

Measurement of procalcitonin levels can be used to support shortening the duration of antimicrobial therapy.

PROCALCITONIN

It is a peptide precursor of the hormone calcitonin, found serendipitously as a marker of infection. PCT levels have a half-life of 25–30 hours, usually rise within 4 hours and peak at 6 hours. It has been useful in diagnosis of bacterial infection and differentiates infectious from noninfectious causes. Bacterial infection is present when PCT levels are between 0.1 and 0.5 ng/mL and usually levels are ≥10 ng/mL in Septic shock.

It is mainly recommended as a biomarker for de-escalation of antibiotics and serial PCT monitoring is recommended. PCT levels decrease by 50% over 24 hours when a proper host response and antibiotic therapy are in place.

SOURCE CONTROL

A specific anatomic diagnosis of infection and emergent source control intervention be implemented as rapidly as possible—as in intra-abdominal abscess, gut perforation, ischemic bowel, volvulus, pyonephrosis, cholangitis, cholecystitis, empyema, and septic arthritis, e.g., drainage of an abscess, the debridement of infected necrotic tissue, the removal of an infected device. Prompt removal of intravascular access devices that are a possible source of sepsis or septic shock after other vascular access has been established.

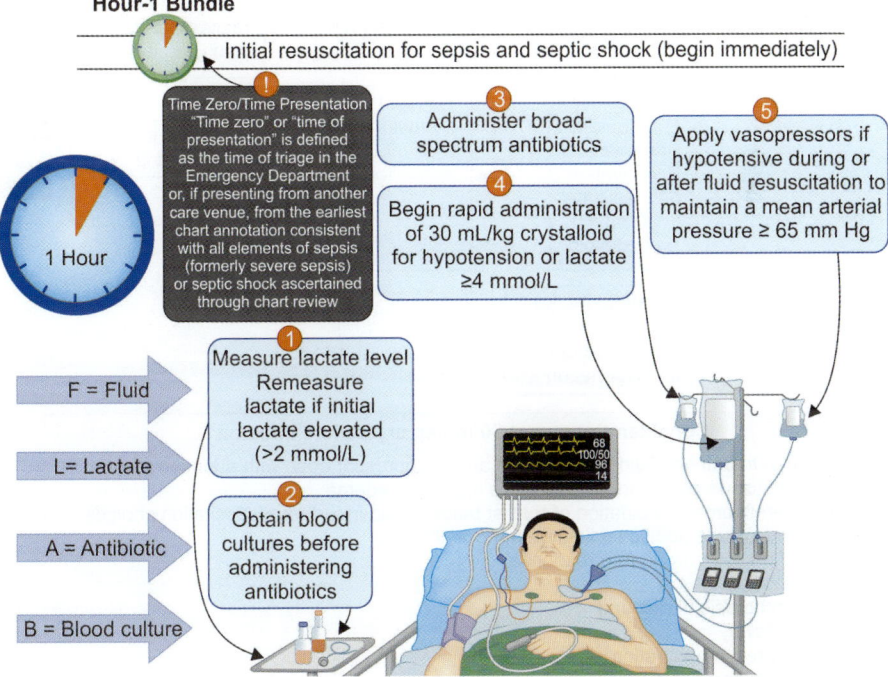

Crystalloids are first-line intravenous fluids.
- Balanced crystalloids instead of normal saline—plasmalyte, ringer's lactate
- Albumin in patients who received large volumes of crystalloids
- Starches, gelatins—not recommended.
- The use of a restrictive versus liberal fluid strategy after the initial fluid resuscitation

For adults with sepsis or septic shock, SSG suggests using balanced crystalloids instead of normal saline for resuscitation.
- Rapid high-volume infusion of normal saline may result in hyperchloremic metabolic acidosis and increased risk of acute kidney injury (AKI).
- The risk of hyperchloremia is reduced with use of balanced/buffered salt solutions (BSS) in which chloride content is reduced.

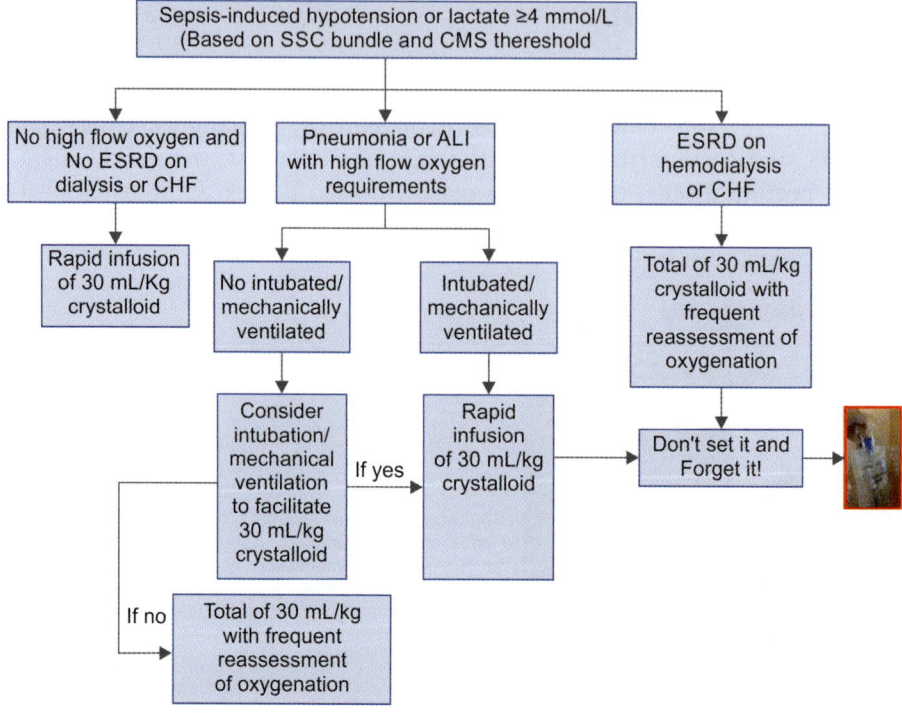

FLOWCHART 2: Application of fluid resuscitation in adult septic shock.

(ALI: acute lung injury; CHF cogestive heart failure; CMS: US Centers for Medicare and Medicaid Services; CVP central venous pressure; ESRD; end stage renal disease; Kg: kilograms; mL: milliliter; ScvO$_2$: superior vena cava oxygen saturatuon)

BSS contains organic anions such as lactate, gluconate, citrate, and acetate which act as physiological buffers and are rapidly converted to bicarbonate upon administration. But firm evidence is lacking.

- Earlier RCTs such as The SMART and SALT-ED trials support the use of balanced crystalloids with a network meta-analysis demonstrating decreased mortality with balanced fluids. They showed that saline solutions are associated with increase in major adverse kidney events—a composite of death, new RRT, or persistent renal dysfunction.

- But, the later SPLIT trial, a cluster RCT of mainly postoperative patients failed to show any advantage of BSS over NS. The most recent PLUS study in 2022 concluded that BSS has not reduced 90 days all-cause mortality or risk of AKI.

ALBUMIN

- It is a natural colloid, safe, and has volume expansion effects in patients with septic shock, spontaneous bacterial peritonitis or other bacterial infections.
- It is expensive and has limited shelf life.
- It may be appropriate to restore hemodynamic endpoints in a more timely and effective manner if substantial amounts of crystalloids fail to achieve hemodynamic endpoints because of lower net fluid balance with early attainment of mean arterial pressure and static filling pressure.
- It is particularly indicated in septic patients with cirrhosis and renal dysfunction.

Treating Fluids as Drugs: The Four Ds

- **D**rug
- **D**ose
- **D**uration
- **D**e-escalation

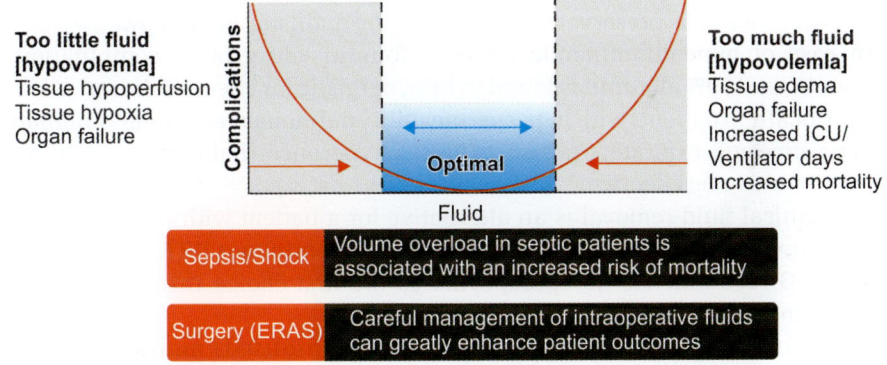

REPLACEMENT FLUIDS AND NUTRITION FLUIDS

Replacement fluids:
- Should mimic fluid that is lost.
- Give saline or NH4Cl in case of Gl losses; Gl losses are the only indication for saline.
- Give isotonic replacement in case of burns.
- Give blood when bleeding.

Nutrition fluids:
- Should cover caloric needs.
- Often overlooked as source of fluid accumulation.

DURATION OF FLUID THERAPY

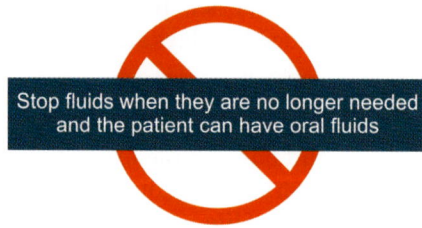

- Restrictive fluid management strategy is found to be beneficial in ARDS, AKI, and "Sepsis".
- Deresuscitation or active fluid removal is a new concept (coined in 2014), being explored in critically ill patients with fluid accumulation syndrome.
- Inappropriate and overzealous fluid administration during resuscitation is a common reason for fluid accumulation.
- De-escalation and de-resuscitation are core components of fluid stewardship which can mitigate the adverse effects of fluid accumulation.
- De-resuscitation is a salvage approach and should start as soon as the resuscitation is completed.
- The first step of de-resuscitation is the assessment of renal function and electrolytes.
- If renal function is preserved, diuretics are the mainstay of therapy.
- In case of hypoalbuminemia (serum albumin <30 g/L)—a combination of diuretic and 20% albumin is found to be synergistic for effective diuresis.
- In critically ill patients with hyperpermeability pulmonary edema, a combination of positive end-expiratory pressure (PEEP), hyperoncotic albumin and diuretics were found to be effective.

Mechanical fluid removal is an alternative for a patient with renal failure-like slow continuous ultrafiltration and intermittent or continuous RRT.

- The SSG recommends norepinephrine as the first-choice vasopressor (strong recommendation, moderate quality of evidence).
- The SSG recommends adding either vasopressin (up to 0.03 U/min) or epinephrine to norepinephrine with the intent of raising MAP to target, or adding vasopressin (up to 0.03 U/min) to decrease norepinephrine dosage.

CIRCI (Critical illness related corticosteroid insufficiency) is defined as inadequate cellular corticosteroid activity for the severity of the patient's critical illness manifested by insufficient glucocorticoid-glucocorticoid receptor-mediated downregulation of proinflammatory transcription factors.

CIRCI is thought to occur in several acute conditions, including sepsis and septic shock, severe CAP, ARDS, cardiac arrest, head injury, trauma, burns, and post-major surgery.

Sepsis Management: Current Update

Vasoactive agent management
Use norepinephrine as first-line vasopressor

For patients with septic shock on vasopressors

 Target a MAP of 65 mm Hg

 Consider invasive monitoring of arterial blood pressure

If central access is not yet available

 Consider initiating vasopressors peripherally*

If MAP is inadequate despite low-to-moderate dose norepinephrine

 Consider adding vasopressin

If cardiac dysfunction with persistent hypoperfusion is present despite adequate volume status and blood pressure

 Consider adding dobutamine or switching to epinephrine

Strong recommendations are displayed in Green and weak recommendations are displayed in Yellow
*When using vasopressors peripherally, they should be administered only for a short period of time and in a vein proximal to the antecubital fossa

■ CORTICOSTEROIDS IN SEPSIS

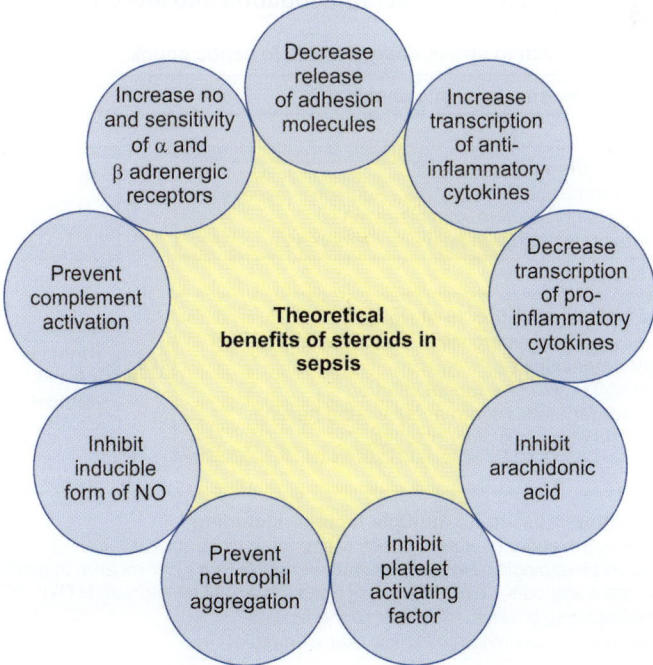

TABLE 1: Putative signs and symptoms of critical illness related corticosteroid insufficiency (CIRCI).

Clinical		
General	• Confusion • Delirium • Coma	
Cardiovascular	• Hypotension refractory to fluid resuscitation • Decreased sensitivity to catecholamines • High cardiac index	
Digestive	• Nausea • Vomiting • Intolerance to enteral nutrition	
Respiratory	• Persistent hypoxia	
Laboratory	• Hypoglycemia • Hyponatremia • Hyperkalemia • Metabolic acidosis • Hypereosinophilia	
Imaging	Hemorrhage or necrosis in hypothalamus, pituitary gland, or adrenal gland	

1. SSG suggests against using IV hydrocortisone to treat septic shock patients if adequate fluid resuscitation and vasopressor therapy are able to restore hemodynamic stability. If this is not achievable, SSG suggests IV hydrocortisone at a dose of 200 mg/day (weak recommendation and low quality of evidence).

Approach to stress dose steroids in septic shock

Vasopressor-dependent septic shock
↓

Strong indication for steroids?
• Chronic adrenal insufficiency (i.e., Addison's disease)
• Chronic systemic steroid administration
• Hypotension refractory to fluid and vasopressor
→ Yes → **Strongly consider steroid**

↓ No

Relative contraindication to steroids?
• Paralytic infusion (synergistic risk of myopathy)
• Diabetic ketoacidosis
• HBV, HIV, TB, invasive fungal infertion
• Recent surgery with conern about wound healing
• Active or recent peptic ulcer disease
→ Yes → **Probably avoid steroid**

↓

Expert judgment based on multiple factors, including:
• How sick is the patient? How are they responding to treatment?
• How much physiologic reserve does patient have? (e.g., low reserve in patients with critical aortic stenosis, severe cardiomyopathy, servere pulmonary HTN)
• Prior exposure to adrenal-suppressive medication?
  (e.g., etomidate, phenytoin, rifampin, ketoconazole)

Sepsis Management: Current Update

MECHANICAL VENTILATION

The SSG recommends:
- Using higher PEEP over lower PEEP in adult patients with sepsis-induced moderate to severe ARDS.
- Using prone over supine position in adult patients with sepsis-induced ARDS and a PaO_2/FIO_2 ratio <150.
- Against the use of HFOV in adult patients with sepsis-induced ARDS.
- Against the use of β-2 agonists for the treatment of patients with sepsis-induced ARDS without bronchospasm.
- Using lower tidal volumes over higher tidal volumes in adult patients with sepsis-induced respiratory failure without ARDS.

GLYCEMIC CONTROL

The SSG recommends a protocolized approach to blood glucose management in ICU patients with sepsis, commencing insulin dosing when two consecutive blood glucose levels are >180 mg/dL. This approach should target an upper blood glucose level <180 mg/dL rather than an upper target blood glucose < 110 mg/dL. (Strong recommendation; high quality of evidence)

It is recommended that blood glucose values should be monitored every 1-2 hours until glucose values and insulin infusion rates are stable, then every 4 hours thereafter in patients receiving insulin infusions.

NUTRITION

The SSG recommends:
- Against the administration of early parenteral nutrition alone or parenteral nutrition in combination with enteral feedings (but rather initiate early enteral nutrition) in critically ill patients with sepsis or septic shock who can be fed enterally.
- Against the administration of parenteral nutrition alone or in combination with enteral feeds (but rather to initiate IV glucose and advance enteral feeds as tolerated) over the first 7 days in critically ill patients with sepsis or septic shock in whom early enteral feeding is not feasible.
- Against routinely monitoring gastric residual volumes in critically ill patients with sepsis or septic shock.
- However, suggests measurement of gastric residuals in patients with feeding intolerance or who are considered to be high risk for aspiration.
- The use of prokinetic agents in critically ill patients with sepsis or septic shock and feeding intolerance.

BLOOD AND BLOOD/PRODUCTS TRANSFUSION

- Transfuse red blood cells when Hb decreases to <7 and target a Hb of 7-9 in adults.
- Higher Hb level may be required in presence of myocardial ischemia, severe hypoxemia, or acute hemorrhage.

- Erythropoietin is not recommended as a treatment of sepsis related severe anemia.
- Fresh frozen plasma (FFP) should only be used to correct clotting abnormalities in the presence of bleeding or planned invasive procedures.
- Antithrombin should not be used for the treatment of severe sepsis.
- Administer platelets in severe sepsis when:
    - Counts are <10,000 regardless of bleeding
    - Counts are <20,000 and the patient has a significant risk of bleeding.
    - Counts are >50,000 but patient having active bleeding or undergoing surgery and invasive procedures.

IV immunoglobulin are *not* recommended in the treatment of severe sepsis.

USE OF BICARBONATE

Do not use sodium bicarbonate for the purpose of improving hemodynamics or reducing vasopressor requirements when treating hypoperfusion induced lactic acidemia with a pH > 7.15.

DEEP VEIN THROMBOSIS PROPHYLAXIS

- Patients with severe sepsis should receive daily pharmacoprophylaxis against VTE.
- Use once daily subcutaneously low-molecular-weight heparins (LMWH) (grade 1B vs. BD dosing of UFH and grade 2C vs. TDS dosing of UFH).
- If CrCl < 30 use dalteparin.
- Whenever possible, treat with a combination of pharmacological therapy and intermittent pneumatic compression.
- Where heparin is contraindicated (low platelets, severe coagulopathy, active bleeding or recent ICH) mechanical prophylactic treatment (compression stocking or devices) should be used.

STRESS ULCER PROPHYLAXIS

- Use H2 bocker or proton pump inhibitor in patients who have bleeding risk factors.
- When stress ulcer prophylaxis is needed use PPI rather than H2 RA. Patients without risk factors should not receive prophylaxis.

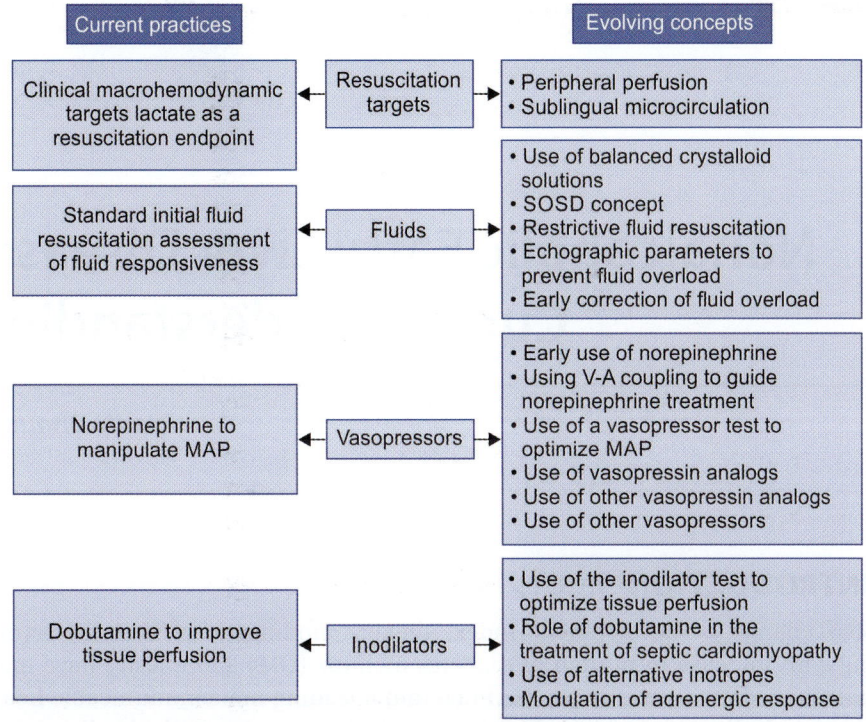

FIG. 2: Some evolving concepts on septic shock resuscitation.

Source: Bakker I, Kattan E, Anneane D, et al. Current practice and evolving concepts on septic shock resuscitation. Intensive Care Med. 2022;48(2):148-63.

CHAPTER 54

Nonalcoholic Fatty Liver Disease: Current Understanding

Pradip Bhaumik

■ INTRODUCTION

Global change of development index, dietary modification, lifestyle changes along with increase in burden of diabetes mellitus (DM) and obesity have made nonalcoholic fatty liver disease (NAFLD) into a leading noncommunicable health problem in India and world. NAFLD has gradually becoming as the leading causes of cirrhosis and hepatocellular carcinoma (HCC). Considering the importance, Government of India included NAFLD in NPCDCS (National Program for Prevention and Control of Cancer, Diabetes, Cardiovascular Disease, and Stroke) a flagship program to prevent noncommunicable disease since 2020.

■ DEFINITION

Nonalcoholic fatty liver disease is defined as the presence of >5% fat in the liver [hepatic steatosis (HS)] either on imaging or on liver histology after excluding other causes of fat accumulation in the liver like significant alcohol intake, drug-induced liver injury, and relevant diseases. NAFLD is divided into two groups:
1. Nonalcoholic fatty liver (NAFL)
2. Nonalcoholic steatohepatitis (NASH)

Nonalcoholic fatty liver is defined as HS with no evidence of hepatocellular injury in the form of hepatocyte ballooning. NASH is defined as the presence of HS and inflammation with hepatocyte injury (ballooning) with or without fibrosis.

The diagnosis of NAFLD is made on the basis of: (1) presence of >5% of fat in liver (steatosis) by imaging or biopsy, (2) absence of significant alcohol use, (3) no other causes of HS like viral hepatitis, and (4) no coexisting cause of chronic liver disease.

Nonalcoholic fatty liver disease is currently renamed as metabolic (dysfunction)-associated fatty liver disease (MAFLD). The new terminology correctly points out the "positive" determinants of the association with metabolic disorders, rather than giving a name what it is not (i.e., nonalcoholic).

Definition of "Significant" Alcohol Use

All guidelines characterize NAFLD by the presence of HS in the absence of significant alcohol consumption. However, there is no international consensus as to the amount of alcohol considered "significant". The Asia Pacific Association of Study of Liver (2017) guideline has given more useful conservative alcohol threshold which is usually followed: men—two standard drinks/day or 140 g/week and women—one standard drink per day or 70 g/week.

■ TERMINOLOGIES OF NONALCOHOLIC FATTY LIVER DISEASE

- *NAFLD*: Indicates fatty infiltration of the liver defined as a fat concentration >5–10% of the liver weight. HS > 5% in biopsy specimens.
- *Simple steatosis*: Fatty infiltration with no or minimal inflammation and no fibrosis
- *NASH*: HS with inflammation, ballooned hepatocytes, and/or fibrosis (which may progress to cirrhosis)
- *Primary NAFLD*: Occasionally used in the literature but not uniformly accepted. Indicates typical disease associated with features of metabolic syndrome but without a specific, additional etiology.
- *Secondary NAFLD*: NAFLD associated with a specific cause implies the absence of insulin resistance (IR). May represent exacerbation of underlying primary NAFLD.
- *Presumed NAFLD*: Presumptive diagnosis of NAFLD used in epidemiological and pediatric studies based on the following:
  - Abnormal liver enzyme levels
  - Negative results from viral studies
  - Exclusion of other common liver disease etiologies
  - Echogenic or bright liver on imaging (often abdominal ultrasound) consistent with fatty infiltration

(Matteoni et al.)

■ HISTORY OF NONALCOHOLIC FATTY LIVER DISEASE

In 1980, the term NASH was first used by Ludwig et al. to describe a histological condition resembling alcoholic steatohepatitis who were not alcoholic. The majority of patients were obese women or many were diabetic. In fact Addison first described fatty liver in 1836. In 1838, the pathologist Rokitansky documented hepatic fat accumulation that might be causative of cirrhosis.

Schaner and Thaler were first to use the name "nonalcoholic fatty liver disease" in 1986.

Presently genetic determinants of disease production and progression are increasingly recognized.

■ EPIDEMIOLOGY

Nonalcoholic fatty liver disease is the most common liver disease worldwide and the leading cause of liver-related morbidity and mortality. It is now almost epidemic across the continent and gradually becoming major public health problem. The overall prevalence of NAFLD worldwide was estimated to be 32.4%. Prevalence increased significantly over time, from 25.5% in or before 2005 to 37.8% in 2016. Overall prevalence of NAFLD was significantly higher in men than in women 39.7 versus 25.6%. Most patients with NAFLD are overweight, obese, and have type 2 diabetes mellitus (T2DM). Some NAFLD patients may have lower body mass index (BMI) within the lean threshold (lean NASH). Nevertheless, the higher the number of components of metabolic syndrome, the higher the risk for adverse outcomes. Prevalence of NAFLD in India ranges from 30 to 48%.

PATHOGENESIS OF NONALCOHOLIC FATTY LIVER DISEASE

The development of NASH is a complex process and is not completely understood. It has been suggested that the development of NASH is a two-step process (two hit). The first step of this process is fat deposition in the liver that will increase IR. The second part of this process is cellular and molecular changes involving oxidative stress, and oxidation of fatty acids in the liver due to a variety of factors (cytokine injury, hyperinsulinemia, hepatic iron and/or lipid peroxidation, variation of the extracellular matrix, energy homeostasis, and change in the immune system function). Various risk factors plays an important role in the pathogenesis of NAFLD **(Box 1)**.

GENETICS OF NONALCOHOLIC FATTY LIVER DISEASE

Like many other metabolic and noncommunicable disorders pathophysiology of NAFLD has a high possibility of inheritability, and the multiple genetic determinants of disease biology including prognosis are being understood very fast. Development of genetic studies of NAFLD passed through two major evolutionary stages: (1) candidate gene approach and (2) genome-wide association studies (GWAS). Candidate genes hypotheses are based on the prior knowledge. Whereas first GWAS in hepatology aimed at investigating the genetic basis of susceptibility to NAFL was described in 2008. Since then, GWAS, whole-genome, and whole-exome sequencing have become the methodology of choice to determine genotype–phenotype associations.

Number of different genes is associated with susceptibility to development and progression of NAFLD. These include: *patatin-like phospholipase domain-containing protein 3* (*PNPLA3*), *transmembrane 6 superfamily member 2* (*TM6SF2*), *glucokinase regulator* (*GCKR*), and *hydroxysteroid 17-dehydrogenase* (*HSD17B13*).

It remains uncertain whether "genetic NAFLD" is perfectly equivalent to "metabolic NAFLD". Presently phenome-wide association study (PheWAS) and exome-wide association study are emerging to consider single phenotype to multiple phenotypes.

It is recently observed that genetic predisposition to NAFLD may vary according to ancestral ethnicity. Recent Indian study reflect that the *TM6SF2* variant (rs58542926) was significantly associated with NAFLD susceptibility among individuals from South Indian ethnicity. *PNPLA3* variant (rs2281135) conferred a higher risk for NAFLD in those of North East Indian ancestry.

BOX 1: Risk factors of hepatic steatosis.

Metabolic syndrome:
- Insulin resistance
- Obesity
- Sedentary lifestyle
- Type 2 diabetes mellitus
- Hypertension
- Dyslipidemia

Drugs:
- Tamoxifen
- Corticosteroids
- Amiodarone
- Methotrexate
- Estrogens
- Valproic acid
- Antiretroviral medications

Nutrition:
- Carbohydrate excess (e.g., diet and total parenteral nutrition)
- Rapid weight loss
- Altered small bowel anatomy
- Obesity surgery (e.g., jejunoileal bypass)
- Pancreaticoduodenal resection
- Short gut

Metabolic diseases (resulting in a NASH-like histology):
- Hypobetalipoproteinemia
- Abetalipoproteinemia
- Wilson's disease
- Lipodystrophies
- Andersen disease
- Weber–Christian syndrome

Infections:
- Chronic hepatitis C virus, mainly genotype 3
- Human immunodeficiency virus and acquired immune deficiency syndrome

Emerging associations:
- Polycystic ovarian syndrome
- Hypothyroidism
- Obstructive sleep apnea
- Hypopituitarism
- Hypogonadism

(NASH: nonalcoholic steatohepatitis)

SPECTRUM AND CLINICAL PRESENTATION

In NAFLD presence of fatty liver is significant for progressive NASH with or without hepatic fibrosis that adds to the significant liver disease and extrahepatic disease burden. It has been described that patients with NAFLD showed histological NASH in >60% of patients and advanced fibrosis (≥ F3) in 35% of patients. The presence of metabolic risk factors also suggests NAFLD to be the predominant cause of cirrhosis and HCC in India. Similarly NAFLD is associated with several nonhepatic conditions, like coronary artery disease (CAD), chronic kidney disease (CKD), polycystic ovarian disease (PCOD), obstructive sleep apnea, vitamin D deficiency, and hypothyroidism **(Fig. 1)**.

SCREENING OF NONALCOHOLIC FATTY LIVER DISEASE

Most of the Leading Scientific Associations recommend that systematic screening for NAFLD in the general populations is not required. American Association for the Study of Liver Diseases (AASLD) currently recommends against screening even in high-risk populations. A "high index of suspicion" for NAFLD is advised in patients with T2DM.

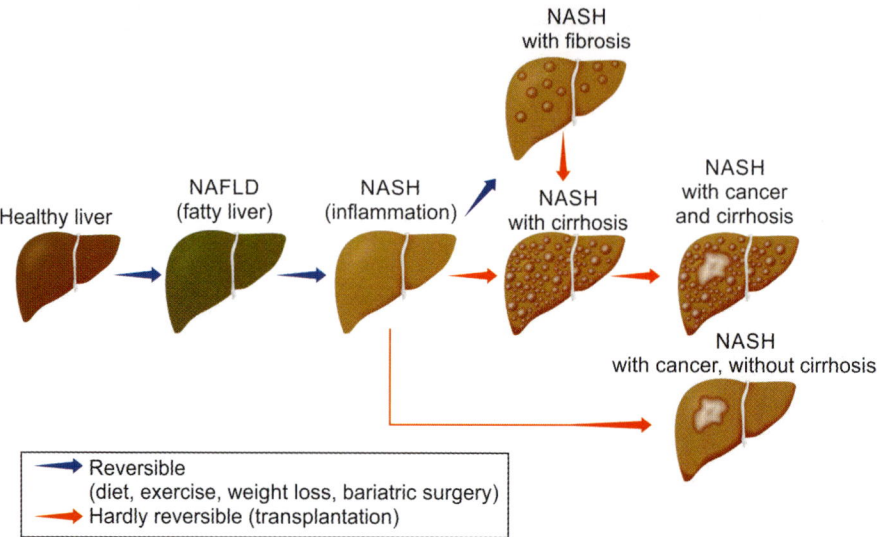

FIG. 1: Spectrum of nonalcoholic fatty liver disease (NAFLD) (American Association for the Study of Liver Diseases, Clinical Liver Disease, 2016).

The European guideline recommends that all patients with obesity or the metabolic syndrome be screened for NAFLD because of the prognostic implications of progressive disease. Screening may be considered in at-risk groups, such as patients with diabetes and obesity. Lean NAFLD is prevalent in Asia, where almost a quarter of patients with NAFLD are not obese. Thus, IR and altered body fat distribution rather than BMI may be better indicators of NAFLD in this group.

Ultrasound is the first-line assessment tool for HS. However, it is less reliable when steatosis is <20% and raises concerns of underestimating the prevalence of NAFLD. Magnetic resonance imaging-derived proton density fat fraction is highly sensitive but is not commonly available, controlled attenuation parameter is available with the fibro scan system and may be more sensitive than ultrasound **(Fig. 2)**.

DIAGNOSIS AND MONITORING

- *Liver histology*: It is an invasive procedure and involves risk as well as high cost. But it is the method of choice for diagnosis, prognostication, and staging. It is basically the gold standard but not followed due to its invasive nature and associated costs. In practice biopsy is considered more for research and only in selected individuals **(Table 1)**.
- *Noninvasive method*: Multiple noninvasive methods are in use for diagnosis and staging of NAFLD. These are used to stratify patients as low or high risk for advanced fibrosis. There are currently no acceptable noninvasive modalities to differentiate between bland steatosis and steatohepatitis. The presence of the metabolic syndrome increases the risk for steatohepatitis.

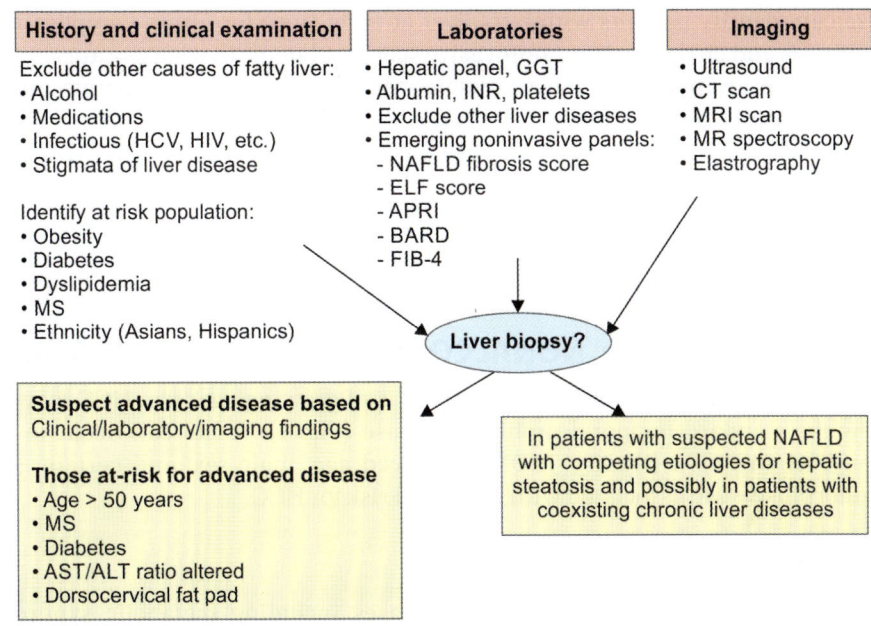

FIG. 2: Workup for nonalcoholic fatty liver disease (NAFLD): Incidentally detected abnormal liver chemistry/imaging (American Association for the Study of Liver Diseases 2012).

(AST: aspartate aminotransferase; ALT: alanine transaminase; APRI: aspartate aminotransferase to platelet ratio index; CT: computed tomography; ELF: enhanced liver fibrosis; FIB-4: fibrosis-4 index; GGT: gamma glutamyl transferase; HCV: hepatitis C virus; HIV: human immunodeficiency virus; INR: international normalized ratio; MS: metabolic syndrome; MRI: magnetic resonance imaging; MR: magnetic resonance)

TABLE 1: Fibrosis score: histological.	
0	None
1a	Mild (delicate) zone 3 perisinusoidal fibrosis
1b	Moderate (dense) zone 3 perisinusoidal fibrosis
1c	Portal/periportal fibrosis only
2	Zone 3 perisinusoidal fibrosis with portal/periportal fibrosis
3	Bridging fibrosis
4	Cirrhosis

NONINVASIVE SCORING SYSTEMS OF NONALCOHOLIC FATTY LIVER DISEASE

Multiple noninvasive (without biopsy) scoring systems have been evolved in current year's. Most of these systems need proper validation particularly for the population it is being considered. Most of these scoring systems compare the severity of the disease, ranging from HS and NASH to fibrosis, by contrasting the corresponding serum markers, clinical associations, and performance metrics.

These can identify patients with fatty liver at early stage for future complications like fibrosis and cirrhosis. Few noninvasive scoring systems in wide use are:
- Aspartate aminotransferase to platelet ratio index (APRI): Aspartate amino transferase to platelet ratio
- The BMI, aspartate aminotransferase (AST)/alanine transaminase (ALT) ratio and Diabetes (BARD)
- The fibrosis-4 index (FIB-4)
- Hepamet fibrosis score (HFS)
- NAFLD fibrosis score (NFS)

KEY OUTCOMES IN NONALCOHOLIC FATTY LIVER DISEASE

Hepatocellular carcinoma related to NAFLD is of growing concern. HCC may not follow the standard temporal profile of disease **(Fig. 1)**, rather can occur in the absence of cirrhosis. Obesity, T2DM, advanced age, male sex, and certain gene polymorphisms are associated with increased risk for HCC.

Treatment

The treatment of NAFLD and related diseases including metabolic syndrome consists of several tiers of conservative medical therapy and surgical intervention. Mostly the treatment of patients with NAFLD consists of a multimodal intervention targeting aspects like weight loss, lifestyle modifications, and possible optimum medical therapy.

Lifestyle modification. Therapeutic lifestyle changes (TLC) are the primary modality for the management of NAFLD and have been shown to improve biochemical and histological features. Target weight loss of 7–10% can be achieved with daily calorie deficit of 500–1,000 and moderate-intensity exercise, preferably in a structured weight loss program. No specific recommendations related to specific macronutrient or diets usually advocated. Mediterranean diet, avoidance of processed foods, and added fructose is routinely required.

Pharmacotherapy: For nondiabetic NASH therapies vitamin E (800 mg/day) is recommended, pioglitazone, a thiazolidinedione is a good choice for NASH and diabetes. More recently, liraglutide, a glucagon-like peptide-1 (GLP-1) receptor agonist, was recommended. Drug controller general of India has approved the use of saroglitazar, a dual peroxisome proliferator-activated receptor α/γ agonist, (4 mg/day) for use in patients with NASH with F1-3 fibrosis. Recent data on vitamin D supplementation, high-potency multistrain probiotic, GLP-1 agonists, and sodium-glucose cotransporter-2 (SGLT-2) inhibitors also have been encouraging in Indian patients with NAFLD. Genetic evaluation and precision medicine in NAFLD is developing very fast with encouraging initial results.

Surgical intervention: Bariatric surgery was found to improve histology of NAFLD, including NAFLD activity score and fibrosis. Among various endoscopic therapies, only intragastric balloon found to induce weight loss. NASH-related decompensated cirrhosis and HCC are leading indications for liver transplant in India.

CONCLUSION

Nonalcoholic fatty liver disease is gradually becoming a significant association of metabolic syndrome. Hence, early diagnosis and multipronged intervention is highly needed. The morbidity and mortality of NAFLD may not be only liver-related complication, rather cardiovascular and other disorder can be equal contributor. With the growing increase in obesity worldwide and the rising coexistence of conditions like DM and NAFLD, the management of this high prevalent condition has become very complex and difficult.

Newer pharmacological agents may address NAFLD and metabolic disorders simultaneously leading to better outcome. NAFLD is one of the very dynamic liver disorder and guideline issued by various leading bodies are being changed very fast. The guideline in use today may become outdated soon. Future guideline updates should emphasize on more practical issues of early diagnosis, cost-effective and minimally invasive staging, and treatment, which will be applicable for maximum number of people. There is also a pressing need of developing community hepatology to reduce the global burden of NAFLD and its complications.

SUGGESTED READINGS

1. Lonardo A, Leoni S, Alswat KA, et al. History of nonalcoholic fatty liver disease. Int J Mol Sci. 2020;21(16):5888.
2. Ando Y, Jou JH. Nonalcoholic fatty liver disease and recent guideline updates. Clin Liver Dis (Hoboken). 2021;17(1):23-8.
3. De A, Duseja A. Nonalcoholic fatty liver disease: Indian perspective. Clin Liver Dis (Hoboken). 2021;18(3):158-63.
4. Riazi K, Azhari H, Charette JH, et al. The prevalence and incidence of NAFLD worldwide: A systematic review and meta-analysis. Lancet Gastroenterol Hepatol. 2022;7(9):851-61.
5. Pouwels S, Sakran N, Graham Y, et al. Non-alcoholic fatty liver disease (NAFLD): A review of pathophysiology, clinical management and effects of weight loss. BMC Endocr Disord. 2022;22(1):63.
6. Puri P, Sanyal AJ. Nonalcoholic fatty liver disease: Definitions, risk factors, and workup. Clin Liver Dis (Hoboken). 2012;1(4):99-103.
7. Segura-Azuara NIÁ, Varela-Chinchilla CD, Trinidad-Calderón PA. MAFLD/NAFLD biopsy-free scoring systems for hepatic steatosis, NASH, and fibrosis diagnosis. Front Med (Lausanne). 2022;8:774079.

CHAPTER 55

Metabolic Syndrome: An Overview

KK Lohani

■ INTRODUCTION

Metabolic syndrome is a group of metabolic abnormalities that increase the risk of type 2 diabetes mellitus (T2DM) and cardiovascular disease (CVD). Syndrome X, insulin resistance syndrome, Reaven's syndrome, and deadly quartet are some of the other names for it.

Metabolic syndrome is characterized by central obesity, hypertriglyceridemia, low high-density lipoprotein (HDL), hyperglycemia, and hypertension.

■ RISK FACTORS

Obesity/Overweight—central (key feature), sedentary behavior, aging—the prevalence rises with age. Diabetes mellitus—approximately 75% of T2DM or impaired glucose tolerance (IGT) suffer from metabolic syndrome. CVD—50% of coronary heart disease (CHD) patients have metabolic syndrome. Premature coronary artery disease (CAD) affects roughly one-third of mitral stenosis (MS) patients. Lipodystrophy, characterized by severe insulin resistance, can be genetic or acquired.

■ CLINICAL FEATURES

A high index of suspicion is required for diagnosis when the patient is asymptomatic. Important clinical findings include an increase in waist circumference, an increase in blood pressure, lipoatrophy, and *Acanthosis nigricans*/skin tags. CVD—increased risk for new-onset CVD, ischemic stroke, peripheral vascular disease (PVD), T2DM increased risk by 3- to 5-fold, nonalcoholic fatty liver disease (NAFLD) and/or nonalcoholic steatohepatitis (NASH), hyperuricemia; PCOS—prevalence 40–50%; and obstructive sleep apnea (OSA)—commonly associated with obesity **(Fig. 1)**.

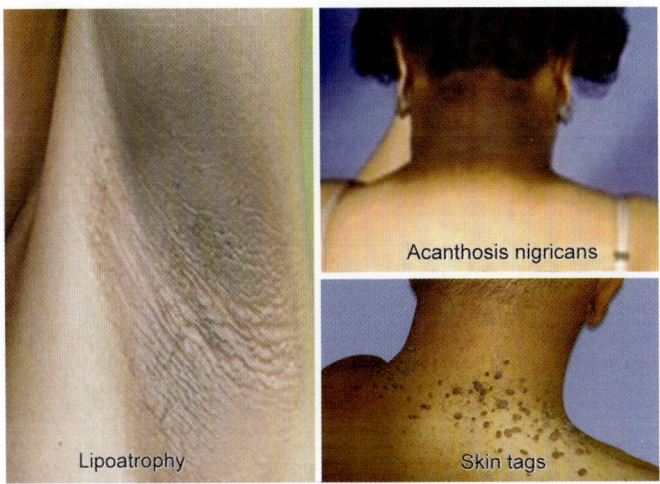

FIG. 1: Clinical features of metabolic syndrome.

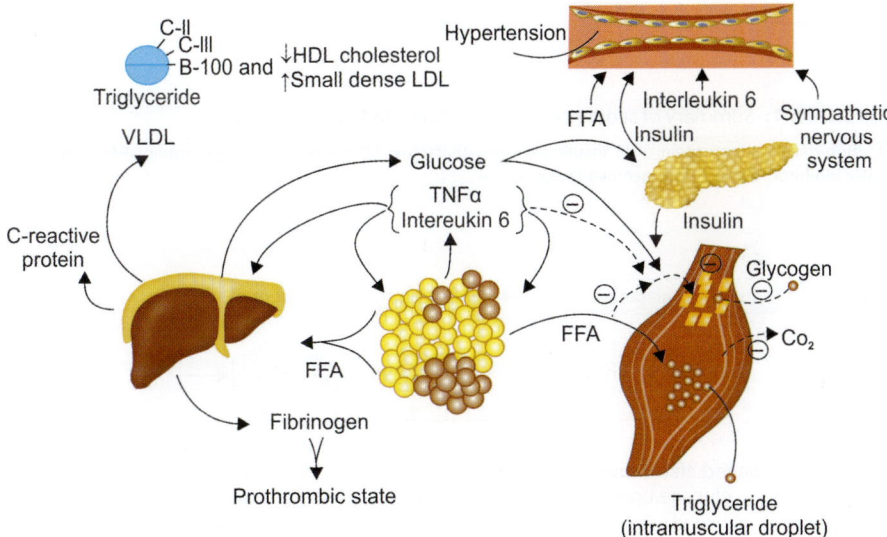

FIG. 2: Pathogenesis of metabolic syndrome.
(FFA: free fatty acid; LDL: low-density lipoprotein; VLDL: very low-density lipoprotein; TNF: tumor necrosis factor)

PATHOGENESIS

Central obesity is a keystone in the pathogenesis of "Metabolic Syndrome." Central obesity causes insulin resistance. Pathogenesis is influenced by a number of factors, including interleukin-1 (IL-1), IL-6, IL-18, resistin, tumor necrosis factor-alpha (TNF-α), and C-reactive protein (CRP). Adiponectin, an anti-inflammatory cytokine, is reduced in metabolic syndrome. Please see **Figure 2**.

The sequence of events shown in **Figure 2** is summarized in **Flowchart 1**.

Metabolic Syndrome: An Overview

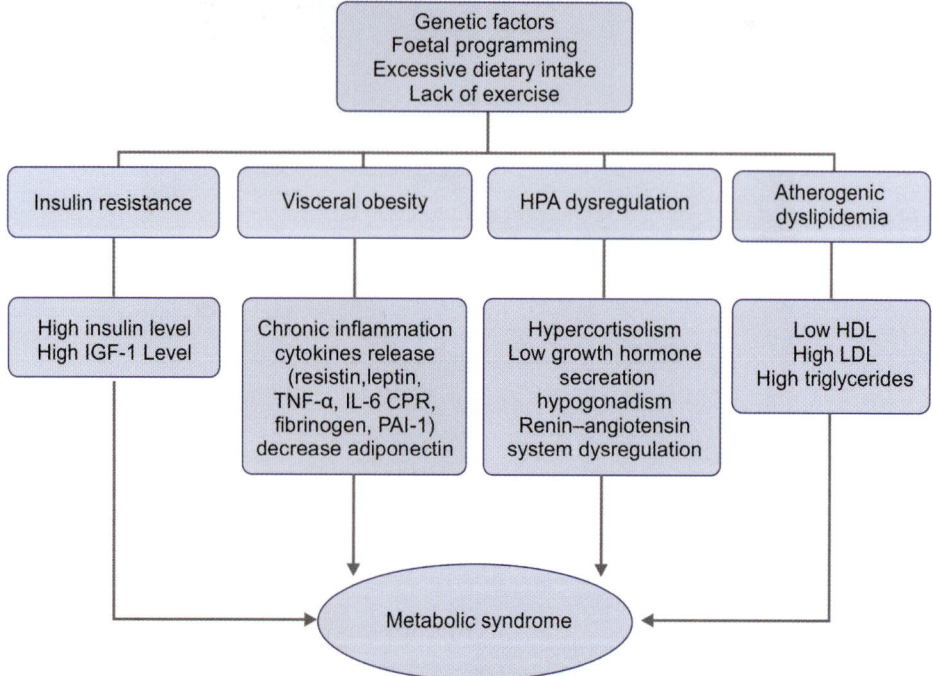

FLOWCHART 1: Summary of sequence of events shown in **Figure 2**.
(HDL: high-density lipoprotein; IGF: insulin-like growth factor; LDL: low-density lipoprotein; PAI: plasminogen activator inhibitor; TNF-α: tumor necrosis factor-alpha)

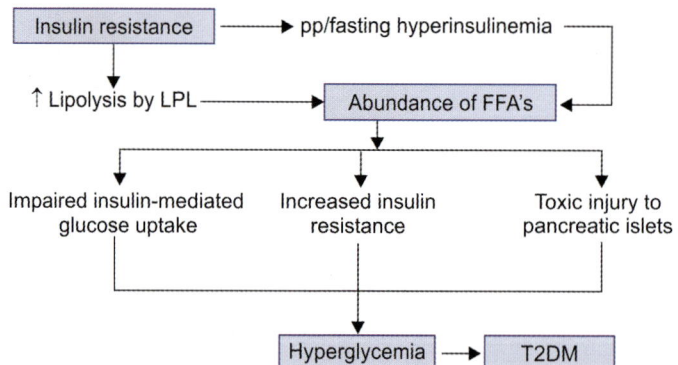

FLOWCHART 2: Pathogenesis of metabolic syndrome and diabetes mellitus.
(FFA: free fatty acid; LPL: lipoprotein lipase; T2DM: type 2 diabetes mellitus)

Metabolic Syndrome and Diabetes Mellitus

There is increased risk of T2DM by 3- to 5-fold. The pathogenesis can be summarized as shown in **Flowchart 2**.

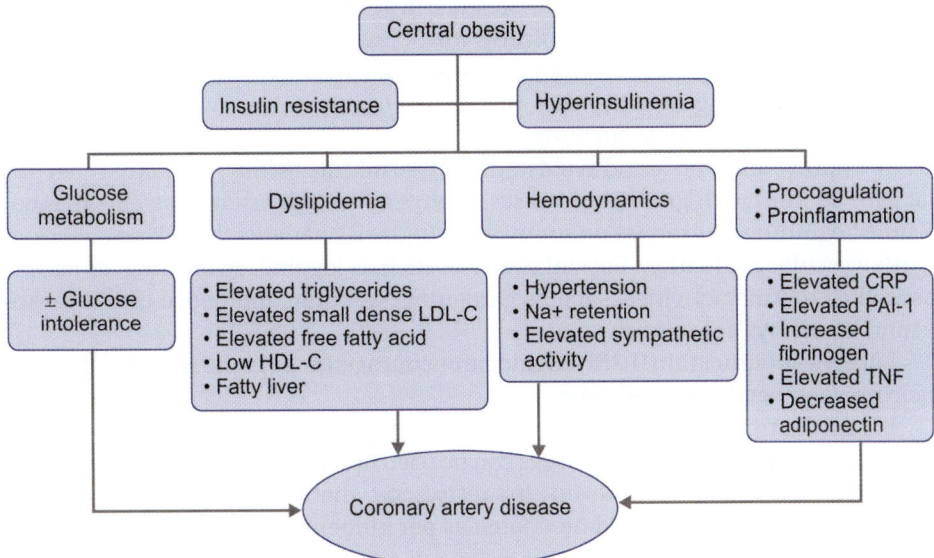

FLOWCHART 3: Pathogenesis of coronary artery disease.

(CRP: C-reactive protein; HDL-C: high-density lipoprotein cholesterol; LDL-C: low-density lipoprotein cholesterol; PAI: plasminogen activator inhibitor; TNF: tumor necrosis factor)

Metabolic Syndrome and Coronary Artery Disease

The deadly quartet of central obesity, hyperglycemia, dyslipidemia, and hypertension play important role in pathogenesis of CAD; insulin resistance being the common factor **(Flowchart 3)**.

■ DIAGNOSIS

How to suspect—history of (H/o) OSA in all patients, H/o polycystic ovary syndrome (PCOS) in premenopausal women, and family H/o CVD and diabetes. Waist circumference and blood pressure measurements have increased values.

Abnormal fasting lipid profile and fasting glucose, liver function test (LFT) suggestive of NAFLD, according to laboratory investigations. On routine USG, fatty liver is a common finding.

Criteria for the International Diabetes Federation (IDF): Waist circumference: 90 cm in men, 80 cm in women, plus two or more of the following—hypertriglyceridemia (defined as 150 TGs or a specific medication), low HDL cholesterol levels of 40 (M) and 50 (F), or specific medication; hypertension is defined as a blood pressure of 130 mm Hg systolic or 85 mm Hg diastolic, or a specific medication, fasting plasma glucose level of 100 mg/dL, or specific medication, or previously diagnosed DM.

■ TREATMENT

Weight loss can be achieved through a combination of caloric restriction, increased physical activity, and behavior modification.

Diet: A 500 kcal restriction per day results in a weekly weight loss of 1 pound. Carbohydrate-restricted diets typically result in rapid initial weight loss. Diet adherence is more important than diet selection. To provide the greatest overall health benefit, a high-quality diet rich in fruits, vegetables, whole grains, lean poultry, and fish should be encouraged.

To improve adherence and avoid injury, 60–90 minutes of physical activity per day (at least 30 min) with gradual increases in physical activity should be encouraged. Before beginning an exercise program, some high-risk patients should have a formal cardiovascular evaluation. Formal exercise, such as jogging, swimming, or tennis, as well as routine activities, such as gardening, walking, and house cleaning, are examples of physical activity.

Lifestyle modification (LSM) should be encouraged at beginning in childhood to help prevent metabolic syndrome.

Bariatric surgery is also an option for patients with BMI >40 kg/m^2 or >35 kg/m^2 with comorbidities. Antiobesity drugs can be tried before planning bariatric surgery.

Different components like insulin resistance, diabetes, dyslipidemia, hypertension and/or NAFLD should be treated as per guidelines if LSM is not enough to manage it.

For symptoms suggestive of OSA opinion of specialist should be sought.

CONCLUSION

Metabolic syndrome is a group of metabolic abnormalities which makes a person prone to T2DM and ASCVD. It is also considered a predisposing factor for NAFLD and CKD. Central obesity, hypertension, impaired fasting glucose, high triglyceride and low HDL are its cardinal features. Insulin resistance is the most important patho physiological abnormality. It is diagnosed on the basis of IDF criteria. Life style modifications consisting of diet, exercise and weight loss are the mainstay of treatment.

SUGGESTED READINGS

1. Kahn R, Buse J, Ferrannini E, et al. The metabolic syndrome: time for a critical appraisal. Joint statement from the American Diabetes Association and the European Association for the Study of Diabetes. Diabetologia. 2005;48:1684-99.
2. Grundy SM. Metabolic syndrome: a multiplex cardiovascular risk factor. J Clin Endocrinol Metab. 2007;92:399-404.
3. Reaven GM. The metabolic syndrome: is this diagnosis necessary? Am J Clin Nutr. 2006;83:1237-47.
4. Huang PL. Unraveling the links between diabetes, obesity, and cardiovascular disease. Circ Res. 2005;96:1129-31.
5. Grundy SM, Cleeman JI, Daniels SR, et al. Diagnosis and management of the metabolic syndrome: an American Heart Association/National Heart, Lung and Blood Institute scientific statement. Circulation. 2005;112:2735-52.
6. Cordero P, Li J, Oben JA. Bariatric surgery as a treatment for metabolic syndrome. JR Coll Physicians Edinb. 2017;47(4):364-8.
7. Chen YY, Fang WH, Wang CC, et al. Association of Percentage Body Fat and Metabolic Health in Offspring of Patients with Cardiovascular Diseases. Sci Rep. 2018;8(1):13831.
8. van der Pal KC, Koopman ADM, Lakerveld J, et al. The association between multiple sleep-related characteristics and the metabolic syndrome in the general population: the New Hoorn study. Sleep Med. 2018;52:51-7.

CHAPTER 56

Erectile Dysfunction

MPS Chawla

INTRODUCTION

Erectile dysfunction (ED) prevalence is more in older men above 40 years of age. The etiology is multifactorial and may be associated with endocrine system or nonendocrine causes. Nonendocrine causes may be vasogenic, involving the abnormalities of arterial inflow or venous outflow, neurogenic or iatrogenic. Reduced testosterone levels have been implicated in the endocrine causes. The importance of ED is now paramount as its role is not only limited to sexual satisfaction alone, it has now been implicated as a measure of systemic endothelial dysfunction. Its presence in a patient is a sign of advent of cardiovascular diseases and associated with major cardiovascular events, therefore, these patients should be thoroughly investigated for organic causes and followed up closely for cardiovascular monitoring. A number of lifestyle diseases are associated with ED, such as hypertension, diabetes mellitus, dyslipidemia, neurological disorders, morbid obesity, stress, depression, anxiety, chronic kidney disease, chronic liver disease, substance abuse and smoking. Various cultural and socioeconomic factors also contribute to the problem. It is imperative to completely comprehend the physiology of erection, the various mechanisms playing a part in this process in order to diagnose accurately and manage the problem. A detailed history, a thorough clinical examination will guide us in determining the line of diagnostics that need to be undertaken to get to the underlying cause and guide the management of the individual patient. With time, there have been several breakthroughs in the management, including pharmacotherapeutics, lifestyle modifications, devices, prostheses and surgical interventions. The discovery of the role of nitric oxide (NO) system in signaling smooth muscle relaxation has fuelled an expansive research focusing on sexual dysfunction in men.

EPIDEMIOLOGY

It has been seen in various studies that the prevalence of ED is higher in the United States, Eastern and Southeast Asian countries as compared to South American and European nations. It also has a strong association with patients presenting with lower urinary tract symptoms in benign prostatic hyperplasia (BPH). Both ED and lower urinary tract symptoms due to BPH are more frequently seen in aging men, possibly due to other common associated risk factors. The Sexual Human Inventory for Males (SHIM) scores are used to assess ED, which is actually an abridged version of the International Index of Erectile Dysfunction (IIEF) aimed to diagnose ED **(Table 1)**. The SHIM questionnaire is a 5 point questionnaire with 5 points ascribed to each question; the final score is calculated by adding the scores of all the questions. A score of 21 or less is considered as ED, and can be further categorized into categories of mild, moderate and severe. The data from the European Male Ageing Study show that ED increases with age. The prevalence of severe ED, which is defined as an international index of erectile function score of between 1 and 7, increases at a higher rate than that of moderate ED (with score of 8 to 11) in men above 60 years of age. Another study showed that 22.1% of men <40 years of age had low (<21) SHIM scores. ED is strongly related to age, general health status and emotional function.

The Sexual Health Inventory for Men further classifies ED severity with the following breakpoints:
- 1–7 severe ED
- 8–11 moderate ED
- 12–16 mild to moderate ED
- 17–21 mild ED

PHYSIOLOGY OF PENILE ERECTION

Penile erection is a neurovascular event that is regulated by hormonal and psychological factors. Nitric oxide (NO) is the primary neurotransmitter responsible for penile erection and is mainly released from the endothelial cells and parasympathetic nerve terminals. Sexual stimulation causes nerve impulses, leading to the release of neurotransmitters from the cavernous nerve terminals and of relaxing factors from the endothelial cells, resulting in the relaxation of cavernosal arterial smooth muscles. This leads to manifold increase in the penile blood flow along with rapid expansion of the sinusoidal system. It causes compression of the subtunical small veins between tunica albuginea and the trabeculae, thus occluding the local venous return. This sequence of events traps the blood within the corpora cavernosa resulting in raising the penis from a dependent position to an erect position, with an estimated intracavernous pressure of almost 100 mm Hg in the phase of full erection. Sexual activity triggers the bulbocavernosus reflex forcing the ischiocavernosus muscles to compress the base of the blood-filled corpora cavernosa leading to the penis becoming even harder, with an intracavernous pressure escalating to much higher than hundred millimeters of mercury in the phase of rigid erection. The inflow and outflow of blood temporarily stops during this phase.

Erectile Dysfunction

TABLE 1: The Sexual Human Inventory for Males (SHIM) questionnaire assessment. (Over The Past 6 Months).

		Very low	Low	Moderate	High	Very high
1. How do you rate your confidence that you could get and keep an erection?		1	2	3	4	5
2. When you had erections with sexual stimulation, how often were your erections hard enough for penetration (entering your partner)?	No sexual activity	Almost never or never	A few times (much less than half the time)	Sometimes (about half the the)	Most times (much more than half the time)	Almost always or always
	0	1	2	3	4	5
3. During sexual intercourse, how often were you able to maintain your erection after you had penetrated (entered) your partner?	Attempt intercourse	Almost never or never	A few times (much less than half the time)	Sometimes (about half the the)	Most times (much more than half the time)	Almost always or always
	0	1	2	3	4	5
4. During sexual intercourse, how difficult was it to maintain your erection to completion of intercourse?	Did not attempt intercourse	Extremely difficult	Very difficult	Difficult	Slightly difficult	Not difficult
	0	1	2	3	4	5
5. When you attempted sexual intercourse, how often was it satisfactory for you?	Did not attempt intercourse	Almost never or never	A few times (much less than half the time)	Sometimes (about half the time)	Most times (much more than half the time)	Almost always or always
	0	1	2	3	4	5

Add the numbers corresponding to questions 1–5.   Total: _____

Penile detumescence occurs with the sympathetic activation of the adrenergic receptors on the surface of cavernous arteries during ejaculation, cessation of the neurotransmitter release and hydrolysis of secondary messengers (cGMP) by phosphodiesterase type-5 (PDE5) in the trabecular smooth muscles. Thus, resulting in the reduction of arterial inflow and causing a collapse of the lacunar spaces and decompression of the drainage venules of the cavernous bodies, thereby resulting in the relief of erection.

Penile flaccidity is maintained by the semi-contracted state of the intracorporeal smooth muscles that results from the intrinsic myogenic activity, adrenergic neurotransmission and endothelium derived contracting factors such as endothelins and PGF-2-alpha. Calcium influx into the cells is regulated by norepinephrine signaling and levels of inositol 1,4,5-trisphosphate, which is produced from Phosphatidylinositol 4,5-bisphosphate by phospholipase-C in the cells. The increased intracellular calcium ions binds to calmodulin, facilitating the formation of the calmodulin–myosin light chain kinase (MLCK) complex leading to the phosphorylation of MLC, causing smooth muscle contraction and flaccid penis. Norepinephrine signaling also inhibits adenylyl cyclase and modulates the RHO-associated protein kinase (ROCK) pathway, which increases the sensitivity of MLC to ionic calcium, which is negatively regulated by testosterone. Endothelins and prostaglandins from the endothelium also trigger an increase in the intracellular calcium ions promoting smooth muscle contraction. There is minimal blood inflow through the cavernous artery when the smooth muscle is contracted and blood outflows freely through the subtunical venous plexus. NO-independent, proerectile mechanisms of androgens also regulate expression of smooth muscle myosin isoforms and sphingosine-1-phosphate (S1P). In endothelial cells, activation of S1P receptors trigger the phosphoinositide 3kinase (PI3K)–AKT pathway, which enables the crosstalk between ROCK and the endothelial nitric oxide synthase (eNOS) pathways. These findings reinforce a beneficial role of androgens on many overlapping NOindependent pathways (S1P, PI3K–AKT and ROCK) favoring erectile response.

■ PATHOPHYSIOLOGIC MECHANISMS OF ERECTILE DYSFUNCTION

Erectile dysfunction can be classified into psychogenic, organic (neurogenic, vascular, hormonal, cavernosal or drug-induced) and mixed (both psychogenic and organic). Mixed variant is usually the most common cause of all mentioned.

Psychogenic Erectile Dysfunction

It is also known as adrenaline-mediated or noradrenaline-mediated or sympathetic-mediated ED, as noradrenaline is the primary erectolytic (antierectile) neurotransmitter.

Performance anxiety, lack of sexual arousability, strained relationship and overt psychiatric disorders such as depression and schizophrenia are some of the usual causes of psychogenic ED. Performance anxiety associated with sexual dysfunction itself leads to avoidance of sex, low self-esteem and depression.

Factors related to the development of psychogenic ED:
Predisposing factors
- Traumatic past/childhood experiences
- Strict upbringing
- Physical and mental health problems
- Inadequate sex education

Precipitating factors
- Acute relationship problems
- Family or social pressures
- Major life events such as pregnancy, childbirth, recent bereavement or loss of a job

Maintaining factors
- Physical or mental health problems
- Relationship problems.
- Absence of knowledge of availability of various treatment options

Religious and cultural differences do also influence the factors that affect the development of psychogenic ED.

Neurogenic Erectile Dysfunction

It is caused by some defect in the nerve signaling or conduction to the corpora cavernosa. Such deficits can occur in neurological conditions such as lumbar disk disease, traumatic brain injury, spinal cord injury, multiple sclerosis, Parkinson's disease, radical pelvic surgery (radical prostatectomy, radical cystectomy or abdominoperineal resection) and diabetes mellitus, etc.

Functional and structural alterations owing to the decreased innervation are usually caused by sacral cord lesions (S2–S4, *nervi erigentes*, being responsible for reflexogenic erections). Reduction of NO load that is available to the effectual smooth muscles results in the functional changes.

Vasculogenic Erectile Dysfunction

The risk factors associated with penile arterial insufficiency include atherosclerosis, hypertension, diabetes mellitus, dyslipidemia, cigarette smoking and pelvic irradiation. It is the secondary arterial wall changes in the form of reduced elasticity, and not hypertension per se, that results in ED. Broadly speaking, endothelial dysfunction is the root cause of vasculogenic ED. When ED occurs in men younger than age 60 years, it is strongly associated with an increase in the risk of future cardiac events when compared with men without ED. Blunt pelvic or perineal trauma (e.g., sustained from bicycling accidents) may result in focal stenosis of the common penile artery causing ED.

Veno-occlusive dysfunction may be caused by the formation of large venous channels draining the corpora cavernosa, degenerative changes to the tunica albuginea (due to Peyronie's disease, old age or diabetes mellitus) or traumatic injury (penile fracture), resulting in ED. Shunts acquired as a result of operative correction of priapism may also cause failure of erection.

Endocrinological Erectile Dysfunction

Androgen deficiency results in diminished nocturnal erections and libido, although erection in response to visual sexual stimulation is preserved in men with hypogonadism, thus indicating that androgen is not fundamentally necessary for penile erection.

The physiological effects of testosterone are well-defined in the regions of the brain that control sexual arousal like – amygdala, medial preoptic area and hypothalamic nuclei, at the spinal cord level (affecting neuronal firing from the pelvic ganglia) and within the penis (regulating endothelial and smooth muscle cell function). Testosterone is known to regulate the release of NO from non-cholinergic and non-adrenergic fibers, and the functioning of NO synthase in the endothelial cells. In the smooth muscle, testosterone modulates the activity of PDE5, the kinase that regulates Ca^{2+} and K^+ levels, and adrenergic receptor sensitivity.

Hyperprolactinemia from any cause results in both reproductive and sexual dysfunction as prolactin inhibits central dopaminergic activity causing diminished secretion of gonadotropin-releasing hormone, thereby resulting in hypogonadotropic hypogonadism.

Thus, prolactin should be considered for screening, together with testosterone and luteinizing hormone in ED.

Drug-induced Erectile Dysfunction

Cigarette smoking is known to cause vasoconstriction and penile venous leakage, due to the contractility of the cavernous smooth muscle. Ethanol in small quantities may improve penile erection and also increases libido because of its vasodilatory effect and allaying anxiety, but larger amounts can lead to central sedation, diminished libido, and transient ED. Chronic alcohol consumption in significant amount may also result in hypogonadism and polyneuropathy, affecting penile nerve function.

Central neurotransmitters such as noradrenergic, serotonergic and dopaminergic pathways are important in the normal sexual functioning and are altered by centrally acting antihypertensive drugs, antipsychotics, and antidepressants.

Beta-adrenergic blockers cause ED by potentiating alpha-1 adrenergic activity in the penis. Thiazide diuretics and digoxin have been implicated in ED, with unknown mechanism. Spironolactone also causes ED as well as gynecomastia with decreased libido.

H2 receptor antagonist, cimetidine, has been reported to reduce libido and cause ED by acting as an antiandrogen and causing hyperprolactinemia. Estrogens and some other drugs with antiandrogenic action, such as ketoconazole and cyproterone acetate, are known to cause ED.

5α–reductase inhibitors used in treatment of benign prostatic hyperplasia, antiandrogens and luteinizing hormone-releasing agonists/antagonists used to treat prostate cancer also cause ED.

Erectile Dysfunction due to Aging and Systemic/Metabolic Diseases

Sexual function declines progressively in healthy aging men. With increasing age, there is a decline in penile sensitivity to tactile stimulation, decrease in concentration of serum testosterone and an increase in the tone of cavernous muscle. Also, the latent period between sexual stimulation and erection increases, erections are less turgid, ejaculation is less forceful, the ejaculatory volume decreases, and the refractory period between erections lengthens with aging.

More than 50% of men with long standing diabetes mellitus have ED. In addition to affecting the smaller blood vessels, diabetes mellitus adversely affects the cavernous nerve terminals and endothelial function, thereby resulting in the deficiency of neurotransmitters.

Chronic kidney disease is frequently associated with diminished erectile function, impaired libido and infertility. The mechanism is multifactorial, involving low serum testosterone levels, vascular insufficiency, polypharmacy, somatic and autonomic neuropathy, and psychological stress. Individuals with coronary artery disease or cardiac failure usually have ED due to depression, anxiety, polypharmacy and associated penile arterial insufficiency.

DIAGNOSIS AND SCREENING

The identification of the causative factors involved in ED is the mainstay of an accurate diagnosis and successful treatment. ED could be the presenting symptom of a variety of diseases, such as diabetes mellitus, coronary artery disease, dyslipidemia, hypertension, pituitary tumor and spinal cord pathology.

The main goals of assessment are to establish whether the disorder is actually ED, to identify the cause of the disorder, and to ascertain the risk factors and potentially life-threatening comorbid conditions associated with ED.

The initial workup includes an assessment of all the aforesaid factors, establishing an accurate medical and sexual history; a detailed general and focused genitourinary examination; and the requisite hormonal and biochemical tests.

A detailed psychosocial history is essential to know any deep-seated psychological problems or relationship conflicts that can be effectively managed only by mental health specialists.

The general physical examination must include the evaluation of the hair distribution and other secondary sexual characters; palpation of peripheral pulses; presence of arterial bruit; blood pressure measurement; examination of local penile deformities such as Peyronie disease, phimosis, frenulum breve and testing of genital and perineal sensations including bulbocavernosus reflex.

Recommended laboratory tests should include urinalysis, complete hemogram, and assessment of serum glucose, thyroid profile, kidney and liver functions, lipid profile and testosterone levels. If the serum testosterone levels are low then serum free testosterone, prolactin, and luteinizing hormone levels should be determined.

Some specific investigations for ED include penile duplex Doppler ultrasonography to assess for vascular function and evaluate for Peyronie disease; nocturnal penile tumescence and rigidity testing using the RigiScan device to differentiate between psychogenic and organic causes. Arteriography and dynamic infusion cavernosometry (measuring cavernosal blood pressure) and cavernosography (to assess for venous leak) are done in young individuals only who may be potential candidates for vascular reconstructive surgery after traumatic arterial insufficiency or venous leakage.

MANAGEMENT

In the absence of any specific reversible etiology, the treatment for ED is mostly empirical and is provided in a stepwise manner. Initial therapy is based on lifestyle modification and psychosexual counseling, followed by first-line therapies primarily PDE5 inhibitors and vacuum erection devices (VEDs). Intraurethral suppository (IUS) of prostaglandin E1 (alprostadil) and intracavernosal injection (ICI) of vasoactive substances constitute the second-line therapy. Surgical intervention is only reserved as the last option after conservative options have been exhausted.

Lifestyle Modifications

They have a significant role in younger individuals with identifiable reversible risk factors which may contribute to the patient's ED, such as precipitating medications, poor dietary habits, lack of physical exercise, endocrinopathies, stress, and anxiety. The major drawback remains the lack of interventional studies assessing the effect of lifestyle changes on ED.

Cessation of cigarette smoking plays a major role in improving ED as there is a direct dose response relationship between greater number of packs of cigarettes smoked or more years of smoking, with increased erectile difficulties. Mild alcohol consumption might improve erectile function by allaying anxiety; however, chronic alcohol use can have deleterious effects on the liver functions, resulting in low testosterone levels and increased levels of estrogen, both of which contribute to ED. Patients with performance anxiety, interpersonal relationship issues and current life stressors may benefit from confidence restoration with erectogenic medications and/or counseling with a psychologist or a mental health expert specializing in sexual dysfunction.

Adults should do atleast 30 minutes of moderate-intensity aerobic exercises or sporting activities on most days of the week. Weight loss in obese or overweight men, and switching over to a Mediterranean diet, plus exercise, has been shown to improve sexual health.

The European Association of Urology recommends that "lifestyle changes and modification of risk factors must precede or accompany any ED therapy", and classifies the level of evidence for lifestyle modifications as 1b with a grade A recommendation.

Nonsurgical Interventions

PDE5-inhibitors

Oral PDE5-inhibitors are the mainstay of the treatment of ED. These drugs facilitate penile erection by inhibiting the PDE5 enzyme, which is responsible for the degradation of cyclic guanosine monophosphate (cGMP) in the cavernous smooth muscles. This inhibition results in the prolonged activity of cGMP resulting in decreased intracellular calcium concentrations and thus maintaining the smooth muscle relaxation, leading to rigid penile erections. Individuals need to be reminded that PDE5-inhibitors still require both physical and mental sexual stimulation, to create arousal and initiate rise in the available NO levels in order to generate cGMP production. They must be administered with adequate time interval before sexual intercourse to allow for peak drug levels at the appropriate time. Patients should be instructed on optimal conditions for the medications to work effectively.

Daily use of PDE5-inhibitors in ED can significantly improve endothelial dysfunction with the potential for a cure. Potential advantages of their daily use include salvage of on-demand PDE5-inhibitor nonresponders, apparent disease modification, and development of a more natural sexual function. PDE5-inhibitors lead to improvement of sexual performance and not increase in libido. PDE5-inhibitors lead to shortening of the refractory period and better ejaculatory control in young and potent individuals. Hypogonadal patients, who do not respond to treatment with PDE5-inhibitors alone, might show clinical response to a combination of testosterone and PDE5-inhibitors.

Phosphodiesterase type 5 inhibitors are contraindicated in nitrate users as they increase the risk of severe hypotension and should be used with caution in patients with serious cardiovascular diseases, uncontrolled hypertension, unstable angina, and in those taking alpha-blockers for blood pressure control. Side-effects related to these drugs are generally mild and well-tolerated such as headache, heartburn, facial flushing, nasal congestion, and myalgias (especially with tadalafil). Occurrence of priapism is also a concern but only rarely seen. There have also been concerns regarding PDE5-inhibitors use and auditory changes like hearing loss and tinnitus. Some vision-related conditions are also cause for increased concerns, including retinitis pigmentosa, macular degeneration and nonarteritic anterior ischemic optic neuropathy. They are contraindicated in patients with vision loss due to nonarteritic anterior ischemic optic neuropathy.

Phosphodiesterase type 5 inhibitors are good first-line therapy but up to 35% of the patients with ED fail to respond adequately to them **(Table 2)**. The common causes of treatment failure include diabetes mellitus and severe neurological and vascular diseases. Although there is no consensus on how to define the failure to PDE5-inhibitors therapy, the inability to attain or maintain adequate penile erection during sexual intercourse on at least four consecutive occasions, despite of optimum drug dosing, is an acceptable definition. Management of PDE5-inhibitor treatment failure is dependent on the underlying cause and includes patient counseling, switching over to another PDE5-inhibitor, intracavernosal injection therapy, intraurethral drug administration, combination therapy, or referral to the expert for further evaluation. Patients not responding to any of the medical treatment options may be candidates for penile implant surgery.

As ED is considered the harbinger of coronary heart disease and a predictor of future silent cardiac events, the use of PDE5-inhibitors and resumption of sexual activities should only be done as per the Princeton III Consensus Recommendations **(Table 3)** for the management of ED and cardiovascular disease. These guidelines help in the risk stratification and cardiovascular evaluation for sexual activity in the patients with ED.

TABLE 2: Characteristic properties of PDE5-inhibitors.

	Sildenafil	Vardenafil	Tadalafil	Udenafil	Mirodenafil
Dosage	25, 50, and 100 mg. Usually start with 50 mg. Maximum dose 100 mg daily	2–5, 5, 10, and 20 mg. Usually start with 10 mg. Maximum dose 20 mg daily	2–5, 5, 10, and 20 mg. Usually start with 10 mg. Maximum dose 20 mg daily	100 mg. Maximum dose 200 mg daily	50 or 100 mg. Maximum dose 100 mg daily
Onset	30–60 min	30 min	45 min	30–60 min	30–60 min
Duration	4–8 h	4–8 h	Up to 36 h	12 h	6–12 h
Efficacy	>65%	>65%	>65%	>65%	>65%
Side effects	Headache, flushing, and dyspepsia	As for sildenafil	Flushing, back pain, and general myalgia	Facial flushing, nasal congestion, ocular hyperemia, and headache	Facial flushing, headache, nausea, and eye redness
Contraindications	Nitrate-containing compounds, recent serious cardiovascular events, non-arteritic ischemic optic neuropathy, and a blockers	As for sildenafil, but also type 1 or 3 antiarrhythmics and congenital prolonged QT syndrome	As for sildenafil	As for sildenafil	As for sildenafil
Food and alcohol interaction	Interacts with food, administer while fasting. No alcohol interaction	Interacts with food, administer while fasting. No alcohol interaction	No food or alcohol interaction	No food or alcohol interaction	No alcohol interaction. Data on food interaction not available

TABLE 3: Princeton III consensus recommendations.

Profile	Description	Sexual activity and PDE5 inhibitor use
Low	• Fewer than three risk factors for coronary artery disease* (excluding sex) • Controlled hypertension • Class I or II stable angina‡ • Successful coronary revascularization • History of uncomplicated myocardial infarction • Mild valvular disease, congestive heart failure without left ventricular dysfunction and/or New York Heart Association class I heart failure	• Cleared to resume sexual activity • Cleared to take PDE5 inhibitors

Continued

Continued

Profile	Description	Sexual activity and PDE5 inhibitor use
Intermediate	• At least three risk factors for coronary artery disease* (excluding sex) • Class I or II stable angina‡ • Recent myocardial infarction (within 2–6 weeks) • Left ventricular dysfunction and/or New York Heart Association class II congestive heart failure • Noncardiac sequela from atherosclerotic disease (stroke and/or peripheral vascular disease)	• Cardiac evaluation necessary prior to resuming sexual activity • No contraindication to PDE5 inhibitor use
High	• Unstable or refractory angina • Uncontrolled hypertension • New York Heart Association class III-IV congestive heart failure • Recent myocardial infarction (within 2 weeks) • High-risk arrhythmias • Severe cardiomyopathy • Moderate to severe vascular disease	Sexual activity delayed until cardiac condition stabilized

*Major cardiovascular risk factors include age, male gender, hypertension, type 1 and type 2 diabetes mellitus, smoking, dyslipidemia, sedentary lifestyle and family history of premature cardiovascular disease.

‡Defined by the Canadian Cardiovascular Society.

Vacuum Erection Devices

Vacuum erection devices (VED) operate by applying continuous negative pressure to the shaft of the penis drawing blood inside lacunar spaces inside the corpora cavernosa causing tumescence. In order to prevent the backflow of blood, a constriction band is placed at the base of the penis in these devices. About 70% of diabetic men, who do not respond to PDE5-inhibitors, are able to have sexual intercourse when using a VED to achieve tumescence. On the other hand, discontinuation rates of nearly 35% are reported owing to bruising on the penis, pivoting at the base of the penis, coldness or numbness of the penis, pain related to the constriction band and/or decreased ability to achieve orgasm. Successful usage of VED requires obtaining a tight seal of the cylinder against the body of the penis using a lubricant and trimming the pubic hair.

Intraurethral Suppository

The use of intraurethral suppository (IUS) involves the placement of a prostaglandin E1-loaded pellet within the urethra before sexual intercourse. The patient should then massage that area of the penis to help disperse the medication. The absorption of the drug through the urethra into the corpora cavernosa increases the intracellular levels of cyclic AMP (cAMP), leading to decreased intracellular Ca^{2+} levels, increased smooth muscle relaxation, and tumescence. It is a second-line therapy to PDE5-inhibitors, showing efficacy in approximately 55% patients with primarily organic ED. The medication may cause localized pain and burning. Some adverse effects include penile pain, urethral pain, dizziness, and priapism. Repeated use with wrong technique may lead to urethral stricture.

Intracavernosal Injection

It involves injecting vasoactive substances directly into the corpora cavernosa via a 28G needle. The vasoactive agents include prostaglandin E1, papaverine and phentolamine (and also, atropine), which work alone or in conjunction to elicit penile erection. Phentolamine is an alpha 1 adrenergic receptor inhibitor that prevents vasoconstriction to maintain tumescence. Papaverine is a nonspecific phosphodiesterase-inhibitor causing increased levels of cAMP and cGMP. Prostaglandin E1 is approved as a single-agent intracavernosal injection (ICI) for ED, increasing cAMP levels.

Priapism is the major concern with ICI. If it occurs, then the patient needs urgent medical attention, requiring local blood aspiration or surgical shunt formation or ICI of phenylephrine to induce cavernosal vasoconstriction. Dropout rates are high because of fear of penile injections, local pain, and occasional bruising.

Surgical Interventions
Penile Prostheses/Implants

Surgical interventions are suitable options in patients who are refractory to medical therapy, have contraindications or adverse effects to first line drug therapy; in patients having troublesome priapism or local infections; have penile fibrosis due to Peyronie disease; and in patients with vascular or anatomical penile defects or in cases of genital or pelvic trauma. The current surgical options include insertion of a penile prosthesis and vascular reconstructive surgery. The corporal tissue is irreversibly altered once the penile prosthesis surgery is done and smooth muscle relaxation is impossible thereafter.

Penile implants consist of malleable or inflatable devices. The malleable penile prosthesis involves two semirigid rods that are placed in the corpora cavernosa. The implant does change in size when it is bent upward before intercourse. Two-piece inflatable penile prostheses (IPPs) consist of two cylinders with a scrotal pump, enabling transfer of fluid to the cylinder chambers whenever an erection is desired. Three-piece inflatable penile prostheses are considered the gold standard. They involve the placement of two inflatable cylinders (in the corpora cavernosa), a pump in the scrotum and a fluid reservoir in the lower abdomen alongside the bladder. The pressure applied to the pump causes a transfer of fluid from the reservoir to the cylinders, leading to penile rigidity. The pump has a release valve or button to transfer the fluid back from the cylinders to the reservoir at the end of intercourse. Maximum girth expansion and penile rigidity occurs with these devices, as and when an erection is desired, alongside maximum flaccidity on deflating.

Penile Revascularization Surgery

Penile revascularization surgery was developed to anastomose the inferior epigastric artery to either the dorsal artery or deep dorsal vein (arterialization), with or without venous ligation to improve penile vascular inflow while reducing venous outflow, on similar principles of coronary artery bypass grafting in coronary artery disease. It is recommended for younger men (<55 years) who are nondiabetic, nonsmokers and have a documented isolated stenotic segment of the internal pudendal artery without concomitant venous leak. Potential complications of penile revascularization procedures include glans hyperemia, shunt thrombosis, and inguinal hernias.

POTENTIAL FUTURE TREATMENT OPTIONS FOR ERECTILE DYSFUNCTION

Only temporary symptomatic relief is provided by the current therapeutic options as they do not halt or slow down the primary disease process. Bioavailability of NO is essential for PDE5 inhibitors, which are the most preferred therapy, to exhibit any effect. Hence, prospective pharmacological interventions will need efficacy in individuals not responding to PDE5 inhibition, particularly in men with neurogenic ED. The site of action may be either the central or the peripheral nervous system controlling the balance between the vasorelaxation and vasoconstriction. The ROCK pathway plays an important part in maintaining the flaccid state of the penis. ROCK phosphorylates and inactivates myosin light chain phosphatase. This allows the myosin light chain to stay phosphorylated and bind to the smooth muscle actin. ROCK inhibition, Maxi-K channel activators and soluble guanylate cyclase activators provide alternative mechanisms that are independent to NO mediated smooth muscle relaxation. Central stimulation signaling with clavulanic acid, dopamine agonists and melanocortin receptor agonists are under investigation for utility in therapy for ED. Stem cell therapy or regenerative medicine might provide definitive symptomatic relief by reversing or halting the disease progression in ED. Regenerative medicine can probably alter the disease course and in many instances possibly regenerate damaged cells, tissues or whole organ systems. Various tools such as gene transfer, stem cells, angiogenic and neurotropic growth factors and tissue engineering can be used to achieve this goal.

CONCLUSION

There has been a significant increment in our knowledge and understanding of the pathophysiology of erectile dysfunction, resulting in numerous treatment options for the patients in the last three decades. Despite of the achievements, there is a greater need for more effective pharmacological options that can provide long-lasting improvements. Therapeutic decision-making should involve both the patient and his partner. Risk factor assessment for cardiovascular disease should be done in all the patients with erectile dysfunction. Future promising therapeutic strategies include gene and cell-based therapy, to provide definitive cure.

SUGGESTED READINGS

1. Andersson KE, Wagner G. Physiology of penile erection. Physiol Rev. 1995;75:191-236.
2. Lue TF, Tanagho EA. Physiology of erection and pharmacological management of impotence. J Urol. 1987;137:829-36.
3. Bacon CG, Mittleman MA, Kawachi I, et al. A prospective study of risk factors for erectile dysfunction. J Urol. 2006;176:217-21.
4. Ghanem HM, Salonia A, Martin-Morales A. SOP: physical examination and laboratory testing for men with erectile dysfunction. J Sex Med. 2013;10:108-10.
5. Corona G, Razzoli E, Forti G, et al. The use of phosphodiesterase 5 inhibitors with concomitant medications. J Endocrinol Invest. 2008;31:799-808.
6. Nehra A, Jackson G, Miner M, et al. The Princeton III Consensus recommendations for the management of erectile dysfunction and cardiovascular disease. Mayo Clin. Proc. 2012:87; 766-78.
7. Levine LA, Dimitriou RJ. Vacuum constriction and external erection devices in erectile dysfunction. Urol Clin North Am. 2001;28:335-41.
8. Hellstrom WJ, Montague DK, Moncada I, et al. Implants, mechanical devices, and vascular surgery for erectile dysfunction. J Sex Med. 2010;7:501-23.

CHAPTER 57

The Untold Story of Acute Encephalitis Syndrome

Jitendra Singh, Anju Dinkar

■ INTRODUCTION

Encephalitis affects all age groups and is an important cause of global morbidity, mortality, and permanent neurologic disability. Encephalitis results from inflammation of part or all of the brain parenchyma associated with clinical and/or investigational evidence of neurological dysfunction. Direct neuronal injury of any part of the central nervous system (CNS) caused by invasion of a pathogen can result in various clinical syndromes, including encephalitis, meningitis, myelitis, and neuritis. The clinical presentation of encephalitis may be acute, subacute, or chronic. Though infectious causes, especially viruses, are common causes of encephalitis. Sometimes, the inflammation of the CNS may be due to indirect immunologically mediated injury rather than infectious.

The burden of acute encephalitis syndrome (AES) depends on seasonal and geographical variation in the causative organism. The outbreak of Japanese encephalitis (JE) in India generally coincides with the monsoon and post-monsoon periods due to the increased density of mosquitoes. Encephalitis due to water-borne diseases, including *Enteroviruses*, is reported throughout the year. In India, the case fatality and morbidity are very high among various viral encephalitis, especially JE or Enterovirus encephalitis.

■ DEFINITION

Acute encephalitis syndrome is a group of clinically similar neurologic manifestations caused by several different viruses, bacteria, fungus, parasites, spirochetes, chemical/toxins, etc.

According to WHO, clinically, a case of AES is defined as a person of any age, at any time of year, with the acute onset of fever and a change in mental status (including symptoms such as confusion, disorientation, coma, or inability to talk) *and/or* new onset of seizures (excluding simple febrile seizures). Other early clinical findings can include an increase in irritability, somnolence, or abnormal behavior greater than that seen with usual febrile illness.

ETIOLOGY

Acute encephalitis syndrome is a severe neurological syndrome due to various infectious agents, including viruses, bacteria, fungi, spirochetes and parasites, and noninfectious causes such as autoimmune disorders. The most important causes remain the infections, especially viruses, and often difficult to identify etiology. This chapter will focus on infections, especially viral etiology. Among viral etiology, primary neurotropic viruses (Arboviruses, Herpesviruses, and Rabies virus) as well as other "incidental" nervous system pathogens (entero-, orthomyxo-, paramyxo-, and adenoviruses) primarily cause disorder elsewhere in the body and involve the CNS only occasionally. Herpes simplex encephalitis (HSE) is the most common sporadic infectious encephalitis. JE is probably the most common cause and epidemics in India, especially in the south and east region. JE was the main agent of AES in a severe epidemic of JE in the Gorakhpur division of Eastern Uttar Pradesh in 2005. Despite comprehensive diagnostic efforts, most cases of AES remain undiagnosed, especially viral etiology. A list of identified causes of AES is depicted in **Table 1**.

CLINICAL FEATURES

Clinical presentations depend on predominantly involved areas of the CNS that are infected and injured, which vary with specific pathogens also. The typical feature of AES in the initial stage include fever, headache, and vomiting lasting for less than a week, followed by altered mental status. The severity of presentation varies widely from mild febrile illness with the headache to a severe form with convulsions, coma, neurologic deficits with or without signs of meningeal irritation, life-threatening rise in intracranial tension, decerebration, or flaccid coma and death. There may be irritability, agitation, screaming spells, confusion, delirium, drowsiness, hallucination, personality changes, behavioral disorders, and at times a frankly psychotic state also. The common neurologic signs include hemiparesis, aphasia, ataxia, cranial nerve palsies, involuntary movements (myoclonus or jerks), and focal or generalized seizures. Other important neurologic findings may be dysregulation of temperature and vasomotor control due to autonomic dysfunction and diabetes insipidus or the syndrome of inappropriate secretion of antidiuretic hormone (SIADH) resulting from hypothalamic dysfunction.

DIAGNOSIS

Based on the clinical presentation, AES is suspected. The diagnostic criteria are shown in **Box 1**. The gold standard, a detailed clinical history and examination, may form the foundation for reaching an etiological diagnosis. Consequently, any event related to the patient, such as epidemiology and risk factors, may help to suspect a specific organism **(Table 2)**. A methodical review of systems is important to elicit the underlying disorder to reach diagnosis **(Table 3)**. Many investigations may be needed as per the differential diagnosis. Preferred samples for diagnosis of encephalitis are blood, cerebrospinal fluid (CSF), sputum, throat swab, skin vesicle, biopsy of skin lesions, and brain tissue. If clinical and epidemiologic clues are suggestive, microscopy, culture, histopathologic examination, and various

TABLE 1: Etiology of acute encephalitis syndrome.

Viral agents	Bacterial agents
1. Herpes viruses: • Herpes simplex virus types 1 and 2 • Varicella-zoster virus • Cytomegalovirus • Epstein–Barr virus • Human herpesvirus type 6 • Herpesvirus B 2. Vector-borne viral infections: • West Nile virus • St Louis encephalitis • Murray Valley encephalitis virus • Eastern equine encephalitis virus • Western equine encephalitis • Venezuelan equine encephalitis • California encephalitis virus • Japanese encephalitis • Colorado tick fever virus • Tick-borne encephalitis virus • Zika virus* • Chikungunya virus* • Dengue virus* 3. Enteroviruses: • Polioviruses • Coxsackie viruses • Echoviruses • Enteroviruses 70 and 71 4. Orthomyxoviruses: • Influenza viruses 5. Paramyxoviruses: • Measles virus • Mumps virus • Parainfluenza viruses • Nipah virus* 6. Rhabdoviridae: • Rabies virus 7. Other emerging encephalitis viruses*: • Coronavirus • Parvovirus B19 • Adenoviruses • Monkeypox virus • Rubella virus • HIV	• *Mycoplasma pneumoniae* • *Listeria monocytogenes* • *Treponema pallidum* • *Leptospira interrogans* • *Streptococcus pneumonia* • *Bacillus anthracis* • *Borrelia burgdorferi* • *Legionella pneumophila* • *Salmonella typhi* • Cat scratch disease (*Bartonellosis*) • *Mycobacterium tuberculosis* *Rickettsia* species: • Rocky mountain spotted fever • Endemic and epidemic typhus • *Coxiella burnetii, Ehrlichiosis* • Scrub typhus (*Orientia tsutsugamushi*) Fungi: • *Cryptococcus species* • *Histoplasma capsulatum* • *Aspergillus species* • *Mucormycosis* • *Candida species* • *Coccidioides* Parasites: • *Naegleria fowleri* • *Acanthamoeba species* • *Balamuthia mandrillaris* • *Toxoplasma gondii* • *Plasmodium falciparum* Non-infectious causes: • Acute disseminated encephalomyelitis • Antibody-associated encephalitis • Collagen vascular disorders

*Emerging encephalitis viruses.

BOX 1: Diagnostic criteria for encephalitis and encephalopathy.

Major criterion
- Patients with altered mental status (decreased or altered level of consciousness, lethargy or personality change) lasting ≥24 hours with no alternative cause identified

Minor criteria
- Documented fever ≥38°C (100.4°F) within the 72 hours before or after the presentation
- Generalized or partial seizures not fully attributable to a pre-existing seizure disorder
- New onset of focal neurologic findings
- CSF WBC count ≥5/mm^3
- Abnormality of brain parenchyma on neuroimaging suggestive of encephalitis that is either new from prior studies or appears acute in onset
- Abnormality on electroencephalography that is consistent with encephalitis and not attributable to another cause

Note: Possible encephalitis = 1 major criterion and 2 minor criteria; Confirmed encephalitis = 1 major criterion and ≥3 minor criteria.

TABLE 2: Epidemiology and risk factors to suspect possible etiologic agents.

Factors	Possible etiology
Epidemiology	
Central and South America	Rabies virus, EEEV, WEEV, VEEV, St Louis encephalitis virus, *Rickettsia rickettsii*, *Plasmodium falciparum*, *Taenia solium*
Australia	Murray valley encephalitis virus; JE virus; Hendra virus
Southeast Asia, China	JE virus, Tick-borne encephalitis, Nipah virus, *P. falciparum*, *Gnathostoma* species, *T. solium*
India, Nepal	Rabies virus, JE virus, Chikungunya virus, *P. falciparum*
Africa	Rabies virus, WNV, Rift Valley fever virus, *P. falciparum*, *T. brucei gambiense*, *T. brucei rhodesiense*
Middle East	WNV, *P. falciparum*
Europe	WNV, tick-borne encephalitis, *A. phagocytophilum*, *B. burgdorferi*
Russia	Tick-borne encephalitis
Age	
Neonates	HSV-2, CMV, Rubella virus, *Listeria monocytogenes*, *Treponema pallidum*, *Toxoplasma gondii*
Infants and children	EEEV, JE virus, Murray valley encephalitis virus, Influenza virus
Elderly persons	EEEV, St Louis encephalitis virus, WNV, sporadic CJD, *L. monocytogenes*
Risk factors	
Occupation	
Physicians and healthcare workers	VZV, HIV, influenza virus, coronavirus, measles virus, MTB
Laboratory workers	WNV, HIV, coronavirus, *C. burnetii*, *Coccidioides* species
Veterinarians	Rabies virus *Bartonella* species, *C. burnetii*
Exposure to animals	Rabies virus, *C. burnetii*, *Bartonella* species

Continued

Continued

Factors	Possible etiology
Exposure to horses	Hendra virus
Person-to-person transmission	HSV (neonatal), VZV, VEEV (rare), poliovirus, enteroviruses, measles virus, mumps virus, rubella virus, EBV, HHV-6, herpesvirus B, WNV (transfusion, transplantation, breast-feeding), HIV, Rabies virus (transplantation), Influenza virus, *M. pneumoniae*, MTB, *T. pallidum*
Ingestions	
Unpasteurized milk	Tick-borne encephalitis virus, *L. monocytogenes*, *C. burnetii*
Raw meat, fish, or reptiles	*Gnathostoma* species
Raw or partially cooked meat	*T. gondii*
Season	
Late summer/early fall	All agents transmitted by mosquitoes and ticks (see above), Enteroviruses
Winter	Influenza virus
Insect contact	
Mosquitoes	EEEV, WEEV, VEEV, St Louis encephalitis virus, Murray Valley encephalitis virus, JE virus, WNV, California encephalitis group, Chikungunya virus, *Plasmodium falciparum*
Ticks	Tick-borne encephalitis; Powassan virus, *Rickettsia rickettsii*, *Ehrlichia chaffeensis*, *Anaplasma phagocytophilum*, *C. burnetii* (rare), *B. burgdorferi*
Sandflies	*Bartonella bacilliformis*
Tsetse flies	*Trypanosoma brucei gambiense*, *Trypanosoma brucei rhodesiense*
Animal contact	
Rodents	EEEV, VEEV, Tick-borne encephalitis, Powassan virus (woodchucks), La Crosse virus (chipmunks and squirrels), Monkeypox, *Bartonella quintana*
Dogs	Rabies virus
Cats	Rabies virus, *Coxiella burnetii*, *Bartonella henselae*, *T. gondii*
Raccoons	Rabies virus, *Baylisascaris procyonis*
Skunks	Rabies virus
Old World monkeys	Herpesvirus B
Horses	EEEV, WEEV, VEEV, Hendra virus
Sheep and goats	*C. burnetii*
White-tailed deer	*Borrelia burgdorferi*
Birds	WNV, EEEV, WEEV, VEEV, St Louis encephalitis virus, Murray Valley encephalitis virus, JE virus, *Cryptococcus neoformans* (bird droppings)
Bats	Rabies virus, Nipah virus
Swine	JE virus, Nipah virus
Recreational activities	
Swimming	Enteroviruses, *Naegleria fowleri*

Continued

Continued

Factors	Possible etiology
Camping/hunting	All agents transmitted by mosquitoes and ticks (see above)
Sexual contact	HIV, *T. pallidum*
Spelunking	Rabies virus, *H. capsulatum*
Other	
Transfusion and transplantation	CMV, EBV, WNV, HIV, Tick-borne encephalitis virus, Rabies virus, Iatrogenic CJD, *T. pallidum, A. phagocytophilum, R. rickettsii, C. neoformans, Coccidioides* species, *H. capsulatum, T. gondii, Plasmodium falciparum*
Agammaglobulinemia	Enteroviruses, *Mycoplasma pneumoniae*
Unvaccinated	VZV, JE virus, Poliovirus, Measles virus, Mumps virus, Rubella virus
Recent vaccination	ADEM
Immunocompromised	VZV, CMV, HHV-6, WNV, HIV, JC virus, *L. monocytogenes*, MTB, *C. neoformans, Coccidioides* species, *Histoplasma capsulatum, T. gondii*

(ADEM: acute disseminated encephalomyelitis; CMV: cytomegalovirus; CJD: Creutzfeldt–Jakob disease; EBV: Epstein–Barr virus; EEEV: Eastern equine encephalitis virus; HHV: human herpesvirus; HIV: human immunodeficiency virus; HSV: herpes simplex virus; JE virus: Japanese encephalitis virus; LCMV: lymphocytic choriomeningitis virus; MTB: *Mycobacterium tuberculosis*; VEEV: Venezuelan equine encephalitis virus; WEEV: Western equine encephalitis virus; WNV: West Nile virus; VZV: varicella-zoster virus)

TABLE 3: Specific clinical findings to suspect possible etiologic agents.

Clinical finding	Possible etiology
Pallor	Parvovirus B19
Icterus	Leptospirosis, malaria, scrub typhus
Lymphadenopathy	HIV, EBV, CMV, measles virus, rubella virus, WNV, *Treponema pallidum, Bartonella henselae* and other *Bartonella* species, MTB, *Toxoplasma gondii, Trypanosoma brucei gambiense*
Rash	VZV, B virus, HHV-6, WNV, rubella virus, some Enteroviruses, HIV, *Rickettsia rickettsii, Mycoplasma pneumoniae, Borrelia burgdorferi, T. pallidum, Ehrlichia chaffeensis, Anaplasma phagocytophilum*, Dengue, chikungunya, EBV, coxsackievirus, parvovirus B19, echoviruses
Grouped vesicles	VZV
Nonhealing skin lesions	*Balamuthia, Acanthamoeba* species
Conjunctivitis	Adenovirus, Zika virus
Retinitis	CMV, WNV, *B. henselae, T. pallidum*
Parotitis, mastitis, orchitis	Mumps virus, LCMV
Hepatitis	*Coxiella burnetii*
Organomegaly	Malaria, dengue, Leptospirosis, HIV
Respiratory tract findings	VEEV, Nipah virus, Hendra virus, influenza virus, adenovirus, *M. Pneumoniae, C. Burnetii*, MTB, *Histoplasma capsulatum*
Urinary symptoms	St Louis encephalitis virus (early)

Continued

Continued

Clinical finding	Possible etiology
Hydrophobia, aerophobia	Rabies virus
Myocarditis, pericarditis	Enterovirus, Mumps virus, CMV
Cerebellar ataxia	VZV (children), EBV, mumps virus, St Louis encephalitis virus, *Tropheryma whipplei, T. brucei gambiense*
Cranial nerve abnormalities	HSV, EBV, *Listeria monocytogenes*, MTB, *T. pallidum, B. burgdorferi, T. whipplei, Cryptococcus neoformans, Coccidioides species, H. capsulatum*
Dementia	HIV, human transmissible spongiform encephalopathies (sCJD and vCJD), measles virus (SSPE), *T. pallidum, T. whipplei*
Myorhythmia	*T. whipplei* (oculomasticatory)
Parkinsonism symptoms	JE virus, St Louis encephalitis virus, WNV, Nipah virus, *T. gondii, T. brucei gambiense*
Poliomyelitis-like flaccid paralysis	JE virus, WEV, tick-borne encephalitis virus; enteroviruses (Enterovirus-71, coxsackieviruses), poliovirus
Rhombencephalitis	HSV, WNV, enterovirus-71, *L. monocytogenes*
Prominent limbic symptoms	Autoimmune limbic encephalitis, HHV6/7
Behavior changes followed by myoclonic spasms/jerks	Measles
Abnormal behavior (temper tantrums, agitation, aggression), psychotic features, seizures or movement disorder	NMDAR encephalitis, rabies virus

(CMV: cytomegalovirus; CJD, Creutzfeldt–Jacob disease; EBV: Epstein–Barr virus; HHV: human herpesvirus; HIV: human immunodeficiency virus; HSV: herpes simplex virus; JE virus: Japanese encephalitis virus; LCMV: lymphocytic choriomeningitis virus; MTB: *Mycobacterium tuberculosis*; NMDA: anti-*N*-methyl-D-aspartate (NMDA) receptor; SSPE: subacute sclerosing panencephalitis; VEEV: Venezuelan equine encephalitis virus; WNV: West Nile virus; VZV: varicella-zoster virus)

serological tests should be performed to identify various viral, bacterial, and fungal etiologies of encephalitis. Polymerase chain reaction (PCR) makes the specific diagnoses of etiological agents. Despite newer techniques, including CSF PCR, up to 70% of cases of encephalitis remain of unknown etiology in modern surveys. Identifying particular etiology may help to prognosticate the clinical course and available treatment options.

Blood tests: Considering many clues from the clinical sense, etiologic specific and routine blood investigations can be sent. Other specific blood investigations may include peripheral smear, various organ function tests, culture, serology, antigen detection by immunofluorescence, nucleic acid detection by PCR, etc.

Radiological tests: Apart from chest X-ray (CXR), ultrasonography and brain imaging may prove very helpful in predicting etiological clues and complications such as raised intracranial pressure. MRI brain may provide the key to concentrating on etiology by imaging features **(Table 4)**.

TABLE 4: Specific neuroimaging findings to suspect possible etiologic agents.

Neuroimaging findings	Possible etiology
Frontal lobe	*Naegleria fowleri*
Temporal lobe	HHV 6/7
Basal ganglia and/or thalamus	Respiratory virus, arbovirus, MTB
Brainstem	Respiratory virus, Arbovirus, *Listeria*, Brucella, MTB
Cerebellum	VZV, EBV
Diffuse cerebral edema	Respiratory virus
Space occupying and/or ring-enhancing lesions	MTB, Fungal infections, *Balamuthia mandrillaris*, *Acanthamoeba* species, *Toxoplasma gondii*
Hydrocephalus and/or basilar meningeal enhancement	MTB, fungal infection, *B. mandrillaris*
White matter lesions	Oligoclonal bands, IgG index, Lyme disease, *Brucella* species
Infarction or hemorrhage	MTB, fungal infections, respiratory virus
Incomplete ring-enhancing lesions	ADEM

(ADEM: acute disseminated encephalomyelitis; EBV: Epstein–Barr virus; HHV: human herpesvirus; IgG: immunoglobulin G; MTB: *Mycobacterium tuberculosis*; VZV: varicella-zoster virus)

EEG: EEG is not routinely indicated in AES as its findings are generally nonspecific and do not help etiologically. In brainstem encephalitis, EEG abnormalities may show diffuse slow-wave activity and intermittent rhythmic activity. In HSE, EEG demonstrates a temporal focus demonstrating periodic lateralizing epileptiform discharges in more than 80% of cases. It can be helpful to detect nonconvulsive seizure activity in patients with a confused, obtunded, or comatose state. It generally has no role in correlation with the severity of disease, but rapidly improving EEG findings often indicate a good prognosis.

CSF analysis: CSF analysis is essential in every patient with encephalitis if there is no contraindicated. The findings differ according to disease etiologies such as virus, bacteria, fungus, and parasite. In VE, CSF evaluation usually revealed normal glucose, increased protein, and a mild-to-moderate mononuclear pleocytosis (predominantly lymphocytic but can be neutrophilic early in the course). Sometimes, eosinophils in CSF may indicate certain etiologic agents, such as more common in helminths and less common in *Treponema pallidum*, *Mycoplasma pneumoniae*, *Rickettsia rickettsii*, *Coccidioides immitis*, and *Toxoplasma gondii* infections. Nucleic acid detection by PCR in CSF samples is now primarily a diagnostic test for herpes simplex virus-1 (HSV-1) and -2, varicella-zoster virus (VZV), cytomegalovirus (CMV), Epstein–Barr virus (EBV), human herpesvirus 6 (HHV-6), and Enteroviruses to confirm the etiological agents. PCR is preferable to serologic testing for acute encephalitis. Serology often requires 2–4 weeks after acute infection to develop a diagnostic rise in antibody titers and is of limited value for viruses with high basal seroprevalence rates. During acute infection, CSF PCR yields positive results because the amount of replicating the virus is maximal. CSF PCR is less invasive than brain biopsy and become the "gold standard" for the diagnosis of many CNS infections **(Table 5)**.

TABLE 5: Preferred laboratory test for etiological agents of AES.	
PCR (Serum/CSF)	Serology (Serum/CSF)
HSV-1, and HSV-2	Arboviruses
CMV	CMV
Cytomegalovirus (CMV)	EBV
Varicella-zoster virus (VZV)	West Nile virus
Human herpes virus 6 (HHV-6)	Measles virus
Enteroviruses (EV)	Mumps virus
Coronavirus	Adenovirus
Nipah virus	Rubella virus
Human immunodeficiency virus (HIV)	Japanese encephalitis virus
Rabies virus	*Treponema pallidum*
Parvovirus	*Leptospira*
Human T-cell lymphotropic virus	*Rickettsia* species
Mycoplasma pneumoniae	*Salmonella typhi*
Borrelia burgdorferi (Lyme disease)	*Cryptococcus*
Toxoplasma	
Mycobacterium tuberculosis	

(AES: acute encephalitis syndrome; CSF: cerebrospinal fluid; EBV: Epstein–Barr virus; HSV: herpes simplex virus)

Brain biopsy: It was used routinely during the days when vidarabine was the only therapeutic option in HSE. All the major treatment trials of HSE conducted by the National Institutes of Allergy and Infectious Diseases Collaborative Antiviral Study Group (NINAIDCASG) in the 1980s were used to take 1 cm^3 of the brain tissue from the anterior portion of the involved inferior temporal gyrus by subtemporal craniectomy under general anesthesia. The HSE brain biopsy had more than 95% sensitivity and specificity greater than 99%. After introducing aciclovir early in the treatment of HSE, brain biopsy has a premise largely unnecessary. Brain biopsy may be considered in patients with encephalitis of unknown etiology, whose clinical condition deteriorates despite treatment, including with acyclovir.

■ MANAGEMENT

Supportive therapy: Management of AES depends on clinical condition and underlying etiology. Though many times it remains supportive. The patient should be monitored according to disease severity in the intensive care unit or general ward. Respiratory or contact isolation can be considered in case of encephalitis of unknown etiology or with rashes until diagnosed, COVID-19, etc. Points for the patient to protect the brain from further insult should care.
- Management of airways, breathing, and circulation
- Control of convulsion and intracranial pressure
- Control of temperature
- Proper hydration and adequate nutrition

- General management, including stable vitals
- Prone/semiprone position to reduce risk of aspiration
- Specific treatment of any treatable cause
- Investigations, samples collection and transportation
- Reporting of a case
- Rehabilitation

Raised intracranial pressure: It should be managed only after correction of dehydration as follows.
- Mannitol 20% intravenous (IV)—5 mL/kg in ½ hour as first dose then 2.5 mL/kg at 6 hours intervals up to 48 hours (eight doses).
- Injection Lasix IV—1 mg/kg up to 40 mg can be given.
- Glycerol solution—oral, 0.5 mL/kg mix with fruit juice can be given by nasogastric tube, three times a day.
- Steroids—use of steroids in VE is debatable. The steroid may be used to relieve a life-threatening rise in intracranial tension but with a risk of flaring up of viral infection. A study did not find the benefit of high-dose dexamethasone in JE.
- Another option is to use hypertonic saline (3%), 0.1-1 mL/kg/h infusion to maintain serum sodium between 145 and 155 mEq/L.
- Hyperventilation while keeping arterial carbon dioxide (CO_2) tension between 25 and 30 mm Hg may also be tried to combat raised intracranial tension.
- Surgical decompression can be life-saving in the case of medical treatment-resistant rapidly increasing intracranial tension.

Specific Therapy

- Based on specific epidemiologic or clinical findings in AES, empirical treatment, i.e., antimicrobial agents presuming either viral, bacterial, fungal, or parasitic etiology therapy, should be initiated, and steroids for autoimmune disorders.
- Acyclovir should be empirically started early in all patients with suspected encephalitis until etiology is confirmed if clinically indicated. Acyclovir resistant is rare (0.5% in immunocompetent).
- Minocycline is a known neuroprotective agent due to its antiviral properties and excellent penetration into CSF, as shown in a trial conducted in Lucknow, showing modest benefit in cumulative mortality at 3 months from the onset and neurologic sequelae.
- Some drugs are effective against specific etiology **(Table 6)**.

CONCLUSION

- Acute encephalitis syndrome should be evaluated in a direction to reach etiology. In addition, empirical therapy should be started early to prevent further neurological damage.
- Different epidemiological and other risk factors can give a clue about etiological agents.
- A thorough examination from head to toes may help for suspicion of etiology.
- A sincere collaboration between microbiologists and clinicians may prove constructive in diagnosing etiology early and estimating the true burden of disease.

TABLE 6: Specific therapy as per etiology.

Etiologic agents	Specific therapy
Virus	
Herpes simplex virus	Acyclovir, foscarnet for aciclovir-resistant HSE
Varicella-zoster virus	Acyclovir, Ganciclovir is alternative
Cytomegalovirus	Ganciclovir or/with foscarnet, if fail to respond—cidofovir is alternative.
Epstein–Barr virus	Corticosteroids may be beneficial
Human herpesvirus 6	Ganciclovir or foscarnet
B virus	Valacyclovir, alternatives—ganciclovir and acyclovir
Influenza virus	Oseltamivir
Measles virus	Ribavirin, intrathecal ribavirin in SSPE
Nipah virus	Ribavirin
West Nile virus	Ribavirin
Japanese encephalitis virus	IFN-α
St Louis encephalitis virus	IFN-2α
California encephalitis virus	IV ribavirin
HIV	HAART
JC virus	Reversal of immunosuppression or HAART in HIV patient
Bacteria	
Bartonella bacilliformis	Chloramphenicol, ciprofloxacin, doxycycline, ampicillin, or trimethoprim–sulfamethoxazole
Bartonella henselae	Doxycycline or azithromycin, with or without rifampin
Listeria monocytogenes	Ampicillin plus gentamicin, trimethoprim–sulfamethoxazole for the penicillin-allergic patient
Mycoplasma pneumoniae	Azithromycin, doxycycline, or a fluoroquinolone
Tropheryma whipplei	Ceftriaxone, followed by either trimethoprim–sulfamethoxazole or cefixime
Mycobacterium tuberculosis	Antituberculous therapy, adjunctive—dexamethasone in meningitis
Rickettsioses and Ehrlichioses	
Anaplasma phagocytophilum	Doxycycline
Ehrlichia chaffeensis	Doxycycline
Rickettsia rickettsii	Doxycycline, alternative—chloramphenicol in pregnancy
Coxiella burnetii	Doxycycline plus fluoroquinolone plus rifampin
Spirochetes	
Borrelia burgdorferi	Ceftriaxone, cefotaxime, or penicillin G
Treponema pallidum	Penicillin G, alternative—ceftriaxone
Fungi	
Coccidioides species	Fluconazole, alternatives—itraconazole, voriconazole, amphotericin B (IV and IT)

Continued

Continued

Etiologic agents	Specific therapy
Cryptococcus neoformans	Amphotericin B deoxycholate plus flucytosine or a lipid formulation of amphotericin B plus flucytosine
Histoplasma capsulatum	Liposomal amphotericin B followed by itraconazole
Protozoa	
Acanthamoeba	Trimethoprim–sulfamethoxazole plus rifampin plus ketoconazole or fluconazole plus sulfadiazine plus pyrimethamine
Balamuthia mandrillaris	Pentamidine combined with a macrolide (azithromycin or clarithromycin), fluconazole, sulfadiazine, flucytosine, and a phenothiazine
Naegleria fowleri	Amphotericin B (IV and IT) and rifampin, combined with other agents
Plasmodium falciparum	Quinine, quinidine, or artemether, alternative—atovaquone-proguanil, exchange transfusion in patients with more than 10% parasitemia or cerebral malaria
Toxoplasma gondii	Pyrimethamine plus either sulfadiazine or clindamycin, trimethoprim-sulfamethoxazole alone and pyrimethamine plus either atovaquone, clarithromycin, azithromycin, or dapsone
Trypanosoma brucei gambiense	Eflornithine, alternative—melarsoprol
Trypanosoma brucei rhodesiense	Melarsoprol
Helminths	
Baylisascaris procyonis	Albendazole plus diethylcarbamazine, adjunctive—corticosteroids
Gnathostoma species	Albendazole or ivermectin
Taenia solium	Albendazole, alternative—praziquantel
Postinfectious/Postvaccination status	
ADEM	High-dose corticosteroids, alternatives—PE, and IVIG
AIE	Methylprednisolone pulse therapy, IVIG, plasmapheresis, rituximab, and azathioprine

(ADEM: acute disseminated encephalomyelitis; AIE: autoimmune encephalitis; HAART: highly active antiretroviral therapy; HSE: herpes simplex encephalitis; IFN: interferon; IT: intrathecal; IV: intravenous; IVIG: intravenous immunoglobulin; PE: plasma exchange; SSPE: subacute sclerosing panencephalitis)

■ SUGGESTED READINGS

1. Kumar R. Understanding and managing acute encephalitis. F1000Res. 2020;9:F1000 Faculty Rev-60.
2. NVBDCP. Government of India. (2009). Guidelines clinical management of acute encephalitis syndrome including Japanese encephalitis. [online] Available from https://nvbdcp.gov.in/WriteReadData/l892s/Revised_guidelines_on_AES_JE.pdf [Last accessed October, 2022].
3. WHO. (2006). WHO-recommended standards for surveillance of selected vaccine preventable diseases. [online] Available from https://apps.who.int/iris/handle/10665/64165 [Last accessed October, 2022].
4. Roos KL, Tyler KL. Encephelitis. In: Jameson JL, Kasper DL, Longo DL, et al. (Eds). Harrison's Principles of Internal Medicine, 20th edition. New York: McGraw Hill; 2018. pp. 991-8.

5. Kumar R. Viral encephalitis and encephalopathies. In: Singh M (Ed). Medical Emergencies in Children. New Delhi: Sagar Publications; 2006. pp. 324-32.
6. Kumar R, Tripathi P, Singh S, et al. Clinical features in children hospitalized during the 2005 epidemic of Japanese encephalitis in Uttar Pradesh, India. Clin Infect Dis. 2006;43(2):123-31.
7. Beckham JD, Tyler KL. Encephalitis. In: Bennett JE, Dolin R, Blaser MJ (Eds). Mandell, Douglas, and Bennett's Principles and Practice of Infectious Diseases, 8th edition. New York: Saunders, an imprint of Elsevier Inc.; 2015. pp. 1144-63.
8. Dinkar A, Singh J. Dengue infection in North India: An experience of a tertiary care center from 2012 to 2017. Tzu Chi Med J. 2020;32(1):36-40.
9. Venkatesan A, Tunkel AR, Bloch KC, et al. International Encephalitis Consortium. Case definitions, diagnostic algorithms, and priorities in encephalitis: consensus statement of the international encephalitis consortium. Clin Infect Dis. 2013;57(8):1114-28.
10. Tunkel AR, Glaser CA, Bloch KC, et al.; Infectious Diseases Society of America. The management of encephalitis: clinical practice guidelines by the Infectious Diseases Society of America. Clin Infect Dis. 2008;47(3):303-27.
11. Debiasi RL, Tyler KL. Molecular methods for diagnosis of viral encephalitis. Clin Microbiol Rev. 2004;17(4):903-25.
12. Venkatesan A, Geocadin RG. Diagnosis and management of acute encephalitis: A practical approach. Neurol Clin Pract. 2014;4(3):206-15.
13. Chaudhuri A, Kennedy PG. Diagnosis and treatment of viral encephalitis. Postgrad Med J. 2002;78(924):575-83.
14. Singh J, Kumar N, Dinkar A. Demographic, clinical, investigational characteristics of COVID-19 related Guillain–Barré syndrome with differences from typical and another virus-related Guillain–Barré syndrome. Infect Disord Drug Targets. 2022. doi: 10.2174/1871526522666220429134113. Epub ahead of print. PMID: 35507796.

CHAPTER 58

Management of Acute Ischemic Stroke: What is New?

TP Singh, Akansha

■ INTRODUCTION

Stroke is a serious global public health problem and second leading cause of death worldwide and the third common cause of disability-adjusted life years in the world, according to the Global Burden of diseases, Injuries, and the Risk Factor Study (GBD 2010). The age standardized incidence of stroke has reduced by 12% in high-income countries whereas in India, it has increased by 12%. India is experiencing a stroke epidemic. The National Commission of Macroeconomics and Health projects the number of stroke cases will increase from 1,081,480 in the year 2000 to 16,667,372 in 2015 (Indian Council of Medical Research, ICMR, Bulletin, 2008). The prevalence of stroke ranges from 84 to 262/100,000 in the rural setting and 334 to 424/100,000 in the urban areas in India. The incidence is about 19 to 145/100,000 based on recent population-based studies.

Since the 1990s, intravenous (IV) tissue plasminogen activator (IV tPA) has been the only evidence-based therapeutic option for improving outcomes for patients with acute ischemic stroke (AIS). Landmark trials such as the NINDS and ECASS III have been important milestone in journey of IV thrombolysis. The NINDS study was the first to report the benefit of administering IV recombinant tissue plasminogen activator (rtPA) (alteplase) to patients with AIS within 3 hours of stroke onset. Subsequently, intra-arterial thrombolysis (IAT) was tested in the Prolyse in Acute Cerebral Thromboembolism II (PROACT II) study, which found potential safety and efficacy of IAT for middle cerebral artery (MCA) occlusions treated within 6 hours. The ECASS III was aimed to extend the treatment window beyond 3 hours and included 821 patients with AIS (18–80 years) who received rtPA 0.9 mg/kg, with a time frame of 3–4 hours that was later extended to 3–4.5 hours. The ECASS III was clearly a positive trial establishing Class 1, Level A evidence of efficacy in the 3- to 4.5-hour window.

Subsequently, the Interventional Management of Stroke (IMS) trial investigated the feasibility and safety of combined IV and intra-arterial therapy in AIS. The ensuing years witnessed the evolution of endovascular procedures, from forcefully injecting thrombolytic agents or saline into the thrombus to mechanically disrupting the clot by microwires and microcatheters, to the advent of energy-emitting endovascular devices and percutaneous angioplasty. These advances led to the development of simple snare devices followed by US Food and Drug Administration (USFDA) approval of the first device for the indication of opening cerebral vessels, the Merci Retrieval System (Concentric Medical, Inc), and subsequently by suction catheters, intracranial stents, and stent retrievers. In parallel to this evolution, the design of AIS trials advanced, and the value of endovascular revascularization was clearly shown after the application of rigorous patient selection criteria. This advancement resulted in the second paradigm shift in AIS care since the initial approval of IV tPA. This shift was attributable partly to the efficacy of stent retrievers in clot extraction but largely to the appropriate selection of patients with salvageable brain tissue based on multimodal imaging.

PREHOSPITAL EVALUATION AND TRIAGE

Educating the public to recognize the symptoms and signs of acute stroke and use of urgent triage and treatment are essential to improve outcomes. This effort requires public service campaigns, emergency medical services (EMS), and development of systems of care for rapid transfer of patients to nearby stroke centers.

Prehospital assessment scales have been developed to identify acute stroke and severity, including the Los Angeles Prehospital Stroke Screen, the Rapid Arterial occlusion Evaluation scale, and the Cincinnati Stroke Triage Assessment Tool. None have shown to be superior to another in identifying large vessel occlusion (LVO). The FAST acronym (face drooping, arm weakness, speech difficulty, time to call emergency services) has been endorsed by multiple professional organizations and has been the centerpiece of recent educational campaigns. Calling EMS (by dialing 9-1-1 in the United States) when stroke is suspected must be emphasized because use of EMS is associated with faster arrival to the emergency department (ED) and higher rates of treatment with reperfusion therapies. Training of dispatch personnel of recognize the urgency of stroke and the use of standardized stroke scales in the prehospital setting are also very important and may increase diagnostic accuracy. Prearrival notification of the ED that a suspected stroke case is being transported has been shown to accelerate times to thrombolysis. As useful as the FAST acronym is, it has considerable limitations, particularly with regard to posterior circulation and right hemispheric stroke symptoms (e.g., hemianopia, diplopia, and neglect).

Although, the role of primary stroke centers (PSCs) has focused on prompt administration of IV tPA, the emergence of recent endovascular trials and mobile stroke units (MSUs) has initiated a debate about bypassing PSCs in patients with severe stroke caused by LVO and transferring these patients directly to comprehensive stroke centers (CSCs) with endovascular capabilities. The American Heart Association Mission: Lifeline Stroke's Severity Based Stroke Triage Algorithm for EMS can be used to identify these patients. MSUs are ambulances equipped with a computed tomography (CT) scanner, point-of-care laboratory, and telemedicine connection and have been reported to be safe and effective in reducing time of thrombolysis. A randomized trial found a considerable reduction in the median time from alarm to therapy decision [35 minutes (interquartile range, 31–39 minutes) vs. 76 minutes (interquartile range, 63–94 minutes); $p < 0.0001$], and treatment with IV tPA increased from 21–33%. Further, transporting patients with severe symptoms directly to CSCs may lead to improved clinical outcomes. In one study, 46% of the 52 candidates for transfer were diagnosed with intracerebral hemorrhage on portable CT, while 54% had AIS with need for thrombectomy. By establishing AIS diagnosis in the MSU, the PSC was bypassed and patients were taken directly to the CSC for further management. Thus, the MSU saves critical time by allowing early triage of patients and differentiation between ischemic and hemorrhagic stroke in the prehospital setting.

OUTSIDE HOSPITAL EVALUATION AND TRIAGE

Primary stroke centers provide timely assessment of patients and can initiate treatment with IV tPA. However, only 7.2% of patients with AIS receive IV tPA within 3 hours of symptom onset at local hospitals. With the advent of telemedicine, patients with stroke can be evaluated promptly by stroke specialists remotely. Indeed, telestroke services are safe and comparable in quality to care provided face-to-face. The National Institutes of Health Stroke Scale (NIHSS), used to assess severity of deficit, can be performed remotely in a reproducible and accurate manner. The implementation of telemedicine increases the use of IV tPA from 5 to 24% and shortens time to treatment (17 minutes vs. 33 minutes; $p = 0.003$). Despite established evidence supporting its use, barriers to telemedicine exist, including licensure and financial sustainability.

EMERGENCY DEPARTMENT EVALUATION

The first step is to verify that the patient is medically stable with a general examination focused on vital signs and the cardiovascular system. Comorbidities are common in this patient population, with most patients having a history of hypertension and about one-third having diabetes mellitus. Peripheral, coronary, and other arterial diseases are also common. The evaluating physician needs to be vigilant to other emergency conditions that can present with stroke.

Every patient with suspected acute stroke should have a focused neurologic examination yielding as NIHSS score, which ranges from 0 (no obvious deficit) to 42 (quadriplegia and deep coma). The NIHSS is a structured and standardized neurologic examination of consciousness, vision, ocular, facial and limb movement, coordination, sensation, language, and awareness.

Immediate brain imaging noncontrast-enhanced computed tomgraphy (NCCT) brain is an essential first step in managing patients with stroke. The American College of Radiology considers either CT angiography (CTA) or magnetic resonance angiography (MRA) to be appropriate. American Heart Association (AHA) guidelines strongly recommend CTA or MRA for patients when endovascular therapy (EVT) is being contemplated to avoid sending patients to the catheter laboratory only to find out they have no clot to extract. American Academy of Neurology guidelines support superiority of diffusion-weighted imaging (DWI) over NCCT for diagnosing cerebral infarction; however, the majority of tissue exhibiting diffusion restriction will ultimately not be salvageable. Thus, the prediction of patients with salvageable ischemic tissue cannot be estimated without supplementation by perfusion imaging.

Intravenous Thrombolysis

Intravenous thrombolysis with alteplase became the first evidence-based short-term treatment for improving outcomes after AIS over 20 year ago. Since then, this treatment has been confirmed to be effective within 4.5 hours of stroke onset in randomized controlled trials and through extensive experience across the globe. Over time, it has also become clear that patients with some of the exclusion criteria from the original trials can safely receive thrombolysis. **Box 1** lists the current indications and contraindications for the use of IV alteplase for AIS.

Intravenous alteplase (at a dose of 0.9 mg/kg, not to exceed 90 mg and with 10% of the dose given as a bolus and the rest as infusion over the following 60 minutes) increases the chances by one-third of recovery to independent function at 3 months when administered within 3 hours of stroke onset. However, the therapeutic benefit decreases rapidly with time. Benefit is greatest in the first 90 minutes from symptom onset and no longer notable after 4.5 hours. Although, outcomes are less favorable in very elderly patients, IV tPA is still beneficial in patients with preexisting cognitive or physical disabilities and in those with very severe neurologic deficits (likely related to proximal vessel occlusion by a larger clot).

The most serious complication from IV tPA in intracranial hemorrhage (ICH). It often occurs in the area of infarction and is caused by reperfusion injury. Although, most of these reperfusion hemorrhages are asymptomatic they can sometimes provoke neurologic decline and, when severe, can be fatal. Hemorrhages remote from the infarction are less common but possible. The reported frequency of symptomatic ICH varies across studies depending on the definition used. When symptomatic ICH is defined as radiologically proven hemorrhage with decline of four or more points on the NIHSS attributable to the hemorrhage, the risk is not higher than 2-3%. Further, because these hemorrhages are more prone to occur in patients with large area of ischemia, they typically make a bad situation worse, rather than harming patients who would have otherwise had a favorable prognosis.

After IV tPA, patients need to be monitored in a dedicated stroke unit for 24 hours. Strict blood pressure control below 180/105 mm Hg is necessary, and antithrombotics should be avoided to reduce the risk of ICH. In case of neurologic worsening, CT should be repeated immediately. The presence of hemorrhage should prompt discontinuation of alteplase infusion if still ongoing. Cryoprecipitate or antifibrinolytics can be used to reverse the fibrinolytic effects of the drug, although the benefit of these interventions remains unproven. In life-threatening cases, surgical evacuation of the hematoma can be considered. Orolingual angioedema is another uncommon complication of IV alteplase. It typically occurs shortly after alteplase administration, and the risk is increased in patients previously taking angiotensin-converting enzyme inhibitors and in those with involvement of the insular region. Treatment consists of methylprednisolone (100–150 mg), diphenhydramine (25–50 mg), and an H_2 blocker. More severe cases may necessitate epinephrine (inhaled or subcutaneous) or even tracheal intubation.

> **BOX 1: Indications and contraindications for intravenous thrombolysis with alteplase.**
>
> *Indications:*
> - Diagnosis of ischemic stroke causing a measurable disabling neurologic deficit
> - Onset of symptoms <4.5 hours before beginning treatment
> - Age ≥18 years
>
> *Contraindications:*
> - Severe head trauma in previous 3 months
> - Symptoms suggestive of subarachnoid hemorrhage
> - Previous ICH
> - Intracranial/spinal surgery in previous 3 months
> - Intracerebral neoplasm
> - Infective endocarditis
> - Aortic arch dissection
> - Elevated blood pressure (systolic >185 mm Hg or diastolic >110 mm Hg) that cannot be lowered safely
> - Active internal bleeding
> - Acute bleeding diathesis, including but not limited to:
>   - Platelet count <1,00,000/mm^3
>   - Heparin received within 48 hours with an elevated aPTT (>40 seconds)
>   - Current use of treatment doses of low-molecular-weight heparin within the previous 24 hours (not applicable to DVT prophylactic dosages of low-molecular-weight heparin)
>   - Current use of anticoagulant with INR >1.7 or PT >15 seconds
>   - Current use of direct thrombin inhibitors or direct factor Xa inhibitors
> - CT demonstrates infarction (hypodensity) >1/3 cerebral hemisphere
> - CT demonstrates an acute ICH
>
> *Relative contraindications:*
> - Mild and nondisabling or rapidly improving stroke symptoms
> - Very severe neurologic deficits (NIHSS score >25) within the 3- to 4.5-hour window
> - Pregnancy
> - Seizure at onset (consider alteplase if neurologic deficits are thought to be caused by a stroke)
> - Arterial puncture at noncompressible site in previous 7 days
> - Untreated intracranial arteriovenous malformation
> - Untreated giant intracranial aneurysm
> - Recent major surgery or serious trauma (within previous 14 days)
> - Recent gastrointestinal or urinary tract hemorrhage (within pervious 21 days)
> - Ischemic stroke within previous 3 months
> - Recent ST-elevation acute myocardial infarction (within previous 3 months)
> - Blood glucose concentration <50 mg/dL (2.7 mmol/L) (consider IV alteplase if deficits still present after glucose normalization)
>
> (aPTT: activated partial thromboplastin time; CT: computed tomography; DVT: deep vein thrombosis; ICH: intracranial hemorrhage; INR: international normalized ratio; NIHSS: National Institutes of Health Stroke Scale; PT: prothrombin time)

Tenecteplase is a bioengineered variant of alteplase with longer half-life, greater fibrin specificity, and more resistance to plasminogen activator inhibitor 1. For many years, it has been the preferred thrombolytic agent for acute myocardial infarction. In one randomized trial, tenecteplase (0.4 mg/kg up to 40 mg as a single IV bolus) had safety and efficacy similar to the standard dose of alteplase among 1,100 patients with AIS treated within 4.5 hours of symptom onset. Although, the results did not meet the superiority criterion, they may be sufficient to consider tenecteplase as a valid alternative to alteplase, particularly given the convenience of its administration as a single bolus. Yet, alteplase remains the only approved thrombolytic agent for treating AIS to date.

Endovascular Therapy

The intra-arterial administration of thrombolytic agents directly into the clot was EVT for AIS in 1980s.

In PROACT I and PROACT II trials, intra-arterial recombinant prourokinase plus heparin versus heparin alone were compared in patients with AIS of <6 hours and angiographically proven LVO. The former had higher recanalization rages (66% vs. 18%) and were significantly more independent at 90 days (40% vs. 25%). The positive results of this trial to other EVT recanalization approaches.

Devices

Mechanical thrombectomy devices are classified into two major groups based on their mechanism of action: those that use an approach distal (retrievers) or proximal to thrombi (aspiration devices). In 2004, the USFDA approved MERCI for mechanical thrombectomy. While the MERCI and multi-MERCI trials showed good recanalization rates, the IMS-III, SYNTHESIS Expansion, and MR RESCUE trial all failed to show benefit of endovascular treatment compared with IV thrombolysis. These devices are outdated by the emergence of newer-generation devices that have shown robust benefits in clinical trials.

Newer-generation Devices

Newer-generation devices include devices that are used proximal to the clot (aspiration devices) and those that are used distal and within the clot (stent retrievers).

Stent Retrievers

Stent retrievers are composed of a distal metallic mesh (usually made out of an alloy such as Nitinol) that is attached to a delivery wire. They are deployed across the clot to form a temporary endovascular bypass; the clot gets engaged in the stent and then is retrieved along with the stent. These are available in different diameters and lengths; the selection of a particular device is based on the size of the vessel that is occluded. As per the latest guidelines, stent retrievers arc currently the preferred primary thrombectomy device. Examples of stent retrievers are:
- Solitaire FR (Medtronic Inc, USA)
- Trevo ProVue (Stryker Neurovascular, USA).

- pRE SET (Phenox GmBH, Germany)
- TIGERtriever (Rapid Medical, Israel)

Aspiration Devices

Aspiration devices are large-bore catheters that can be navigated to the occluded artery proximal to the clot and then used to aspirate the clot. Examples of aspiration devices include the Penumbra System (Penumbra Inc), QuickCat (DSM Inc, PA, USA), and PRONTO (Vascular Solutions Inc, MN, USA) extraction devices. Aspiration is done either manually or by an aspiration pump. Recent studies have shown comparable recanalization rates with aspiration as compared with stent retrievers.

The MR CLEAN was the first study completed in 2014. Patients with documented anterior circulation Large Artery Occlusion on Computed Tomographic Angiogram presenting within 6 hours from stroke onset were enrolled to receive EVT or usual care alone. Stent retrievers were used in 81.5% patients, and tPA was administered in 90.6% where positive outcomes of modified Rankin scale (mRS) score 0-1 was found in favor of intervention. The positive results precipitated an early interim analysis of the remaining four EVT trials: (1) ESCAPE, (2) REVASCAT, (3) EXTEND-IA trial (Extending the Time for Thrombolysis in Emergency Neurological Deficits-Intra-Arterial), and (4) SWIFT PRIME, which were subsequently prematurely stopped because of positive outcomes.

The DEFUSE 3 trial and DAWN trial investigating about mechanical thrombectomy in patients with an internal carotid artery or proximal MCA occlusion and presenting between 6 and 16 hours and 6-24 hours from last known normal time, many of whom are wakeup stroke patients, using penumbra-core mismatch on perfusion imaging and clinical imaging mismatch to identify stroke patients with salvageable tissue who could benefit from intervention.

■ MANAGEMENT OF MALIGNANT INFARCTION

Although, most hemispheric infarctions reach their maximal swelling after 3-5 days, infarctions involving the entire MCA territory (with or without anterior cerebral artery territory involvement) can produce live-threatening swelling within the first 48 hours. These "malignant" infarctions demand treatment in the intensive care unit. Medical therapies (including osmotic agents, such as mannitol and hypertonic saline) are at best supportive or merely temporizing. Without decompressive surgery, the mortality in these cases exceeds 60-70%.

Decompressive hemicraniectomy with dural expansion is very effective in reducing mortality in patients with malignant hemispheric brain infarctions. However, functional outcomes after surgery are highly dependent on age and rehabilitation potential. In randomized trials, 55% of survivors aged 60 years or younger had regained the ability to walk, and 18% were functionally independent at 1 year. However, the outcomes were much poorer among survivors older than 60 years (11% were able to walk, while none were functionally independent at 1 year). Thus, clinicians should carefully discuss the expected postsurgical prognosis with patient and families before proceeding with the decompression, especially when contemplating the intervention for older patients. If surgery is pursued, it should ideally take place within the first 48 hours or very shortly after neurologic decline from swelling begins to ensue.

Large cerebellar infarctions—typically involving the posterior inferior cerebellar artery territory—can lead to death by occluding the fourth ventricle, causing obstructive hydrocephalus and brainstem compression. In such cases, emergency ventriculostomy and suboccipital craniectomy with dural expansion can save lives. Many of these patients can ultimately regain good function. Although, there is a clear correlation between the size of the cerebellar infarction and the risk of secondary neurologic decline from swelling, there is no accurate method to predict which patients will require surgical intervention, and therefore, close neurologic monitoring in the intensive care unit is indispensable.

■ ANTITHROMBOTIC THERAPY

In patients who undergo thrombolysis, aspirin and other antithrombotic agents should not be given alone or in combination for the first 24 hours following treatment with IV tPA. Otherwise, in the absence of contraindications, antiplatelet agents should be started as soon as possible after the diagnosis of ischemic stroke is confirmed. According to the AHA, oral administration of aspirin (initial dose is 325 mg) within 24-48 hours after stroke onset is recommended for treatment of most patients. Dual antiplatelet therapy in the form of aspirin (160-325 mg loading dose, followed by 50-100 mg daily) plus clopidogrel (300 mg loading dose, followed by 75 mg once daily) is recommended for patients with minor ischemic stroke, defined by an NIHSS score ≤3. For patients who are on anticoagulation, it should be stopped at least for the short term. There is no indication to use full-dose parenteral anticoagulation with heparin except in select patients with acute cardioembolic ischemic stroke due to intracardiac thrombus in the left ventricle or thrombus associated with mechanical or native heart valves who are neurologically stable. Timing of starting anticoagulation after AIS is controversial and largely depends on clinical (neurological status, bleeding risk) and radiological (hemorrhagic transformation and size of infarct) evaluation. The AHA recommends that it is reasonable to initiate oral anticoagulation (OAC) within 14 days for most patients with stroke with atrial fibrillation (AF), and delay anticoagulation for >14 days in patients with high risk for hemorrhagic transformation at initial CT.

■ CONCLUSION

Acute stroke management has evolved tremendously over the years and will likely continue to improve with individualized patient care and careful selection criteria. In addition to IV tPA, EVT is now a standard of care in patients with LVO of the anterior circulation. Extending the therapeutic window to 16 and 24 hours has recently been established by the DEFUSE 3 and DAWN trial for selected patients based on imaging identification of salvageable brain tissue. Despite these paradigm shifts in stroke management, disability from AIS remain pervasive, and there is still need for developing criteria for revascularization of posterior circulation and basilar artery occlusions (BAOs). Improvements are also needed for developing systems in the prehospital and posthospitalization settings and for rapid transfer of patients to appropriate stroke centers for timely management.

SUGGESTED READINGS

1. Pandian JD, Sudhan P. Stroke epidemiology and stroke care services in India. J Stroke. 2013;15:128-34.
2. National Institute of Neurological Disorders and Stroke rt-PA Stroke Study Group. Tissue plasminogen activator for acute ischemic stroke. N Engl J Med. 1995;333(24):1581-7.
3. del Zoppo GJ, Higashida RT, Furlan AJ, et al. PROACT: a phase II randomized trial of recombinant pro-urokinase by direct arterial delivery in acute middle cerebral artery stroke. PROACT Investigators. Prolyse in Acute Cerebral Thromboembolism. Stroke. 1998;29(1):4-11.
4. Broderik JP, Palesch YY, Demchuk AM, et al.; Interventional management of Stroke (IMS) III Investigators. Endovascular therapy after intravenous t-PA versus t-PA alone for stroke. N Engl J Med. 2013;368(10):893-903.
5. Kidwell CS, Starkman S, Eckstein M, et al. Identifying stroke in the field; prospective validation of the Los Angeles Prehospital Stroke Screen (LAPSS), Stroke. 2000;31(1):71-6.
6. Perez de la Ossa N, Carrera D, Gorchs M, et al. Design and validation of a prehospital stroke scale to predict large arterial occlusion; the Rapid Arterial oCclusion Evaluation scale. Stroke. 2014;45(1):87-91.
7. McMullan JT, Katz B, Broderick J, et al. Prospective Prehospital Evaluation of the Cincinnati Stroke Triage Assessment Tool. Prehosp Emerg Care. 2017;21(4):481-8.
8. American Stroke Association. (2017). Stroke symptoms. [online] Available from http;//www.strokeassociation.org/STROKEORG/WarningSigns/Stroke-Warning-Signs-and-Symptoms_UCM_308528_SubHomePage.jsp [Last accessed October, 2022].
9. Ekudayo OJ, Saver JL, Fonaraw GC, et al. Patterns of emergency medical services use and its association with timely stroke treatment: findings from Get With the Guidelines-Stroke. Circ Cardiovasc Qual Outcomes. 2013;6(3):262-9.
10. Kothari RU, Pancioli A, Liu T, et al. Cincinnati Prehospital Stroke Scale: reproducibility and validity. Ann Emerg Med. 1999;33(4):373-8.
11. Lin CB, Peterson ED, Smit EE, et al. Emergency medical service hospital prenotification is associated with improved evaluation and treatment of acute ischemic stroke. Circ Cardiovasc Qual Outcome. 2012;5(4):514-22.
12. MoccoJ, Fiorella D, Albuquerque FC. The mission lifeline severity-based stroke treatment algorithm: We need more time. J Neurointerv Surg. 2017;9(5):427-8.
13. Fassbender K, Grotta JC, Walter S, et al. Mobile stroke units for prehospital thrombolysis, triage, and beyond: benefits and challenges. Lancet Neurol. 2017;16(3):227-37.
14. Walter S, Kostopoulos P, Haass A, et al. Diagnosis and treatment of patients with stroke in a mobile stroke unit versus in hospital: a randomized controlled trial. Lancet Neurol. 2012;11(5):397-404.
15. Ebinger M, Winter B, Wendt M, et al.; STEMO Consortium. Effect of the use of ambulance-based thrombolysis on time to thrombolysis in acute ischemic stroke: a randomized clinical trial. JAMA. 2014;311(16):1622-31.
16. Schlemm E, Ebinger M, Nolte CH, et al. Optimal transport destination of ischemic stroke patients with unknown vessel status: use of prehospital triage scores. Stroke. 2017;48(8):2184-91.
17. Zafar A, Udeh B, Reimer A, et al. Abstract TP249: Hospital Transfer Cost Savings From Triaging Selected Stroke Patients Directly to the Comprehensive Stroke Centers (CSCs) Courtesy of the Mobile Stroke Treatment Unit (MSTU). Stroke. 2017;48(suppl 1):ATP249.
18. Adams HP Jr, del Zoppo G, Alberts MJ, et al. Guidelines for the early management of adults with ischemic stroke: a guideline from the American Heart Association/American Stroke Association Stroke Council, Clinical Cardiology Council, Cardiovascular Radiology and Intervention Council, and the Atherosclerotic Peripheral Vascular Disease and Quality of Care Outcomes in Research Interdisciplinary Working Groups: the American Academy of Neurology affirms the value of this guideline as an educational tool for neurologists. Stroke. 2007;38(5):1655-711.
19. Audebert HJ, Boy S, Jankovits R, et al. Is mobile teleconsulting equivalent to hospital-based telestroke services? Stroke. 2008;39(12):3427-30.

20. Müller-Barna P, Schwamm LH, Haberl RL. Telestroke increases use of acute stroke therapy. Curr Opin Neurol. 2012;25(1):5-10.
21. Salmela MB, Krishna SH, Martin DJ, et al. All that bleeds is not black: susceptibility weighted imaging of intracranial hemorrhage and the effect of T1 signal. Clin Imaging. 2017;41:69-72.
22. Schellinger PD, Bryan RN, Caplan LR, et al.; Therapeutics and Technology Assessment Subcommittee of the American Academy of Neurology. Evidence-based guideline: The role of diffusion and perfusion MRI for the diagnosis of acute ischemic stroke: report of the Therapeutics and Technology Assessment Subcommittee of the American Academy of Neurology. Neurology. 2010;75(2):177-85.
23. Hacke W, Kaste M, Bluhmki E, et al.; ECASS Investigators. Thrombolysis with alteplase 3 to 4.5 hours after acute ischemic stroke. N Engl J Med. 2008;359(13):1317-29.
24. Demaerschalk BM, Kleindorfer DO, Adeoye OM, et al; American Heart Association Stroke Council and Council on Epidemiology and Prevention. Scientific Rationale for the Inclusion and Exclusion Criteria for Intravenous Alteplase in Acute Ischemic Stroke: A Statement for Healthcare Professionals From the American Heart Association/American Stroke Association. Stroke. 2016;47(2):581-641.
25. Fugate JE, Rabinstein AA. Update on intravenous recombinant tissue plasminogen activator for acute ischemic stroke. Mayo Clin Proc. 2014;89(7):960-72.
26. Seet RC, Rabinstein AA. Symptomatic intracranial hemorrhage following intravenous thrombolysis for acute ischemic stroke: a critical review of case definitions. Cerebrovasc Dis. 2012;34(2):106-14.
27. Saver JL. Hemorrhage after thrombolytic therapy for stroke: the clinically relevant number needed to harm. Stroke. 2007;38(8):2279-83.
28. Frontera JA, Lewin JJ III, Rabinstein AA, et al. Guideline for reversal of antithrombotics in intracranial hemorrhage: a statement for healthcare professionals from the Neurocritical Care Society and Society of Critical Care Medicine. Neurocrit Care. 2016;24(1):6-46.
29. Myslimi F, Caparros F, Dequatre-Ponchelle N, et al. Orolingual angioedema during or after thrombolysis for cerebral ischemia. Stroke. 2016;47(7):1825-30.
30. Logallo N, Novotny V, Assmus J, et al. Tenecteplase versus alteplase for management of acute ischaemic stroke (NOR-TEST): a phase 3, randomized, open-label, blinded endpoint trial. Lancet Neurol. 2017;16(10):781-8.
31. Furlan A, Higashida R, Wechsler L, et al. Intra-arterial prourokinase for acute ischemic stroke. The PROACT II study: a randomized controlled trial. Prolyse in Acute Cerebral Thromboembolism. JAMA. 1999:282(21):2003-11.
32. Balasubramaian A, Mitchell P, Dowling R, et al. Evolution of endovascular therapy in acute storke: implications of device development. J Stroke. 2015;17:127-37.
33. Kidwell CS, Jahan R, Gornbein J, et al. Atrial of imaging selection and endovascular treatment for ischemic stroke. N Engl J Med. 2013;368(10):914-23.
34. Jovin TG, Chamorro A, Cobo E, et al. Thrombectomy within 8 hours after symptom onset in ischemic storke. N Engl J Med. 2015;372:2296-306.
35. Albers GW, Thijs VN, Wechsler L, et al.; DEFUSE Investigators. Magnetic resonance imaging profiles predict clinical response to early reperfusion: the diffusion and perfusion imaging evaluation for understanding stroke evolution (DEFUSE) study. Ann Neurol. 2006;60:508-17.
36. Vahedi K, Hofmeijer J, Juettier E, et al.; DECIMAL, DESTINY, and HAMLET investigators. Early decompressive surgery in malignant infarction of the middle cerebral artery: a pooled analysis of three randomised controlled trials. Lancet Neurol. 2007;6(3):215-22.
37. Juttler E, Unterberg A, Woitzik J, et al.; DESTINY II Investigations. Hemicraniectomy in older patients with extensive middle-cerebral-artery stroke. N Engl J Med. 2014;370(12):1091-100.
38. Wijdics EF, Ssheth KN, Carter BS, et al; American Heart Association Stroke Council. Recommendations for the management of cerebral and cerebellar infarction with swelling: a statement for healthcare professionals from the American Heart Association/American Stroke Association. Stroke. 2014;45(4):1222-38.
39. Datar S, Rabinstein AA. Cerebellar infarction. Neurol Clin. 2014;32(4):979-91.

40. Clark WM, Albers GW, Madden KP, et al. The rtPA (alteplase) 0- to 6-hour acute stroke trial, part A (A0276g) : results of a double-blind, placebo-controlled, multicenter study. Thromblytic therapy in acute ischemic stroke study investigators. Stroke. 2000;31(4):811-6.
41. Anderson CS, Robinson T, Lindley RI, et al, Low-dose versus standard-dose intravenous alteplase in acute ischemic stroke. N Engl J Med. 2016;374(24):2313-23.
42. Thomalla G, Simonsen CZ, Boutitie F, et al. MRI-guided thrombolysis for stroke with unknown time of onset. N Engl J Med. 2018;379(7):611-22.

CHAPTER 59

Advances in Epilepsy Management and Current Perspectives

Man Mohan Mehndiratta, Vasundhara Aggarwal

INTRODUCTION

Major advances in epilepsy management have surfaced in recent years. In recent years, there have been many improving definitions, guidelines, diagnostic, and treatment protocols that have come to the fore. The causes and consequences of epilepsy have been more deeply explored. It is very important to fine tune our knowledge and keep updated. It is rightly said "staying updated is our commitment to our patients".

DEFINITION AND CLASSIFICATION: RECENT CHANGES

The first step toward accurate diagnosis, therapy, and prognostication of epilepsy is adequate knowledge of its definition and classification. One of the most important international organization dedicated to epilepsy care, education, and research is the International League Against Epilepsy (ILAE). **Table 1** describes the 2014 ILAE operational (practical) definition of epilepsy.

TABLE 1: 2014 ILAE operational (practical) definition of epilepsy.			
Epilepsy is a disease of the brain defined by any of the three following conditions			
A least two unprovoked (or reflex) seizures occurring >24 hours apart	One unprovoked (or reflex) seizure and a probability of further seizures similar to the general recurrence risk (at least 60%) after two unprovoked seizures, occurring over the next 10 years	Diagnosis of an epilepsy syndrome	Epilepsy is considered to be resolved for individuals who had an age-dependent epilepsy syndrome but are now past the applicable age or those who have remained seizure-free for the last 10 years, with no seizure medicines for the last 5 years

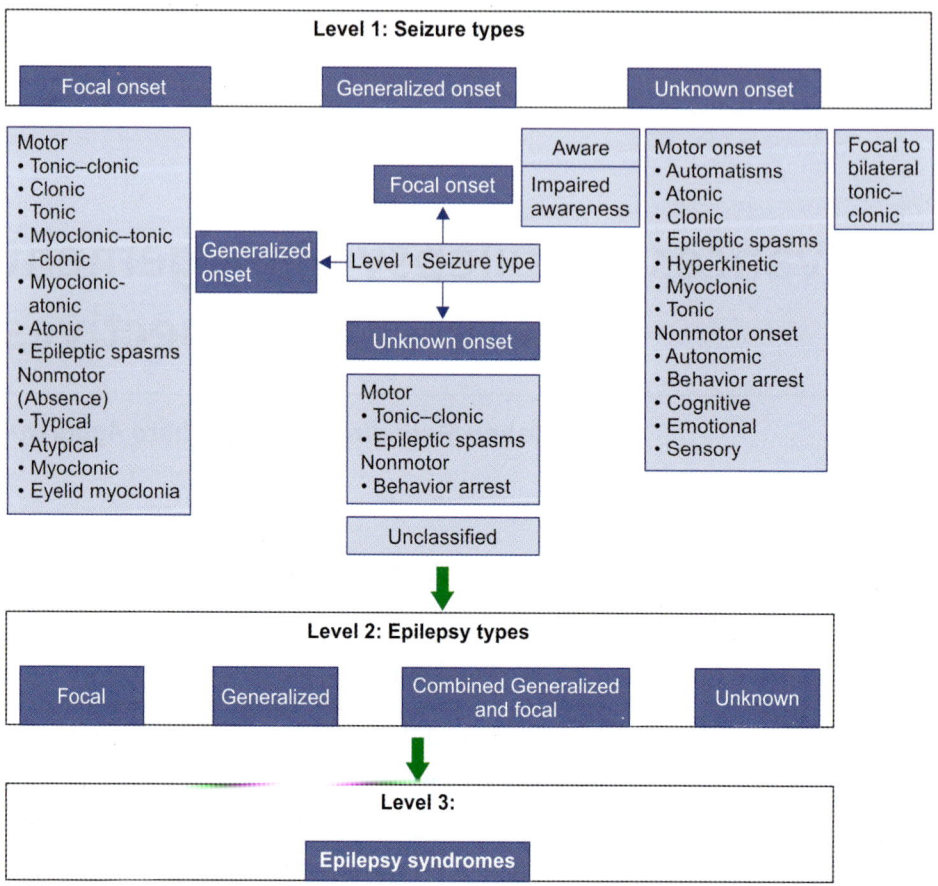

FLOWCHART 1: New multilevel classification of approach to diagnosis of epilepsy.

Seizure is defined as "transient occurrence of signs and/or symptoms due to abnormal excessive or synchronous neuronal activity in the brain."

International League Against Epilepsy published "position papers" on a new classification of epilepsies and seizures, as well as an "instruction manual" for use in the operational classification of seizures in 2017. ILAE classification of the epilepsies: Position paper of the ILAE Commission for Classification and Terminology 2017 states a new multilevel classification **(Flowchart 1)** which requires a diagnosis at all three levels. Assuming that the patient is having epileptic seizures as defined by the new 2017 ILAE seizure classification it starts with level 1: Seizure type diagnosis. The next step is level 2: Epilepsy type diagnosis, including focal epilepsy, generalized epilepsy, combined generalized, and focal epilepsy, and also an unknown epilepsy group. The next is level 3: epilepsy syndrome diagnosis.

It also incorporates and emphasizing the requirement to considering etiology at each step of diagnosis. The *etiology* is broken into six subgroups **(Fig. 1)**, keeping in mind the potential therapeutic consequences. It lays special emphasis on diagnosing a genetic cause of Epilepsy. It also emphasizes to consider *comorbidities*, such as depression, anxiety disorder, migraine, and cognitive impairment, which can affect

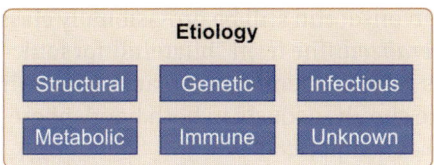

FIG. 1: Six broad subgroups of etiology of epilepsy.

the course and treatability. There are certain drugs to be preferred and avoided in epilepsy with comorbidity. The understanding of etiology and comorbidities will help targeted therapies to the specific type of disease and etiology.

■ NEW REGARDING THE CLASSIFICATION OF EPILEPSY

- Combined generalized and focal epilepsy type added (it cannot be just focal or generalized)
- "Benign" are now termed "self-limiting" or "pharmacoresponsive" (it can spontaneously resolve or respond to therapy).
- New term added epileptic encephalopathy (seizure burden by itself leads to encephalopathy) and developmental and epileptic encephalopathy (both seizure burden and metabolic, structural, or genetic alterations lead to encephalopathy).
- Psychosocial and other comorbidities included

■ NEW REGARDING THE CLASSIFICATION OF SEIZURES

- Newly added types and terms in ILAE 2017 classification:
  - New focal seizure types include automatisms, autonomic, behavior arrest, cognitive, emotional, hyperkinetic, sensory, and focal to bilateral tonic–clonic seizures. Atonic, clonic, epileptic spasms, myoclonic, and tonic seizures can be either focal or generalized.
  - New generalized seizure types include absence with eyelid myoclonia, myoclonic absence, myoclonic-tonic-clonic, myoclonic-atonic, and epileptic spasms
- The discontinued terms are:
  - Simple/complex partial
  - Convulsions
  - Dyscognitive
  - Psychic
  - Secondarily generalized
- *Changed terms*:
  - Partial seizure—focal (onset) seizure
  - Secondarily generalized clonic—focal to bilateral tonic-clonic
  - Simple—aware
  - Complex—impaired awareness
  - Hypermotor—hyperkinetic
  - Psychic/experiential—cognitive

- Seizures of unknown onset can still be provisionally classified.
- *Bilateral versus generalized*: The term "bilateral" for tonic–clonic seizures is used when it propagates to both hemispheres and "generalized" for seizures that apparently originate simultaneously in both hemispheres.
- *Classifiers used in the classification*:
    - Onset:
        - Decides focal/generalized if there is 80% confidence level.
        - The first prominent sign/symptom is used to classify seizure type.
    - Awareness: Used as classifier of focal seizures
    - Motor/nonmotor
    - Additional descriptors: After classifying seizure type based on initial manifestations, it is encouraged to add descriptions of other signs and symptoms, suggested descriptors or free text. These do not alter the seizure type.

APPROACH TO MANAGEMENT OF EPILEPSY

Pharmacological Management

Antiepileptic drugs (AEDs) are the mainstay of treatment. Two key questions WHEN AND WHAT TO START??

When to start AEDs: Treatment indicated??

Definitions:
- Unprovoked seizure —unknown etiology as well as one that occurs in relation to a preexisting brain lesion or progressive nervous system disorder (often referred to as a remote symptomatic seizure)
- Provoked seizures are due to an acute condition such as a toxic or metabolic disturbance, head trauma, or acute stroke (i.e., acute symptomatic seizures)

First unprovoked seizure:
- Decision should be individualized and guided by following factors:
    - Sufficiently high risk of seizure recurrence to meet criteria for epilepsy according to ILAE
    - Increased risk clinical variables
    - Clinical history or neuroimaging reveals remote symptomatic cause, as identified by (e.g., brain tumor, brain malformation, head injury with loss of consciousness, prior central nervous system infection, or scarring from a prior brain injury or brain surgery)
    - Prior brain insult
    - An electroencephalogram (EEG) with epileptiform abnormalities
    - A significant brain imaging abnormality
    - A nocturnal seizure
    - Abnormal neurologic examination, including focal findings and intellectual disability
    - Individual patient comorbidities and age considering the side-effect profiles
    - Patient values and preferences, e.g., social consequences

What to start? Which and how many antiepileptic drugs?
Start with a single AED introduced at a small dose (except status epilepticus or frequent seizures). Monotherapy advantages being:
- Decreases the likelihood of adverse effects
- Avoids drug interactions
- Less expensive than polytherapy

To minimize adverse effects, the dose gradually increased to the lowest effective maintenance dose.

Tailored to *factors such as disease related factors, drug-related factors and individual person characteristics*—no single AED that is ideal for all patients.

First-generation AEDs remain valuable first-line therapies which included **(Table 2)**.

Second-generation AEDs **(Table 3)** offer advantages in terms of drug resistance, fewer drug interactions, and improved tolerability and tailoring treatment **(Table 3)**.

Antiepileptic drugs can also be divided based on their mechanisms **Table 4**.

TABLE 2: First generation antiepileptic drugs (AEDs).	
First generation AEDs	Valproic acid
	Benzodiazepines
	Phenobarbital
	Primidone
	Carbamazepine
	Phenytoin
	Ethosuximide

TABLE 3: Second-generation antiepileptic drugs (AEDs).	
Second generation AEDs	Lamotrigine
	Levetiracetam
	Topiramate
	Zonisamide
	Oxcarbazepine
	Perampanel
	Vigabatrin
	Rufinamide
	Felbamate
	Eslicarbazepine acetate
	Lacosamide
	Pregabalin
	Gabapentin
	Tiagabine
	Brivaracetam
	Everolimus
	Stiripentol

TABLE 4: Antiepileptic drugs (AEDs) based on mechanism of action.

Mechanism	Name
Blockers of repetitive activation of the sodium channel	Phenytoin, carbamazepine, oxcarbazepine, eslicarbazepine, lamotrigine, topiramate, and cenobamate
Enhancers of slow inactivation of the sodium channel	Lacosamide and rufinamide
N-methyl-D-aspartic acid (NMDA) receptor blockers	Felbamate
Gamma-aminobutyric acid (GABA)–A receptor enhancers	Phenobarbital, benzodiazepines, and clobazam
T-calcium channel blockers	Ethosuximide and valproate
Alpha-amino-3-hydroxy-5-methyl-4-isoxazole propionic acid (AMPA) receptor blockers	Perampanel and topiramate
H-current modulators	Gabapentin and lamotrigine
N- and L-calcium channel blockers	Lamotrigine, topiramate, zonisamide, and valproate
Blockers of unique binding sites	Gabapentin, levetiracetam, and perampanel
Neuronal potassium channel (KCNQ [Kv7]) opener	Ezogabine
Carbonic anhydrase inhibitors	Topiramate and zonisamide
Other anticonvulsants	Cannabidiol and stiripentol

For example, if carbamazepine fails to control the seizures, lamotrigine, topiramate, tiagabine, gabapentin, levetiracetam, oxcarbazepine, pregabalin, and zonisamide are considered for second- or third-line therapy.

New anticonvulsants are considered second-line therapy, however, can be used as first-line therapy in some patients.

If seizures persist on the first AED despite optimal uptitration to the maximally tolerated dose, exclude noncompliance should be and re-appraise the diagnosis and treatment.

If an AED change is required switch to an alternative monotherapy.

Polytherapy is usually offered after failure of two or three sequential monotherapies (except in a difficult to treat form of epilepsy unlikely to respond fully to monotherapy).

Drug-resistant epilepsy: ILAE defined drug-resistant epilepsy as "failure of adequate trials of two tolerated, appropriately chosen and used AED schedules (whether as monotherapies or in combination) to achieve sustained seizure-freedom."

Factors Influencing Choice of Antiepileptic Drugs

Disease-related factors: Anticonvulsants for specific seizure types.
Absence seizures:
- If only absence seizures are present—ethosuximide.
- If absence seizures are present along with other seizure types (e.g., generalized tonic–clonic seizures, myoclonic seizures)—valproic acid or lamotrigine or

topiramate. *Caution*: Drugs may exacerbate absence seizures—carbamazepine, gabapentin, or tiagabine
- Lennox-Gastaut syndrome with seizures—broad-spectrum drugs (e.g., valproic acid, lamotrigine, and topiramate) or felbamate as a last resort
  – As adjunctive therapies for seizures associated with Lennox-Gastaut syndrome, Dravet syndrome, or tuberous sclerosis complex—rufinamide, clobazam, extended-release topiramate, cannabidiol, and stiripentol.
- Juvenile myoclonic epilepsy (JME) and myoclonic seizures—valproic acid, lamotrigine, and topiramate (JME has a high recurrence rate)
- As adjunctive therapy of JME—levetiracetam
- Primary generalized tonic-clonic seizures—valproic acid, topiramate, or lamotrigine
- As adjunctive therapy for these seizures—levetiracetam and perampanel

Generalized and unclassified epilepsies:
- Valproate should remain the drug of first choice for many patients except in women of childbearing age.
- Focal-onset seizures monotherapy—carbamazepine, cenobamate, lacosamide, lamotrigine, oxcarbazepine, and topiramate.
- Adjunctive therapy with levetiracetam, tiagabine, gabapentin, pregabalin, lacosamide, cenobamate, or ezogabine
- In elderly subjects (patients aged ≥60 years), lamotrigine as first-line

Standard and New Antiepileptic Drugs (SANAD) trial: The largest individual randomized trial examining different antiseizure drugs as monotherapy for the initial treatment of epilepsy **(Fig. 2)**.

Drug-related Factors
Refer **Box 1**.

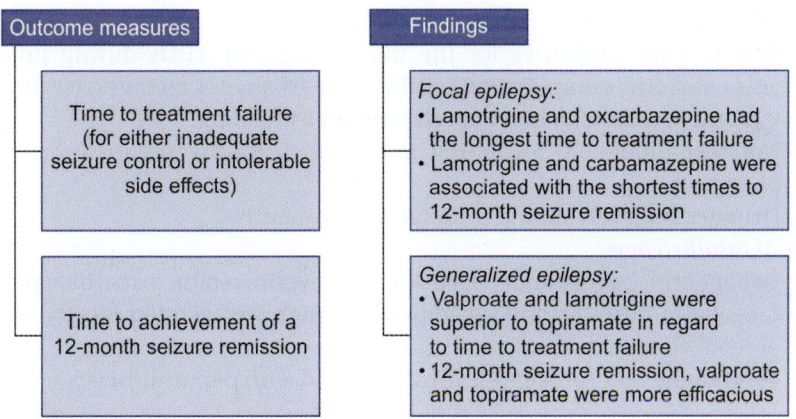

FIG. 2: Standard and New Antiepileptic Drugs (SANAD) trail.

> **BOX 1: Drug-related factors influencing choice of antiepileptic drugs (AEDs).**
>
> - Comparative efficacy
> - Dosing frequency
> - Drug interactions
> - Aging
> - Neurocognitive side effects
> - Hypersensitivity reactions: Stevens–Johnson syndrome (SJS), toxic epidermal necrolysis (TEN)
> - Suicidality
> - Weight gain or loss
> - US Food and Drug Administration (FDA) indications
> - Cost of medications

Individual-related Factors

Specific patient populations and conditions-related considerations:
- *Neonates and children*:
    - Doses per kilogram of body weight
    - Tend to metabolize the drugs faster than adults.
    - Rapid increases in the total volume of distribution.
- *Elderly patients*:
    - Need lower initial and maintenance doses (slowed hepatic metabolism, decreased renal clearance, and decreased volumes of distribution)
- *Women on contraceptive agents*:
    - Efficacy of oral contraceptive pills decreased with AEDs that induce hepatic enzymes (carbamazepine, phenytoin, phenobarbital, primidone, felbamate, lamotrigine, topiramate, and oxcarbazepine)
    - High-dose estrogen-progesterone contraceptive to counteract this effect
    - Second method of contraception
- *Women of childbearing age and pregnant women*:
    - 2009, the American Academy of Neurology and the American Epilepsy Society new guidelines for the management of AEDs during pregnancy cover obstetric complications and seizure frequency changes, teratogenesis, vitamin K, folic acid, blood levels, and breastfeeding.
    - Not recommended: Switching medications during pregnancy and polypharmacy
    - Drug serum levels should be obtained frequently.
- *Renal insufficiency*:
    - Gabapentin, zonisamide, lacosamide, levetiracetam, oxcarbazepine, and pregabalin doses should be adjusted as they are excreted mostly by means of renal clearance.
    - Topiramate and zonisamide are associated with nephrolithiasis.

- *Hepatic disease*:
  - Levetiracetam, gabapentin, pregabalin, and vigabatrin do not undergo hepatic metabolism and are less problematic for use in patients with chronic liver disease.
  - Phenytoin, carbamazepine, valproic acid, and felbamate have been associated with acute hepatic injury.
- *Poststroke epilepsy*:
  - Consider impact of the antiseizure drug on poststroke functional recovery and the potential for drug interactions with warfarin and salicylates.
- *Brain tumors*:
  - Consider potential drug interactions with chemotherapeutic agents and increased potential for allergic cutaneous reactions during radiotherapy.
- *Psychiatric disorders*:
  - Depression correlates more strongly with a poor quality of life than the frequency of the seizures.
  - Some antiseizure drugs appear to have mood stabilizing properties.
  - In contrast, some antiseizure drugs cause or exacerbate a depressed mood.
- *Migraine*:
  - Valproate, gabapentin, and topiramate are antiseizure drugs that have demonstrated efficacy for migraine prevention in placebo-controlled trials.
- *Osteoporosis risk*:
  - Antiseizure drugs in chronic use have been associated with bone loss. Particularly problematic for patients with epilepsy, as seizures are associated with falls and bone fractures. Monitor of bone density, routine supplementation of calcium and vitamin D, and a consistent exercise regimen.

Discontinuing Antiepileptic Drugs

Many consider discontinuing AEDs after a person has been seizure free for typically 2-5 years. Many outgrow many epileptic syndromes of childhood.

The recurrence rate during adulthood for patients with JME is about 80-90% in 2 years.

Risk of Seizure Recurrence

Risk of relapse after drug discontinuation, increase if there are:
- Epileptiform or focal abnormalities on an EEG or abnormalities on a brain magnetic resonance imaging (MRI) scan significantly the relapse risk.
- Long duration of epilepsy before the seizures were controlled
- High number and frequency of seizures
- *Seizure type*: Tonic or atonic seizures are present.
- Short duration of freedom from seizure

During tapering and for at least 3 months after discontinuation, advise patients to observe strict seizure precautions (including not driving).

NONPHARMACOLOGICAL THERAPY

There have been rapid advances in surgical technology and neuroimaging and parallel understanding of developments in epilepsy neurobiology.

Surgical Procedures

The types of surgery performed in patients for refractory epilepsy include:
- *Anterior temporal lobectomy (ATL)*: The most common surgical procedures performed in temporal lobe epilepsy in adolescents and adults.
- *Extratemporal resection*: In infancy and early childhood, this is the most common type of epilepsy surgery performed with etiologies being malformations of cortical development, vascular malformations, and low-grade tumors.
- *Lesionectomy*: Lesionectomy involves the resection of circumscribed epileptogenic lesions, including tumors, vascular malformations, and well-delineated malformations of cortical development.
- *Hemispherectomy*: When the entire hemisphere is considered epileptogenic and little or no functional cortex remains. For example in Rasmussen's encephalitis, Sturge–Weber syndrome, hemi anencephaly or large hemispheric infarction.
- *Corpus callosotomy (CC)*: The procedure is performed in patients with symptomatic generalized epilepsy who are poor candidates for resective surgery. Occasionally, done in the treatment of frequent secondary generalized tonic-clonic, tonic and atonic seizure leading to falls and injuries.
- *Multiple subpial transection (MST)*: Occasionally used in the treatment of focal epilepsy arising in or around eloquent areas.
- *Thermal ablation*: Minimally invasive type of laser surgery treatment. Laser destroys the small well defined seizure focal point in brain tissue without damaging the surrounding tissue.

Devices

- *Devices for brain stimulation*:
    - Intracranial systems (Implant device): Deep brain stimulation (DBS) and responsive neurostimulation (RNS)
    - Extracranial systems (implant device):
        - Focal cooling and uncaging
        - RTM—repetitive transcranial magnetic stimulation
        - TDC—transcranial direct current stimulation
        - TNS—trigeminal nerve stimulation TNS
        - VNS—vagus nerve stimulation
- *Devices detecting seizures*, alerting family members and caregivers thus helps in controlling the seizure behavior. These devices also have their own limitations.
    - Wearable device—accelerometer, Medpage ST-2, SeizAlert, Protective Headwear's
    - Sensor implant device—BrainGate™ neural interface system
    - Mobile phone-based device—Epdetect and Epilert
    - Watch-based device—SmartWatch alert
    - Software-based multichannel sensor device—NeuroPort system

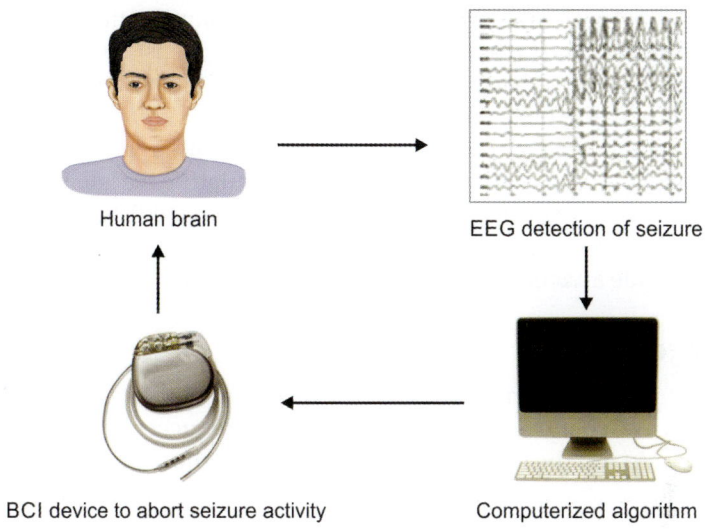

FIG. 3: Responsive neurostimulation (RNS).

- Cortical stimulators and mapping—Rehabilicare
- Working mats—Safety Place Mat®
- *Devices for surgery*:
    - Cyber knife functional MRI, gamma knife—high-resolution brain SPECT magnetoencephalography, NIRS—near-infrared spectroscopy, SIGFRIED—signal modeling for real-time identification, and event detection tractography and diffusion tensor imaging
    - Responsive neurostimulation **(Fig. 3)** is the first generation "closed loop" device using brain computer interface (BCI).
    - Once the device is set to particular EEG depending on the patients individual EEG and response, then this implant helps in detecting, collecting and recording the brain's EEG. Whenever, the implant identifies a seizure, it sends an electrical signal to control or disrupt the seizure activity.

In November 2013, the US Food and Drug Administration (FDA) approved the NeuroPace RNS System for the reduction of seizures in patients with drug-resistant epilepsy particularly in patients with partial-onset epilepsy in whom other antiepileptic treatment approaches have failed and that the benefits outweigh the risks.

Transcranial magnetic stimulation (TMS) is another method for brain stimulation magnetic field-induced brain currents were introduced with the help of magnetic stimulator coil from a safe distance to stimulate focally and deeply in the brain tissues.

Vagal Nerve Stimulation

Vagal nerve stimulation is FDA approved to treat medically refractory focal-onset epilepsy in patients older than 12 years. Candidates for VNS should meet the following criteria—(1) medically refractory seizures, (2) adequate trials of at least 2 or 3 AEDs (preferably with different mechanism of action), (3) exclusion of nonepileptic events, and (4) not a good candidate for epilepsy surgery. If the patient is a good candidate for focal resective surgery, them it should be preferred over VNS, as this procedure has a superior seizure-free rate.

Transcutaneous vagus nerve stimulation (tVNS) is a noninvasive brain stimulation technique used to treat epilepsy by stimulating the left auricular branch of the vagus nerve at the ear conch. It is a newly developed tVNS (NEMOS®) device certified by CE (Cerbomed GmbH, Erlangen, Germany). It is an external device with a bipolar electrode attached to the skin of the left ear conch.

Radiosurgery

Radiosurgery is a promising alternative to respective surgery and drug-resistant epilepsy, such as CyberKnife® and Gamma Knife® are successful up to some extent but often the safety of the normal tissues surrounding the lesion is at risk due to the radiosensitivity.

Diet Therapy

Ketogenic diet (KD)—diet is strictly prescribed with high fat and low carbohydrates + proteins (3:1 or 4:1) ratio by weight, in patients with drug-resistant epilepsy and where surgery is not possible.

Modified Atkins diet (MAD) is a modified traditional KD. Diet consists of approximately 1:1 [fat: (carbohydrate + protein) weight ratio]. It is highly efficient in both children and adults as it is less complex and more palatable compared to KD. Efficacy in children with refractory epilepsy is similar to KD.

Software

Analysis of user-defined seizure events over a given time period and all the events will be logged in a database for creating customizable reports and graphs of aggregate seizure data. Emergency mobile phone alerts to high-tech seizure pattern analysis software tools are presently available. For example, include EpiTrax eemagine EEG Epivista Epilexia iPlan® Net IdentEvent™ Leonardo Brainmap

Neuroport Software System NeuroScore NeuroGuide Deluxe QEEG 2.5.5 Net Station 4.3

ACTIVITY MODIFICATION AND RESTRICTIONS

Seizure Lifestyle Precautions

- *Driving-motorized vehicles*: Driving laws vary from country to country. Generally, it is not advisable for persons with epilepsy to drive during the first 2 years of treatment. USA permits a person to drive if she/he has been free of seizures between 3 and 18 months. In the UK, a driving license can be granted if the person has been free from seizures for 1 year. In Australia, driving licenses are issued to those who've been seizure-free for a period of 6 months–2 years. As of today, the Government of India has no provision to issue special driving licenses to people with epilepsy (PWE), no matter how long they have been free of seizure.

- *Water precautions*: Should not swim alone, adult lifeguard, wearing a life jacket in a boat is important. Even as simple as taking a bath may be risky.
- *Heights, fire, and power tools*: Use of safety devices, e.g., an automatic shut off switch, is recommended.

CONCLUSION

- There has been tremendous advancement on the diagnostic and therapeutic front of epilepsy. Better education level and awareness is of immense help to reduce the treatment gap in the low- and middle-income countries.
- Video capture of events through the mobile phones and closed circuit TV helps to define the semiology of seizures and accordingly treatment. There are more than 20 antiseizure medicines available in the market with latest introductions have safer and less drug–drug interaction profile.
- Newer devices are immensely not only helpful in early detection of the event but also in drug delivery to terminate the seizures.
- Surgery for epilepsy is becoming available even in relatively smaller cities in addition to the facilities available in Metropolis.

SUGGESTED READINGS

1. Fisher RS, Acevedo C, Arzimanoglou A, et al. ILAE official report: a practical clinical definition of epilepsy. Epilepsia. 2014;55(4):475-82.
2. Scheffer IE, Berkovic S, Capovilla G, et al. ILAE classification of the epilepsies: Position paper of the ILAE Commission for Classification and Terminology. Epilepsia. 2017;58(4):512-521.
3. Fisher RS, Cross JH, French JA, et al. Operational classification of seizure types by the International League Against Epilepsy: Position Paper of the ILAE Commission for Classification and Terminology. Epilepsia. 2017;58(4):522-30.
4. Regg S. The new classification of epilepsy and seizures of the International League Against Epilepsy (ILAE) 2017. Swiss Arch Neurol Psychiatr Psychother. 2019;170:w03059.
5. Liyanagedera S, Williams RP. The new classification of seizures: an overview for the general physician. J R Coll Physicians Edinb. 2017;47(4):336-8.
6. Perucca P, Scheffer IE, Kiley M. The management of epilepsy in children and adults. Medical Journal of Australia. 2018;208(5):226-33.
7. Schachter SC. Uptodate. (2010). [online]. Available from: https://www.uptodate.com/contents/overview-of-the-management-of-epilepsy-in-adults.
8. Ko DY. (2022). Epilepsy and Seizures Treatment and Management: Approach Considerations, Anticonvulsant Therapy, Anticonvulsants for Specific Seizure Types. [online] Available from https://emedicine.medscape.com/article/1184846-treatment [Last accessed October, 2022].
9. Yasam V, Jakki S, Senthil V. An Overview of Non-drug Therapies for the Treatment of Epilepsy. Indian J Pharm Sci. 2018;80:223-34.
10. http://www.epilepsyindia.org/documents/EpilepsyLawIndia_Book.pdf

CHAPTER

60

Changing the Course of Allergic March

Pradyumn Sharma

■ WHAT IS ALLERGIC MARCH?

The term "allergic march" (also called "atopic march") refers to the natural history of atopic manifestations, which is characterized by a typical sequence of immunoglobulin E (IgE) antibody responses, and clinical symptoms which may appear early in life, persist over years or decades, and often remit spontaneously with age **(Fig. 1)**.

■ INTRODUCTION

The development of atopic dermatitis (AD) in infancy and subsequent allergic rhinitis and asthma in later childhood is known as the atopic march. This progressive atopy is

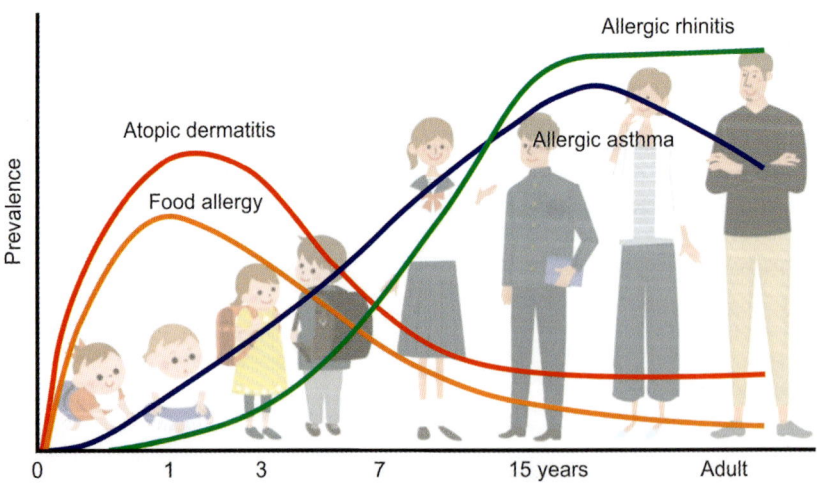

FIG. 1: Allergic march.

dependent on various underlying factors such as the presence of filaggrin mutations as well as the time of onset and severity of AD. Clinical manifestations vary among individuals. Previously, it was thought that atopic disorders may be unrelated to sequential development. Recent studies support the idea of a causal link between AD and later onset atopic disorders. These studies suggest that a dysfunctional skin barrier serves as a site for allergic sensitization to antigens and colonization of bacterial superantigens. This induces systemic Th2 immunity that predisposes patients to allergic nasal responses and promotes airway hyper-reactivity. While AD often starts early in life and is a chronic condition, new research signifies that there may be an optimal window of time in which targeting the skin barrier with therapeutic interventions may prevent subsequent atopic disorders. In this chapter, we highlight recent studies describing factors important in the development of atopic disorders and new insights into our understanding of the pathogenesis of the atopic march.

▉ WHAT CAUSES ALLERGIC MARCH?

The development of AD in infancy and subsequent allergic rhinitis and asthma in later childhood is known as the atopic march. This progressive atopy is dependent on various underlying factors such as the presence of filaggrin mutations as well as the time of onset and severity of AD.

Atopic diseases, including AD, allergic rhinitis, and asthma, have increased in frequency in recent decades and now affect approximately 20% of the population worldwide. The concept of the atopic march was developed to describe the progression of atopic disorders from AD in infants to allergic rhinitis and asthma in children.

Patients with AD may develop a typical sequence of AD, allergic rhinitis, and asthma at certain ages. Some may have disease that persists for several years, whereas others may see improvement or resolution with increasing age.

Studies have suggested a link between eczema and later onset allergies. In addition, scientists believe that a dysfunction in the skin barrier can cause eczema and predispose children to developing food allergies and general immune hyper-reactivity.

Eczema affects 3% of adults and 30% of children.

One study found that of kids with eczema, 50% of them developed a food allergy by the age of 1.3 years.

Eczema and other allergies are caused by a combination of environmental and genetic factors. However, scientists believe that the increase in allergic asthma prevalence may also be linked to lifestyle factors and changes in environmental situations, such as dust mites and outdoor air pollution.

▉ ROLE OF FOOD ALLERGY IN THE ATOPIC MARCH

Early sensitization to food and the presence of a filaggrin mutation in infants with early onset eczema each increased the risk for persistent eczema and for subsequent asthma **(Fig. 2)**.

A prospective 10-year follow-up study investigated whether the atopic march theory could be applied to local allergic rhinitis, a newly described entity in which patients demonstrate elevated local specific IgE and markers of allergic inflammation with positive nasal provocation tests but exhibit no systemic sensitization with negative skin prick testing (SPT) and serum specific IgE levels **(Fig. 3)**.

Course of allergy march can be changed by:
- Allergen-specific immunotherapy
- Anti-IgE therapy—omalizumab

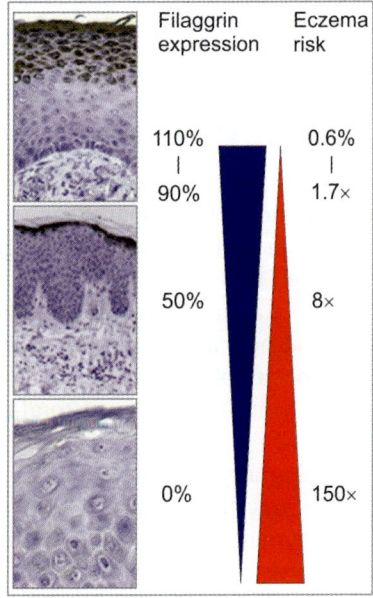

FIG. 2: Filaggrin—skin barrier formation and hydration.

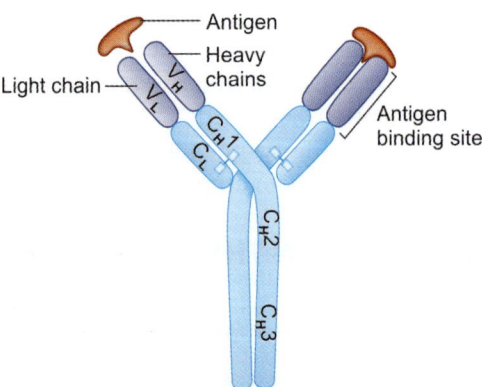

FIG. 3: Immunoglobulin.

Allergen-specific Immunotherapy

Allergen-specific immunotherapy (also known as allergy shots) is an effective treatment used by allergists and immunologists for common allergic conditions, particularly allergic rhinitis/conjunctivitis, allergic asthma, and stinging insect hypersensitivity.

This form of therapy typically involves the subcutaneous administration of gradually increasing quantities of the patient's relevant allergens until a dose is reached that is effective in inducing immunologic tolerance to the allergens. The primary objectives of allergen-specific immunotherapy are to decrease the symptoms triggered by allergens and to prevent recurrence of the disease in the long term. Currently, it is the only identified disease-modifying intervention for allergic diseases **(Fig. 4)**.

Successful immunotherapy has been associated with a shift from T helper cell type-2 (Th2) immune responses, which are associated with the development of atopic conditions, to Th1 immune responses. It is also associated with the production of T regulatory cells that produce the anti-inflammatory cytokine, interleukin-10 (IL-10), amongst others such as transforming growth factor-beta (TGF-β). IL-10 has been shown to reduce the levels of allergen-specific IgE antibodies, increase the levels of immunoglobulin G (IgG) (blocking) antibodies that play a role in secondary immune responses, and reduce the release of pro-inflammatory cytokines from mast cells, eosinophils, and T cells. Allergen-specific immunotherapy has also been found to decrease the recruitment of mast cells, basophils, and eosinophils to the skin, nose, eye, and bronchial mucosa after exposure to allergens and reduce the release of mediators, such as histamine, from basophils and mast cells.

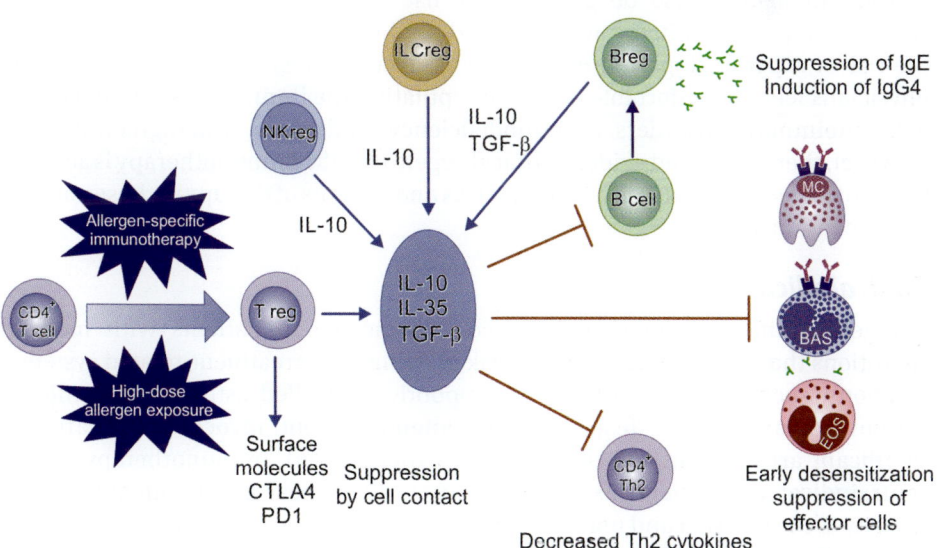

FIG. 4: Mechanisms of allergen-specific immunotherapy and allergen tolerance.

Indications

Allergen-specific immunotherapy is indicated in patients with allergic rhinitis/conjunctivitis and/or allergic asthma who have evidence of specific IgE antibodies to clinically relevant allergens. SPT is the preferred method of testing for specific IgE antibodies. Allergen-specific IgE testing which provides an in vitro measure of a patient's specific IgE levels against particular allergens is a reasonable alternative to SPT. However, SPTs are generally considered to be more sensitive and cost effective than allergen-specific IgE tests.

Patients with allergic rhinitis/conjunctivitis or allergic asthma who may be good candidates for immunotherapy include those who have symptoms that are not well controlled by pharmacological therapy or avoidance measures; require high doses of medication, multiple medications, or both to maintain control of their disease; experience adverse effects of medications; or wish to avoid the long-term use of pharmacological therapy.

Special Considerations

Special consideration should be given to the use of allergen-specific immunotherapy in children under 6 years of age, pregnant women, the elderly, and patients with malignancy or immunodeficiency/autoimmune diseases.

Immunotherapy is effective in children and is often well tolerated. However, children less than 6 years of age may have difficulty cooperating with the immunotherapy regimen and injections and, therefore, physicians need to weigh the risks and benefits of therapy in this patient population. Immunotherapy is generally not initiated in pregnant women; however, it can be safely continued in women who have been on treatment prior to becoming pregnant. Special consideration must also be given to the use of immunotherapy in the elderly since these patients often have comorbid medical conditions that may increase the risk of experiencing immunotherapy-associated adverse events. Finally, some physicians feel uncomfortable about manipulating the immune system in patients with autoimmune disorders, immunodeficiency syndromes, or malignant disease. However, there is no solid evidence that allergen-specific immunotherapy is actually harmful to these patients, provided the risks and benefits of therapy in these patients have been considered.

Contraindications

Allergen-specific immunotherapy is contraindicated in patients with medical conditions that increase the patient's risk of dying from treatment-related systemic reactions, such as those with severe or poorly controlled asthma or significant cardiovascular diseases (e.g., unstable angina, recent myocardial infarction, significant arrhythmia, and uncontrolled hypertension). Immunotherapy is also contraindicated in patients using beta-blockers since these agents can amplify the severity of the reaction and make the treatment of systemic reactions more difficult. Immunotherapy should be considered, however, in patients with life-threatening stinging insect hypersensitivity, even if they also require beta-blocker medications, because the fatal risk associated with an insect sting is greater than the risk of an immunotherapy-related systemic reaction.

TYPES OF IMMUNOTHERAPY

Immunotherapy is of two types:
1. Subcutaneous immunotherapy (SCIT)
2. Sublingual immunotherapy (SLIT)

Subcutaneous Immunotherapy

Subcutaneous immunotherapy is a form of SIT, whereby small doses of specific allergens are administered by injection, and refers to what is commonly known as an "allergy shot." It is currently the standard in allergen desensitization and provides symptomatic relief for patients with allergic rhinitis and asthma **(Fig. 5)**.

Safety

Allergen-specific immunotherapy is generally safe and well tolerated when used in appropriately selected patients. However, local and systemic reactions may occur. Local reactions, such as redness or itching at the injection site, can generally be managed with local treatment (e.g., cool compresses or topical corticosteroids) or oral antihistamines. Systemic reactions occur in approximately 1–4% of patients on allergen immunotherapy and can be mild-to-severe. The most severe reaction is anaphylaxis. Fatal anaphylactic reactions are rare, occurring in an estimated 1 in every 8 million doses of immunotherapy administered

Sublingual Immunotherapy

Immunotherapy treats the cause of allergies by giving small doses of what a person is allergic to, which increases "immunity" or tolerance to the allergen and reduces the allergic symptoms. Unlike injection immunotherapy, which is given as shots, SLIT is given as drops under the tongue **(Fig. 6)**.

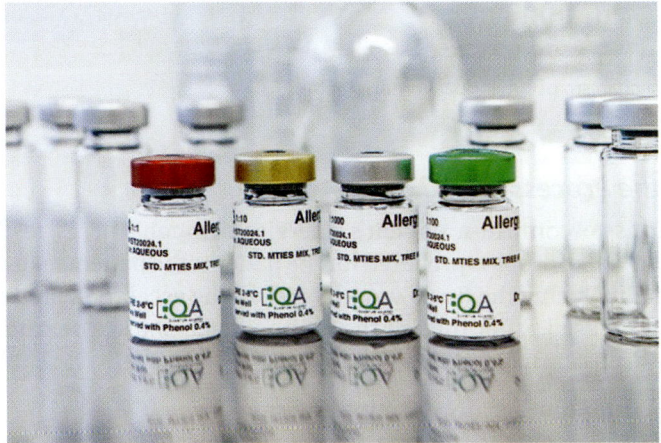

FIG. 5: Subcutaneous immunotherapy.

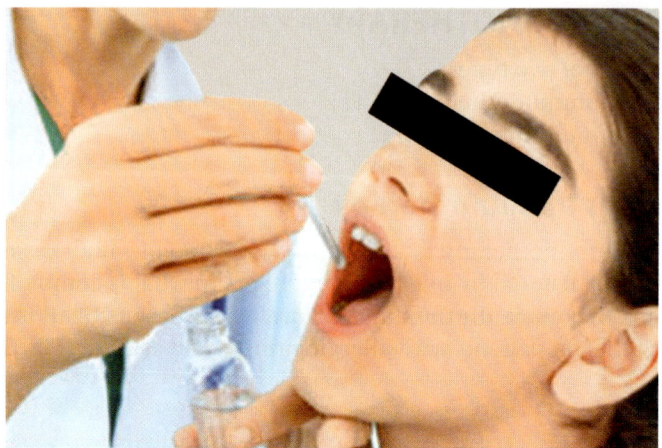

FIG. 6: Sublingual immunotherapy.

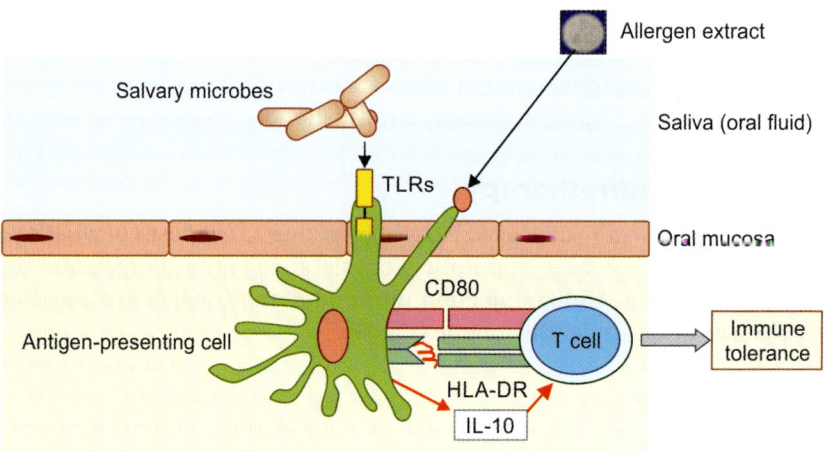

FIG. 7: Mechanism of sublingual immunotherapy.

How does the Process Work?

The first step is to confirm a patient's allergies through allergy testing. Then, a custom-mixed vial of drops is prepared for the patient. The patient takes drops under the tongue daily. During the first 4 months, called the escalation phase, the dosage is gradually increased. After that, in the maintenance phase, the patient takes the same dose of drops each day **(Fig. 7)**.

Is sublingual immunotherapy effective and safe?

Most clinical trials and surveys published over at least 20 years show that SLIT is relatively safe and effective for the treatment of rhinitis and asthma caused by allergies to dust mites, grass, ragweed, cat dander, and tree pollens. Evidence is emerging that SLIT may be effective for treating the red, itchy eyes caused by pollen during hay fever season. In addition, it might prove an effective therapy for children with mild eczema and is currently being studied for its potential in treating food allergies.

Side effects among both children and adults are usually local and mild, most often occur early in treatment, and include itching in the mouth or stomach problems. These can usually be managed by dose adjustments. Very rarely, severe allergic reactions (anaphylaxis) have been reported using SLIT. Therefore, this treatment is best prescribed by an allergist.

■ KEY TAKE-HOME MESSAGES

Allergen-specific immunotherapy is a potentially disease-modifying therapy that is effective for the treatment of allergic rhinitis/conjunctivitis, allergic asthma, and stinging insect hypersensitivity.

Allergen immunotherapy is contraindicated in patients on beta-blockers, those with uncontrolled or severe asthma, or those with significant comorbid cardiovascular disease.

The decision to proceed with allergen immunotherapy should be made on a case-by-case basis, taking into account individual patient factors such as disease severity, efficacy of avoidance measures and pharmacological therapy, and patient preferences.

Allergen immunotherapy carries the risk of anaphylactic reactions and, therefore, should only be prescribed by physicians who are adequately trained in the treatment of allergy.

Injections must be given under medical supervision in clinics that are equipped to manage life-threatening anaphylaxis.

■ ANTI IGE THERAPY: OMALIZUMAB

Omalizumab binds with free IgE and prevents free IgE from attaching to high-affinity IgE receptor (Fc epsilon RI) on effector cells such as mast cells, basophils, and dendritic cells. The result is a blocking of mediator release from these cells and the inhibition of antigen presentation by dendritic cells.

Omalizumab prevents early and late phase allergic reactions of skin and lungs. It has been investigated extensively in moderate-to-severe asthma in adults and children. It effectively reduces rates of asthma exacerbation, emergency visits for asthma, and hospital admissions among these patients. Currently, omalizumab is primarily indicated for patients, age 6 years and over, with moderate-to-severe asthma (GINA step 4). Omalizumab was investigated in patients with seasonal allergic rhinitis (to ragweed, birch, and grass pollens) and has been found to improve rhinitis symptoms and to reduce medication use among these patients. Administered together with allergen immunotherapy, omalizumab reduced the incidence of side effects and rates of anaphylaxis from allergen immunotherapy. Omalizumab has been investigated in the treatment of food allergy, AD, and urticaria.

Biologic therapy drugs for treating allergy and asthma
- Xolair® (omalizumab)
- Nucala® (mepolizumab)
- Cinqair® (reslizumab)
- Fasenra® (benralizumab)
- Dupixent® (dupilumab)

CONCLUSION

Allergen-specific immunotherapy along with omalizumab has very promising results in changing the course of allergic march.

SUGGESTED READINGS

1. Spergel JM, Paller AS. Atopic dermatitis and the atopic march. J Allergy Clin Immunol. 2003;112:S118-27.
2. Spergel JM. Epidemiology of atopic dermatitis and atopic march in children. Immunol Allergy Clin North Am. 2010;30:269-80.
3. World Allergy Organization. The allergic march. [online] Available from https://www.worldallergy.org › education [Last accessed October, 2022].
4. Filipiak-Pittroff B, Schnopp C, Berdel D. Value of food sensitization and filaggrin mutations in children with eczema. J Allergy Clin Immunol. 2011;128:1235-41.
5. Abramson MJ, Puy RM, Weiner JM. Allergen immunotherapy for asthma. Cochrane Database Syst Rev. 2003;CD001186.
6. Abramson MJ, Puy MR, Weiner JM. Is allergen immunotherapy effective in asthma? A meta-analysis of randomized controlled trials. Am J Respir Crit Care Med. 1995;151:969-74.
7. Ross RN, Nelson HS, Finegold I. Effectiveness of specific immunotherapy in the treatment of allergic rhinitis: an analysis. Clin Ther. 2000;22:342-50.
8. Ross RN, Nelson HS, Finegold I. Effectiveness of specific immunotherapy in the treatment of asthma: a meta-analysis of prospective, randomized, double-blind, placebo-controlled studies. Clin Ther. 2000;22:329-41.
9. Frew AJ. Allergen immunotherapy. J Allergy Clin Immunol. 2010;125:S306-13.
10. Canadian Society of Allergy and Clinical Immunology: Immunotherapy Manual. Fall. 2010
11. Joint Task Force on Practice Parameters, American Academy of Allergy, Asthma and Immunology, American College of Allergy, Asthma and Immunology, Joint Council of Allergy, Asthma and Immunology: Allergen immunotherapy: a practice parameter second update. J Allergy Clin Immunol. 2007;120 (3 Suppl):S25-85.
12. D'Amato G, Liccardi G, Noschese P, et al. Anti-IgE monoclonal antibody (omalizumab) in the treatment of atopic asthma and allergic respiratory diseases. Curr Drug Targets Inflamm Allergy. 2004;3(3):227-9.

CHAPTER 61

Recent Advances in Management of Interstitial Lung Disease

Prashant Prakash, SK Kushwah

■ INTRODUCTION AND CLASSIFICATION

Interstitial lung diseases (ILDs) are a "heterogenous group of more than 150 disease entities that differ significantly with respect to prevention, therapy, and prognosis." The current classification scheme of ILDs is shown in **Flowchart 1**. The "multidisciplinary classification of the idiopathic interstitial pneumonias (IIPs) has been updated by an official American Thoracic Society (ATS)/European Respiratory Society (ERS) statement in 2013 by which IIPs have been classified into major IIPs,

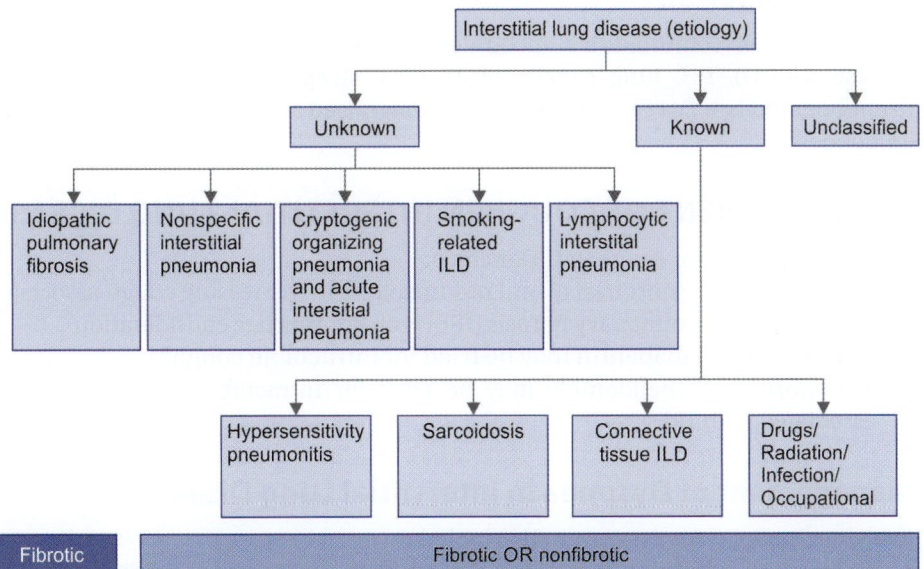

FLOWCHART 1: Classification of ILD on the basis of known or unknown etiology.
(ILD: interstitial lung disease)

TABLE 1: Categorization of major idiopathic interstitial pneumonias.		
Category	Clinical-radiological-pathologic diagnosis	Associated radiologic and/or pathologic-morphologic patterns
Chronic fibrosing interstitial pneumonia (IP)	• Idiopathic pulmonary fibrosis • Idiopathic nonspecific IP	• Usual IP • Nonspecific IP
Smoking-related IP*	• Respiratory bronchiolitis-interstitial lung disease • Desquamative IP	• Respiratory bronchiolitis • Desquamative IP
Acute/Subacute IP	• Cryptogenic organizing pneumonia • Acute IP	• Organizing pneumonia • Diffuse alveolar damage

*Desquamative IP can occasionally occur in nonsmokers.

rare IIPs, and unclassifiable cases. The major IIPs are grouped into chronic fibrosing, smoking-related, and acute/subacute IIPs **(Table 1)**".

The diagnostic strategy in a patient with ILD is based on considerations regarding the dynamic time course (acute, subacute, chronic), cause (known or unknown), and context of the disease at presentation (presence of extrapulmonary/systemic disease manifestations).

The management of ILDs can be broadly divided into general management of common comorbidities, management of symptoms such as cough, dyspnea, and pulmonary hypertension (PH), and specific therapies.

■ MANAGEMENT OF COMORBIDITIES IN INTERSTITIAL LUNG DISEASE

"Most common comorbidities encountered in ILD are gastroesophageal reflux disease (GERD), PH, lung cancer, obstructive sleep apnea (OSA), and venous thromboembolism (VTE), which have to be diagnosed and managed as per existing guidelines".

■ MANAGEMENT OF COUGH IN INTERSTITIAL LUNG DISEASE

Evolving therapies for cough in ILD include:
- *Prednisolone*: "A short trial of oral prednisolone in distressing cough associated with idiopathic pulmonary fibrosis (IPF) is an appropriate consideration".
- *Gabapentin*: "Gabapentin may be tried for intractable cough".
- *Thalidomide*: "Thalidomide may be tried for intractable/distressing cough associated with IPF".

Management of Dyspnea in Interstitial Lung Disease

Evolving therapies for dyspnea in ILD include:
- *Pulmonary rehabilitation*: It is advocated in dyspneic patients with ILD. Pulmonary rehabilitation has no beneficial effects on survival. The effects last as long as the program is continued.

- *Supplemental oxygen*: It is recommended in "patients with documented resting hypoxemia and/or exercise-induced hypoxemia, and desaturation while sleeping. Long-term oxygen therapy (LTOT) is indicated for patients with ILD who have persistent resting hypoxemia".
- *Nebulized opioid therapy*: "Nebulized opioid therapy is not beneficial to relieve dyspnea in all ILD patients and may be used only for patients receiving comfort and palliative care".

VACCINATION IN INTERSTITIAL LUNG DISEASES

According to a "consensus statement of Indian Chest Society (ICS) and National College of Chest Physicians (NCCP) on management of ILDs, vaccinations (influenza and pneumococci) are advocated for all patients with ILD".

MANAGEMENT OF PULMONARY HYPERTENSION IN INTERSTITIAL LUNG DISEASE

Evolving therapies for PH in ILD include:
- "The consensus statement of ICS and NCCP on management of ILDs endorses the guidelines for management of chronic PH, specific therapy for patients with PH, and the treatment of underlying lung disease as the mainstay of therapy and supplemental oxygen in cases of hypoxemia".
- "Ambrisentan is contraindicated in patients with PH related to IPF. The therapeutic benefits of other PH-specific therapy in ILD-related PH remains unknown".

ROLE OF NONINVASIVE VENTILATION AND MECHANICAL VENTILATION IN INTERSTITIAL LUNG DISEASE

- "Consideration of noninvasive ventilation (NIV) is advocated as early as possible in patients who require high-flow supplemental oxygen at rest, especially in patients manifesting acute exacerbation (AE) ILD with respiratory failure as it has been associated with better short-term outcomes".
- "The consideration of mechanical ventilation (MV) in patients with AE ILD with respiratory failure should be made only after proper counseling".

ROLE OF LUNG TRANSPLANTATION IN INTERSTITIAL LUNG DISEASE

- "Lung transplantation is the only treatment with clearly proven survival benefit in advanced ILD, especially IPF, and should be considered in carefully selected patients".
- "Posttransplant survival is variable in lung transplant programs. While the 5-year survival in most experienced lung transplant programs is about 70%, less experienced programs have lesser survival rates".

MANAGEMENT OF IDIOPATHIC INTERSTITIAL PNEUMONIAS

The diagnosis of IIPs requires exclusion of known causes of ILD such as drug or inhalational exposure and connective tissue disease (CTD)–ILD. The major IIPs are grouped into chronic fibrosing, smoking-related, and acute/subacute IIPs **(Table 1)**. The doses, side effects, and management of side effects of commonly used drugs in ILDs are outlined in **Table 2**.

Chronic Fibrosing Idiopathic Interstitial Pneumonias

Idiopathic Pulmonary Fibrosis

Idiopathic pulmonary fibrosis is defined as a specific form of "chronic, progressive fibrosing interstitial pneumonia of unknown cause, occurring primarily in older

TABLE 2: Doses, side effects, and management of side effects of commonly used drugs in the treatment of ILD.

Drug	Dose	Side effect	How to manage side effect
Pirfenidone	1,800–2,400 mg/day in divided doses, 200 mg three tablets thrice a day	Nausea, vomiting photosensitivity, rash, elevated liver enzymes	• Reduce or stop the drug, PPI • Cover exposed skin, sunscreen • Monitor LFT monthly for 6 months, thereafter 3 monthly
Nintedanib	150 mg twice a day	Diarrhea, nausea, vomiting, elevated liver enzymes	• Reduce or stop drug, Imodium • Reduce or stop drug, PPI • Monitor LFT monthly for 3 months, thereafter 3 monthly
N-acetylcysteine	600 mg thrice a day	Nausea, vomiting, diarrhea	Self-limiting, reduce or stop the drug
Prednisolone	1 mg/kg BW tapered to 0.25 mg/kg BW*	• Hyperglycemia • Hypertension • Swelling face • Osteoporosis • Reduced immunity • Weight gain	• Bring to the lowest dose possible, sugar avoidance, oral hypoglycemics (if the patient develops diabetes mellitus), exercise salt avoidance, calcium, bisphosphonates, exercise • Bring to the lowest dose possible, PCP prophylaxis, influenza vaccine (once steroid dose is <7.5 mg/day), avoid crowded places • Dietary modification, exercise, bring to lowest dose
Azathioprine	50 mg twice a day	Cytopenias Infections Nausea, vomiting	• Reduce or stop drug, monitor CBC monthly till 6 months, thereafter 3 monthly • Reduce dose, avoid crowded places, PCP prophylaxis • Reduce or stop the drug, PPI

Continued

Continued

Drug	Dose	Side effect	How to manage side effect
Methotrexate[†]	10 mg/week may be increased to 20 mg/week and brought down to 5 mg/week	• Hematological neutropenia, thrombocytopenias • Gastrointestinal • Hepatic • Pulmonary toxicity • Teratogenicity	• Reduce or stop the dose • Folic acid is added once a week • Give with food • PPI • Split the dose • Stop or reduce dose • Monitor LFT • Stop the drug • Birth control till 6 months after stopping the drug
MMF	1.5–3 mg/day	• Leucopenia • Diarrhea	• Reduce or stop the drug • Reduce dose, hydration
Cyclophosphamide	500–1,000 mg IV per 4 weeks or 1–2 mg/day orally	• Hemorrhagic cystitis • Neutropenia • Infertility	• Mesna • Hydration • Less with intermittent dosing • Monitoring CBC • Leuprorelin
Infliximab	3 mg/kg at 0, 2, 6, 12, 18, 24 weeks	• Allergic reactions • Infections	• Slow infusion, antiallergics, paracetamol corticosteroid loading • Rule out pulmonary tuberculosis prior to initiation, PCP prophylaxis, monitoring
Rituximab	1,000 mg IV repeat at 2 weeks	• Allergic reactions • Cytopenias • Infections	• Stop infusion • Antiallergic medications, paracetamol corticosteroid loading • CBC monitoring • PCP prophylaxis, monitoring

[*]In Scleroderma ILD the dose of prednisolone should be kept <10 mg/day.
[†]Patients on methotrexate should be followed up with monthly CBC, LFT and RFT for 6 months followed by 3 monthly testing.
(BW: body weight; CBC: complete blood count; ILD: interstitial lung disease; IV: intravenous; LFT: liver function test; MMF: mycophenolate mofetil; PCP: *Pneumocystis carinii*; PPI: proton-pump inhibitor)

adults (sixth to seventh decade), limited to the lungs, and associated with the histopathologic and/or radiologic pattern of usual interstitial pneumonia (UIP) defined".

The diagnosis of "IPF requires (1) exclusion of other known causes of ILD, (2) the presence of a UIP pattern on high-resolution computed tomography (HRCT) in patients not subjected to surgical lung biopsy (SLB), and (3) specific combinations of HRCT and SLB patterns in patients subjected to SLB".

The consensus statement of the ICS and NCCP on the management of ILDs outline the following management protocols in IPF:

- "All symptomatic IPF patients with forced vital capacity (FVC) of >50% predicted should be initiated on pirfenidone".
- "The patients on pirfenidone developing ≥10% subsequent decline in FVC in any 6–12 months period should be given a choice of continuation of therapy or switch to an alternative therapy depending on case-to-case basis".
- "All symptomatic IPF patients with FVC of >50% predicted should be initiated on nintedanib".
- "The patients on nintedanib developing ≥10% subsequent decline in FVC in any 6–12 months period should be given a choice of continuation of therapy or switch to an alternative therapy on case-to-case basis".
- "Either pirfenidone or nintedanib may be chosen for patients with IPF based on patient preference and tolerability".
- "Duration of treatment is lifelong".
- "N-acetylcysteine (NAC) is currently not recommended for routine treatment of IPF and may be considered in certain subgroups on a case-to-case basis".
- "More evidence is needed to recommend the use of pirfenidone in combination with nintedanib or NAC and the dose of individual drugs to be used in such therapy in patients with IPF".

"Pirfenidone has been associated with slowing of the absolute decline in FVC, increases progression-free survival, and reduces mortality. Nintedanib has been associated with reduction in decline in predicted FVC, acute exacerbation and risk of all cause, and respiratory-related and on treatment mortality".

Idiopathic Nonspecific Interstitial Pneumonia

The typical clinical presentation in idiopathic nonspecific interstitial pneumonia (NSIP) was breathlessness and cough of 6–7 months' duration, predominantly in women, in never-smokers, and in the sixth decade of life. Importantly, "the NSIP pattern occurs not only as an idiopathic condition but also in a variety of settings including CTD–ILD, hypersensitivity pneumonitis (HP), and drug toxicity, and in some patients with familial pulmonary fibrosis".

The consensus statement of the ICS and NCCP on the management of ILDs outlines the following management protocols in NSIP:
- "Oral corticosteroids are recommended for the treatment of NSIP".
- "Immunosuppressants, for example, cyclophosphamide, might be utilized as add-on treatment in patients not receptive to steroids".

"Corticosteroids improve symptom score and lung function with response more pronounced in cellular NSIP, concomitant consolidation, seronegative antinuclear antibody (ANA), and shorter disease duration. In asymptomatic or mildly symptomatic cases, close observation is often done as the risk of treatment outweighs the benefits. In symptomatic patients, oral corticosteroids are the mainstay of therapy".

Smoking-related Idiopathic Interstitial Pneumonias

Respiratory Bronchiolitis—Interstitial Lung Disease

Histologic respiratory bronchiolitis (RB) "is always present in current smokers and can be viewed as a physiological response to smoking, which in a few individuals becomes extensive enough to result in an ILD (RB-ILD)". The only proven therapy for RB-ILD is smoking cessation. Only those who continue to be symptomatic in spite of smoking cessation should be considered for corticosteroid therapy.

Desquamative Interstitial Pneumonia

"Desquamative interstitial pneumonia (DIP) has been recognized in nonsmokers, perhaps reflecting extension of childhood DIP into adult life [with the latter often due to surfactant protein (SP) gene mutations]. The 10-year survival remains approximately 70%, with resistance to treatment in a significant minority". There is clinical response to smoking cessation alone or in combination with corticosteroid therapy, as well as some possible spontaneous resolution.

Acute or Subacute Idiopathic Interstitial Pneumonias

Cryptogenic Organizing Pneumonia

"Patients with cryptogenic organizing pneumonia (COP) typically present with a subacute illness of relatively short duration (median, <3 months) with variable degrees of cough and dyspnea. The majority of patients recover completely with oral corticosteroids, but relapse is common". Cytotoxic drugs and steroid-sparing agents are used in addition to corticosteroid where there is slow response to steroids alone. A small group (10–15%) may progress to pulmonary fibrosis and one-third of the patients can relapse. Factors that may predict poor outcome include the lack of lymphocytosis on bronchoalveolar lavage (BAL), predominantly interstitial pattern of imaging, and histological features of scarring and remodeling of lung parenchyma.

Acute Interstitial Pneumonia

"Acute interstitial pneumonia (AIP) is a distinct IIP characterized by rapidly progressive hypoxemia, mortality of 50% or more, and no proven treatment. Survivors usually have a good long-term prognosis [similar to adult respiratory distress syndrome (ARDS) survivors] but some experience recurrences or chronic, progressive ILD. AIP is idiopathic and should be distinguished from ARDS with known cause". Since there is no proven treatment, supportive care with oxygen supplementation and MV is indicated. Early corticosteroid therapy and combination therapy with intravenous cyclophosphamide and vincristine have been reported.

■ MANAGEMENT OF HYPERSENSITIVITY PNEUMONITIS

"Hypersensitivity pneumonitis appears to be more common in men and during middle age, although it is not known whether this reflects host predisposition or merely frequency of exposure to relevant antigens. The disease is sometimes progressive and the development of lung fibrosis is associated with an increased mortality. Inhalation of organic particles is the most common cause of HP, but it can occur following inhalation of inorganic chemicals and, occasionally, ingestion of drugs".

Traditionally, "HP is categorized as acute, subacute, or chronic. Acute HP presents 4–8 hours after often heavy exposure with fever, malaise, cough, dyspnea, and chest tightness. The symptoms remit over 24–48 hours in the absence of further exposure. The subacute and chronic forms usually occur with ongoing lower-level exposure. Dyspnea, cough, and fatigue develop insidiously, and weight loss is a common feature. Patients with chronic HP typically do not give a history of acute symptoms but present with diffuse pulmonary fibrosis, which must be distinguished from other conditions including IPF and fibrotic NSIP".

The consensus statement of the ICS and NCCP on management of ILDs outline the following management protocols in HP:
- Oral corticosteroids
- Azathioprine
- Mycophenolate (MMF)

"Oral corticosteroids for 4–12 weeks are an appropriate treatment option for patients with acute/subacute HP with monitoring of lung function parameters and side effects. Prolonged use of oral steroids, azathioprine, and MMF should be based on clinical response and tolerance. In patients with acute HP, there is improvement in symptoms and lung functions with oral corticosteroid. However, this benefit is not sustained over long term".

"There is a lack of evidence pertaining to duration and dose of corticosteroids for long-term therapy in HP. Prolonged use of corticosteroids and other immunosuppressants should be prescribed after weighing benefit of individual response and side effects associated with the drugs. Inability to identify the inciting antigen is associated with worse survival. Thereby, every effort should be made to identify the inciting antigen".

MANAGEMENT OF CONNECTIVE TISSUE DISEASE-ASSOCIATED INTERSTITIAL LUNG DISEASE

Connective tissue disease may be associated with pleura-parenchymal disease or sometimes interstitial tissue involvement of the lung. The ILD in CTD may either be an initial manifestation or may manifest after a long-standing autoimmune illness. The presentation of CTD-associated ILD is challenging due to the occurrence of a variety of interstitial pneumonia patterns, and the presentation of ILDs is also variable. The prevalence of CTD–ILD is the highest in systemic sclerosis (SSc) and the least in systemic lupus erythematosus (SLE). An acute presentation of ILD is more common in SLE and polymyositis/dermatomyositis (PM/DM).

The management protocols of individual connective tissue lung diseases associated with ILD as per the consensus statement of the ICS and NCCP are as follows:

Rheumatoid Arthritis-associated Interstitial Lung Disease

- "Corticosteroids might be utilized in the treatment of rheumatoid arthritis (RA)-ILD. They are anti-inflammatory drugs which help suppress disease activity, leading to improvement in symptoms and lung functions".
- In case of "poor response to corticosteroids, cyclophosphamide, mycophenolate mofetil, and rituximab might be utilized in the treatment of RA-ILD".

- The following other drugs have a role in "RA patients who develop ILD":
  - "Methotrexate ought to be stopped in patients of RA determined to have ILD".
  - "Leflunomide can be given in patients determined to have RA–ILD".
  - "Other antitumor necrosis factor (TNF) agents might be utilized with caution".

Scleroderma-associated Interstitial Lung Disease

- "Low-dose steroids may be continued in the treatment of scleroderma-associated ILD (SSC–ILD). High-dose steroids should be avoided in scleroderma as it is associated with the risk of renal crisis. Immunosuppression and secondary infection are a dreaded complication of these drugs. Effect lasts till the drugs are taken and there is no long-lasting benefits".
- "Treatment in SSC–ILD may be initiated in cases with progressive disease with either cyclophosphamide or mycophenolate mofetil".
- "Mycophenolate mofetil has better tolerability and lesser side effects, though more expensive".
- "Azathioprine is an alternate drug for maintenance therapy in SSC–ILD".
- "Rituximab could be considered in patients with refractory scleroderma. It should be administered at tertiary care level after evaluating for the pros and cons of treatment".
- "Nintedanib, an antifibrotic drug, has been shown to reduce the annual decline in lung functions associated with SSC–ILD. However, there was no advantage on the other manifestations of the SSC".

Sjögren's Syndrome

The treatment of Sjögren's syndrome and ILD remains empiric, since no controlled studies have been performed. In symptomatic patients with Sjögren's syndrome and ILD and functional deterioration, the standard treatment is oral prednisone in the dosage of 1 mg/kg/day with subsequent tapering, continued for at least 6 months. The patients who do not improve with systemic glucocorticoids should receive azathioprine, cyclophosphamide, and cyclosporine.

Dermatomyositis and Polymyositis

Treatment of ILD in patients with myositis almost always requires glucocorticoids, regardless of whether pulmonary or muscle disease is the predominant feature of the patient's illness. No controlled trials of glucocorticoids have been undertaken; about 50% myositis patients with ILD respond to corticosteroids.

Since ILD is a fatal disease, a second agent is added from the beginning of therapy in patients with DM or PM complicated by ILD. Options for this second agent in patients with mild ILD include azathioprine and methotrexate; azathioprine is preferred because of its favorable side effect profile. In patients with moderate-to-severe ILD, cyclophosphamide is given. In patients with inexorable disease, rituximab and intravenous immunoglobulin (IVIG) are the most commonly used treatment options.

The commonly employed drugs for CTD-related pulmonary diseases are listed in **Box 1**.

> **BOX 1: Common drugs employed for the treatment of connective tissue disease (CTD)-related lung diseases.**
> - Corticosteroids, cyclophosphamide, methotrexate and azathioprine, and biological agents are the main drugs used for CTD-related lung diseases
> - Rheumatoid arthritis-related interstitial lung disease responds to corticosteroids and methotrexate
> - Corticosteroids are not useful in scleroderma-related lung disease; cyclophosphamide is the drug of choice
> - Acute lupus pneumonitis responds to corticosteroids
> - Collagen vascular disease-related OP/CP has good prognosis and responds to corticosteroids
> - Polymyositis-dermatomyositis-related lung disease is fatal; corticosteroids and cyclophosphamide should be used

MANAGEMENT OF SARCOIDOSIS

The consensus statement of the ICS and NCCP on the management of ILDs outline the following drugs for management in sarcoidosis:
- *Corticosteroids*: "They improve dyspnea score, lung functions, and radiology in sarcoidosis. Corticosteroids have no significant benefits for asymptomatic stage 0/1 sarcoidosis. Moreover, the effects last as long as they are used. There are no long-term benefits in terms of lung functions. Immunosuppression is another concerning feature not only for corticosteroids but also for other immunosuppressants".
- *Methotrexate*:
- *Azathioprine*:
- *Leflunomide*:

"May be tried in patients not responding to oral steroids or with associated steroid toxicity"

- *Hydroxychloroquine*:
- *Infliximab*:

"May be tried after carefully weighing the risk-benefit ratio in patients with refractory pulmonary sarcoidosis".

Management Protocols in Sarcoidosis
- "Observe patients without pharmacological interventions in patients who are asymptomatic stage 0/1 pulmonary sarcoidosis".
- "Treat patients with symptomatic stage 1 and all stage 2, 3, and 4 pulmonary sarcoidosis with oral corticosteroids".

CONCLUSION

To conclude, pirfenidone/nintedanib seem to have a prominent role in IPF. In other ILDs, the role of these two drugs is limited. Corticosteroids are advocated in most ILDs except IPF and chronic HP. The role of other immunosuppressants is limited in IPF but they seem to have a role in other ILDs, especially in case of no response to corticosteroids or where the use of corticosteroids is limited by their side effects. Identification of inciting agent is of paramount importance in the management of HP.

SUGGESTED READINGS

1. Singh S, Sharma BB, Bairwa M, Gothi D, Desai U, Joshi JM, et al. Management of Interstitial Lung Diseases: A consensus statement of the Indian Chest Society (ICS) and National College of Chest Physicians (NCCP). Lung India 2020;37:359-78.
2. An Official American Thoracic Society/European Respiratory Society Statement: Update of the International Multidisciplinary Classification of the Idiopathic Interstitial Pneumonias. Am J Respir Crit Care Med 2013;188 (6): 733-48.
3. Klinger JR, Elliott CG, Levine DJ, et al. Therapy for pulmonary arterial hypertension in adults: update of the CHEST guideline and expert panel report. Chest. 2019;155:565-86.
4. Jindal SK. Textbook of Pulmonary and Critical Care Medicine, 2nd edition. New Delhi: Jaypee Brothers Medical Publishers; 2017. pp.1017-30.
5. Wells AU and Hirani N. Intersitital lung disease guideline: the British Thoracic Society in collaboration with the Thoracic Society of Australia and New Zealand and the Irish Thoracic Society. Thorax 2008; 63: v1-58.
6. Castelino FV, Varga J. Interstitial lung disease in connective tissue diseases: evolving concepts of pathogenesis and management. Arthritis Res Ther. 2010;12:213.

CHAPTER 62

Approach to Undiagnosed Pleural Effusion

DP Singh

INTRODUCTION

Pleural effusion (PE) is caused by >60 different pleuropulmonary or systemic etiologies. A total of 25-40% of patients remains undiagnosed even after diagnostic thoracentesis and/or blind pleural biopsy. However, there is no universally accepted definition of undiagnosed pleural effusion (UPE).

Diagnosis of pleural effusion usually begins with detailed history, physical examination, and chest X-ray. Pleural fluid expression and biochemical, cytological, microbiological and molecular test are the investigations of choice to determine the etiology of pleural effusion.

Pleural effusion may be transudate or exudates. Transudate PE may be caused by CCF or hepatic hydrothorax or other causes of low oncotic pressure, while exudative PE is chiefly due to tuberculosis, malignancy, parapneumonic effusion and pulmonary thromboembolism **(Table 1)**.

DISEASES CAUSING UPE

During the past several decades' differentiation of transudate and exudate has been done by measuring the protein and LDH levels in pleural fluid and serum [Light Criteria]. If one or more criteria are met the fluid is exudates otherwise transudate **(Box 1)**.

Transudative Pleural Effusion

Congestive heart failures, cirrhosis of liver and nephrotic syndrome are three important causes of transudative pleural effusion, which should be considered in revealing the cause of undiagnosed pleural effusion **(Table 2)**.

TABLE 1: Showing diseases causing undiagnosed PE.

Exudative pleural effusion (EPE)	Transudative pleural effusion (TPE)
Tuberculosis	Congestive heart failure
Pneumonia	Cirrhosis of liver
Malignancy	Nephrotic syndrome
Pulmonary embolism	Myxedema
Fungal infection	
Intra-abdominal abscess	
Pancreatic pseudocyst	
Postcardiac injury syndrome	
Meigs' syndrome	
Rheumatoid pleuritis	
SLE	
Drug-induced pleural disease	
Asbestos pleural effusion	
Yellow nail syndrome	
Uremia	
Chylothorax	
Pseudochylothorax	

BOX 1: Showing Light's criteria.

- Pleural fluid protein/serum protein >0.5
- Pleural fluid LDH/serum LDH >0.6
- Pleural fluid LDH >0.67 the normal upper limit for serum

(LDH: lactic dehydrogenase).

TABLE 2: Showing transudative pleural effusion with salient features.

Congestive heart failure	Cirrhosis of liver with PE	Nephrotic syndrome
Most common cause: • DOE, orthopnea, PND • Basal crackles, S3 gallop pedal edema • Pleural fluid BNP level <1,000 pg/mL	Cirrhosis with massive ascites diagnosis of hepatic hydrothorax is easy	• >20% of patients with nephritic syndrome have bilateral PE • Serum protein and urinary protein should be measured for hypoproteinemia and proteinuria

Exudative Pleural Effusion

Among the causes of exudative pleural effusion tuberculosis, malignancy, and pulmonary embolism should be considered in every patient with an undiagnosed pleural effusion. Other causes such as fungal pleural effusion, chronic pancreatic pleural effusion, rheumatoid arthritis, and drug-induced pleural diseases should also be investigated for differential diagnosis.

Tuberculous Pleural Effusion

Tuberculosis remains one of the most common causes of exudative pleural effusion. If it is left untreated the effusion resolves but 50% of patients develop active pulmonary tuberculosis or extra-pulmonary tuberculosis. Therefore, all cases of undiagnosed pleural effusion should be tested for tuberculosis.

1. If pleural ADA level is >40 IU/L and pleural χ-interferon is >140 pg/mL, diagnosis is most likely tuberculosis.
2. Pleural fluid should also be sent for CBNAAT (cartridge based nucleic acid amplification test), which confirms the bacteriological diagnosis.
3. A needle pleural biopsy, finding of tubercle, and confirmation by CBNAAT clinch the diagnosis.
4. Wherever available, thoracoscopy should be done in undiagnosed cases.

Malignant Pleural Effusion

Malignant pleural effusion is one of the most common causes of undiagnosed exudative PE. There are four clinical characteristics suggestive of malignancy.

1. Any patient having symptoms for more than 1 month
2. Fever not present
3. Hemoptysis
4. Chest CT showing features of malignancy

Lung cancer is most common cause of PE. Second highest number of pleural effusion is caused by breast cancer and third highest by lymphoma and leukemia. If there is a history of exposure to asbestos mesothelioma should be the diagnosis. In patients of AIDS with lymphocytic PE diagnosis is primary lymphoma.

PULMONARY THROMBOEMBOLISM

In a case of undiagnosed PE pulmonary embolism should be considered in every patient. A total of 30% cases of PTE present with exudative PE. Spiral CT and CT pulmonary angiogram should be done to confirm the diagnosis of PTE.

Approach to a patient of undiagnosed pleural effusion should be done systematically in the following steps:

1. History
2. Physical Examination
3. Laboratory Investigation
4. Imaging Procedures
5. Needle Biopsy of Pleura
6. Thoracoscopy
7. Bronchoscopy
8. Open Pleural Biopsy

History

History is the first step in revealing the etiology of undiagnosed PE. If a patient has TPE attention should be paid to the history of dyspnea on exertion, paroxysmal nocturnal dyspnea, or orthopnea. If the patient has history of cirrhosis of liver or alcoholism hepatic pleural effusion may be diagnosed.

In a patient of EPE history of malignancy should be sought **(Table 3)**.

Physical Examination

A careful physical examination is needed to find out the signs indicating the diagnosis of UPE as shown in **Table 4**.

TABLE 3: Showing history unveiling etiology of undiagnosed PE.	
History	**Suggesting diagnosis**
Exposure to asbestos	Mesothelioma
History of fever	Tuberculosis, chronic anaerobic or fungal infection/Intra-abdominal abscess
History of alcoholism/pancreatic disease	Pancreatic Pleural Effusion
History of CABG surgery/PCI	Post CABG PE
History of rheumatoid arthritis	Rheumatoid PE
History of drugs	Nitrofurantoin, amiodarone drugs causing SLE, methotrexate, phenytoin, beta-blocker
Hemoptysis	Malignancy, pulmonary embolism, tuberculosis

TABLE 4: Showing transudative PE and exudative PE.	
Signs	**Suggesting diagnosis**
Transudative PE	
Basal crackles, S3 gallop, engorged neck veins	Congestive heart failure
Pedal edema	Congestive heart failure, cirrhosis with hepatic PE, nephrotic syndrome, pericardial disease, yellow nail syndrome
Ascites	Cirrhosis of liver
Exudative PE	
Lymph adenopathy, breast lump	Malignant PE
Distant heart sounds, pericardial friction rub, Kussmaul's sign	Pericardial disease with PE
Ascites with pelvic mass	Meigs' syndrome
Deformities of joints with subcutaneous nodules	Rheumatoid PE
Unilateral lower extremity swelling	Pulmonary embolism
Weight loss	Malignancy tuberculosis
Hepatosplenomegaly	Malignancy

Laboratory Examination

Several blood tests may be done to determine the etiology of undiagnosed PE. Liver and kidney function tests will confirm the diagnosis of cirrhosis of liver and nephritic syndrome. A Positive Serum ANA tests will clinch the diagnosis of SLE. Pleural fluid ADA or interferon gamma measurement is suggestive of pleural tuberculosis. The pleural fluid is milky, pleural fluid cholesterol should be measured. Pleural fluid LDH level should be measured every time thoracentesis is done.

Imaging Procedures

Spiral CT scan of chest helps in the diagnosis of pulmonary thromboembolism. In addition, pleural masses, mediastinal lymphadenopathy and lung infiltrate/masses may also be identified. An echocardiogram may reveal pericardial effusion and cardiac images.

Needle Biopsy of Pleura

During the last five decades diagnosis of tuberculous pleural effusion used to be confirmed with a needle biopsy of pleura. But pleural fluid ADA and g-interferon have become significant markers of tuberculosis. A needle biopsy of pleura also establishes the diagnosis of pleural malignancy.

Thoracoscopy

Medical thoracoscopy also known as pleuroscopy today remains the gold standard to diagnose and manage UPE. It is a safe procedure and has good diagnostic yield in patients with undiagnosed pleural effusions. It is an important tool for undiagnosed malignant and tuberculous PE [Indian J Chest Dis Allied Sci. 2011;53:21-24], when thoracentesis with cytology and makers of tuberculosis have not yielded a diagnosis thoracoscopy in the investigation of choice. In malignant pleural effusion thoracoscopy establishes diagnosis of 90% of cases. Overall diagnostic yield of thoracoscopic pleural biopsy is 70–80% in patients with undiagnosed pleural effusions. One of the studies of pleural malignancy was diagnosed in 48.6% of patients and tuberculosis in 22.8% of patients. There may be few complications such as empyema in this procedure.

Bronchoscopy

Bronchoscopy should be done in the following circumstances:
1. A case of PE with parenchymal infiltrate in chest X-ray or chest CT.
2. Hemoptysis with pleural effusion—hemoptysis indicates the likelihood of malignancy or pulmonary embolism. Malignancy can be diagnosed with bronchoscopy.
3. Massive pleural effusion—if it is caused by malignancy.
4. If the mediastinum is shifted toward the side of effusion an obstructive endobronchial lesion is suspected. This can be identified and biopsy can be done to confirm the diagnosis.

Open Biopsy

The chief indication for open pleural biopsy is progressive undiagnosed pleural disease in a place where thoracoscopy is not available or contraindicated. Even with an open biopsy of pleura a diagnosis is not always obtained. In one study of 21 patients no diagnosis obtained in seven cases.

■ CONCLUSION

Approach a patient of undiagnosed pleural effusion should be taken stepwise.
1. First step is whether the patient has transudate or exudates. This can be easily done by Light's criteria. If it is clinically transudate but Light's exudative criteria are met, a serum/pleural fluid protein gradient >3.1 indicates transudative pleural effusion.
2. Pleural fluid ADA and g-interferon are valuable markers of tuberculosis. CBNAAT of pleural fluid may clinch the diagnosis of tuberculosis but it is not positive in majority of cases.
3. If the pleural fluid BNP level is >1,500 pg/mL diagnosis of congestive heart failure is strongly suggestive.
4. CT chest is a valuable imaging for the diagnosis of malignant pleural effusion and pulmonary thromboembolism.
5. Needle biopsy of pleura and thoracoscopy are useful procedures to unveil the diagnosis of undiagnosed pleural effusion specially tuberculosis and malignant pleural effusion.
6. In some cases bronchoscopy with biopsy may show the path of final diagnosis.

■ SUGGESTED READINGS

1. Light RW. The undiagnosed pleural effusion. Clin Chest Med. 2006;27(2):309-19.
2. Saguil A, Wyrick K, Hallgren J. Diagnostic approach to pleural effusion. Am Fam Physician. 2014;90(2):99-104.
3. Romero S, Candela A, Martin C, et al. Evaluation of different criteria for the separation of pleural transu-datesfromexudates. Chest. 1993;104(2):399-404.
4. Skouras V, Kalomenidis I. Effusions due to drugs. In: Light RW, Lee YC (Eds). Textbook of pleural diseases. 2016. pp. 382-93.
5. Spiral CT for pulmonary embolism. Semin Respir Crit Care Goodman PC 2000.
6. Menzies R, Charbonneau M. Thoracoscopy for the diagnosis of pleural disease. Ann Intern Med. 1991;114(4):271-6.
7. Mootha VK, Agarwal R, Singh N, et al. Medical thorascoscopy for undiagnosed pleural effusion: experience from a tertiary care hospital in North India. Indian J Chest Dis Allied Sci. 2011;53(1):21-4.
8. Chang SC, Perng RP. The role of fiberoptic bronchoscopy in evaluating the causes of pleural effusions. Arch Intern Med.1989;149(4):855-7.

CHAPTER

63

A Clinical Approach to Patient with Joint Pain

Tarun Satija, Samarth Loomba

■ INTRODUCTION

Joint pain is a cardinal symptom in rheumatology. It is important to recognize and find the cause of joint pain by good history taking, physical examination, and judicious use of investigations to ensure proper management of the patient.
Here is a stepwise approach to evaluate a patient with joint pain:

- *Articular or nonarticular:* It is important to realize all joint pains may not arise from articular surface of joint, periarticular structures such as bursa, tendons, muscles, bones, and ligaments may be culprits for the symptoms. One must also remember non-rheumatic conditions such as depression, neuropathic pain, and hypothyroidism may cause symptoms which might be perceived by patient as pain arising from the joint. So, first step in evaluating a patient is to differentiate between articular and nonarticular pain.

  In general, pain arising from a joint is diffuse and deep-seated, can be associated with joint swelling and increases with both active and passive movements. Whereas periarticular pain increases more with active movements than with passive movements and is not associated with joint swelling. Pain due to a bursitis has localized point tenderness away from joint line. In tendinitis, patient has a tender linear swelling of tendon and may have an audible or palpable rub and stretching the tendon increases the pain. Muscle pain is more diffuse, less localized, and is associated with muscle tenderness. Enthesitis is characteristic of spondyloarthropathy (SpA) and is associated with inflammation at site of tendon insertion. Paresthesia's, numbness and constant burning pain unrelated to movement suggest a neurologic cause.

- *Inflammatory or noninflammatory:* Arthritis can be inflammatory or noninflammatory (degenerative). The presence of joint swelling, erythema, and morning stiffness of >1 hour and symmetric pain even at rest is suggestive of inflammatory. Condition. A symmetric presentation suggests an underlying inflammatory arthritis.

Rheumatoid arthritis (RA), systemic lupus erythematosus (SLE), Spondyloarthropathy's, and Vasculitis are some common causes of inflammatory arthritis. Noninflammatory arthritis may present with swelling and tenderness but is not associated with warmth, redness over the joint, and morning stiffness. Osteoarthritis (OA) of knee is an example of noninflammatory joint involvement where weight bearing joint of lower limb is involved in asymmetrical pattern and associated with pain worsening with movement and relief with rest whereas pain in inflammatory arthritis worsens after rest. Crepitations on joint movement without warmth and erythema suggest degenerative process like OA.

It is also important to realize patient may complain of joint pain but may have no signs of inflammation, e.g., fibromyalgia or early stages of rheumatic diseases where joint inflammation may not be evident clinically. When signs of inflammation are absent in patient with joint pain, it is called arthralgia.

- *Pattern of pain:* Joint pains occur in many rheumatological diseases but the pattern of joint involvement can help a clinician to reach a reliable diagnosis in most of cases. Here are the things one should look for:
    - *Mode of onset of joint pain*: Acute onset is seen in infective arthritis (bacterial or viral), trauma, and gout. Insidious onset is seen in RA, OA, and SpA.
    - *Duration of joint pain*: If duration of symptoms is < 6 weeks, it is classified as acute and if symptoms have been present for > 6 weeks, the disease is classified as chronic. Less than 6 weeks symptoms may be a result of viral arthritis or other self-limiting illnesses and may not require detailed evaluation unless the patient has definite systemic or multiorgan involvement.
    - *Number of joints involved*: Monoarthritis is involvement of one joint and this occurs in trauma, gout, and septic arthritis. In oligoarthritis, two to four joints are involved and this is a feature of SpA and psoriasis. Polyarthritis is involvement of five or more joints and is seen in RA, SLE, and Systemic Sclerosis (SSc). However, it is important to remember number of joints involved may vary as disease progresses, e.g., gout may be monoarticular initially but may have multijoint involvement in later stages.
    - *Symmetry*: RA, SLE, and SSc result in symmetrical arthritis whereas Gout and SpA cause asymmetrical arthritis. Psoriasis can cause both asymmetrical or symmetrical arthritis. In symmetrical arthritis, there is involvement of same joints both sides but mirror image symmetry is not essential. However, initially in RA one may have asymmetrical involvement and typical symmetrical pattern is seen as disease evolves.
    - *Small or large joint involvement*: RA, SLE, SSc, and Psoriasis affect both small and large joints whereas SpA affects mainly large joints of lower limbs.
    - *Type of joint involvement*: RA typically involves small joints of hands symmetrically such as metacarpophalangeal (MCP) joints and proximal interphalangeal (PIP) joints sparing distal interphalangeal (DIP) joint in contrast to OA, psoriasis, and SSc where DIP joint is involved. SLE affects similar joints as RA, however, joint destruction is rare.

    Inflammatory low back pain is typical of SpA whereas spinal involvement is rare in RA except for cervical spine.

- *Upper or lower limb joint involvement:* RA, SLE, and Psoriasis involve both upper and lower limbs joints in contrast to SpA and gout which involve lower limb joints.
- *Sequence of involvement*: Joint involvement may be called additive when one or more joint are affected with time, as a new joint is involved the pain and swelling in previous joint persists, examples include RA, SLE, SpA, and Psoriasis. In intermittent arthritis, patient is totally asymptomatic in between episodic periods of joint involvement. Gout and Behçet's syndrome cause intermittent arthritis. In migratory arthritis, joint involvement in a specific joint starts rapidly and subsides in 24–36 hours and then new joints get involved. This pattern is seen in rheumatic fever, gonococcal arthritis, and viral diseases. However, it is important to realize that one may not see the typical patterns because of the medication patient has received.
- *Type of musculoskeletal involvement*: Enthesitis (inflammation of entheses), dactylitis (sausage digits), and low backache are seen typically in SpA. Gout involves tendon sheaths and bursa and leads to superficial inflammation.
- *Extra-articular involvement*: An extra-articular involvement detected on history and examination may help in narrowing in on the diagnosis. Constitutional symptoms suggest a systemic disorder and rule out degenerative arthritis.
    - Weakness, fever, and weight loss may be a sign of intensive inflammation present in SLE and systemic vasculitis.
    - Skin and nails—Psoriatic arthritis may be accompanied by classic nail findings such as hyperkeratosis and pitting besides characteristic skin lesion. Slapped-cheek rash described as lacy, erythematous, and maculopapular in appearance can indicate previous parvovirus B-19 infection. SLE is associated with light sensitive rash classically involving the face but can also be seen in between joints. Skin lesions may help in narrowing down diagnosis in diseases like dermatomyositis, scleroderma, erythema nodosa, etc. Nodules may be part of RA and Gout.
    - Eye—anterior uveitis can be seen in SpA, Pan Uveitis or Posterior Uveitis is seen in Behçet's disease while granulomatous uveitis is seen in tuberculosis and sarcoidosis. Dry eye is seen in Sjögren's syndrome. Episcleritis and scleritis can be associated with RA. Conjunctivitis may be due to reactive arthritis.
    - Peripheral lymphadenopathy can be a feature of rheumatic diseases like SLE, Adult Onset Still's Disease (AOSD), and Sjögren's syndrome beside lymphoma. Hepatosplenomegaly can be found in SLE and ASD.
    - Urogenital involvement—in a patient who has polyarthritis with renal failure or glomerular involvement (suggested by hematuria and proteinuria), SLE and Systemic Vasculitis must be considered. Urogenital infections can cause reactive arthritis.
    - Gastrointestinal system—Dysphagia may be seen in Scleroderma and Polymyositis. Infective diarrhea can be a cause for reactive arthritis whereas diarrhea and perianal disease present as part of inflammatory

A Clinical Approach to Patient with Joint Pain

bowel disease. Systemic vasculitis may present with mesenteric ischemia. All these diseases can cause polyarthritis.
- Cardiovascular system—Aortic dilatation and Aortic insufficiency may develop in ankylosing spondylitis (AS). Absence of peripheral pulses may be an indication of Aortitis. Syphilis can cause polyarthritis along with aortic insufficiency.
- Pulmonary features such as pleuritis, effusions, lung nodules, interstitial lung disease, pulmonary hypertension, and hemorrhage in patients with polyarthritis may suggest infection, rheumatic disease, or malignancy.
- Widespread musculoskeletal pains with multiple soft tissue tender points along with features of anxiety and depression may be suggestive of fibromyalgia.

Miscellaneous causes of arthritis—infections like Syphilis, Lyme's disease, Urogenital and Gastrointestinal infections can cause polyarthritis. One may need to investigate for the same if features of infection are present. Polyarthritis can occur with malignancies as paraneoplastic syndrome. Hematolymphoid malignancies along with adenocarcinoma of lung and breast may cause polyarthritis. One should investigate for malignancies in presence of weight loss, fever and lymphadenopathy.

Certain drugs, such as Nivolumab, Durvalumab, clindamycin, INH, and Antithyroid drugs can cause polyarthritis and so drug history should be taken in all patients with polyarthritis **(Flowchart 1)**.

■ LABORATORY STUDIES

Laboratory investigations should be used as an adjunct to good history and physical examination to reach a diagnosis and should not be the sole criterion for the same. Standard tests, such as complete blood count, urine analyses, and renal and liver function tests rule out systemic organ involvement and then some specific tests which may be done are:
- Inflammatory markers—Erythrocyte Sedimentation Rate (ESR) and C-reactive protein (CRP) are nonspecific indicators of inflammation and may help in differentiating between inflammatory and noninflammatory state. ESR can be raised in inflammatory conditions but it is important to keep in mind it may be increased in wide variety of infections, malignancies, renal failure, diabetes, and dysproteinemia besides rheumatological diseases. One should also remember ESR may be normal even in rheumatological conditions like RA.
- Rheumatoid factor (RF)— RF has a limited diagnostic value for diagnosis of RA as up to one third of patient may remain seronegative throughout their course. RF may be positive with bacterial infections like Bacterial Endocarditis, Tuberculosis, Leprosy, Syphilis, Viral infections like hepatitis B besides Parasitic infections, Sarcoidosis, and malignancies. Higher RF factor titers may have a better predictive value for diagnosis and may also predict poorer outcomes in RA.
- Anticyclic citrullinated peptide (anti-CCP) antibody testing is more specific than RF for diagnosis of RA and may predict erosive disease more effectively.
- Antinuclear antibody (ANA) has high sensitivity but low specificity for SLE as it may be positive in normal people, many rheumatic and non-rheumatic illnesses besides SLE. Thus positive ANA in a patient who has no symptoms of SLE

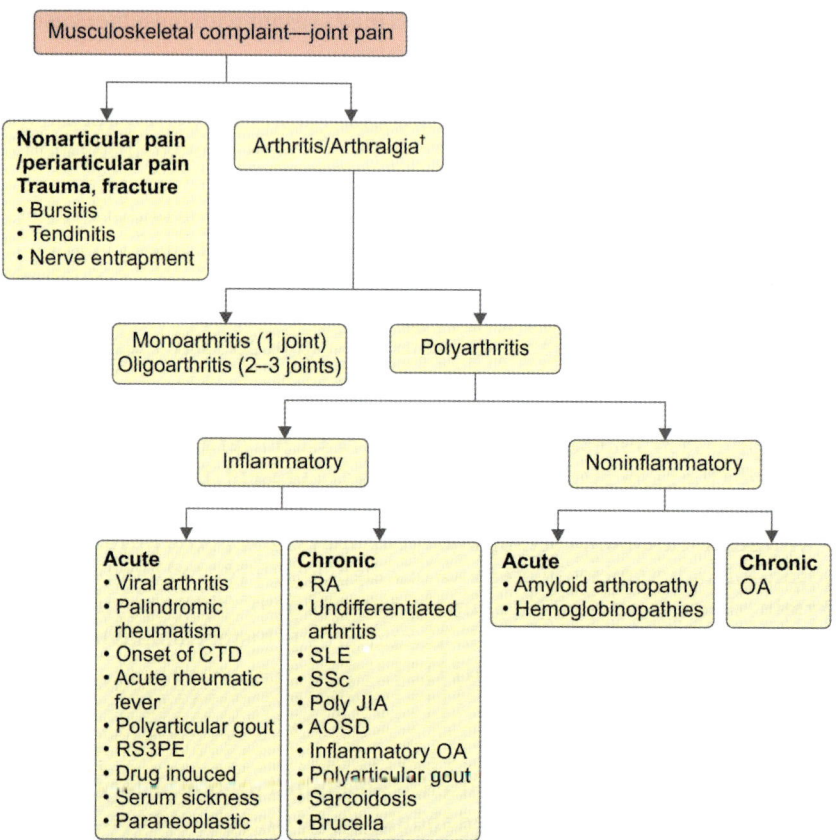

†See text on how to differentiate arthritis from periarticular/nonarticular pain.

FLOWCHART 1: Approach to patient with joint pain and differential diagnosis of polyarthritis.

(AOSD: adult onset still's disease; CTD: connective tissue disease; OA: osteoarthritis; Poly JIA: polyarticular juvenile idiopathic arthritis; RA: rheumatoid arthritis; RS3PE: remitting seronegative symmetrical synovitis with pedal edema; SLE: systemic lupus erythematosus; SSc: systemic sclerosis)

probably has no significance. The higher the titer of ANA, more are the chances that patient has SLE. Additional serologic tests such as anti-double-stranded DNA antibodies may help in reaching a diagnosis.
- Serum uric acid (UA) also a limited diagnostic utility as asymptomatic hyperuricemia has high prevalence in general population and it may be normal in attack of gout, including patients with poly articular involvement.
- Synovial fluid analysis can be used to make a diagnosis of infective arthritis, crystal induced arthritis and hemarthrosis besides it helping to differentiate between inflammatory and noninflammatory arthritis. The white cell count and its differential, cultures, gram stain, and polarized light microscopy of synovial fluid are done.

Noninflammatory causes like OA have < 2,000 white blood cell's (WBC's) per microliter in synovial fluid with <25% neutrophils, inflammatory causes like RA have between 2,000 to 20,000 WBC's per microliter with 50–75% neutrophils and septic arthritis have > 20,000 WBC's per microliter with >75% neutrophils. With

most bacterial organisms, synovial WBC count is typically >50,000 per microliter (and often > 1,00,000 cells per microliter) but lower counts (in the inflammatory range) may be seen in setting of septic arthritis, especially in disseminated gonococcal infection or prior antibiotic use. Monosodium urate crystals in synovial fluid are diagnostic of gout. Synovial fluid culture, if positive, confirms septic arthritis.
- The following imaging studies may be useful in evaluation of arthritis:
  - Plain X-ray films can confirm diagnosis and severity of OA but one must remember they can be normal in OA and occasionally finding of OA may not relate to patent's symptoms. They can pick up marginal erosions in RA and erosions with overhanging edge in chronic gout besides ruling out fractures and osteomyelitis.
  - Ultrasound of joints can detect subtle synovitis and early erosions in RA and other causes of inflammatory arthritis, and also pick up UA crystal deposition in gout and calcium pyrophosphate crystals in calcium pyrophosphate crystal deposition disease.
  - Magnetic resonance imaging (MRI) is more sensitive than plain X-ray to pick up early sacroiliac involvement in SpA.
  - Positron emission tomography-computed tomography (PET-CT) may be used rarely in ruling out malignancy and large vessel vasculitis as cause of arthritis.
- Occasionally, synovial biopsy may be required to confirm diagnosis of tuberculosis and sarcoidosis. Tissue biopsy may be required to diagnose cutaneous lupus or skin vasculitis (skin), glomerulonephritis (kidney), and pulmonary vasculitis (lung).

CONCLUSION

Evaluating a patient with joint pain is a challenge and requires a good history, clinical examination, and correlation with relevant investigations.

SUGGESTED READINGS

1. American College of Rheumatology Ad Hoc Committee on Clinical Guidelines. Guidelines for the initial evaluation of the adult patient with acute musculoskeletal symptoms. Arthritis Rheum. 1996;39(1):1-8
2. El-Gabalaway HS, Duray P, Goldbach-Mansky R. Evaluating patients with arthritis of recent onset. JAMA. 2000;284(18):2368-73.
3. Mies Richie A, Francis ML. Diagnostic approach to poly-articular joint pain. Am Fam Physician. 2006;73(7):1153.
4. West S. Musculoskeletal signs and symptoms B. Polyarticular joint disease. In: Klippel JH (Ed). Primer on the Rheumatic Diseases, 13th edition. New York: Springer; 2008:47-57.
5. Shmerling RH. (2022). Evaluation of the adult with polyarticular pain. [online] Available from https://www.uptodate.com/contents/evaluation-of-the-adult-with-polyarticular-pain [Last accessed October, 2022].
6. Meador R, Schumacher HR. Evaluating and treating patients with polyarthritis of recent onset. Hosp Physician. 2003;39(3):37-45.
7. Chaturvedi V, Thabah MM. Approach to the patient with polyarthritis. Assoc Physici India. 2014;32:169-73.

CHAPTER 64

New Concepts in Systemic Lupus Erythematosus

S Bhavana, RN Tejaswini, Vijaya Prasanna, G Narsimulu

■ INTRODUCTION

Systemic lupus erythematosus (SLE) is a prototype systemic autoimmune disorder characterized by organ damage mediated by autoantibodies and immune complexes. Polyclonal B cell activation is the immunological hallmark in SLE. The first clinical description of SLE was by Biett and Cazenave in 1833, when they referred to it as erythema centrifugum. The characteristic "butterfly skin rash" simile for malar rash was described in 1846. The first criteria for SLE were formulated by the American College of Rheumatology (ACR) in 1971. Extensive research and updating of knowledge continue to this day in all facets pertaining to SLE such as immunopathogenesis, diagnostic/classification, biomarkers of prognosis, and management.

■ IMMUNOPATHOGENESIS

Reduction in quantity and functional capacity of cluster of differentiation (CD8) T cells, B cells, and natural killer (NK) cells has been described. Defective production of transforming growth factor beta (TGF-β) causes abnormal inhibition of immunoglobulin production by B cells hence leading to increased autoantibody production. TGF-β is being studied as a target for gene therapy in SLE to help restore normal T cell functions. Autologous stem cell transplantation following intensive immunosuppression with cyclophosphamide helps reset T-lymphocyte population and has been noted to lead to clinical remission of disease.

■ GENOMICS

The human leukocyte antigens (HLA) region at 6p21.3 has shown strongest association with SLE and is involved in both B cell and T cell signaling. IRF5 is the most consistent non-major histocompatibility complex (*MHC*) gene in SLE and is important for transactivation of type 1 interferons (IFNs). Impaired deoxyribonucleic acid (DNA) methylation in CD4+ T cell, caused by environmental influences, contributes to SLE pathogenesis.

CLASSIFICATION CRITERIA

In 2019, SLE classification criteria were updated by ACR/European League Against Rheumatism (EULAR) and included positive antinuclear antibodies (ANA) as an obligatory entry criterion, followed by weighted criteria in clinical and immunological domains. Those scoring ≥10 points would be classified as SLE. Seven clinical domains included are—constitutional, hematologic, neuropsychiatric, mucocutaneous, serosal, musculoskeletal, renal, and three immunological domains are—antiphospholipid antibodies, complement protein levels, and SLE-specific antibodies. These new criteria have a sensitivity of 96.1% and specificity of 93.4% compared to the sensitivity of 82.8% and specificity of 93.4% of 1997 ACR criteria, and sensitivity of 96.7% and specificity of 83.7% of the Systemic Lupus International Collaborating Clinics (SLICC) 2012 criteria. Placing emphasis on autoantibodies in SLE, positive ANA has been made an entry criterion.

BIOMARKERS OF SLE

Serum proteins such as B lymphocyte stimulator (BLyS), IFN-γ-induced protein 10 (IP-10), monocyte chemoattractant protein-1 (MCP-1), TNF-α, type I interferon signature, or increased Th17, and plasma cell populations have been proposed as SLE specific markers of disease. However, further research is necessary to include these biomarkers as part of disease classification criteria or treatment algorithms.

SLE DAMAGE ASSESSMENT

In 1996, the SLICC–ACR damage index (SDI) was developed to quantify irreversible organ dysfunction. It assessed 41 items in 12 organ systems. SDI has prognostic value and helps predict morbidity and mortality. It is necessary for a manifestation to be present for at least 6 months duration for it to be valid for scoring. This index is undergoing an update in order to modernize it.

SLE RESPONSE MEASURES

An attempt has been made to define rigorous response criteria such as remission and lupus low-disease activity state (LLDAS). LLDAS is a clinically relevant outcome, taking into consideration that (i) remission in SLE is desirable, but not always achievable and (ii) patients who spend >50% of their observed time in LLDAS have significantly reduced damage accrual.

NEWER THERAPIES

Targeting B Cell

B cell depleting drugs like rituximab have a well proven and established role in therapy of major organ involvement in SLE.

- *Obinutuzumab*, anti-CD20 antibody has been studied in lupus nephritis and has encouraging results. Complete renal response was achieved in 40% patients on obinutuzumab.
- *Belimumab* has positive results in those with lupus nephritis and secondary failure to rituximab.
- *Obexelimab* is an antibody targeting CD19 molecule on B cells. It simultaneously binds the Fcγ receptor IIb (FcγRIIb), the inhibitory receptor on B cell surface.

Targeting T Cells

- *Belatacept* is an Fc segment containing fusion protein that targets CTLA-4 extracellular domain, similar to abatacept, blocks costimulation and has been studied in lupus nephritis postrenal transplantation.
- Lulizumab is an anti-CD28 monoclonal antibody which blocks T cell costimulation.
- Rigerimod or Lupuzor is a peptide fragment of small nuclear ribonucleoprotein U1-70K. It is thought to act as an immunomodulator by binding MHC class II and hence inhibiting T-cell reactivity. Costimulation blockade, however, has not shown very rewarding results in SLE, perhaps pointing to importance of other pathways in pathogenesis

Targeting Plasma Cells

Daratumumab, an immunoglobulin G (IgG1k) antibody against CD38 causes depletion of plasma cells. Treatment with daratumumab resulted in remarkable clinical outcomes not only of severe manifestations but also on less severe manifestations and was associated with favorable serologic responses.

Targeting Dendritic Cells

- VIB7734 is an antibody that binds to ILT7, a surface molecule of plasmacytoid dendritic cells (pDCs), resulting in their elimination.
- BIIB059 is a humanized IgG1 monoclonal antibody that binds the specific receptor of pDC BDCA2 (blood dendritic cell antigen 2), and inhibits the production of IFN-I.

Targeting Cytokines

- *Belimumab* is a specific BLyS inhibitor which has been introduced into standard treatment regimen of patients of lupus with nephritis.
- *Telitacicept* is a recombinant TACI-Fc fusion protein which binds BLyS and a proliferation-inducing ligand (APRIL) and inhibits their activities. Without affecting early and memory B cells, it inhibits the development and survival of mature B cells and plasma cells
- Anifrolumab is a fully human monoclonal Antibody that binds to the type I interferon receptor, blocking the activity of type I interferons such as interferon-α and interferon-β. Anifrolumab also led to a reduction of the glucocorticoid dosages and in an improvement of skin involvement.

- Low levels of IL-2 may result in disruption of immune tolerance and lupus is a low IL-2 disease. Low-doses of IL-2 might be a beneficial and safe choice in the treatment of patients with SLE.

INHIBITION OF INTRACELLULAR PATHWAYS

- *Voclosporin* is a novel cyclosporine analog, the most potent and least toxic among all known calcineurin inhibitors.
- Sirolimus is an immunosuppressive macrolide which blocks T cell and B cell activation through mTOR inhibition.
- *Baricitinib* is an oral inhibitor of Janus kinase (JAK), blocking the subtypes JAK1 and JAK2, reduces SLE disease activity.

ONGOING TRIALS

Several drugs are being studied for efficacy in SLE.

Dapirolizumab pegol is an anti-CD40L pegylated Fab fragment that blocks costimulation of T cells. Itolizumab (EQ001) is a monoclonal antibody targeting the CD6 receptor on the surface of T cells inhibiting immune responses. CC-220 is a cereblon modulator causing potent degradation of Ikaros and Aiolos leading to suppressed B cell proliferation and cytokine production.

Cenerimod is a selective agonist for the G-protein-coupled sphingosine-1-phosphate receptor 1 (S1P receptor 1 or S1P1) is an immunomodulator with effects on both T and B cells.

CONCLUSION

Patients with SLE are now enjoying longer, near normal lives, thanks to the ever expanding knowledge on pathophysiology and newer tools in therapeutic armamentarium.

Ongoing research will further help discover aspects in immunology and targeted management of the disease.

SUGGESTED READINGS

1. Ohtsuka K, Gray JD, Stimmler MM, et al. Decreased Production of TGF-beta by Lymphocytes from Patients with Systemic Lupus Erythematosus. J Immunol. 1998;160(5):2539-45.
2. Traynor AE, Schroeder J, Rosa RM, et al. Treatment of severe systemic lupus erythematosus with high-dose chemotherapy and haemopoietic stem-cell transplantation: A phase I study. Lancet. 2000;356(9231):701-7.
3. Johnson S, Hinchcliff M, Asano Y. Controversies: molecular vs. clinical systemic sclerosis classification. SAGE Open. 2017;1(3):277-85.
4. Staveri C, Karokis D, Liossis SNC. New onset of lupus nephritis in two patients with SLE shortly after initiation of treatment with belimumab. Semin Arthritis Rheum. 2017;46(6):788-90.
5. Morand EF, Furie R, Tanaka Y, et al. Trial of Anifrolumab in Active Systemic Lupus Erythematosus. N Engl J Med. 2020;382(3):211-21.
6. Rovin BH, Solomons N, Pendergraft WF, et al. A randomized, controlled double-blind study comparing the efficacy and safety of dose-ranging voclosporin with placebo in achieving remission in patients with active lupus nephritis. Kidney Int. 2019;95(1):219-31.
7. Strasser DS, Froidevaux S, Sippel V, et al. Preclinical to clinical translation of cenerimod, a novel S1P1 receptor modulator, in systemic lupus erythematosus. 2020;6(2):e001261.

CHAPTER 65

Changing Landscape of Rheumatoid Arthritis Management

Uma Kumar, Israrul Haque

■ INTRODUCTION

Rheumatoid arthritis (RA) is the most common female predominant autoimmune inflammatory arthritis, affecting about 0.5-1% of the population. Delayed or suboptimal treatment of RA can result in dysfunction, deformities, disability, development of multiple comorbidities, and reduced life-span. In the past two decades, there has been considerable advancement in the understanding of the pathogenesis of RA which has resulted in the development of new promising therapeutic agents. The expansion of the therapeutic armamentarium and availability of various validated objective disease activity assessment tools have resulted in a paradigm shift in the management of RA. Now, the focus is on achieving remission or low disease activity (if remission is not achievable because of certain factors) in RA. Here, we will discuss the principles of management of RA in current times.

■ EARLY DIAGNOSIS OF RA—"THE THERAPEUTIC WINDOW OF OPPORTUNITY"

The concept of early disease has evolved from 12-24 months in the 1990s to 6 months from symptom onset in current times. This is driven by the fact that significant joint damage is incurred within the first year of symptom onset and more so in the first 6 months. Further evidence shows that disease within the first 12 weeks may be immunopathologically distinct from later disease, thus leading to a transition from resolving arthritis to chronic persistent arthritis.

The 1987 American Rheumatology Association (ARA) revised criteria for the classification of RA (sensitivity—76% and specificity—76%) failed to diagnose some patients with early disease who might benefit most from the early aggressive treatment. Accordingly, in 2010 the American College of Rheumatology (ACR) and the European League Against Rheumatism (EULAR) put forward revised classification criteria (sensitivity—97% and specificity—55%) which took into account early disease characteristics and anti-citrullinated protein antibodies (ACPAs), a biomarker that predicts aggressive disease. The domains of the 2010 ACR/EULAR criteria are grouped into four classifications, with point scores for each: Joint symptoms, serology [rheumatoid factor (RF) and/or ACPA], symptom duration (whether <6 weeks or >6 weeks), and acute-phase reactants [C-reactive protein (CRP) and/or erythrocyte sedimentation rate (ESR)].

■ EARLY TREATMENT WITH DISEASE-MODIFYING ANTIRHEUMATIC DRUGS

In a meta-analysis of 12 early RA trials (<2 years at presentation), it was concluded that radiographic progression after 3 years was 33% less in patients who received early treatment than those in whom treatment was delayed. Disease duration of less than 3 months at the time of starting treatment is the strongest predictor of remission at 6 months. The therapeutic window of opportunity hypothesis in early RA has evolved and suggests that there is a stage during which the disease may be potentially altered or even reversed with a complete return to normality.

■ "TREAT-TO-TARGET" AND "TIGHT CONTROL OF DISEASE ACTIVITY" APPROACH FOR BOTH EARLY AND ESTABLISHED DISEASE

The principle of treat-to-target has proved its importance in many medical illnesses such as hypertension and diabetes. Treat-to-target has several distinct components: Choosing the right target and a method for measuring it, assessing the target at a prespecified time point, changing the therapy if the target is not achieved, and shared decision-making. This concept has become more relevant in RA with the availability of biologic disease-modifying antirheumatic drugs (DMARDs) [tumor necrosis factor (TNF) inhibitors, interleukin 6 (IL-6) inhibitors, rituximab, abatacept, etc.) and targeted synthetic DMARDs (tofacitinib, baricitinib), defined target (remission or at least minimal disease activity), and validated disease activity assessment indices (DAS 28ESR/DAS 28 CRP, SDAI, CDAI, RAPID3). In routine clinical practice, methotrexate (MTX) remains the first choice among available conventional synthetic DMARDs (csDMARD) and MTX can be combined with other csDMARDs (hydroxychloroquine, sulfasalazine, or leflunomide) if required. A landmark COmbinatie therapy Bij Rheumatoide Arthritis (COBRA) study showed that combination therapy was superior to sulfasalazine monotherapy in terms of clinical efficacy and inhibiting the progression of structural damage and reducing mortality in early RA patients. Another trial Finnish Rheumatoid Arthritis Combination Therapy (FIN-RACo) and NEO-RACo study reiterated that early and aggressive treatment is more important than a specific drug to control the disease activity of RA and has long-term beneficial effects. Also, combination DMARDs therapy is more effective in controlling RA disease activity.

The TIght COntrol of Rheumatoid Arthritis (TICORA) trial compared tight control of disease activity with routine care and found that the remission rate was much higher in the aggressive treatment group.

The BehandelStrategieën (BeSt), The Computer Assisted Management for Early Rheumatoid Arthritis (CAMERA) study, Cyclosporine, MEthotrexate, STeroid in Rheumatoid Arthritis (CIMESTRA) study, and the Treatment of Early Aggressive RA (TEAR) study emphasized the fact that tight control of disease activity in RA patients results in significantly better clinical outcome than the usual care. The concept of the treat to target implies that clinical remission or minimal disease activity (if remission cannot be achieved due to certain limitations) as per any of the ACR recommended measures of disease activity is the goal of therapy in RA.

Rheumatoid arthritis patients with poor prognostic factors [presence of one or more of the following features: functional limitation (e.g., Health Assessment Questionnaire [HAQ] disability index [DI] or similar valid tools), extraarticular disease (e.g., presence of rheumatoid nodules, RA vasculitis, Felty's syndrome), positive RF or anti-cyclic citrullinated peptide antibodies or bony erosions by radiograph] are to be treated aggressively in particular. In order to achieve remission or LDA, patients need to be followed up more frequently (typically every 1–3 months) to assess disease activity and if moderate or high disease activity persists, then using a combination of csDMARD or biologic DMARD with or without csDMARD is recommended to achieve the goal. Regular follow-up and assessment of disease activity ensure that bDMARDs and tsDMARD (which increase the risk of infection and cost of therapy) are only continued if they are effective to achieve the goal of therapy. In case of primary failure or secondary failure, discontinuation of the drug and changing to another drug is recommended.

Thus, the treat-to-target approach and tight control aiming for remission or LDA is a promising option to treat early RA patients. This strategy is less expensive in comparison to newer drugs.

Biosimilars remain a hot topic in rheumatology, and some physicians are cautious about their application in the real world. With many biosimilar products in the market, it is important to understand their real clinical and economic potential in the treatment of RA.

It is important to remember that using a targeted therapy does not mean that a treat-to-target strategy is being followed.

ROLE OF SYSTEMIC GLUCOCORTICOIDS

Systemic glucocorticoids (GC) improve disease activity and functional status and reduce radiographic progression to some extent. But due to their systemic toxicity, the EULAR 2022 guidelines recommend the use of only low-dose GC for the shortest possible duration typically as a bridge therapy for quick symptomatic relief when DMARDs are started/changed. It also states that the steroid should be tapered and discontinued as rapidly as clinically feasible.

DEFINING SPECIFIC SUBSETS OF DISEASE SUCH AS REFRACTORY RA AND DIFFICULT-TO-TREAT RA FOR BETTER THERAPEUTIC MANAGEMENT

EULAR defines difficult-to-treat (D2T) RA as (1) failure of ≥2 biologic/tsDMARDs with different mechanisms of action after failing on csDMARDs (unless contraindicated) AND (2) active moderate disease activity/progressive disease based on signs and/or symptoms' inability to taper GC below 7.5 prednisolone or equivalent, rapid radiographic progression, presence of RA symptoms that reduce the quality of life despite good disease control, and (3) management of symptoms is perceived as problematic by the rheumatologist and/or patient.

Approximately 30% of patients fit into the category of D2T RA. It has been observed that approximately 16.8% of RA patients suffer from depression.

Treatment of D2T RA patients should be individually tailored and specific aspects such as comorbidities, fatigue, pain, and functional disability must be addressed appropriately. Existent concomitant fibromyalgia and osteoarthritis can mimic active RA.

One must remember that lifestyle factors (lack of exercise, smoking, alcohol consumption, and dietary habits) play an important role in D2T disease.

CONCLUSION

The last two decades have witnessed huge changes in the management of RA. Patients are treated more aggressively to achieve remission within the defined period of time. Early diagnosis and effective treatment strategies comprising csDMARDs, biologics, and targeted synthetic DMARDs with constant monitoring for the development of comorbidities have resulted in improved quality of life of RA patients. However, DMARDs-free long-term remission in RA is still elusive.

SUGGESTED READINGS

1. Hochberg M, Gravallese E, Smolen S, et al. (Eds). Rheumatology, 8th edition. Philadelphia: Elsevier; 2022.
2. Van Vollenhoven R. Treat-to-target in rheumatoid arthritis — are we there yet? Nat Rev Rheumatol. 2019:15;180-6.
3. Radu AF, Bungau SG. Management of rheumatoid arthritis: An overview. Cells. 2021;10:857-90.
4. Fraenkel L, Bathon JM, England BR, et al. 2021 American College of Rheumatology Guideline for the Treatment of Rheumatoid Arthritis. Arthritis Care Res (Hoboken). 2021;73(7):924-39.
5. Nagy G, Roodenrijs NMT, Welsing PMJ, et al. EULAR points to consider for the management of difficult-to-treat rheumatoid arthritis. Ann Rheum Dis. 2022;81(1):20-33.

CHAPTER 66

Familial Hypercholesterolemia

Raman Puri, Rashmi Nanda

■ INTRODUCTION

One baby is born with familial hypercholesterolemia (FH) every minute. FH is underdiagnosed and undertreated globally. Over 90% of FH patients were characterized by the presence of cardiovascular disease at the time of death. Three out of four FH patients had experienced one or more myocardial infarctions prior to death. Classical risk factors were more prevalent in FH patients who died at a younger age.

What is familial hypercholesterolemia?
Familial hypercholesterolemia is an inherited condition leading to severely elevated serum low-density lipoprotein cholesterol (LDL-C) that leads to premature atherosclerotic cardiovascular disease (ASCVD) and accounts for 2–3% of the cases of myocardial infarction in patients aged <60 years.

What is the cause of familial hypercholesterolemia?
It is caused by mutations in the genes of the LDL-receptor (LDL-R), Apolipoprotein B (Apo B) or proprotein convertase subtilisin/kexin type-9 (PCSK-9) that interferes with the clearance of LDL-C by the liver. Elevated circulating markers of vascular inflammation and endothelial dysfunction are present in children with FH, reflecting early atherogenesis.

What are the types of familial hypercholesterolemia and how common are they?
Clinically, the heterozygous (HeFH) phenotype is encountered most often (1 in 250–500) while the rarely encountered homozygous (HoFH) phenotype has much worse sequelae (1 in 300,000).

Considering the Indian population of 1.35 billion and a ratio of HeFH of 1 in 500 there will be approximately 2.6 million population of HeFH and 4,500 cases of HoFh. Most of these patients are undiagnosed and are responsible for premature coronary artery disease in India.

What are the characteristics of heterozygotes familial hypercholesterolemia (HeFH) and homozygotes familial hypercholesterolemia (HoFH)?

HeFH is seen when the individual inherits one mutant gene and is characterized by a three- to four-fold higher LDL-C concentration. Lipid stigmata including corneal arcus **(Fig. 1)** and tendon xanthomata **(Figs. 2A and B)** can be seen and patients develop premature cardiovascular disease in their fourth decade, although women may develop these later. Untreated HeFH cases experience fatal or nonfatal coronary events in their 40s and 50s but can be readily treated with cholesterol-lowering medication in addition to lifestyle modifications. In addition to statins, agents like bile acid sequestrants, cholesterol absorption inhibitors (e.g., ezetimibe), bempedoic acid, or PCSK9i may be required.

In contrast, patients with HoFH inherit the defective genes from both parents, have four to eightfold higher LDL-C concentration than the general population, and develop cutaneous stigmata and atherosclerotic cardiovascular disease in their teens. LDL values in HeFH cases are generally between 350 and 550 mg/dL, whereas in HoFH, this value is between 650 and 1,000 mg/dL. Tendon xanthomas are pathognomonic of FH, especially HoFH. Accelerated atherosclerosis of the

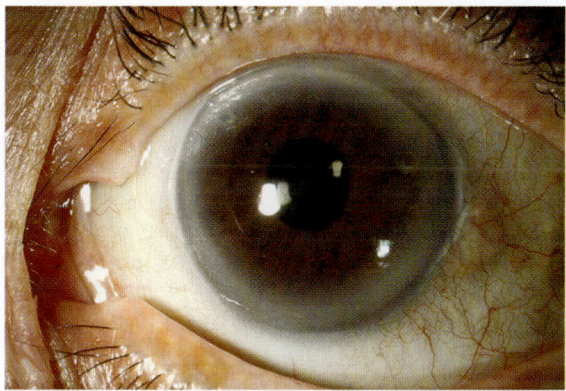

FIG. 1: Corneal arcus.

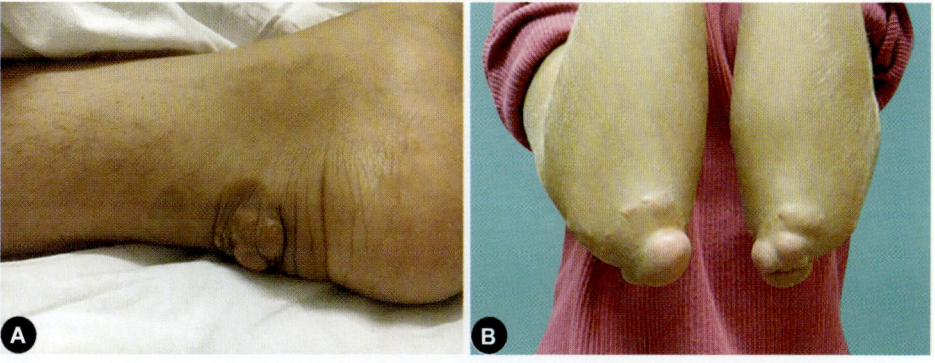

FIGS. 2A AND B: Tendon xanthoma over ankle and elbows.

coronary, carotid, and lower limb arteries leading to cardiovascular diseases, recurrent transient ischemic attacks, strokes, intermittent claudication, or gangrene is commonly seen at a younger age. Calcific aortic valve disease is also seen in these patients. Severe coronary artery disease requiring percutaneous interventions or coronary bypass surgery is common and the disease has high mortality in the second decade of life.

How do you diagnose familial hypercholesterolemia?
The Lipid Association of India (LAI) recommends the Simon Broome criteria for diagnosis of FH because of the ease of applying and diagnosing cases based on the criteria. The Simon Broome Criteria takes into consideration total cholesterol and LDL-C concentrations, the presence of tendon xanthomata **(Figs. 2A and B)**, the presence of a family history of premature vascular disease, and the total cholesterol and LDL-C concentration in the family members.

■ TYPICAL PHYSICAL FINDINGS (STIGMATA) OF FAMILIAL HYPERCHOLESTEROLEMIA

The clinical diagnosis of homozygous familial hypercholesterolemia is typically based on the presence of cutaneous xanthomas before 10 years of age and an untreated LDL-C >500 mg/dL. Interdigital xanthomas **(Fig. 3)** are pathognomonic for homozygous familial hypercholesterolemia, particularly between the thumb and index finger.

What is the significance of family history?
The family history of premature ischemic heart disease helps to identify an autosomal dominant mode of inheritance. If both parents have very high LDL-C (>190 mg/dL) and/or a history of heart disease before age of 55–65 years, this may suggest that they both have FH and can each pass a mutated gene to their children. When each parent has HeFH, by chance, 1 of 4 children will have a normal cholesterol level, 2 of 4 children will have HeFH, and 1 of 4 children will have HoFH. LAI recommends Simon Broome's criteria for the diagnosis of FH.

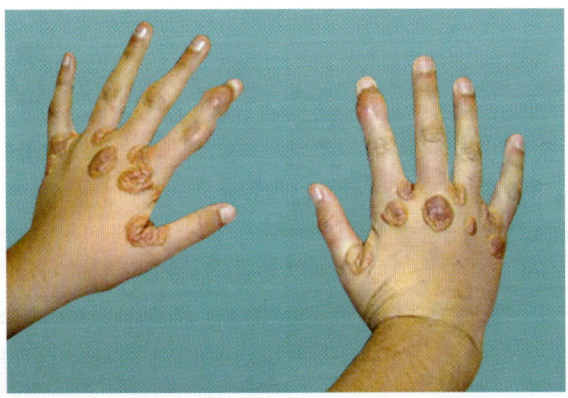

FIG. 3: Interdigital xanthoma.

SIMON BROOME DIAGNOSTIC CRITERIA FOR FAMILIAL HYPERCHOLESTEROLEMIA

Definite FH if the following are present:
- Total cholesterol > 260 mg/dL or LDL-C > 155 mg/dL in a child <16 years or total cholesterol > 300 mg/dL and LDL-C > 190 mg/dL in an adult with tendon xanthomas or evidence of these signs in a first- or second-degree relative.
or,
- DNA-based evidence of an LDLR mutation, familial defective Apo B-100, or a PCSK-9 mutation.

Possible FH if the following are present:
- Cholesterol concentrations defined as above and at least one of the following:
  - Family history of MI in a first-degree relative younger than 60 years or a second-degree relative younger than 50 years, or
  - Family history of raised total cholesterol >300 mg/dL in an adult first- or second-degree relative or >260 mg/dL in a child, brother, or sister aged younger than 16 years.

The Dutch criteria use a point system for LDL-C concentration, presence of xanthomata, and presence of CVD, and a total score of over 8 is considered as definite FH and 6–8 as probable FH. The US Make Early Diagnosis to Prevent Early Deaths (MEDPED) criteria uses age and relative-specific LDL-C concentration for diagnosing FH.

What is cascade testing?
It involves performing the lipid profiles on the relatives of the "index" patient. It helps in the identification of new cases and in the institution of early therapy. The index patient is diagnosed clinically through history, physical examination, lipid profile, or molecular diagnosis. Subsequently, the cascade testing of the family can be carried out similarly using lipid profiles followed by molecular testing in those meeting the criteria for FH. Training health professionals in the construction of the genetic tree is an important aspect of cascade testing. The updated 2020 risk stratification approach as recommended by the Lipid Association of India is described in **Figure 4**.

What is the significance of molecular diagnosis?
A diagnosis of FH can be confirmed by genetic testing. However, it should be understood by healthcare providers that failure to detect a mutation does not exclude a diagnosis of FH, and intervention with lipid-lowering therapy is required even if the diagnosis is clinical. Remember to "Treat the Phenotype and Counsel the Genotype". Financial restrictions due to the additional expense of genetic testing to families need to be kept in mind.

What is the management of FH?
Lifestyle issues such as physical activities, dietary modifications, smoking cessation, alcohol restriction, and stress management should be addressed, and other ASCVD risk factors should be meticulously looked for and treated. Based on the LAI risk algorithm, identify ASCVD risk categories and LDL-C targets.

Risk factors/markers		
Major ASCVD risk factors • Age ≥45 years in males and ≥55 years in females • Family history of premature ASCVD • Current cigarette smoking or tobacco use • High blood pressure • Low HDL-C	**Other high-risk features** • Diabetes with 0–1 other major ASCVD risk factors and no evidence to targets organ damage • CKD stage 3B or 4 • Familial hypercholesterolemia (other than familial homozygous hypercholesterolemia) • Extreme of a single risk factor • Coronary calcium score >300 HU • Nonstenotic carotid plaque • Lipoprotein (a) ≥50 mg/dL	**Moderate risk nonconventional risk factors** • Coronary calcium score 100–299 HU • Increased carotid IMT • Lipoprotein (a) 20–49 mg/dL • Impaired fasting glucose • Increased waist circumference • Apolipoprotein B ≥110 mg/dL • hsCRP ≥2 mg/L

Risk group					
Low risk	Moderate risk	High risk	Very high risk	\multicolumn{2}{c}{Extreme risk}
0–1 major ASCVD risk factor and life-time CVD risk <30%	• Two major ASCVD risk factors • Low risk group with ≥1 moderate risk nonconventional risk factor • Life-time CVD risk ≥30%	• ≥3 major ASCVD risk factors • Two major ASCVD risk factors with ≥1 moderate risk nonconventional risk factor • ≥1 other high-risk features	• Preexisting ASCVD • Diabetics with ≥2 other major ASCVD risk factors or evidence of target organ damage • Familial homozygous hypercholesterolemia	Category A ↓ CAD with ≥1 features of *high risk group*	Category B ↓ CAD with ≥1 features of *very high risk group* or recurrent ACS (within 1 year) despite LDL-C ≤50 mg/dL or polyvascular decrease

Clinical judgment to be used if the patient has atherosclerotic peripheral arterial disease instead of coronary artery disease. "A fasting blood sugar level from 100 to 125 mg/dL. It should be confirmed by repeating testing," Waist circumference is to be measured at the superior border of the iliac crest just after expiration. Increased waist circumference is defined as >90 cm in men and >80 cm in women. If increased waist circumference is the only risk factor, it should again be measured after 6 months after initiating heart healthy lifestyle measures, on two occasions at least 2 weeks apart. For reclassifying moderate risk group only.

FIG. 4: Updated 2020 risk stratification approach recommended by the Lipid Association of India.

(ASCVD: atherosclerotic cardiovascular disease; CAD: chronic kidney disease; CVD: cardiovascular disease; HDL-C: high-density lipoprotein cholesterol; LDL-C: low-density lipoprotein cholesterol)

Statins at high doses are the mainstay of therapy. Other drugs like ezetimibe may need to be added. Bile acid resins are now available in India. Both mipomersen and lomitapide have the potential for use in HoFH. PCSK-9 inhibitors lower LDL-C levels by up to 60% in patients already on statins and have been recommended in heterozygotes. Evolocumab (Repatha) is presently available in India though cost remains a constraint.

LDL apheresis, a standard therapy until now used routinely in HoFH in many developed countries is now available in a few centers in India.

For the treatment of homozygous familial hypercholesterolemia (HoFH) in patients 12 years of age and older, the Food and Drug Administration (FDA) has approved evinacumab injection. It is expensive and presently not available in India.

What are the implications of early diagnosis?
The diagnosis of FH is important not only for the prognosis of the patient but also has implications for the family members who may have inherited the same disorder. The contribution of FH to premature CVD in Indians is unknown, mainly due to the lack of awareness of this condition among both healthcare providers and the general population.

Homozygous FH is a serious medical condition and is life-threatening if not treated at a young age, preferably beginning in early childhood. A child or adult with HoFH needs life-long medications and other specialized treatments to lower the LDL-C and prevent heart attacks. This requires the expertise of a lipid specialist.

What is the need for the maintenance of a Registry?
Keeping in mind the lack of awareness of the seriousness of FH among the medical fraternity and the general population, creating a registry may be an eye-opener to the incidence and prevalence of this entity in Indian Society. We need to remember that FH contributes to premature coronary events. Timely intervention may help to reduce the existing and ever-expanding trend of cardiovascular disease among Indians.

■ LIPID ASSOCIATION OF INDIA RECOMMENDATIONS

- Lipid profile estimation of children to be done at 2 years of age in those with a family history of FH and premature ASCVD.
- Universal screening of lipids to be carried out at age 20 years or at the time of college admission including Lp(a).
- LAI recommends the Simon Broome criteria for the diagnosis of FH.
- In an established case of FH, LAI recommends estimation of Lp(a) levels.
- Genetic testing **(Flowchart 1)** and cascade screening should be performed wherever feasible.
- Look for other ASCVD risk factors and manage them appropriately.
- Based on the LAI risk algorithm, identify ASCVD risk categories and LDL-C targets.
- Strict dietary recommendations and lifestyle modifications as advised.
- Drug therapy to be started at the age of 8 years or earlier in individualized cases.
- LDL-C targets to be achieved: <70 mg/dL for HoFH, <100 mg/dL for HeFH in children and in adults <50 mg/dL in HoFH and <70 mg/dL in HeFH without ASCVD and ≤50 mg/dL for HoFH and ≤70 mg/dL for HeFH in children and in adults ≤ 30 mg/dL in HoFH and ≤50 mg/dL in HeFH with ASCVD.

Familial Hypercholesterolemia

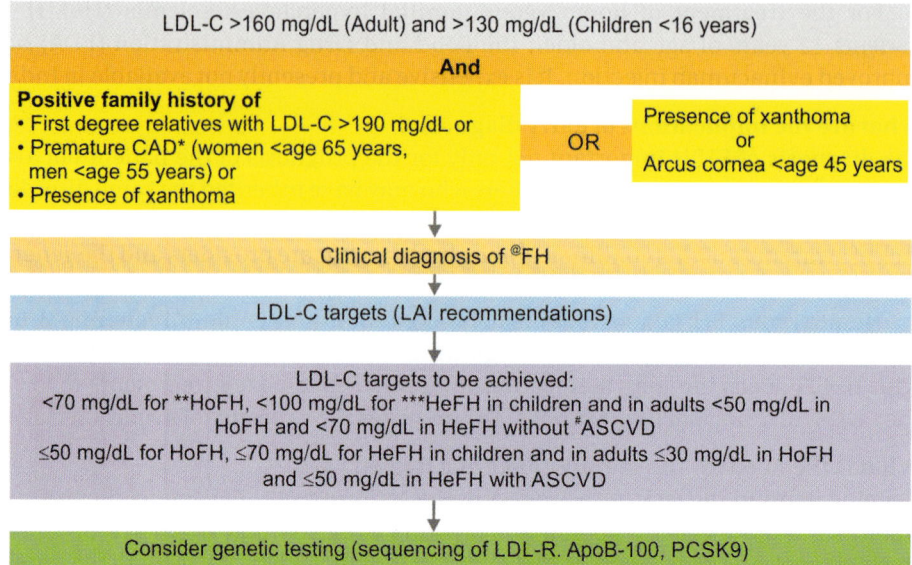

***HeFH (Heterozygous Familial Hypercholesterolemia), **HoFH (Homozygous Familial Hypercholesterolemia), #Atherosclerotic Cardiovascular Disease (ASCVD), @FH familial Hypercholesterolemia, *CAD Coronary artery disease

FLOWCHART 1: A simplified algorithm for detecting and treating Indians with high LDL-associated genetic risk (LAI recommendation).

■ SUGGESTED READINGS

1. Youngblom E, Pariani M, Knowles JW. Familial Hypercholesterolemia. In: Adam MP, Ardinger HH, Pagon RA, et al. (Eds). GeneReviews® [Internet]. Seattle (WA): University of Washington, Seattle; 2014 [Updated 2016]. 1993-2018.
2. Austin MA, Hutter CM, Zimmern RL, et al. Genetic causes of monogenic heterozygous familial hypercholesterolemia: a HuGE prevalence review. Am J Epidemiol. 2004;160:407-20.
3. Jameson JL, Fauci A, Kasper D, et al. Harrison's principles of internal medicine, 19th edition, Vol 2: Ch 421;2441. India: McGraw-Hill Education/Medical; 2017.
4. Trump TR, Hartgers ML, Hooving GK, et al. Worldwide prevalence of homozygous familial hypercholesterolemia: retrospective cohort study. Lancet. 2022;399:719-28.
5. Cuchel M, Bruckert E, Ginsberg HN, et al. Homozygous familial hypercholesterolemia: new insights and guidance for clinicians to improve detection and clinical management. A position paper from the Consensus Panel on Familial Hypercholesterolemia of the European Atherosclerosis Society. Eur Heart J. 2014;35:2146-57.
6. Durrington P. Dyslipidaemia. Lancet. 2003;362:717-31.
7. Versmissen J, Oosterveer DM, Yazdanpanah M, et al. Efficacy of statins in familial hypercholesterolemia: a long-term cohort study. Brit Med J. 2008;337:a2423.
8. Goldberg AC, Hopkins PN, Toth PP, et al. Familial hypercholesterolemia: screening, diagnosis, and management of pediatric and adult patients. J Clin Lipidol. 2011;5:S1-8.
9. Risk of fatal coronary heart disease in familial hypercholesterolemia. Scientific steering committee on behalf of the Simon Broome registers group. Br Med J. 1991;303:893-6.
10. Dutch Lipid Network. World Health Organization. Familial hypercholesterolemia—report of a second WHO Consultation. Geneva, Switzerland: World Health Organization, 1999. (WHO publication no. WHO/HGN/FH/CONS/99.2).

11. Williams RR, Hunt SC, Schumacher MC, et al. US Med Ped. Diagnosing heterozygous familial hypercholesterolemia using new practical criteria validated by molecular genetics. Am J Cardiol. 1993;72:171-6.
12. Setia N, Sawhney JP, Saxena R, et al. Successful role of cascade screening in familial hypercholesterolemia in Indian population. Cardiology. 2015;131:251.
13. Iyengar SS, Puri R, Narasingan SN, et al. Lipid Association of India expert consensus statement on management of dyslipidemia in Indians. part 2. Clin Lipidol. 2017;12(1):56-109.
14. Rader DJ, Kastelein JJ. Lomitapide and mipomersen: two first-in-class drugs for reducing low-density lipoprotein cholesterol in patients with homozygous familial hypercholesterolemia. Circulation. 2014;129:1022-32.
15. Raal FJ, Stein EA, Dufour R, et al. PCSK9 inhibition with evolocumab (AMG 145) in heterozygous familial hypercholesterolemia (RUTHERFORD-2): a randomized, double-blind, placebo-controlled trial. Lancet. 2015;385:331-40.
16. Thompson GR, Catapano A, Saheb S, et al. Severe hypercholesterolemia: therapeutic goals and eligibility criteria for LDL apheresis in Europe. Curr Opin Lipidol. 2010;21:492-8.
17. Kuehn BM. Evinacumab Approval Adds a New Option for Homozygous Familial Hypercholesterolemia with a Hefty Price Tag. Circulation. 2021;143:2494-6.

Antimicrobial Resistance: What the Clinician Should Know?

Dipanjan Bandyopadhyay, Santanu Hazra, Samarth Loomba

■ INTRODUCTION

Antimicrobial resistance (AMR) remains the world's most urgent public health concern. According to the WHO, antibiotic resistance is rising to dangerously high levels in all parts of the world, leading to increased morbidity and mortality. The choice of the best therapeutic option for the treatment of bacterial infections relies on the results of antibiotic sensitivity test (AST). An appropriate selection of antibiotic is the first step toward ensuring infection control in the clinical setting as well as preventing the emergence of resistance with the unrestricted use of newer and stronger antibiotics. Herein lies the importance of the clinician's understanding of a report of antimicrobial resistance testing.

■ INAPPROPRIATE ANTIBIOTICS

In hospital settings, studies suggest that approximately 50% of patients receive at least one antibiotic during their inpatient stay, 30% of which includes broad-spectrum antibiotics. The inappropriate use of antibiotics has been reported to be as high as 50%, although estimates can vary by institution and how "appropriate" is defined. Inappropriate use may lead to increased adverse effects, secondary infections, drug interactions, additional costs, prolonged lengths of stay, and hospital readmissions. Furthermore, bacterial resistance may develop, which can lead to treatment failure.

Conventional culture sensitivity testing consists of performing Gram stain followed by bacterial identification and antibiotic susceptibility testing. The process from start to finish can take up to 5 days, which can delay time to antibiotic de-escalation. Antibiotic susceptibility standards in the United States are determined by the Food and Drug Administration (FDA), which mostly refers to standards, set by the Clinical and Laboratory Standards Institute (CLSI). Standards may vary in other countries, which can lead to discrepancies in the definition of antibiotic susceptibility; this has led to the creation of the National Antimicrobial Susceptibility Testing Committee for the USA (USCAST). This committee works with the European Union Committee for Antimicrobial Susceptibility Testing to normalize standards on an international level.

Quantitative testing is typically performed by identification of the minimum inhibitory concentration (MIC). The MIC is the lowest concentration of antibiotic needed to inhibit the growth of an organism. The lowest MIC does not always correlate with the most effective treatment, as different antibiotics achieve different concentrations in different sites. To determine qualitative categories, specific MIC values, also known as breakpoints, are used to classify bacteria as susceptible, intermediate, or resistant to a specific antibiotic. To determine breakpoints, the CLSI uses pharmacokinetic, pharmacodynamic, resistance mechanisms, and clinical data.

The **MIC is the** *lowest concentration (in µg/mL) of an antibiotic that inhibits the growth of a given strain of bacteria*. Next to each antibiotic is the susceptibility interpretation: S (sensitive), I (intermediate), or R (resistant), followed by the MIC in µg/mL. Sensitive implies that the organism is inhibited by the serum concentration of the drug that is achieved using the recommended dosage; intermediate includes isolates with MICs that approach usually attainable blood and tissue levels and for which response rates may be lower than for susceptible isolates and implies clinical efficacy in body sites where the drug is physiologically concentrated or when a higher than normal dosage of the drug can be used; and resistant implies that the organisms are resistant to the usually achievable serum drug levels.

An antibiotic breakpoint is the dilution where bacteria begin to show resistance. **Breakpoints are** *the concentrations at which bacteria are susceptible to successful treatment with an antibiotic* **and below which exhibits resistance**. Breakpoints are discriminatory antimicrobial concentrations used in the interpretation of results of susceptibility testing to define isolates as susceptible, intermediate, or resistant. Clinical, pharmacological, microbiological, and pharmacodynamic considerations are important in setting breakpoints. The ideal mix of these factors is under constant discussion. Different countries have different approaches to this problem but, by and large, their approaches have much in common which has allowed for the recent progress in setting European breakpoints through the European Committee on Antimicrobial Susceptibility Testing (EUCAST).

Looking at **Table 1**, it appears that this strain of *Escherichia coli* has an MIC of 2 µg/mL for amoxicillin and an MIC of 8 µg/mL for cephalexin. However, we must incorporate the knowledge of the respective breakpoints, to elicit clinically relevant information. Looking at the breakpoints for amoxicillin **(Table 2)**, at 2 µg/mL this strain of *E. coli* is four dilutions away from the breakpoint. For cephalexin, the same strain of *E. coli* at an MIC of 8 µg/mL is two dilutions away from the breakpoint. So, based on MICs, this strain of *E. coli* is more susceptible to amoxicillin than cephalexin. Other factors to take into consideration are the site of the infection, the concentration achieved by that antibiotic at the site of infection, other comorbidities modulating the drug dosing, frequency, and route of administration, and cost of the

TABLE 1: Example of MIC of commonly used antibiotics for *Escherichia coli*.

Organism	MIC for *E. coli*	*E. coli* susceptibility
Amoxicillin	S 2 µg/mL	Sensitive
Amox/Clav acid	S 8 µg/mL	Sensitive
Piperacillin	S ≤ 4 µg/mL	Sensitive
Cephalexin	S 8 µg/mL	Sensitive
Cefpodoxime	S ≤ 0.25 µg/mL	Sensitive
Ceftiofur	S ≤ 1 µg/mL	Sensitive
Cefovecin	S ≤ 1 µg/mL	Sensitive
Amikacin	S ≤ 2 µg/mL	Sensitive
Gentamicin	S ≤ 0.5 µg/mL	Sensitive
Tobramycin	S ≤ 1 µg/mL	Sensitive
Enrofloxacin	S 0.5 µg/mL	Sensitive
Marbofloxacin	S 0.5 µg/mL	Sensitive
Tetracycline	R ≥ 16 µg/mL	Resistant
Nitrofurantoin	S 32 µg/mL	Sensitive
Chloramphenicol	S 8 µg/mL	Sensitive
Trimethoprim/Sulfa	S ≤ 10 µg/mL	Sensitive

(MIC: minimum inhibitory concentration; R: resistant; S: sensitive)

TABLE 2: Example of breakpoints of two antibiotics against *Escherichia coli*.

Tested concentrations of amoxicillin–clavulanic acid							Intermediate	Resistant
Sensitive							Intermediate	Resistant
S	S	S	(S)	S	S		i	r
0.25	0.5	1	(2)	4	8		16	32
								Breakpoint

Tested concentrations of cephalexin (µg/mL)				Intermediate	Resistant
Sensitive				Intermediate	Resistant
S	S	(S)		i	r
2	4	(8)		16	32
					Breakpoint

Note: Circles denote MIC.

antibiotic. Last but not the least, breakpoints have evolved over time and continue to change as more and more resistance drugs appear on the horizon and more and more antibiotics are pumped into the ecosystem. **Table 3** highlights the change in breakpoint values over time.

TABLE 3: Breakpoint changes over time.						
	Breakpoint changes over time for the *Enterobacteriaceae*					
	Historical CLSI			Current CLSI		
	Sensitive	Intermediate	Resistant	Sensitive	Intermediate	Resistant
Cefazolin	≤8	16	≥32	≤2	4	≥8
Cefotaxime	≤8	16–32	≥64	≤1	2	≥4
Ceftriaxone	≤8	16–32	≥64	≤1	2	≥4
Ceftazidime	≤8	16	≥32	≤4	8	≥16
Aztreonam	≤8	16	≥32	≤4	8	≥16
Doripenem	<0.5	–	–	≤1	2	≥4
Ertapenem	≤2	4	≥8	≤0.25	0.5	≥1
Imipenem	≤4	8	≥16	≤1	2	≥4
Meropenem	≤4	8	≥16	≤1	2	≥4

(CLSI: Clinical and Laboratory Standards Institute; I: intermediate; R: resistant; S: susceptible)

ISSUES BEYOND MINIMUM INHIBITORY CONCENTRATION AND BREAKPOINTS

When selecting an antibiotic, it is important to keep in mind that other factors in addition to the MIC are important. The location of the infection must be considered because lipid-soluble drugs reach higher levels in the tissue than they do in serum. Drugs excreted by the kidney reach much higher bladder levels than serum levels. The best example is the susceptibility of *E. coli* causing urinary tract infection (UTI) to Amoxicillin; even if the sensitivity report shows susceptibility of the organism, it is wise to use a Fluoroquinolone or chose another beta lactam such as cefixime which achieves higher urinary concentrations than Amoxicillin or Cephalexin.

Several questions remain on the horizon of susceptibility testing. For example, does a vancomycin MIC of <1 µg/mL predict a better outcome in a patient with a staphylococcal infection than an MIC of 2 µg/mL? More importantly, how have these practices impacted the "art of medicine" as practiced by infectious disease (ID) clinicians? Is information regarding the new breakpoints with associated therapeutic comments ever communicated to physicians and pharmacists who may make use of the information? How are such "Rx" comments in the documents addressed when results are used to direct outpatient therapy by non-ID physicians and in the absence of input from ID pharmacists? That brings us to the issue of comments in clinical microbiology reporting (CMR).

Majority of the Indian microbiology laboratories generate a basic level culture and antimicrobial susceptibility testing (C and AST) report, which comprise only identification of the organism isolated with a list of antimicrobials and their susceptibility results. It is essential that the laboratory microbiologists of India uplift themselves to clinical microbiologists and foster their CMR to higher standards by incorporating specific comments, suggestions, and advices in the C and AST report. Comments such as sterile at 48 hours, sterile at 7 days, sterile (false positive), contaminant, pathogen and pathogenicity uncertain would go a long way in making C and AST reports clinically relevant. Moreover, the microbiologists should communicate with the clinicians at every stage of culture report, with a note on what part of the report is awaited. Stagewise reporting with comment for inprogress reports not only helps in early institution of directed therapy but also gives a clear message to the clinicians to review the report subsequently for further action.

■ CONCEPT OF THERAPEUTIC INDEX

When the test isolate is susceptible to more than one antimicrobials of a similar spectrum, it is often difficult to choose the most appropriate antimicrobial for directed therapy. In this situation, the antimicrobial with a higher therapeutic index should be preferred for therapy. The therapeutic index of an antimicrobial for an organism is defined as the ratio of susceptible breakpoint to minimum inhibitory concentration (MIC) of the test isolate. The lower the therapeutic index, the better the therapeutic efficacy. If laboratories report only the raw MIC values, the clinicians get misguided and select the antimicrobial with the lowest MIC for therapy. For example, if *Klebsiella pneumoniae* is reported by a laboratory with amikacin MIC of 2 µg/mL and meropenem MIC of 0.5 µg/mL, it appears as if meropenem having lower MIC is more effective than amikacin. However, in reality, amikacin is more effective in this case, as it has a higher therapeutic index (susceptible breakpoint is 16 µg/mL; therefore, therapeutic index is 16/2 = 8) as compared to that of meropenem (susceptible breakpoint is 1 µg/mL; therefore, therapeutic index is 1/0.5 = 2). For that reason, it is always advisable for the microbiologists to report therapeutic index along with the raw MIC values.

Comments related to site-specific issues are growing in clinical importance. In a blood culture report, it is essential to mention about the time to positivity (TTP). TTP refers to the time taken for the blood culture bottle to flag positive by the automated blood culture equipment. The clinicians must be aware that the lower the TTP, the higher the organism load in the specimen, and therefore, worse is the clinical outcome. It is also important for the microbiologist to report when a catheter-related bloodstream infection is diagnosed, the laboratory criteria of which are fulfilled when a central line blood culture specimen is flagged more than 2 hours earlier than the venepuncture specimen. The utility of organism-specific comments is mentioned in **Table 4** and susceptibilityrelated comments are mentioned in **Table 5**.

The clinician will be better equipped if we remember the following thumb rules:
- Always start with a beta-lactam if possible, especially in severe infections. They have the best data supporting their use and are in general excellent drugs. *Exception*: Atypical infections.
- Do not compare MICs between drugs; each has different Pk (tissue vs. serum concentrations) and Pd (time vs. concentration vs. AUC/MIC dependent) parameters

Antimicrobial Resistance: What the Clinician Should Know?

TABLE 4: Organism specific comments in a C and AST report.

Category	Organism	Antimicrobial	Result	Comments
MSSA	Staphylococcus aureus	Oxacillin or cefoxitin	S	Antistaphylococcal beta lactams (e.g., cloxacillin) are much superior to vancomycin for the treatment of MSSA infection
MRSA	S. aureus	Oxacillin or cefoxitin	R	MRSA has grown in culture. Kindly avoid all beta lactams except fifth-generation cephalosporins such as ceftaroline and ceftobiprole
MS-CONS	Coagulase-negative Staphylococcus	Oxacillin or cefoxitin	S	Antistaphylococcal beta lactams (e.g., cloxacillin) are much superior to vancomycin for the treatment of MS-CONS infection
MR-CONS	Coagulase-negative Staphylococcus	Oxacillin or cefoxitin	R	Avoid all beta lactams in MR-CONS infection Vancomycin is the drug of choice
CefepimeENB	Enterobacteriaceae	Cefepime	Any	When cefepime is reported for *Enterobacteriaceae* • If MIC is ≤2 μg/mL, it is considered susceptible and the recommended dose of cefepime is 1 g twice daily • If MIC is 4 μg/mL, it is considered susceptible dose dependent (SDD) and the recommended dose of cefepime is 1 g thrice daily or 2 g twice daily • If MIC is 8 μg/mL, it is considered SDD and the recommended dose of cefepime is 2 g thrice daily • If MIC is ≥16 μg/mL, it is considered resistant and therefore is not recommended for treatment
VRE	Enterococcus	Vancomycin	R	VRE has been isolated. Kindly ensure appropriate infection control measures
MRSA/ vancomycin MIC >1 μg/mL	MRSA	Vancomycin	S and MIC 2 μg/mL	In MRSA infection, therapeutic failure may be encountered if vancomycin MIC is >1 μg/mL, even if it is tested susceptible. Therefore, consider alternate therapy

Continued

Continued

Category	Organism	Antimicrobial	Result	Comments
Colistin warning comments	• Enterobacteriaceae Pseudomonas aeruginosa • Acinetobacter baumannii complex	Colistin	MIC ≤ 2 µg/mL	If planning for colistin as therapeutic option, then please keep the following points in mind • Clinical and PK/PD data demonstrate that colistin is of limited clinical efficacy • If available, alternative nonpolymyxin agents are strongly preferred. If these agents are not available, this breakpoint presumes use of colistin in combination with one or more additional, active antimicrobials • Colistin (methane sulfonate) should be given with a loading dose and maximum renal adjusted doses • When given systemically, this drug is unlikely to be effective for pneumonia
Inducible clindamycin	*S. aureus*	Clindamycin	S	Clindamycin should not be given for serious skin and soft-tissue infections as constitutive resistance is likely to develop during such longterm therapy

(C and AST: culture and antimicrobial susceptibility testing; MIC: minimum inhibitory concentration; MRSA: methicillin-resistant *Staphylococcus aureus*; MSSA: methicillin-susceptible *Staphylococcus aureus*; MR-CONS: methicillin-resistant coagulase-negative *Staphylococcus* species; VRE: vancomycin-resistant enterococci)

TABLE 5: Prediction-specific comments in a C and AST report.

Organism	Antimicrobial	Result	Comments
Enterobacteriaceae	Ceftriaxone	Any	Ceftriaxone susceptibility test result can be extrapolated for cefotaxime for *Enterobacteriaceae* family
Staphylococcus	Erythromycin	Any	Erythromycin susceptibility test result of *Staphylococcus* species can be extrapolated for azithromycin or clarithromycin
Enterococcus	Ampicillin	S	Enterococci susceptible to ampicillin are predictably susceptible to amoxicillin, ampicillin–sulbactam, amoxicillin–clavulanate, and piperacillin–tazobactam for nonbeta-lactamase-producing enterococci
Enterococcus	Penicillin	S	Enterococci susceptible to penicillin are predictably susceptible to ampicillin, amoxicillin, ampicillin–sulbactam, amoxicillin–clavulanate, and piperacillin–tazobactam for non-beta-lactamaseproducing enterococci

Continued

Continued

Organism	Antimicrobial	Result	Comments
Streptococcus pneumonia	Oxacillin (disk diffusion)	S	For nonmeningitis isolates of S. pneumonia, if oxacillin is found susceptible, the result can be extrapolated for penicillin, ceftriaxone, cefotaxime, and meropenem
S. pneumonia	Levofloxacin	S	S. pneumonia isolates susceptible to levofloxacin are predictably susceptible to gemifloxacin and moxifloxacin
• Enterobacteriaceae Pseudomonas aeruginosa • Acinetobacter baumannii	Colistin	Any	Colistin susceptibility test result and the MIC value can be extrapolated for polymyxin B for Enterobacteriaceae, Pseudomonas aeruginosa and A. baumannii complex
Any	Tetracycline	S	Organisms that are susceptible to tetracycline are also considered susceptible to doxycycline and minocycline
Enterobacteriaceae	Ampicillin	Any	Ampicillin susceptibility test result of Enterobacteriaceae can be extrapolated for amoxicillin
Staphylococcus aureus	Vancomycin	S	S. aureus isolates susceptible to vancomycin can be predicted susceptible to dalbavancin and oritavancin and MRSA isolates susceptible to vancomycin can be predicted susceptible to telavancin
S. aureus	Linezolid	S	S. aureus isolates susceptible to linezolid can be predicted susceptible to tedizolid
Staphylococcus	Norfloxacin	S	Staphylococcus isolates susceptible to norfloxacin can be predicted susceptible to ciprofloxacin, levofloxacin, moxifloxacin and ofloxacin

(C and AST: culture and antimicrobial susceptibility testing; MRSA: methicillin-resistant *Staphylococcus aureus*)

- If "≤" you can use the drug, provided the following exceptions are kept in mind:
  - Drug does not get to the site of action
  - Drug does not achieve its goal pharmacodynamics parameters
  - Drug does not have inducible resistance
  - Patient-specific factors
  - Drug cost

As new resistance mechanisms develop, laboratories need to develop new ways to detect resistance. One example of this is the detection of extended-spectrum beta lactamase (ESBL) and/or AmpC beta-lactamase. ESBLs are enzymes that break down many beta-lactam antibiotics, rendering them ineffective. They are more likely to be present in gram-negative bacteria that are associated with healthcare-related infections. To detect ESBL, screening is performed by testing certain antibiotics such as cefotaxime and then adding clavulanic acid. If ESBL screening is performed using broth microdilution, the MIC is compared between cefotaxime and cefotaxime plus clavulanic acid. If there is a threefold dilution change in MIC when clavulanic acid is added, ESBL is present. For example, if the MIC is 2 μg/mL with cefotaxime alone and decreases to 0.5 μg/mL when clavulanic acid is added, this suggests that ESBL is present.

CONCLUSION

The interpretation of culture sensitivity reports and their incorporation into our clinical practice need an orientation which we have tried to highlight here. In today's practice, a simple mention of sensitive or resistant is insufficient to guide therapeutic trials. A fundamental idea of MIC and breakpoints is needed to meaningfully interpret a culture sensitivity report, along with basic concepts of pharmacokinetics and drug distribution. Once we begin to read between the lines of a CST report and get our microbiology colleagues on board the prescription team, our antibiotic usage are likely to change for the better.

SUGGESTED READINGS

1. Gajic I, Kabic J, Kekic D, Jovicevic M, Milenkovic M, Mitic Culafic D, et al. Antimicrobial Susceptibility Testing: A Comprehensive Review of Currently Used Methods. Antibiotics 2022;11:427.
2. Kowalska-Krochmal B, Dudek-Wicher R. The Minimum Inhibitory Concentration of Antibiotics: Methods, Interpretation, Clinical Relevance. Pathogens 2021;10:165.
3. Mouton JW, Muller AE, Canton R, Giske CG, Kahlmeter G, Turnidge J. MIC-based dose adjustment: facts and fables. J Antimicrob Chemother. 2018;73:564-8.
4. Deepashree R, Bhat S, Sastry AS. Use of comments in clinical microbiology reporting: The need of the hour. J Acad Clin Microbiol. 2020;22:67-75.

INDEX

Page numbers followed by *b* refer to box, *f* refer to figure, *fc* refer to flowchart, and *t* refer to table.

A

Abdominal compartment syndrome 365
Abductor pollicis 97
Absolute reticulocyte count 389
Acanthosis nigricans 462
Acarbose 236, 263
Accommodate dorsal deformity 250
Achalasia-cardia 285
Achlorhydria, absence of 358
Acid-base disorders, mixed 133
Acotiamide 339
Acquired immunodeficiency syndrome 109, 380, 381, 385, 393
Acrokeratosis paraneoplastica 108
Acro-osteolysis 100
Activated partial thromboplastin time 498
Active urinary sediments 197
　presence of 259
Acute chest pain
　causes of 51*b*
　syndromes 51
Acute encephalitis syndrome 481, 489, 490
　etiology of 483*t*
Acute ischemic stroke 494
　management of 494
Acute myocardial infarction 39, 91
　complications of 52
Acute pancreatitis 340, 341*t*
　causes of 341*t*
　complications of 346, 346*t*
　differential diagnosis of 342*t*
　management of 340
　scoring system for 343
Addison's disease 109, 121, 121*f*, 130, 282, 285, 358
　clinical challenges 282
　treatment 282
Adenosine
　monophosphate-activated protein kinase 36
　triphosphate 202
Adenovirus 19
Adrenal disease 121, 356
Adrenal gland
　function 283*f*
　structure 283*f*
Adrenal hormone secretion, regulation of 284*f*
Adrenal hyperplasia, congenital 284, 285
Adrenal insufficiency 151, 284, 288
　causes of 283

　primary 283, 284, 286, 294
　signs of 285
　symptoms of 285
Adrenal medulla 283
Adrenocorticotropic hormone 283
　raised 358
　stimulation test 287
Adult respiratory distress syndrome 533
Advanced glycation products 194
Aerobic exercise 315, 325
Aflibercept 216
Africans American Study of Kidney Disease and Hypertension 416
Agammaglobulinemia 486
Agra Preventive Intervention Diabetes Study 213
Airways, management of 489
Alanine transaminase 459, 460
Albumin 447
　creatinine ratio 9, 182, 196, 265
　excretion rate 196
Albuminuria 10, 196, 261, 261*f*
　detection of 196
Alcohol
　cessation of 348
　consumption 404, 472
　intoxication 150
　septal ablation 37
Aldosterone 287
Alfa pump system 369
Allergen
　immunotherapy 525
　tolerance 521*f*
Allergic march 518, 518*f*
Allergic reaction, severe 228, 525
Allergic rhinitis 519, 521-523
　subsequent 519
　treatment of 525
Allergy 168, 523
Allylamines 431
Alpha-tropomyosin 31
Alprostadil 474
Alteplase, intravenous 497
Amebic colitis 355
Amebic dysentery 359
American Association of Clinical Endocrinologists Guidelines 279*fc*
American Association of Endocrinology 275, 278

American College of Cardiology 3, 25, 404, 417
American Diabetes Association 204, 208, 239, 256, 262, 275, 279
American Gastroenterological Association 345
American Heart Association 3, 25, 329, 404
American Thyroid Association 304
Aminoglycosides 168
Amlodipine 418
Amoxicillin 569
 clavulanic acid 568
Amyloidosis 38, 285, 356, 357
 cardiac 34
Analgesics 350
Anandamaya kosha 319
Anaphylactic reactions, risk of 525
Anasarca 363
Anemia, aplastic 386
Angiofollicular lymph node hyperplasia 381
Angiogenic growth factors 479
Angiotensin-aldosterone system 283
Angiotensin-converting enzyme 217, 265, 267, 410
 inhibitors 3, 25, 266, 404, 418
Angiotensin-receptor
 blocker 3, 25, 214, 265-267, 404, 407, 418, 421
 neprilysin inhibitor 25, 217
Anidulafungin 432
Anion gap 129
Ankylosing spondylitis 547
Annamaya kosha 319
Anorexia 364
Anthracyclines, cardiotoxicity of 37
Antiarrhythmic therapy 28
Antibiotics 157, 158, 162, 168, 346, 567
 rational for 156
 resistance 159
 sensitivity test 566
 spectrum 165
 therapy 163fc
  rational prescription of 169fc
 timeout 427, 428
Anti-citrullinated protein antibodies 555
Anticoagulation 28
Antidiabetic therapy 263
Antiepileptic drugs 508-510, 510t, 511f, 512b, 513
 first-generation 509t
 second-generation 509t
Antifibrotic drugs 215
Antifungal prophylaxis 433
Antihypertension 405
Antihypertensive drugs 418
Anti-inflammatory cytokine 521
Anti-lymphocyte globulin 390
Antimetabolites 431

Antimicrobial stewardship program 423-425
 core elements of 426
Antimicrobial susceptibility testing 569
Anti-N-methyl-D-aspartate receptor 487t
Antinuclear antibody 358, 388, 532
Antioxidants 350
Antiphospholipid antibodies 285
Antiplatelet therapy 15
Antipsychotics 273, 351
Antiretroviral drugs 401
 classes of 393t
 sites of action of 392f
Antiretroviral therapy 391-393, 393t, 395-397, 402
 regimen, first-line 395t
Antirheumatic drugs 555
 disease-modifying 555
Antisaccharomyces cerevisiae antibody 358
Antithrombotic therapy 501
Antithyroid antibody, positive 298
Anti-thyroid peroxidase 300
Antitransglutaminase 358
Antitumor necrosis factor 535
Anxiety 467
 disorder 506
 reduce 328
Aortic dissection 61, 62fc, 62t
Apert syndrome 100
Apolipoprotein B 558
Arginine vasopressin 205
Arrhythmias 23
 ventricular 87b
Arrhythmogenic right ventricular cardiomyopathy 86
Arterial blood gases 125
Arterial carbon dioxide 490
Arterial diseases 496
Arterial stiffness 277
Arteriography 474
Arthritis 357
Asana 320
Ascites 363
 causes of 363t
 cirrhotic 368
 diagnosis of 364
 etiology of 364t
 rapid reaccumulation of 366
Ascitic fluid 367
 analysis of 366
 depth of 366
 examination 365
 exudative 367
 transudative 367
Aspartate aminotransferase 459, 460
Aspergillosis, invasive 432

Index

Aspiration devices 499, 500
Aspirin 501
Asthma 519, 523
    allergic 521, 525
Atelectasis, X-ray of 79*f*
Atherosclerotic cardiovascular disease 264-266, 562, 564
Athlete's heart 34
Atkins diet, modified 516
Atlanta classification revision 341*t*
Atopic dermatitis, development of 518
Atopic diseases 519
Atopic disorders 519
    development of 519
Atopic march 518
Atrial fibrillation 32, 501
Atrial septal defect 109
Australian Carbohydrate Intolerance Study in Pregnant Women 222
Autoantibodies 270
Autoimmune
    adrenalitis 284
    diseases 122, 522
    disorders 490
    polyendocrinopathy ectodermal dystrophy 284
    polyglandular syndrome 284
Avastin 216
Ayurvedic tonics 218
Azathioprine 534, 536
Azithromycin 168
Azotemia 149
Azygos vein joins 111

B

B lymphocyte stimulator 551
Babesia 377, 378
Bacteria, gram-negative 165
Bacterial infections 156, 157*f*, 355
    clinical manifestations of 156
Bactericidal therapy 166
Bacteriostatic therapy 166
Balamuthia mandrillaris 483, 492
Balanoposthitis 107
Balthazar–Ranson's grading system 343*t*
Bariatric surgery 206, 371
    long-term outcomes of 206
Baricitinib 553
Barium enema 361
Bartonella bacilliformis 485, 491
Bartonella henselae 491
Basal insulins 240
Basilar artery occlusions 501
Baylisascaris procyonis 485, 492
Bazex syndrome 108

Beau's lines 96
Beckwith-Weidemann syndrome 118
Behandelstrategieën 556
Behçet's syndrome 113, 119
Belatacept 552
Belimumab 552
Benralizumab 526
Benzodiazepines 509
Beta-adrenergic blockers 472
Beta-blocker 4, 26, 35, 214, 266, 419
    medications 522
Beta-carotene 350
Beta-cell
    dysfunction 276
    failure 187
    redifferentiation 207
    volume, loss of 277
Beta-lactam 161, 165
    antibiotic 157, 165
    inhibitor 165
Bevacizumab 216
Bicarbonate
    gastrointestinal loss of 129
    use of 452
Biconjugal diabetic couples, offspring of 213
Bigsby's classification 112
Biguanides 263
Bilateral hypoglossal nerve palsy 121*f*
Bile aid malabsorption 354
Biliary pancreatitis 346
Biochemical tests 473
Biochemistry 358
Bionic pancreas 245
Biopsy 361
Biothesiometer 249
Blastomycoses 430
Bliss, body of 319
Bloating, abdominal 364
Blood
    dendritic cell antigen 2 552
    glucose 175, 270
        acceptable 206
        control 201
        preoperative control of 175
        self-monitoring of 242
    lipids 216
    pressure 143, 265, 267, 403, 407, 414, 416
        control 14, 214
        diastolic 404, 411
        lower 259
        measurement of 415
        raised 262
        target 416
    smear 372
        examination, peripheral 378
        peripheral 371, 372, 376

Index

stained saliva 401
sugar, fasting 185
tests 487
Bloody aspirate 366
Bluish discoloration 101
Blunt
　cardiac trauma 61
　pelvic trauma 471
Body
　component of 319
　fluids 401
　mass index 185, 191, 244, 276, 304, 314, 456
　weight 531
Bone mineral density 289
Borrelia burgdorferi 19, 485, 489, 491
Boutonniere deformity 106
Bowel
　diarrhea, chronic small 357
　obstruction 366
Bradyarrhythmias
　causes of 84b
　classification of 84b
Bradycardia 84
Brain
　biopsy 489
　computer interface 515
　injury, traumatic 471
　malformation 508
　natriuretic peptide 2
　stimulation, devices for 514
　tumor 508, 513
Breast milk 401
Brisk walking 279, 325
Brivaracetam 509
Broad-spectrum drugs 511
Bronchiectasis 93
Bronchoalveolar lavage 533
Bronchoscopy 540, 542
Bronchus, carcinoma of 93
Brugada and Wereckei criteria 85fc
Brugia malayi 378
Buccal mucosa 117
Budd-Chiari syndrome 363, 367
Bundle branch block 85, 217
Butaconazole 432
Butenafine 432

C

Café-au-lait spots 387
Calcium
　channel blocker 265, 266, 405, 407, 418
　influx 470
Calmodulin-myosin light chain kinase 470
Calorie restriction 207, 280
Canagliflozin 421

Candida 119, 121
　albicans 119
　infection 123
　paronychia 107
Candidiasis 119
Cannabinoids 351
Caput medusa 365
Carbamazepine 509, 511, 512
Carbohydrate 192
　calorific contribution of 209
　diet, moderate 209
　low 278
　malabsorption 356
　predominant dietary habits 257
Carbon dioxide 128
　breath test 360
Carbonic anhydrase inhibitors 510
Carcinoembryonic antigen 368
Carcinoid
　syndrome 357
　tumor 354
Carcinoma
　bronchogenic 113
　hepatocellular 365
　pancreas 108
　　high-risk of 272
　prostate 389
　stomach 108
Cardiac catheterization 23
Cardiac chamber synchronization 217
Cardiac failure 217
　congestive 354
Cardiac insufficiency bisoprolol study 4
Cardiac involvement, detection of 216
Cardiac resynchronization therapy 6
Cardiac tamponade 57, 114
Cardiomyopathy 16
　causes of 18
　classification of 18
　clinical presentations of 18
　diabetic 37
　diagnosis 16
　dilated 6, 18, 20, 21, 29, 87
　familial 37
　hypertrophic 83
　hypertropic 30
　idiopathic 37
　management 16
　types of 17, 18
Cardiovascular care 344
Cardiovascular disease 2, 11, 192, 196, 255, 268, 276, 277, 306, 404, 462, 479, 562
Cardiovascular outcomes trial 217
Cardiovascular risk
　factors, presence of 10f
　high carbohydrate 195

Cardiovascular system 321
Carnett's sign 336
Carnitine palmitoyltransferase 36
Carolina 203
Carotid artery, internal 500
Carpal tunnel syndrome 98
Caspofungin 432, 433
Castleman's disease 114, 381
Cavernosal blood pressure 474
Cavernosal vasoconstriction 478
Cavernosography 474
Cavernous bodies 470
Cavernous muscle, tone of 473
Celiac disease 355, 357, 361
Cell-based therapy 479
Cenobamate 511
Centers for Disease Control and
    Prevention 231
Central hypothyroidism 293
    treatment of 298
Central nervous system infections 488
Cephalexin 568, 569
Cerebellar infarctions, large 501
Cerebral artery
    anterior 500
    middle 494
    proximal middle 500
Cerebral salt wasting 145, 154
Cerebral thromboembolism, acute 494
Cerebrospinal fluid 166, 167, 489
    analysis 488
Cervical lymphadenopathy 122
Chagas' disease 19
Chédiak-Higashi syndrome 110
Chemoport catheter 112
Chemotherapeutic agents 19
Chennai Urban Population Study 231
Chennai Urban Rural Epidemiology Study 231
Chest
    computed tomography 114
    radiograph 23, 114, 342
    trauma 60
        penetrating 60
    wall, anterior 114f
    X-ray 68t, 487
Cholangiopancreatography 351
    endoscopic retrograde 343
Cholecystectomy 346
Cholecystokinin 350
Cholesterol, total 262
Chron's disease 356, 357, 361
Chronic kidney disease 2, 108, 195, 204, 261,
    264, 267, 404, 414-417, 419, 457, 467, 473,
    562
    management of 260
    pathophysiology of 414

Chronic liver disease 95, 467
    presence of 108
Chronic obstructive pulmonary disease 1
Chronic pancreatitis 270, 348, 355, 358
    management of 352fc
Cicatricial alopecia 110
Cilnidipine 407, 409
    pharmacology of 408f
Ciprofloxacin 346
Circulation
    infection of 249
    maintenance of 249
Cirrhosis 366, 369
    absence of 364
Clindamycin 168
Clonidine 351
Clopidogrel 501
Clostridioides difficile 425
Clostridium
    colitis 361
    difficile 161
        toxins 360
Coccidioides 483
    immitis 488
Coccidiomycoses 430
Coenzyme Q supplementation 217
Colitis
    collagenous 362
    ischemic 359
    microscopic 354, 355
Colon cancers 324
Combination therapy 165, 210
Combined pituitary hormone deficiency 285
Complete blood count 287, 337, 388, 531
Complete urinalysis, three components
    of 197b
Compression atelectasis 79f
Computed tomography 342, 349, 382
    high-resolution 365
Concentration 321
Conjunctivitis 521, 522, 525
Connective tissue disease 109, 380, 530, 548
    management of 534
    mixed 380
    treatment of 536b
Connective tissue disorders 108, 109
Continuous glucose monitoring systems 189,
    242, 265
Contraceptive agents 512
Contusion, cardiac 61
Conventional culture sensitivity testing 566
Cool compresses 523
Corneal arcus 559f
Cornell voltage criteria 83
Coronary artery
    bypass graft 216

disease 1, 9, 10, 52b, 109, 216, 457, 465, 473
  pathogenesis of 465fc
  occlusion 20
  right 88, 89
Coronary syndrome, acute 3, 179
Coronary thrombosis, hemodynamic effects of 64
Coronavirus disease 243
Corpora cavernosa 471, 477, 478
  blood filled 468
Corporal tissue 478
Corpus callosotomy 514
Corrosions 120
Corticosteroids 273, 449, 536
  insufficiency 448, 450t
Corticotropin-releasing hormones 283
Cough, management of 528
Covaxin 227
COVID-19 227
  vaccine 227
Covishield 227
Coxiella burnetii 483, 491
Coxsackie 19
C-peptide 209, 270
  normal 272
C-reactive protein 337, 358, 438, 463, 465, 547, 555
Creutzfeldt-Jacob disease 486, 487
Crohn's disease 108, 119, 361
Cryptococcal disease 123
Cryptococcosis 430, 432
Cryptococcus neoformans 492
Cryptosporidiosis 362
Crystalloids 445
Cullen sign 341
Cushing's syndrome 109, 114, 273
Cyanosis 107
Cyclic guanosine monophosphate 474
Cyclosporine 556
Cyproterone acetate 472
Cystatin C 215
Cystic fibrosis 114
Cytogenetics 389
Cytokines 277, 552
Cytomegalovirus 355, 360, 380, 381, 386, 389, 486-489, 491

D

Dapagliflozin 279
Daratumumab 552
Dark knuckles 99
Deep brain stimulation 514
Deep dorsal vein 479
Deep vein thrombosis 498
  prophylaxis 452

Dehydration 268
  risk of 203
Dehydroepiandrosterone 283
  replacement 291
Dendritic cells 552
Dentifrices 214
Deoxyribonucleic acid 158, 374, 551
Depression 467
Dermatitis
  artefacta 110
  herpetiformis 110
Dermatomyositis 535
Descending artery, left anterior 86, 89, 90, 179
Dexamethasone implants 216
Dharana 321
Dhyana 321
Diabetes
  drug-induced 270, 273
  malnutrition-modulated 270
  mellitus 107, 121, 130, 178, 185, 187, 270, 271, 276, 276f, 278, 304, 353, 356, 358, 421, 454, 464, 464fc, 467, 471, 473
  autoimmune 185
  care 244, 280
  gestational 175, 219, 220, 220fc, 221, 222fc, 223, 270, 272, 276
  impending global epidemic of 280
  management 184
  neonatal 270
  permanent neonatal 271
  secondary 270, 273
  steroid-induced 186
  subsequent 277
  transient neonatal 271
  type 1 186, 195, 225, 238, 244, 259, 265, 269, 271, 304, 353
  type 2 3, 178, 184, 191, 195, 201, 206, 219, 220, 223, 225, 244, 255, 259, 265, 269, 276, 277, 280, 314, 327, 352, 456, 462, 464
  type 3 213
  prevention program 236, 277
  types of 269, 273
  wellness clinic 314
  work group 260
Diabetic foot 249
  offloading of 249
  specialist 252
  ulcers 249
    management of 249
Diabetic footwear 250
Diabetic hand syndrome 103
Diabetic kidney disease 194, 215, 259, 263, 264, 266
  management, care of 260f
  occurrence of 268

pathophysiological interactions of 259
prevention of 262
progression of 262
stages of 195*f*
treatment of 267*fc*
Diabetic nephropathy 178, 194, 215, 268
progression of 263
Diabetic retinopathy 215
detection of 216
Diabetic temporary tattoos 246
Dialysis 420
Diarrhea
chronic 354
continuous 355
diabetic 355
functional 354
inflammatory 355
secretary 354
Diet 215
high-calorie 192
high-carbohydrate 209
modification of 259, 416
therapy 516
Differential leukocyte count 438
Diffusion-weighted imaging 496
Digestive system 322
Digital
clubbing 109
technology, scope of 246
Digitalis
glycosides 27
investigation group 5
Digoxin 5
Dihydropyridine 418
Dilated cardiomyopathy 6, 18, 20, 21, 29, 87
clinical features 20
incidence 21
laboratory findings 21
major causes of 19
prognosis 21
proven therapeutic option 24
treatment 23
Dipeptidyl peptidase-4 175, 203, 214, 264, 353
inhibitors 186
Diphenhydramine 497
Diphtheria 228
Diplopia 495
Dipstick albumin 198
Disability index 556
Discoid lupus erythematosus 110
Disopyramide 35
Disseminated intravascular coagulation 346, 366, 371
Distal metallic mesh 499
Distensibility index 67

Diuretics 369, 419
dose of 368
therapy 24, 30
Diurnal variation 355
Diverticulitis 355
Dolutegravir 394
Dorsal artery 479
Doty and Standford's classification 112
Down syndrome 118
Doxycycline 168
Dravet syndrome 511
Drug
administration 217
drug interaction profile 517
therapy 207
Dry weight reduction 420
Dual endothelin receptor 421
Duodenal mucosa, flattening of 361
Dupilumab 526
Duplex ultrasound 114
Dupuytren's contracture 95
D-xylose absorption test 360
Dysglycemia 213
Dyslipidemia 255, 278, 467, 471
atherogenic diabetic 255-257
management of 266
presence of 262
Dyspepsia 334, 338*fc*
differential diagnosis of 336*b*
functional 335*b*
Dyspnea, management of 528

E

Echocardiographic methods 62, 63*f*
Echocardiography 23, 33, 41, 58*b*, 62, 66*f*, 68*f*
abnormalities 54, 54*t*
guided cardiac output optimization 64, 65*f*
parameters, static two-dimensional 64*f*
role of 51
sector probe for 42*f*
signs 58*f*
Echo-Doppler 38
Eczema 519
persistent 519
Edema 107
cardiogenic pulmonary 67
Efavirenz 394
Egg allergy 228
Ehrlichia chaffeensis 491
Ehrlichioses 483, 491
Eisenmenger's syndrome 93
Ejection fraction 2
Electrocardiogram 39, 81, 314, 365

Electrolyte
  deficiencies 19
  resuscitation 344
Electromyography 322
Electronic health records 243
Electrophysiological studies 85
Emergency
  medical services 495
  ventriculostomy 501
Empirical therapy 164, 490
Encephalitis 484*b*
  autoimmune 492
  viruses 483
Encephalomyelitis, acute disseminated 486, 488, 492
Encephalopathy 484*b*
  acute febrile 435
Endarteritis, presence of 361
Endobronchial ultrasound-guided transbronchial needle aspiration 382
Endocarditis 93
Endocrine disorders 109, 121
Endocrinopathy 474
Endomyocardial diseases 38
Endopeptidases 410
Endoscopic ultrasound 343, 351
Endoscopy, gastrointestinal 361
Endosonography 361
Endothelial cells 468, 470
Endothelial dysfunction 10, 277
Endothelial nitric oxide synthase 470
Endovascular therapy 496, 499
Energy, lack of 285
Enterobacteriaceae 569
Enterotoxins, bacterial 354
Enteroviruses 483, 486
Enzyme-linked immunosorbent assay 436
Eosinophilia 357
Epigastric pain syndrome 335, 337
Epilepsy 271, 505, 505*t*, 511, 516
  classification of 507
  diagnosis of 506*fc*
  drug-resistant 510
  etiology of 507*f*
  focal 506
  juvenile myoclonic 511
  management of 505, 508
  prognostication of 505
  syndrome diagnosis 506
Epinephrine 497
Eplerenone 25
Epstein-Barr virus 380, 386, 389, 486-489, 491
Equine encephalitis virus 486
Erectile dysfunction 467, 473, 479
  drug-induced 472

endocrinological 472
pathophysiologic mechanisms of 470
Erythema nodosum 109
Erythrocyte sedimentation rate 337, 547, 555
Escherichia coli 567, 568*t*
Eslicarbazepine acetate 509
Ethosuximide 509
Ethylene vinyl acetate 250
Ethylenediaminetetraacetic acid 367, 372
European Society of Cardiology 26, 405
European Society of Hypertension 403, 405
Euvolemic hyponatremia 145, 146
Euvolumia, clinical 153
Everolimus 509
Evolocumab 562
Exacerbation, acute 529
Excision biopsy 382
Exercise 327
  anaerobic 325
  benefits of 328
  lack of 269
  moderate 326
  stress test 314
  types of 325
Extended spectrum beta-lactamases 161, 573
Extracellular fluid 144
Extracorporeal shock wave lithotripsy 351
Extracranial systems 514
Extratemporal resection 514

F

Fabry disease 37
False lumen 61*f*
Fanconi's anemia 387, 389
Fasicular block 85
Fatty acids 191
  oxidation, partial 36
Fatty diarrhea 354
Fecal calprotectin level 359
Fecal elastase-1 359
Fecal lactoferrin 359
Fecal osmolar gap 354
Felbamate 509
Felty's syndrome 385, 556
Fertility 306
Fever, acute undifferentiated 435, 437
Fibrocalculous pancreatic diabetes 270, 272
Fibrosis
  idiopathic pulmonary 528, 530
  score 459*t*
Filaggrin mutation, presence of 519
Fine needle aspiration 382
Finnish rheumatoid arthritis combination therapy 555

Fissured tongue 118, 119f
Fixed ankle brace 253
Flapping tremors 104
Flat mucosa 361
Flocculation 361
Fluconazole 432
Fluid
  abnormal accumulation of 363
  adenosine deaminase 367
  glucose 367
  protein level 367t
  resuscitation 288
  therapy, duration of 448
Fluorodeoxyglucose positron emission
    tomography-computed tomography 382
Fluoroquinolones 346
Food allergy
  role of 519
  treatment of 525
Foot, inspection of 249
Footwear
  prescription 250, 251, 252, 253
  selection of 249
Fragmentation 361
Frank-Starling law 16
Free fatty acid 186, 463, 464
Free-wall rupture 52, 53
Fresh frozen plasma 366, 452
Friedreich ataxia 34
Fungal infection 95
Fungi 483, 491
Furosemide, combination of 368

G

Gabapentin 509, 511, 528
Gallbladder 305
Gamma-aminobutyric acid 510
Gamma-glutamyl transferase 459
Gastric cancer 364
Gastroenteritis, eosinophilic 357
Gastroesophageal reflux disease 335, 336, 528
Gastrointestinal disease 108
Gastrointestinal loss 145
Gastrointestinal system 546
Gastrointestinal tract 322
Gaucher's disease 37
Genital secretions 401
Geographic tongue 118, 119f
Giardia 361
Gland, destruction of 285
Glasgow coma
  scale 136, 440
  score 438
Gliclazide 203, 204
Glimepiride 202-204

Glipizide 204
Gliptins 263
Glitazones 263
Glomerular basement membrane 195
Glomerular filtration rate 167, 195, 259, 261, 404
  estimation of 4, 178, 182, 194, 215, 259, 265, 267
Glomerular hematuria 198t
Glomerulonephritis 549
Glomerulosclerosis, focal segmental 197, 421
Glucagon-like peptide 174, 175, 208, 246, 264, 353
  receptor agonist 185, 203, 264, 265, 267
Glucagonoma 108, 273
Glucocorticoids 556
  replacement 288-290
Glucokinase regulator 456
Glucose
  6-phosphate dehydrogenase 374
  fasting 465
  flash monitoring of 245
  monitoring apps 245
  transporter 246
Gluten-sensitive enteropathy 110
Glyburide 272
Glycemic control 14, 203, 451
Glycopeptide 165
Goiter, presence of 298
Gottron's papules 109
G-protein beta-polypeptide 3 334
Granulocyte colony macrophage colony
    stimulating factor 390
Granuloma annulare 102
Granulomatous inflammatory disease 19
Graves' disease 109, 295, 300
Gray Turner sign 341
Growth factor beta, transforming 550, 521
Guanosine monophosphate 5
Guanylyl cyclase stimulators, soluble 3, 5
Guideline-directed medical therapy 2, 3
Guillain-Barré syndrome 228, 229
Gynecomastia 365

H

H2 receptor antagonists 337
Haemophilus influenza type B 229
Hairy tongue 119
Half-and-half nails 108
Hansen's disease 110
  presence of 109
Hashimoto's thyroiditis 300, 308
Head injury 508
Heart 213, 216

disease
  coronary 303, 462, 475
  ischemic 84, 87
  risk of 329
  failure 1, 2, 2*t*, 3, 4, 6, 7*f*, 68*f*, 147, 204, 303, 404
    acute decompensated 3
    chronic systolic 23
    congestive 94, 446
    management of 1
    right-sided 357
    signs of 20
    states 3
    symptoms of 364
    treatment of 29
  major abnormality of 31
  outcomes prevention evaluation 13
  rate 143
    maximum 326
Heavy proteinuria 198
Helicobacter pylori 334
Heliotrope rash 109
Helminths 492
Hematological disorders 120
Hematological malignancy 119
Hematoma, abdominal wall 366
Hematuria 259
  microscopic 197
Hemianopia 495
Hemicraniectomy, decompressive 500
Hemispherectomy 514
Hemochromatosis 20, 285
Hemodialysis, long-term 34
Hemoglobin 389
  glycated 175, 244, 259, 265, 267, 275, 279, 316
  glycosylated 214
Hemorrhage
  intracranial 497, 498
  pituitary 285
Henderson-Hasselbalch equation 125
Hendra virus 485
Henoch-Schönlein purpura 108
Hepamet fibrosis score 460
Heparin therapy, chronic 130
Hepatic
  disease 108, 513
  failure 147
  function 168
  glucose production 277
  malignancy 368
  steatosis 454
    risk factors of 457*b*
  vein thrombosis 368
Hepatitis
  A 229
  B 227, 386, 402
    infection 225
  C 19, 386
    virus 459
Hepatorenal syndrome, high-risk of 366
Hernia, abdominal wall 369
Herpes simplex
  encephalitis 492
  virus 119, 360, 486-489, 491
Herpes viruses 483
Herpes zoster 228
Hickman catheter 112
High anion gap metabolic acidosis 132
High-density lipoprotein 222, 276, 315, 328, 462, 464
  cholesterol 465, 562
  low 255, 257
Highly active antiretroviral therapy 393, 492
Histamine-2 blockers 296
Histoplasma capsulatum 483, 492
Histoplasmoses 430
Holter monitor 85, 217
Holt-Oram syndrome 109
Hormone, antidiuretic 146
Human herpesvirus 486-489, 491
Human immunodeficiency virus 109, 175, 226, 276, 355, 380, 381, 393, 459, 486, 487, 489
  infection 122
    feature of 122
  prophylaxis, pre-exposure 399
Human leukocyte antigens 550
Human papillomavirus 226, 228
Human T-lymphotropic virus 380
Hydralazine 5, 27
Hydration 489, 520*f*
Hydrochlorothiazide 410
Hydrogen breath test 360
Hydrothorax, hepatic 369
Hydroxychloroquine 536, 555
Hydroxysteroid 17-dehydrogenase 456
Hyperbaric oxygen 215
Hypercholesterolemia 560
  familial 558, 560, 561
  heterozygous familial 564
  homozygous familial 563, 564
  management of 561
Hyperglycemia 221, 317
  management of 263
  therapies 217
Hyperhomocystinemia 218
Hyperinsulinemic-euglycemic clamp 191
Hyperkalemia 266
Hyperlipidemia 110, 271
Hyperplasia, benign prostatic 468
Hyperprolactinemia 472

Hypersensitivity
  Arthus-type 229
  pneumonitis 532, 533
  syndromes 380
Hypersplenism 386
Hypertension 1, 13, 178, 216, 234f, 265, 271, 276, 278, 324, 403, 404, 418, 467, 522
  management of 266, 403, 404, 414, 420
  secondary 417
  uncontrolled 1, 23
Hyperthyroidism 356, 358
Hypertonic saline 500
Hypertriglyceridemia 257
  treatment of 257
Hyperuricemia 462, 472
Hypoalbuminemia 363
Hypoglossal nerve palsy, left 121f
Hypoglycemia 217, 316
  neonatal 272
  risk of 204
Hyponatremia 144, 150, 153, 154, 366
  acute 144
  chronic 144, 147
  differential diagnosis of 148fc
  diuretic-induced 154
  duration of 151
  hyperosmolar 155
  hypertonic 145
  hypervolemic 145, 146
  hypotonic 145
  hypovolemic 145
  isotonic 145
Hypoparathyroidism 356
Hypotension 54
Hypothalamic nuclei 472
Hypothyroidism 23, 121, 298
  central 293
  congenital 294
  treatment of 293
Hypovolemia 52, 368
Hypoxemia 42

I

Icterus 107
Idiopathic interstitial pneumonias 528t, 532, 533
  management of 530
Idiopathic thrombocytopenic purpura 110
Ileal pathology 355
Imatinib 296
Immune
  reconstitution inflammatory syndrome 395
  thrombocytopenic purpura 110
Immunoglobulin 520f
  E 518
  G 488, 552
    levels of 521
  intravenous 492, 535
Immunotherapy 522, 523
  allergen specific 520, 521, 521f, 522, 523, 525
  type of 523
Impaired fasting glucose 213, 231
  presence of 275
Impaired glucose tolerance 213, 223, 231, 275, 462
Implantable cardioverter defibrillator 6, 29, 88
Implantable loop recorders 85
Indian Council of Medical Research 269
Indian Guidelines on Hypertension 403
Indian Hypertension Guidelines 405
Infectious Diseases Society of America 424
Inferior vena cava 66f, 112, 367
Infertility 297, 307
Inflammation, allergic 520
Inflammatory bowel disease 108, 355
Infliximab 536
Influenza
  infection 225
  vaccine 227
Infusate sodium 153
Insoles, types of 253f
Insulin 238, 263
  action 277
  delivery
    apps 245
    devices 244
  dose adjustment apps 245
  infusion, continuous 176, 245
  pump 245
  receptor substrate 220, 221
  regimens 239
  resistance 255
  secretion 277
Intellectual disability 508
Intelligence, body of 319
Intensive care unit 286
Intensive glycemic treatment group 263
Intensive lifestyle modification
  therapies 280
Intercellular adhesion molecule 1 216
Interdigital xanthoma 560f
Interferons 551 552
Interleukin 463, 555
International Diabetes Association 269
International Society of Hypertension 403
Interstitial lung disease 527-529, 531, 532, 534
  management of 527
  scleroderma-associated 535
Interstitial pneumonia
  chronic fibrosing idiopathic 530
  desquamative 533

Intra-abdominal adhesions 366
Intra-arterial therapy 494
Intracardiac shunts 23
Intracavernosal injection therapy 474, 475
Intracellular fluid 144
Intracellular pathways, inhibition of 553
Intracranial pressure, raised 490
Intracranial systems 514
Intraurethral drug administration 475
Intravenous albumin, simultaneous infusion of 368
Intravenous thrombolysis 497
  contraindications for 498b
  indications for 498b
Intrinsic muscle paralysis 252
Invasive fungal infection
  diagnosis of 431
  treatment of 431
Iron deficiency anemia 117, 120
Irritable bowel syndrome 335, 355
Ischemic optic neuropathy, nonarteritic anterior 475
Islet cell autoantibody 185
Iso-osmolar hyponatremia 155
Isosorbide dinitrate 5
Itchy eyes 524
Itolizumab 553
Itraconazole 432, 433
Ivabradine 5, 27

J

Jak stat inhibitor baricitinib 215
Janeway lesion 104
Janus kinase 553
Japanese encephalitis virus 486, 487
Jaundice, obstructive 147
Jejunoileal bypass 357
Jelly fish sign 72
Joint
  involvement, type of 545
  number of 545
  pain 544, 545, 548fc
    duration of 545
Jugular venous pressure, raised 365

K

Kaposi's sarcoma 109, 123, 123f, 381
Kawasaki disease 122, 123f, 380, 381
Kearns-Sayre syndrome 19
Ketamine 351
Ketoacidosis
  diabetic 43, 130, 174, 187, 203, 271
  fears of 217
Ketoconazole 432, 472

Ketogenic diet 516
Kexin type 9 inhibitor 265
Kidney 213, 214
  biopsy, clinical indications for 199
  disease 194, 195, 199, 260, 262, 267, 416
    causes of 194, 200
    chronic 2, 108, 195, 204, 261, 264, 267, 404, 414-417, 419, 457, 467, 473, 562
    diabetic 194, 215, 259, 263, 264, 266
    diagnosis of 199
    end-stage 203
    progressive 195
    screening for 194
  failure 199
  function
    abnormalities of 261
    test 21, 199
  injury
    acute 195, 445
    molecule 215
  structure, abnormalities of 261
  transplantation 420
Kikuchi-Fujimoto disease 380, 381
Kimura disease 380, 382
Klebsiella pneumoniae 161, 162, 570
Knuckle pigmentation 110
Koilonychia 94, 107
Kumamoto study 263
Kussmaul's sign 365

L

Lac phalanges 101
Lacosamide 351, 509, 511
Lactate dehydrogenase 367
Lactic acidosis 142
Lamina propria 361
Lamivudine 396
Lamotrigine 509-511
Langerhans cell histiocytosis 380, 382
Laparoscopy 368
Laparotomy 368
Laser photocoagulation 215
Latent autoimmune diabetes 270
Lead pipe appearance 361
Leflunomide 536, 555
Left bundle branch block 6, 86, 91
Left ventricular
  aneurysm 52
  assist device 6
  ejection fraction 2, 28
  hypertrophy 83
  mass index 419
Leishmaniasis 389
Lennox-Gastaut syndrome 511
Lesionectomy 514

Leukemia 108, 120
  acute 387
    myeloid 374f
  chronic myeloid 378
Leukocytosis 358, 371
Leukonychia 94
Levetiracetam 509
Levothyroxine sodium 293, 296
Lichen planus 102, 120, 120f
Lifeline stroke's severity 495
Light's criteria 539b
Linezolid 168
Lipid 303
  abnormalities 255
  assessment 270
  lowering therapy 266
Lipolysis 277
Lipoprotein
  cholesterol, low-density 217, 265, 266, 465, 562
  high-density 222, 276, 315, 328, 462, 464
  lipase 464
  low-density 201, 222, 262, 303, 328, 463, 464
    receptor 558
  very low-density 463
Listeria monocytogenes 491
Liver 213, 217, 305
  biopsy 256
  cirrhosis 364
  disease 94
    chronic 95, 467
    end-stage 368
    stigmata of 365
  fibrosis 459
  function 270
    test 358, 465, 531
  histology 458
  protective foods 218
  transplantation 369
Lobectomy, anterior temporal 514
Loeffers endomyocarditis 38
Loop recorders 85
Low blood pressure 285
Low carbohydrate diet 208, 209, 209t, 234
Lower limb joint involvement 546
Low-molecular-weight heparins 452
L-thyroxine absorption 308
Lucentis 216
Lung
  abscess 93
  diseases 536b
  injury, acute 446
  transplantation, role of 529
Lung ultrasound 41, 68f, 69f, 71f, 73f, 74, 74f
  accuracy of 68t

  normal 70f
  performance of 67
Lupus low-disease activity state 551
Lyme disease 19, 489
Lymph node 379
  biopsy 389
  supraclavicular 365
Lymphadenopathy 107, 357, 379
  acute 381
  causes of 380t
  chronic 381
  peripheral 379
Lymphocyte 375
Lymphocytic choriomeningitis virus 486, 487
Lymphocytosis 371
Lymphohistiocytosis, hemophagocytic 114, 380, 382
Lymphoid tissue
  mucosa-associated 380
  nasal-associated 380
Lymphomas 108, 285
Lymphopenia 357
Lymphoproliferative disorders 389

M

Macrocytic anemia 358
Macroglossia 109, 118, 118f, 121f
Macrovascular complications, spectrum of 277
Macrovascular disorders 278
Malabsorption syndrome 371
Malarial gametocyte 377f
Malignancy 368, 369
  colonic 364
Malignant cells, presence of 366
Malignant infarction, management of 500
Malnutrition 96
  severe 363
Manomaya kosha 319
Marfan's syndrome 103, 109
Massive liver metastases 367
Massive pulmonary embolism 58
Mast cells, recruitment of 521
Matrix metalloproteinase 215
Maturity onset diabetes of young 270, 272
Meal replacement 280
Measles 229
  virus 487
Mechanical thrombectomy 500
Mechanical ventilation 451, 529
Median nerve syndrome 98
Mediastinal syndromes 114
Mediastinum 112
Medical nutrition therapy 271
Medical therapy 28, 478

Medically refractory seizures 515
Mediterranean style 278
Mees' lines 108
Megaloblastic anemia 110, 385
Menstrual abnormality 298
Mental body 319
Mental health problems 471
Mepolizumab 526
Merci retrieval system 495
Mesenteric ischemia 354
Metabolic acidosis 125, 127, 131
    diagnosis 125
    management 125
    mixed 133
Metabolic adaptations 220
Metabolic alkalosis 133
Metabolic disease 118, 473
Metabolic fatty liver disease 454
Metabolic memory 263
Metabolic rate 321
Metabolic syndrome 192, 459, 462, 464, 465
    clinical features of 463f
    pathogenesis of 463f, 464fc
Metacarpophalangeal joint 97
Metallo-beta-lactamases 161
Metastasis 285
Metastatic deposits secrete protein-rich fluid 364
Metformin 234, 272, 279
Methicillin-resistant
    coagulase-negative *Staphylococcus* species 572
    Staphylococcus aureus 572, 573
Methicillin-susceptible *Staphylococcus aureus* 572
Methotrexate 536, 555, 556
Methyl donors 218
Methylprednisolone, treatment consists of 497
Metronidazole 346
Metyrapone test 361
Micafungin 432
Microalbuminuria 9, 11f, 12-14
    concentrations of 12f
    development of 263
Microcellular polymer 250
Microcellular rubber 250
Microcytic hypochromic anemia 357, 373f
Microglossia 118
Microvascular damage 209
Mid foot offloading footwear 252f
Migraine 513
Migratory glossitis, benign 118
Mimic endogenous cortisol secretion 289
Mimicking hypertrophic cardiomyopathy 33
Mineralocorticoid antagonists 214, 217

Mineralocorticoid deficit 145
Mineralocorticoid receptor antagonist 3, 4, 265, 419
Mineralocorticoid replacement 290
Minocycline 490
Mirodenafil 476
Mitochondrial diabetes 270, 273
Mitral regurgitation 44
    ischemic 52, 53, 53f
Mitral stenosis 462
Mitral valve level 47, 47f
Mobile foot deformity 250
Mobile phone-based device 514
Mobile stroke units 495
Molecules, role for upcoming 256
Monocyte chemoattractant protein 551
Mononucleosis, infectious 380
Monotherapy 165
Morbid obesity 467
Motor neuron disease 120
Movements, abnormal 120
Mucocutaneous lymph node disease 122
Mucopolysaccharidoses 37
Mucormycosis 121, 483
Mucosal bleeding 120
Multifaceted metabolic disorder 206
Multifactorial disorder 207
Multiorgan failure, fever with 435
Multiple myeloma 108, 120, 389
Multiple pituitary hormone deficiencies 298
Multiple sclerosis 471
Multiple subpial transection 514
Mumps 226
Muscles, ischiocavernosus 468
Musculoskeletal body 319
Musculoskeletal involvement, type of 546
Musculoskeletal system 322
Mycobacterium tuberculosis 159, 162, 169, 486-489, 491
Mycophenolate 534
    mofetil 531
Mycoplasma pneumoniae 486, 488, 489, 491
Myelodysplastic syndrome 387
Myocardial depression
    alcohol-induced 23
    drug-induced 23
Myocardial infarction 3, 86, 90, 96
    acute 39, 91
        inferior wall 88
    anterior wall 89
    inferior wall 88, 89
    localization of 88
Myocardial ischemia 23
Myocardial metabolic efficiency 36
Myocarditis, inflammatory 19

Index 589

Myoclonic seizures 510, 511
Myosin
	activation 5
	binding protein C 31
Myxedema 109

N

N-acetylcysteine 532
Naegleria fowleri 483, 492
National AIDS Control Organisation 394
National Institute for Clinical Excellence 181
National Kidney Foundation 262
National Urban Diabetes Survey 275
Nebulized opioid therapy 529
Neck vein distension 113
Necrotic foot 253
Neisseria
	gonorrhoeae 162
	meningitidis 157
Neoplastic diseases 124
Nephropathy 416, 421
	diabetic 178, 194, 215, 268
	presence of 199
	salt losing 145
Nephrotic range proteinuria 199
Nephrotic syndrome 363, 365, 367
Nephrotoxic
	agents 214
	substances 268
Nervi erigentes 471
Neuroendocrine tumor 354
Neurogenic erectile dysfunction 471
Neurological disorders 109, 121, 467
Neurological status 501
Neuromuscular electrical stimulation 209
	therapy 209
Neuropathic ulcer 251
Neuropathy, autonomic 473
Neurosyphilis 120
Neurotropic growth factors 479
New-onset ascites 365
Nicotinamide adenine dinucleotide phosphate 36
Night sweats 364
Nitrates 27
Nitric oxide 11, 468
	role of 467
Niyam 320
N-methyl-D-aspartic acid 510
Nocturnal diarrhea 355
Nocturnal therapy 420
Non-adrenergic fibers 472
Nonalcoholic fatty liver disease 255, 305, 454, 462, 456, 458*f*, 459, 459*f*, 460
	history of 455
	pathogenesis of 456
	score 257
	screening of 457
	terminologies of 455
Nonalcoholic steatohepatitis 454, 457, 462
Non-anion-gap metabolic acidosis 130
Nonbacterial infections, antibiotics for 160
Noncaseating granuloma, presence of 361
Non-cholinergic fibers 472
Nondiabetic kidney disease 194
Nondiabetic renal disease 259
Non-fatal stroke 13
Nonglomerular hematuria 198*t*
Non-Hodgkin's lymphoma 114, 380
Noninvasive glucose monitoring 246
Noninvasive scoring systems 459
Noninvasive ventilation 529
	role of 529
Non-nucleoside reverse transcriptase inhibitors 393
Nonoxidative glucose disposal 191
Nonpharmacological therapy 417, 514
Nonproteinuric diabetic kidney disease 215
Nonsteroidal anti-inflammatory drugs 24, 130, 214, 268, 336, 350
Nontraumatic resuscitation 59
Norepinephrine reuptake inhibitors 350
Normal anion gap acidosis, causes of 129
Normal glucose regulation, restoration of 280
Normocytic anemia 358
Normoglycemia 208
Normogram 127
Nucleic acid detection 431, 487
Nucleoside reverse transcriptase inhibitor 393, 397
Nutrition 234, 278, 345, 451
	apps 245
	fluids 447
	practice guideline 209
Nutritional anemia 371
Nutritional deficiencies 19

O

Obesity 304, 324*f*, 330, 357
	abdominal 280
Obeticholic acid 256
Obexelimab 552
Obinutuzumab 552
Obstructive atelectasis 79*f*
Obstructive sleep apnea 415, 462, 528
Octopus trap 38
Ocular fluid 166
Offloading footwear 251*f*
Ofloxacin 346
Omalizumab 520, 525, 526

Omega-3-fatty acids 257
Onycholysis 95
Open biopsy 540, 543
Opponens brevis 97
Opponens pollicis 97
Opportunistic infections 391
Optimal antibiotic therapy, principles of 423
Oral anticoagulation 501
Oral antidiabetic
   agents 240
   medications 273
Oral antihyperglycemic agents 176
Oral corticosteroids 534
Oral glucose tolerance test 231, 275
Oral hairy leukoplakia 123f
Oral hypoglycemic agent 185
Oral Kaposi sarcoma occurs 122
Organ failure assessment
   quick sequential 438, 440
   sepsis-related 437
Organic body 319
Orthomyxoviruses 483
OrthoWedge surgical shoes 253
Osler's nodes 101, 109
Osler-Rendu-Weber syndrome 110
Osmotic diarrhea 354, 359
Osteoarthritis 97, 545, 548
Osteoarthropathy, hypertrophic 108
Osteoporosis 324, 513
Ovarian diseases 363
Overt hypothyroidism, treatment of 293
Oxacillinases 161
Oxcarbazepine 509, 511
Oxygen
   supplemental 529
   therapy, long-term 529
Oxytocin increases 322

P

Pain
   abdominal 20, 285, 365
   management of 349
   medical management for 350
   pattern of 545
Pallor 107
Palmar erythema 95, 365
Pancreatic ascites 364
Pancreatic cancer, screening for 353
Pancreatic diabetes, management of 352
Pancreatic enzyme 350
   replacement therapy 189, 352
Pancreatic exocrine insufficiency, management of 351
Pancreatic pseudocyst 346
Pancreaticojejunostomy 351

Pancreatitis
   acute 340, 341t
      necrotizing 344f
   chronic 270, 348, 355, 358
   etiology of 342t
Pancytopenia 384, 387, 388
   causes of 385, 385b
   drug-induced 387
   etiopathogenesis of 385
Panencephalitis, subacute sclerosing 487, 492
Papillary muscle
   level 47, 48f
   rupture 52, 53
Paracentesis
   abdominal 365
   catheter 366
   complications of 366
   site of 366
Paracoccidiomycoses 430
Paramyxoviruses 483
Paraquat ingestion corroded tongue 120f
Parasites 483
Parasternal long-axis view 43, 44f, 45, 47
Parasternal short-axis view 46f-48f
Parkinson's disease 471
Paronychia 96
Parotid gland, enlarged 365
Paroxysmal atrial fibrillation 217
Paroxysmal nocturnal
   dyspnea 32
   hemoglobinuria 387, 389
Patellar tendon bearing 253
Pathogen-directed therapy 170
Pathophysiologic defects 277
Pedal edema 548
Pediatric Infectious Diseases Society 424
Pefloxacin 346
Pemberton's sign 113
Pemphigus 119
Penicilliosis 430
Penile
   detumescence occurs 470
   duplex Doppler ultrasonography 473
   erection, physiology of 468
   fracture 471
   injections 478
   prostheses 478
   revascularization surgery 479
Pentoxifylline 256
Perampanel 509
Performance anxiety 470
Pericardial effusion
   clinical features of 57
   size of 57
Pericardial fluid 61

Pericardial tamponade 57, 57fc, 58f
  pathophysiology 57
Pericarditis, constrictive 363
Perineal trauma 357, 471
Perinuclear antineutrophil cytoplasmic
  antibody 358
Periodic acid-Schiff 361
Peripancreatic inflammation 344f
Peripartum cardiomyopathy 20, 30
Peripheral vascular disease 278, 462
Peritoneal carcinomatosis 364
Peritoneal disease 364
Periungual fibroma 104
Pernicious anemia 118f
Peroxisome proliferator-activated receptor 220, 221, 407
Person's diabetes mellitus 280
Personality disorders 110
Pertussis 228
Peyronie's disease 471, 473
Pharmacological agent 234, 278
Pharmacological therapy 522
Pharmacotherapeutics 467
Pharmacotherapy 207, 460
Pharmacy 426
Phenobarbital 509, 512
Phentermine 278
Phenylephrine 478
Phenytoin 509, 512
  use, chronic 95
Pheochromocytoma 34
Phosphodiesterase inhibitors 470, 475
Phosphoenolpyruvate carboxykinase 186
Phospholipase
  C 470
  domain-containing protein 3 456
Physical activity 234, 263, 278, 314, 323
  apps 245
  moderate-intensity 278, 279
  plan 314
  risk of 331
Physical exercise, lack of 474
Pill-rolling tremor 105
Pitting nails 96
Pituitary infiltration 285
Pituitary tumors 285
Plantar pressure assessment 249
Plasma
  cells 361, 552
    disorder 147
  exchange 492
  glucose 275, 280
    fasting 239, 275, 280
  insulin 270
  osmolality, basis of 145
  renin 287

Plasmacytoid dendritic cells 552
Plasmalyte 445
Plasminogen activator inhibitor 464, 465, 499
Plasmodium 377, 378, 436
  falciparum 436, 483, 492
  knowlesi 377
  malariae 377
Plastazote 251
Platelet 376
  ratio index 459, 460
Pleura, needle biopsy of 540, 542
Pleural effusion, malignant 540
Pleural fluid 61
Pneumococcal infection 225
Pneumococcal vaccine 226
Pneumocystis
  carinii 531
  jirovecii 430
Pneumonia
  acute interstitial 533
  cryptogenic organizing 533
  interstitial 527, 528, 531
Pneumothorax 74f
Pneumovax 226
Point-of-care laboratory 495
Polyarthritis, differential diagnosis of 548fc
Polyarticular juvenile idiopathic arthritis 548
Polycystic ovary syndrome 276, 465
Polymerase chain reaction 487
Polymicrobial infections 165
Polymorphonuclear neutrophil 369
Polymyositis 535
Polypharmacy 160
Polytetrafluoroethylene 115
Poor glycemic control 262
Portal hypertension 363, 364, 367
  presence of 365
Posaconazole 432, 433
Positive end-expiratory pressure 448
Posterior wall myocardial infarction 91
Postexposure prophylaxis 391, 401
Postinfectious status 492
Postparacentesis circulatory dysfunction, risk of 366
Postpercutaneous transluminal coronary angioplasty 178
Postprandial distress syndrome 335
Postprandial hyperglycemia 186
Poststreptococcal infection 109
Poststroke epilepsy 513
Postural hypotension 285
Postvaccination status 492
Potassium 267
Potential arbitrators 34
Pranamaya kosha 319
Pranayama 320

Pratyahara 320
Prayer's hand 103
Preauthorization 427
Prediabetes 230, 275, 275t, 276, 277, 280
    complications of 233, 233f, 277, 277f
    diagnosis of 231, 275
        macrovascular complications of 278
    management of 234, 278
    reversal of 280
    types of 231
Prednisolone 289, 528
Pre-eclampsia 223
Pregabalin 509
Pregestational diabetes 223
    preexisting 272
Pregnancy 301
Primidone 509, 512
Procalcitonin 444
Prominent E wave 38
Prophylactic therapy 164
Prophylaxis, pre-exposure 391, 399
Proprotein convertase subtilisin 265
Prostaglandin E1 474
Protease inhibitors 393
Protein
    excretion rate 196
    kinase, rho-associated 470
    losing enteropathy 363
Proteinuria 196t, 198, 409
    onset of 198
Proton pump inhibitors 296, 337, 338, 531
Protozoa 492
Proximal interphalangeal joint 97
Pseudohyponatremia 150
Pseudomonas aeruginosa 162
    resistance mechanisms of 162t
Pseudoxanthoma elasticum 37
Psoriasis 95
Psychiatric disorders 513
Psychogenic erectile dysfunction 470
Pubertal hormones 271
Pulmonary congestion 20
Pulmonary edema 55fc
Pulmonary embolism, acute 58
Pulmonary hypertension 83, 368
    management of 529
Pulmonary rehabilitation 528
Pulmonary thromboembolism 540
Pulmonary thrombosis 65f
    hemodynamic effects of 64
Pulmonary trauma 112
Pulmonary valve
    annulus 46
    pathology 46
Pulmonary vasculitis 549

Pulse
    rate 340
    wave
        Doppler imaging 64, 65f
        velocity 407
Pulseless electrical activity 42
Pyuria 199

Q

QT syndrome, long 87
Quality-adjusted life-years 204
Quinolone-resistant enterobacter 161

R

Radial artery, absent 103
Radiation
    colitis 355
    enterocolitis 356
    therapy 115
Radical cystectomy 471
Radical pelvic surgery 471
Radical prostatectomy 471
Radioactive iodine 295
Radiological tests 487
Radiosurgery 516
Ramipril efficacy 416
Randomized controlled trials 5, 175, 393, 437
Ranibizumab 216
Ranolazine 216
Rapamycin, nutrient-sensing mammalian
    target of 191
Rapid arterial occlusion evaluation scale 495
Rapid diagnostic tests 436
Ravanna syndrome 213
Raynaud's phenomenon 101, 109
Reactive oxygen species 213, 239
Reaven's metabolic syndrome 213
Recombinant erythropoietin 390
Recombinant tissue plasminogen activator 494
Red beefy tongue 117f
Red blood cell 357, 372
    morphology of 198, 372
Red cell distribution width 21
Reflex, bulbocavernosus 473
Refractory ascites 365, 369
Refractory hypertension 419
Regional wall motion abnormality scoring 51, 52t
Regurgitation, aortic 109
Renal bicarbonate loss 129
Renal denervation therapy 421
Renal disease 178, 179, 182, 257, 259, 268, 416
    end-stage 178, 179, 194, 195, 259, 446

Renal disorders 194
Renal end-stage disease, prevention of 12
Renal failure 195
  chronic 226
Renal fibrosis 215
Renal function 168, 270
Renal insufficiency 181, 512
Renal replacement therapy 179
Renal tuberculosis 213
Renal tubular acidosis 130, 131
  proximal 129
Renin-angiotensin system 214
  blockers 267
  inhibition 4
Renin-angiotensin-aldosterone system 3, 11, 148, 266, 364, 409, 410fc, 414
  inhibitors of 25, 30
Renoprotection 14, 409
Repaglinide 263
Repetitive transcranial magnetic stimulation 514
Replacement fluids 447
Reproductive abnormalities 304
Resistance exercise 315, 316
Resistant *Escherichia coli* 162
Respiration 321
Respiratory acidosis 132
Respiratory alkalosis 134
Respiratory bronchiolitis 532
Respiratory care 344
Respiratory distress, fever with 435
Respiratory failure 76f, 77f
Respiratory rate 143, 340, 440
Respiratory symptoms, acute 67
Responsive neurostimulation 515
Restrictive cardiomyopathy 37
Retina 213, 215
Retinopathy, diabetic 215
Reverse transcriptase polymerase chain reaction 360
Rhabdoviridae 483
Rheumatic fever, acute 109
Rheumatoid arthritis 97, 98, 110, 534, 545, 548, 554, 556
  early 556
  management 554
  tight control of 556
Rheumatoid factor 547, 555
Rheumatoid nodules 98, 556
Rheumatological disorders 108
Rho kinase inhibitors 216
Rhythm disorders 84
Ribonucleic acid 158, 374
Rickettsia rickettsii 488, 491
Rickettsioses 491
Right bundle branch block 86, 90

Right main bronchus 112
Right ventricular
  hypertrophy 83
  inflow view 45, 45f, 46f, 58
  myocardial infarction 88
Rigiscan device 473
Ringer's lactate 445
Rituximab 555
Robust glycated hemoglobin 201
Rocker bottom shoes 253
Romhilt-Estes point score system 83
Rosai-Dorfman disease 382
Rosiglitazone 236
Routine urinalysis, components of 197
Rubella 226, 229
Rufinamide 509
Rule out hypothyroidism 151

S

Sacroiliitis 357
Sacubitril 25
  valsartan combinations 217
S-adenosyl methionine 218
Salmonella typhi 169
Salvageable brain tissue 501
Sarcoidosis 109, 110, 381
  management of 536
Saturated fatty acid, restrict intakes of 262
Saxagliptin 263
Scars, severe 252
Schilling test 360
Scleredema diabeticorum 107
Sclerodactyly 97
Scleroderma 37
Scleromyxedema 108
Scrotal tongue 118
Scrub typhus 436f
Secondary adrenal insufficiency 283, 286, 291
  causes of 285
  symptoms of 286
Seizure 508, 516
  absence 510
  acute symptomatic 508
  classification of 507
  focal 508
  monotherapy, focal-onset 511
  partial 507
  recurrence, risk of 513
  type 513
    diagnosis 506
Select appropriate antibiotic therapy 163
Selenium 350
  homocholic acid taurine 360
Semaglutide 208
Semilunar valves 45, 47f

Semmes-Weinstein monofilament 249
Senile keratosis 99
Sensitive potassium 202
Sensor implant device 514
Sepsis 440, 449
    management 440, 442, 442fc
    severe 55
Septic shock 43, 446fc
    resuscitation 453f
Serine protease inhibitor 273
Serological tests 358
Serotonin 350
Serum
    amylase 342
    ascitic albumin gradient 367
        facilitate calculation of 367
    glutamic pyruvic transaminase 201
    lipase 342
    osmolality 149
    protein electrophoresis 359
    sodium 153
    testosterone levels, low 473
Sexual dysfunction 467
Sexual health inventory 468
Sexually transmitted infection 400
Sgarbossa's criteria 92f
Sharpen memory 329
Shock 55fc, 56fc
    cardiogenic 55f
    hypovolemic 55f
    types of 54, 54t
Shoe closure system 250
Shortened villi, presence of 362
Sildenafil 476
Simon Broome criteria 560, 561
Simple echocardiography 60b
Simple steatosis 455
Simpson-Golabi-Behmel syndrome 118
Sinus rhythm 6
Sinusoidal obstruction syndrome 367
Sitagliptin 263
Sjögren's syndrome 122, 535, 546
Skin
    barrier formation 520f
    prick testing 520
    rash, fever with 435
    vasculitis 549
Small bowel syndrome 354
Small cell carcinoma, recurrent 114f
Small dense low-density lipoprotein 255
Small intestine
    bacterial overgrowth 352
    dilatation of 361
Small vessel disease 216
Smart blood pressure 244

Smart electrocardiogram 244
Smart socks 244
Smart watches 244
Smart weighing scales 244
Smooth muscle relaxation 475, 478
Smooth tongue 117
Sodium 144
    channel blocker 35
    fractionated excretion of 152
    restriction of 214
Sodium-glucose cotransporter 2 28, 175, 203, 264, 265, 421, 460
    inhibitors 3, 4, 6, 28, 185, 267
Sokolow-Lyon criteria 83
Somatic neuropathy 473
Sorafenib 296
Sphingosine-1-phosphate receptor 1 553
Spinal cord
    injury 471
    level 472
Spirochetes 491
Spironolactione 25, 368
Splinter hemorrhage 95
Spondyloarthropathy 544, 545
Spontaneous bacterial
    infection 369
    peritonitis 365, 369
Staphylococcus aureus 158, 161, 424
Statin
    role of 256
    therapy 29, 256
Steatohepatitis 255
ST-elevation myocardial infarction 81
Stem cell therapy 479
Stenosis, aortic 83
Sterile necrosis 344f
Sterile pyuria 199
Sternum 112
Steroid 556
    nucleus 288
Still's disease 546, 548
    adult-onset 380, 382
Stimulating hormone 300
Stiripentol 509
Stool
    fat screening 360
    frequency of 355
    tests 359
Strawberry tongue 123f
Streptococcus pneumoniae 161, 169
Streptococcus pyogenes 158
Stress
    cardiomyopathy 38
    level of 269
    reduce 328, 404
    ulcer prophylaxis 452

Stroke 303
 centers, primary 495
 management of 494, 501
Strongyloidiasis 357
Structural heart disease 87
Subclinical hypothyroidism 293, 298, 300, 301
 consequences of 302
 treatment of 297
Subcutaneous calcification 100
Subcutaneous immunotherapy 523, 523f
Subcutaneous nodules 109
Sublingual immunotherapy 523, 524, 524f
Submucosa, inflammation of 361
Suboccipital craniectomy 501
Sudden cardiac death 6
Sulfasalazine 555
Sulfonylureas 201-204, 263
 classification of 202, 202t
 mechanism of action of 202
Superbugs 160, 161
Superior vena cava
 obstruction, management of 115
 oxygen saturatuon 446
Superior vena cava syndrome 81, 111, 114, 114f, 115
 classification of 112
 clinical features of 113
 differential diagnosis of 114
Supportive therapy 489
Surfactant protein 533
Surgery, devices for 515
Surgical lung biopsy 531
Surgical myectomy 36
Swan neck deformity 105
Sweet syndrome 108
Syndrome of inappropriate secretion of anti-diuretic hormone 146
Syphilis, secondary 103
Systemic antifungal agents 119
Systemic congestion 20
Systemic coronary risk estimation 14
Systemic diseases 365
 clues suggestive of 107
 presence of 109
 several 117
Systemic disorders, skin signs of 109
Systemic fungal infections 430
Systemic glucocorticoids, role of 556
Systemic inflammatory response syndrome 344, 437, 438, 441
Systemic lupus
 erythematosus 109, 130, 380, 387, 534, 545, 548, 550
 international collaborating clinics 551
Systemic nervous system 415
Systemic nitric oxide 364

Systemic sclerosis 356, 534, 545, 548
Systolic blood pressure 404, 411

T

Tachyarrhythmia
 supraventricular 86
 ventricular 85, 86
Tachycardia
 supraventricular 85
 ventricular 34, 85, 87
Tadalafil 476
Taenia solium 492
Takotsubo 38, 39
 clinical presentation 39
Target organ damage, consequences of 218
Taurodeoxycholic acid 216
T-cells 552
Telangiectasias 110
Telemedicine 243
Telitacicept 552
Telmisartan 410
Telogen effluvium 110
Temporary readymade shoe 251
Temporary symptomatic relief 479
Tendon
 xanthoma 98, 110
  over ankle and elbows 559f
Tenecteplase 499
Tenofovir 394
Tenosynovitis 105
Terbinafine 432
Terminal ileum, short resection of 357
Terminal interphalangeal joint, involvement of 97
Terminal phalanges
 cystic lesion of 100
 X-ray of 100
Terry's nails 94
Tertiary adrenal insufficiency 285
Testicular atrophy 365
Testosterone 472
 modulates 472
Tetanus 226, 228
Thalidomide 528
Thenar compartment, wasting of 97
Therapeutic footwear, selection of 250
Therapeutic index 570
Thermal ablation 514
Thiazolidinediones 24, 201, 218, 234
Thoracentesis 369
Thoracoscopy 540, 542
Thrombocytopenia 120, 366, 435
Thrombocytosis 357
Thromboembolism 32
Thrombophlebitis migrans 108

Thrombosis 113
Thyroid
  acropachy 109
  binding globulin 301
  disease 121
  hormone 293
    replacement, effect of 305
Thyroiditis, chronic autoimmune 300
Thyroid-stimulating hormone 201, 293, 296
  low 358
Thyrotoxicosis 120, 357
Thyrotropin-releasing hormone 293
Thyroxin 308, 322
Tiagabine 509
Tidepool 243
Time-varying albuminuria 13*f*
Tirzepatide 208
Tissue
  penetration 166
  peripheral 191
  plasminogen activator 494
Tongue 117
  lichen planus of 120*f*
Tonic-clonic seizures 508, 510
  primary generalized 511
Topical corticosteroids 523
Topiramate 509, 511, 512
  extended-release 278
Total leukocyte count 438
Toxemia 223
Toxoplasma 489
  gondii 483, 492
Toxoplasmosis 19
Tracheal intubation 497
Traditional cardiovascular disease, risk factors 278
Transcranial direct current stimulation 514
Transcranial magnetic stimulation 515
Transcutaneous vagus nerve stimulation 516
Transient apical ballooning 38
Transjugular intrahepatic portosystemic shunt 368
Transthoracic echocardiography, focus-assessed 43*f*
Transudative pleural effusion 538, 539, 543
Traumatic injury 471
Treponema pallidum 488, 491
Tricuspid regurgitation 45, 363
Tricyclic antidepressant 338, 350
Triglyceride 201, 265
  high level of 255, 366
  medium chain 349
Triiodothyronine 293, 300
Trimetazidine 216
Trimethoprim-sulfamethoxazole 168
Triple A syndrome 285

Troisier sign 108
Tropheryma whipplei 491
Trophozoite, presence of 361
Tropical fever 434, 438*fc*
Trousseau's syndrome 108
True lumen 61*f*
Trypanosoma brucei
  gambiense 485, 492
  rhodesiense 485, 492
Trypanosomiasis 19
Tubercular enteritis 356
Tubercular peritonitis 363
Tuberculosis 109, 355, 364, 366, 368, 381, 393
  abdominal 363
  chronic 111
Tuberculous pleural effusion 540
Tuberous sclerosis complex 511
Tubular necrosis, acute 145
Tumor
  necrosis factor 215, 364, 463-465, 555
  rupture 366
Turbid fluid 366
Typhoid fever 110

U

Udenafil 476
Ulcerative colitis 108, 357, 361
Ulcers 119
  aphthous 123
Ultrasonography, abdominal 342
University Group Diabetes Program 201
Unrelieved biliary obstruction 368
Upper gastrointestinal endoscopy 361
Upper limb joint involvement 546
Upregulation efflux pumps 162
Uric acid 548
Urinary albumin 178
  excretion 12, 407
Urinary bladder, distended 366
Urinary free cortisol 289
Urinary protein 195
  total 198
Urinary sodium level 153
Urinary tract
  infection 215, 268, 569
  symptoms 468
Urinary voiding symptoms 198
Urine
  albumin creatinine ratio 196, 201
  dipstick analysis 197
  interpretation of 194
  osmolality 153
  routine 365
  sample, twenty four-hour timed 9
  sediments 197
Urticaria pigmentosa 357

V

Vacuum erection devices 474, 477
Vagal nerve stimulation 514, 515
Valproic acid 509-511
Valsartan 25
Valvular lesions 23
Vancomycin 168
    resistant enterococci 572
Vardenafil 476
Varicella 229
Varicella-zoster virus 486-489, 491
Vascular disease 201
Vascular endothelial growth factor 215
Vascular end-stage disease, prevention of 12
Vascular insufficiency 473
Vascular stiffness 415
Vasculogenic erectile dysfunction 471
Vasoactive intestinal peptide 358
Venezuelan equine encephalitis virus 486, 487
Venogram 114
Ventricular fibrillation 87
Ventricular paced rhythm 91
Ventricular premature beat 87
Ventricular septal
  defect 43
  rupture 52, 53
Verapamil 35
Vibrio cholerae 354
Vigabatrin 509
Vigorous exercise 326
Vijnanamaya kosha 319
Vildagliptin 263
Vipoma 354
Viral agents 483
Viral infections, vector-borne 483
Virchow's node 108, 336, 365
Virological monitoring 395
Visceral obesity 280
Visibly engorged cutaneous vessels 366
Vitamin
  B6 215
  C 350
  E 218, 256, 350
Voclosporin 553
Voriconazole 432, 433

W

Waldeyer's ring 380
Watery diarrhea 354
Wearing eye protection 216
Weight, gradual loss of 355
West Nile virus 486, 487
Western diet 192
Western equine encephalitis virus 486
Whipple's disease 354, 355, 357, 361
White blood cell 358, 359, 548
    morphology 374
White nails 94
Whooping cough 228
Wolcott-Rallison syndrome 271
Wrist
  drop 99
  X-ray of 103
Wuchereria bancrofti 378, 386

X

X-linked adrenoleukodystrophy 285

Y

Yersinia enterocolitis 355
Yoga 319, 322
  eight limbs of 320
  elements of 320
  physiology of 319
  purpose of 319
Yogasutra 319
Yu's classification 112

Z

Zidovudine 392
Zimmer frames 253
Zona
  fasciculata 283
  glomerulosa 282
  reticularis 283
Zonisamide 509, 512
Zygomycosis 430